Physical Therapy for the Pelvic Floor

Bridging Science and Clinical Practice

For Elsevier:

Publisher: Heidi Harrison
Associate Editor: Siobhan Campbell
Production Manager: Frances Affleck
Text Design: Charles Gray
Cover Design: Stevart Larking
Illustrations: Cactus and David Gardner
Illustration Manager: Merhyn Harvey

Evidence-Based Physical Therapy for the Pelvic Floor

Edited by

Kari Bø, *PT, MSc, PhD*
PT, Exercise Scientist Professor, Department of Sports Medicine, Norwegian School of Sports Sciences, Oslo, Norway

Bary Berghmans, *PT, MSc, PhD*
Health Scientist and Clinical Epidemiologist, Pelvic Care Center Maastricht, University Hospital Maastricht, Maastricht, The Netherlands

Siv Mørkved, *PT, MSc, PhD*
Associate Professor, Clinical Service, St Olavs Hospital, Trondheim University Hospital and Department of Community Medicine & General Practice, Norwegian University of Science and Technology, Trondheim, Norway

Marijke Van Kampen, *PT, MSc, PhD*
Professor, Rehabilitation Scientist, Katholieke Universiteit Leuven,
Faculty of Kinesiology and Rehabilitation Science, University Hospital GHB, Leuven, Belgium

Forewords by

Walter Artibani, International Continence Society

Paul A. Riss, Past President, International Urogynecology Association

Sandra Mercer Moore, World Confederation of Physical Therapy

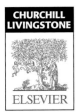

CHURCHILL LIVINGSTONE

ELSEVIER

EDINBURGH LONDON NEW YORK OXFORD PHILADELPHIA ST LOUIS SYDNEY TORONTO 2007

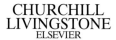

CHURCHILL
LIVINGSTONE
ELSEVIER

An imprint of Elsevier Limited

© 2007, Elsevier Ltd

ISBN 9780443101465

First published 2007
 Reprinted 2008

British Library Cataloguing in Publication Data
A catalogue record for this book is available from the British Library.

Library of Congress Cataloging in Publication Data
A catalog record for this book is available from the Library of Congress.

Note

Neither the Publisher nor the Authors assume any responsibility for any loss or injury and/or damage to persons or property arising out of or related to any use of the material contained in this book. It is the responsibility of the treating practitioner, relying on independent expertise and knowledge of the patient, to determine the best treatment and method of application for the patient.

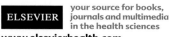

Working together to grow
libraries in developing countries

www.elsevier.com | www.bookaid.org | www.sabre.org

ELSEVIER   BOOK AID International   Sabre Foundation

ELSEVIER your source for books, journals and multimedia in the health sciences

www.elsevierhealth.com

The publisher's policy is to use **paper manufactured from sustainable forests**

Printed in China

Contents

Contributors

Paul Abrams MD, FRCS
Professor of Urology, Bristol Urological Institute, Bristol, UK

Dianne Alewijnse MSc, PhD
Patient Education Communication Advisor, Gelre Hospitals, Apeldoorn and Zutphen, The Netherlands

Arve Aschehoug MSc Sports Science
Department of Sports Medicine, Norwegian School of Sport Sciences, Oslo, Norway

James A. Ashton–Miller PhD
Research Professor, Director, Biomechanics Research Laboratory, Department of Mechanical Engineering, University of Michigan, Ann Arbor, Michigan, USA

James Balmforth MRCOG
Subspecialty Trainee in Urogynaecology, Department of Urogynaecology, Kings College Hospital, London, UK

Mohammed Belal MA, MRCS
Specialist Registrar in Urology, London Deanery, UK

Bary Berghmans PhD, MSc, PT
Health Scientist and Clinical Epidemiologist, Pelvic Care Center Maastricht, University Hospital Maastricht, Maastricht, The Netherlands

Nol Bernards MD
Physician, Dutch Institute for Allied Health Care, Amersfoort, The Netherlands

Espen Berner MD
Department of Surgery, Hamar Hospital, Hamar, Norway

Kari Bø PT, MSc, PhD
Professor, Department of Sports Medicine, Exercise Scientist, Norwegian School of Sports Sciences, Oslo, Norway

Richard C. Bump MD
Senior Medical Fellow, Lilly Research Laboratories and Clinical Professor of Obstetrics and Gynecology, Indiana University, Indiana, USA

Wendy Bower BAppSc, PhD
Associate Professor, Department of Surgery, The Chinese University of Hong Kong, Hong Kong

Pauline Chiarelli Dip Physio, Grad Dip, H Soc Sc, M Med Sc, PhD
Senior Lecturer, School of Health Sciences, University of Newcastle, New South Wales, Australia

Jacques Corcos PhD
Department of Urology, McGill University, Montreal, Quebec, Canada

Rob de Bie PhD, MSc, PT
Professor of Physical Therapy Research, Department of Epidemiology and Center of Evidence Based Physiotherapy (CEBP) Maastricht, Maastricht University, Maastricht, The Netherlands

John O. L. DeLancey MD
Norman F. Miller Professor and Associate Chair for Gynecology, University of Michigan Women's Hospital, University of Michigan, Ann Arbor, Michigan, USA

Hans Peter Dietz MD, PhD, FRANZCOG, DDU, CU
Associate Professor, Department of Obstetrics and Gynaecology, University of Sydney, Sydney, Australia

Grace Dorey PhD, FCSP
Professor Faculty of Health and Social Care, University of West of England, Bristol, UK

Chantale Dumoulin PhD, PT
Assistant Professor, École de Réadaptation, Faculté de Médecine, Université de Montréal, Canada

Helena Frawley PT, BAppSc, GradCertPhysio
Lecturer, Research Fellow, School of Physiotherapy, The University of Melbourne, Australia

Alessandra Graziottin MD
Director, Center of Gynecology and Medical Sexology, H. San Raffaele Resnati, Milano, Italy
Consultant Professor, School of Obstetrics and Gynecology, University of Florence and University of Parma, Italy
Co-director, Postgraduate Course in Medical Sexology, University of Florence, Italy

Rob Herbert BAppSc, MAppSc, PhD
Associate Professor, School of Physical Therapy and Centre for Evidence-Based Physiotherapy, University of Sydney, Australia

Erik Hendriks PhD, MSc, PT
Senior Researcher and Lecturer, Department of Epidemiology, Maastricht University, Maastricht, The Netherlands
Co-director, Department of Epidemiology and Center of Evidence Based Physiotherapy (CEBP) Maastricht, Maastricht University, Maastricht, The Netherlands
Health Scientist and Clinical Epidemiologist, Dutch Institute for Allied Health Care, Amersfoort, The Netherlands

Anders Mattiasson MD, PhD
Professor, Department of Urology, Clinical Sciences, Lund University, Lund, Sweden

Ilse E. P. E. Mesters PhD
Associate Professor, Department of Health Education and Health Promotion, University of Maastricht, Maastricht, The Netherlands

Job F. M. Metsemakers MD, PhD
Department Chair and Professor of General Practice/Family Medicine, University of Maastricht, Maastricht, The Netherlands

Siv Mørkved PT, MSc, PhD
Associate Professor, Clinical Service, St Olavs Hospital, Trondheim University Hospital and Department of Community Medicine & General Practice, Norwegian University of Science and Technology, Trondheim, Norway

Mélanie Morin MSc, PT
PhD Student, Montréal Rehabilitation Institute/Research Centre, Université de Montréal, Canada

Dudley Robinson MRCOG
Consultant Urogynaecologist, Department of Urogynaecology, King's College Hospital, London, UK

Ylva Sahlin MD, PhD
Chief surgeon, Department of Surgery, Hamar Hospital, Hamar, Norway

Margaret Sherburn PT
Lecturer and Research Fellow, Rehabilitation Science Research Centre, School of Physiotherapy, The University of Melbourne, Melbourne, Australia

H. W. van den Borne PhD
Professor of Patient Education, Department of Health Education and Promotion, University of Maastricht, Maastricht, The Netherlands

Marijke Van Kampen PT, MSc, PhD
Professor in Rehabilitation Science, Katholieke Universiteit Leuven, Faculty of Kinesiology and Rehabilitation Science, University Hospital GHB, Leuven, Belgium

David B. Vodušek MD, PhD
Professor of Neurology, Medical Faculty, University of Ljubljana, and Medical Director, Division of Neurology, University Medical Centre, Ljubljana, Slovenia

Jean F. Wyman PhD, APRN, BC, FAAN
Professor and Cora Meidl Siehl Chair in Nursing Research, School of Nursing, University of Minnesota, USA
Professor, Department of Family Medicine and Community Health, School of Medicine, Minneapolis, MN, USA

Foreword – International Continence Society

Walter Artibani

Conservative treatment, and namely physical therapy, is one of the mainstays of management of pelvic floor disorders and urinary incontinence. To transform clinical practice into science, and vice-versa to elect evidence-based medicine as the ground for clinical practice, is a challenge and this is what this wonderful book aims to reach.

Every single related topic is comprehensively dealt with, from anatomy, to neurophysiology, to assessment, to strategies of treatment. All possible clinical situations in which physical therapy can be effectively used are extensively covered including the existing evidence.

The editors and authors are to be commended for their efforts. The outcome is remarkable and this book is going to become THE reference book in regards with physical therapy to all those who are involved in pelvic floor disorders.

Walter Artibani
General Secretary
International Continence Society

Foreword – International Urogynecology Association

Paul A Riss

The science and clinical practice of the diagnosis and treatment of pelvic floor disorders has changed dramatically over the last few years. While previously most researchers and clinicians often focused on a particular problem and remained within their sometimes small area of expertise it has become apparent that the study of the pelvic floor requires a holistic approach. This is true for the different specialties – gynaecology, urology, physiotherapy, physiology – but even more because of the fact that it is not enough to look at a particular, well-circumscribed problem; many different aspects of a pelvic floor dysfunction have to be considered.

In this respect the role of physical therapy has become increasingly important. Originally physical therapy often was considered a minor adjunct in the treatment of pelvic floor disorders for highly motivated women. Today, however, the central role of physical therapy in the prevention and treatment of pelvic floor disorders and lower urinary tract symptoms is recognized. Without doubt it has been the work and experience of our colleagues from Scandinavia which has pioneered these developments.

We owe the Scandinavians a great debt: they not only popularized and implemented physical therapy in their countries but they also put physical therapy on a solid scientific basis. They addressed the questions of epidemiology, they conducted trials, and several reviews – for example in the Cochrane database – demonstrate the usefulness and effectiveness of physical therapy.

What has been lacking, however, is an overview bringing together the different aspects of physical therapy and putting them in context with medical and physiological research. This is what Professor Kari Bø and her colleagues from Norway and Belgium have done with this book. On one hand it almost feels like a textbook on pelvic floor disorders, on the other hand it shows how concepts of physical therapy are relevant for all kinds of problems and should be integrated into therapeutic concepts.

When reading this book one will immediately notice two particularly noteworthy aspects:

Firstly, as the title implies it is evidence-based physical therapy. This means that it is not just the narrative and anecdotal evidence of experienced physical therapists and clinicians but the results of studies and trials which form the basis of what is presented in this book. It goes without saying that in this respect special chapters of the book are devoted to methodology, to the design and the conduction of trials, and to the evaluation of data and the results of trials.

The second noteworthy feature of the book is the fact that it covers every aspect of pelvic floor dysfunction: male and female, sexual and urinary function, urinary and fecal incontinence, incontinence and prolapse, and of course the role of pregnancy and childbirth.

In this respect it is a very modern textbook. It is based on evidence, it brings together physical therapists, clinicians and researchers, and it focuses on what really matters – namely the problem of the patient which impacts on her or his quality of life. Dr Kari Bø, Dr Bary Berghmans, Dr Siv Morkved and Dr Marijke Van Kampen are to be congratulated on having brought together such a distinguished list of contributors. They will open our eyes and give us a new understanding of physical therapy of the pelvic floor.

Professor Dr Paul A Riss
Past President
International Urogynecology Association

Foreword – World Confederation of Physical Therapy

Sandra Mercer Moore

The World Confederation for Physical Therapy (WCPT) postulates that physical therapists have a duty and responsibility to use evidence to inform practice and to ensure that the care of clients, their carers and communities is based on the best available evidence. WCPT also believes that evidence should be integrated with clinical experience, taking into consideration beliefs and values and the cultural context of the local environment. In addition, physical therapists have a duty and responsibility not to use techniques and technologies that have been shown to be ineffective or unsafe.

It therefore follows that physical therapists should be prepared to critically evaluate their practice. In addition they need to be able to identify questions arising in practice, access and critically appraise the best evidence, and implement and evaluate outcomes of their actions (WCPT 2003).

Evidence-Based Physical Therapy for the Pelvic Floor takes us on a wonderful journey where three core themes of *synthesizing*, accessing and implementing evidence are intertwined. Throughout the wealth of information in the book is the constant reminder that in order to provide quality care using the best available evidence, the practitioner must have detailed knowledge of relevant sciences such as anatomy, physiology, pathology and measurement as well as a good understanding of critical appraisal and review of the effects of physical therapy interventions. The book contains an eclectic mix of physical therapy assessment and intervention for a range of conditions from childhood to older age and I am pleased to note that attention is given to both male and female patients.

On behalf of WCPT, I congratulate the authors and editors of *Evidence-Based Physical Therapy for the Pelvic Floor – Bridging Science and Clinical Practice* and commend them for their efforts in contributing to the body of knowledge in this important discipline.

Sandra Mercer Moore DBA MPhty
President
World Confederation of Physical Therapy

WCPT Declarations of Principle – Evidence Based Practice
Approved at the 15th General Meeting of WCPT, June 2003

Preface

Kari Bø, Bary Berghmans, Siv Mørkved and Marijke Van Kampen

It is with great pleasure and excitement that we present this new textbook! We hope it will attract all physical therapists interested in the broad area of function and dysfunction of the pelvic floor. The editors of this book have more than 20 years' experience in clinical practice and research in the prevention and treatment of symptoms of pelvic floor dysfunction. Between us our experience covers most areas of physical therapy for the pelvic floor, from children, women and men, to special groups such as pregnant and postpartum women, athletes, the elderly and patients with special health problems. In addition, we also have extensive background in other areas of physical therapy such as sports physiotherapy, neurology, rehabilitation, musculoskeletal, ergonomics, exercise science, health promotion, biomechanics, motor control and learning and implementation of guidelines.

Prevention and treatment of pelvic floor dysfunction is truly a multidisciplinary field in which every profession should play its own evidence-based role for the highest benefit of the patients. With this in mind, we are very proud that so many leading international clinicians, researchers and opinion leaders from different professions have participated in the realization of this book. Our sincere and warmest thanks to all of you for your unique contribution and the time and effort you have put in to making this book a truly evidence-based and up-to-date textbook.

We sincerely hope to have created a special and important book for the physical therapy profession for pelvic floor dysfunction. We anticipate that it will be useful for physical therapy schools and will be found in scientific libraries worldwide. Moreover, we hope this book will become the base for postgraduate studies in pelvic floor physical therapy. We hope that the multidisciplinary nature of the authorship of this book will be reflected in the readership, serving nurses and other health professionals working in conservative treatment and pelvic floor muscle training, as well as those in the physical therapy field.

As in the medical profession, clinical practice of physical therapy in pelvic floor has built up from a base of clinical experience, through small experimental studies to clinical trials. Today clinicians can build on protocols from high-quality randomized clinical trials (RCTs) showing sufficient effect size (the difference between the change in the intervention group and the change in the control group). A quick search on PEDro (the Physiotherapy Evidence Database, Sydney, Australia, www.pedro.fhs.usyd.edu.au) shows that physical therapy is changing rapidly from being a non-scientific field to a profession with a strong scientific platform. In February 2007 there were 8859 RCTs, 1478 systematic reviews and 461 evidence-based clinical practice guidelines in different areas of physical therapy listed in the database. While this book recognizes that much more research is needed into the prevention and treatment of many conditions in the pelvic floor area, there are already more than 50 RCTs evaluating the effect of pelvic floor muscle training for stress and mixed incontinence. Hence, in good clinical practice the physical therapist should adapt individual patient training programmes according to the protocols from these studies rather than using theories or models which are not backed by clinical data. In addition, good clinical practice always should be individualized and should be based on a combination of clinical experience, knowledge from high-quality RCTs and patient preferences. Next to this, good clinical practice should always be based on respect, empathy and strong ethical grounding.

In 2001, Lewis Wall, Professor of Urogynecology, wrote an editorial in the International Urogynecology Journal describing 7 stages in the life of medical innovations:

1. Promising report, clinical observation, case report, short clinical series
2. Professional and organizational adoption of the innovation
3. The public accepts the innovation – state or third party pays for it
4. Standard procedure – into textbooks (still no critical evaluation)
5. **RCT !**
6. Professional denunciation
7. Erosion of professional support, discredit.

He stated that by the time stage 7 is concluded, or even before the RCT has started, the procedure may already have given way to a new procedure or method which has grown in its wake. This cycle continues with these new methods and procedures being prescribed to patients without patients being informed about the effect, risk factors or complications. It is also noteworthy that, in most cases, patients are unaware of the fact that there is no scientific base for the proposed treatment. While Wall's description of the lifecycle applies specifically to medical innovations, we are subject to the same scrutiny and criticism in physical therapy.

Although physical therapy modalities, in comparison with surgery, rarely produce serious side effects or complications, we suggest that Wall's 7 stages also may be very useful to show how different theories, and not science, impact on physical therapy practice. We are keenly aware and concerned that in the long run such un-scientific evolution of practice will damage patients, the physical therapy profession itself and parties responsible for compensation. In particular, the use of such untested models and theories as a background for implementing new interventions when there is in fact evidence available for alternative and proven treatment strategies, must be considered bad clinical practice, and may even be considered unethical. Hence, it is our hope that this book will be a big step towards evidence-based practice in all symptom areas of pelvic floor dysfunction.

This does not mean that we should not treat conditions for which there are no or only few/weak controlled studies to support clinical practice. However, we sincerely believe that all physical therapists should be aware of the different level and value of statements, theories, clinical experience, knowledge from research designs other than RCTs and knowledge from high-quality research. It is a duty to openly explain to patients and other parties that the proposed treatment is not based on high-quality studies, but only on the best available knowledge at that time. The profession should never confuse statements, clinical experience and theories with evidence from high-quality RCTs, and optimally, we should not use new modalities in regular clinical practice until they have proved to be effective in RCTs. In this book we have tried our best to differentiate between the different levels of knowledge and evidence and to be very clear about the limitations of the research underlying the recommendations for practice. In line with this, we have left out those areas that were not convincing because of lack of evidence. These areas include:

- The role or effect of PFMT on core stability to prevent/treat low back and pelvic girdle pain
- The effect of 'functional training'
- The role of motor control training as the sole treatment of pelvic floor dysfunction
- The definition, assessment and treatment for 'hypertone pelvic floor'
- The effect of body posture on the pelvic floor
- The effect of respiration on the pelvic floor and vice versa.

Our aim is to continue updating the evidence in all areas of research in pelvic floor physical therapy. Therefore, we hope that the next edition will already include more areas because of the continuing growth of knowledge based on high-quality research.

The evidence presented in this book is based on reviews from the Cochrane Library, the three International Consensus Meetings on Incontinence, other systematic reviews and updated searches on newer RCTs. However, the conclusions of these high-quality systematic reviews can differ because they are a product of how the authors have posed their research questions, what type of studies they have included, what choice of outcome measures they have made, and how they have classified the studies. Therefore, not all conclusions in this book are in line with other conclusions. The goal of the editors of this book is to evaluate only clinically relevant research questions. Moreover, our selection procedure and strategy for the in- and exclusion of studies should be transparent and easy to understand for the readers of the book.

Active exercise is the core of physical therapy interventions. Passive treatments may be used to stimulate non-functioning muscles and to manage pain so that active exercise becomes possible. The following is a quote from Hippocrates which elegantly lends itself to the philosophy of physical therapy:

'All parts of the body which have a function, if used in moderation and exercised in labours in which each is accustomed, become thereby healthy, well-developed and age more slowly, but if unused and left idle they become liable to disease, defective in growth, and age quickly.' It is the role of the physical therapist to motivate patients and to facilitate exercise and adapted physical activity throughout the lifespan.

We hope that new students in this exciting and interesting field will find enough guidance in this book to begin to prevent, assess and treat pelvic floor dysfunction effectively in their clients/patients, but they must also learn to be critical of new theories and modalities that have not yet been tested sufficiently. For experienced physical therapists we hope that providing contemporary scientific evidence to support or contradict clinical practice will effect changes in practice and will push for more high-quality clinical research projects.

Hopefully, you will enjoy reading the book just as much as we have enjoyed working with it. Through working on the book we have certainly become aware of many unanswered questions, and have identified many new research areas that need to be addressed in this challenging area. We encourage the readers interested in research to continue with formal education in research methodology (MSc and PhD programs) and join us in trying to make high-quality clinical research in the future. We appreciate any constructive feedback for chapters to be changed or included for the next edition.

Kari Bø, Professor, PhD, MSc PT
Bary Berghmans, Researcher, PhD, MSc PT
Marijke Van Kampen, Professor, PhD, MSc PT
Siv Mørkved, Associate Professor, PhD, MSc PT

Chapter 1

Overview of physical therapy for pelvic floor dysfunction

Kari Bø

PELVIC FLOOR DYSFUNCTION

The framework of this book is based on the approach to disorders of the pelvic floor in women described by Wall & DeLancey (1991). Wall & DeLancey (1991) stated that 'pelvic floor dysfunction, particularly as manifested by genital prolapse and urinary or fecal incontinence, remains one of the largest unaddressed issues in women's health care today' (p. 486). In their opinion lack of success in treating patients with pelvic floor dysfunction is due to a professional 'compartmentalization' of the pelvic floor.

Each of the three outlets in the pelvis has had its own doctor and medical specialty, with the urethra and bladder belonging to the urologist, the vagina and female genital organs belonging to the gynaecologist, and the colon and rectum belonging to the gastroenterologist and the colorectal surgeon (Fig. 1.1).

Wall & DeLancey (1991) argue that instead of concentrating on the three 'holes' in the pelvis, one should look at the 'whole pelvis' with the pelvic floor muscles (PFM), ligaments and fasciae as the common supportive system for all the pelvic viscera.

The interaction between the PFM and the supportive ligaments was later elaborated by DeLancey (1993) and Norton (1993) as the 'boat in dry dock theory'. The ship is analogous to the pelvic organs, the ropes to the ligaments and fasciae and the water to the supportive layer of the PFM (Fig. 1.2).

DeLancey (1993) argues that as long as the PFM or levator ani muscles function normally, the pelvic floor is supportive and the ligaments and fascia are under normal tension.

When the PFM relax or are damaged, the pelvic organs must be held in place by the ligaments and fasciae alone. If the PFM cannot actively support the organs, over time the connective tissue will become stretched and damaged.

Bump & Norton (1998) also used this theoretical framework in their overview on the epidemiology and natural history of pelvic floor dysfunction. They suggested that pelvic floor dysfunction may lead to the following conditions:

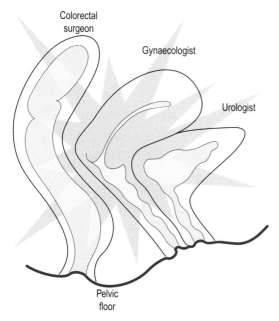

Fig. 1.1 Gynaecologists, urologist, and colorectal surgeons concentrate on their areas of interest and tend to ignore the pelvic floor common to them all.

- urinary incontinence (stress, urge and mixed incontinence);
- fecal incontinence;
- pelvic organ prolapse;
- sensory and emptying abnormalities of the lower urinary tract;
- defecatory dysfunction;
- sexual dysfunction;
- chronic pain syndromes.

Bump & Norton (1998) also described three stages in the development of pelvic floor dysfunction:

1. a perfect pelvic floor that is anatomically, neurologically, and functionally normal;
2. a less than perfect, but well-compensated pelvic floor in an asymptomatic patient;
3. a functionally decompensated pelvic floor in the patient with end-stage disease with urinary incontinence, anal incontinence, or pelvic organ prolapse.

A model describing etiological factors possibly leading to or causing pelvic floor dysfunction in women has been developed, classifying the factors into:

- predisposing factors (e.g. gender, genetic, neurological, anatomical, collagen, muscular, cultural and environmental);
- inciting factors (e.g. childbirth, nerve damage, muscle damage, radiation, tissue disruption, radical surgery);
- promoting factors (e.g. constipation, occupation, recreation, obesity, surgery, lung disease, smoking, menstrual cycle, infection, medication, menopause);
- decompensating factors (e.g. ageing, dementia, debility, disease, environment, medications).

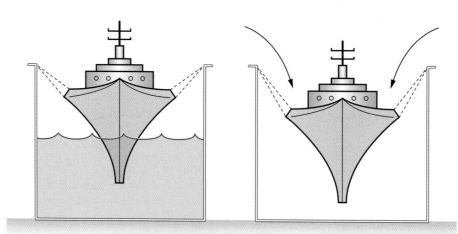

Fig. 1.2 'Boat in dry dock'. (From Norton 1993, p 927.)

Wall & DeLancey (1991) argued that progress in the treatment of pelvic floor dysfunction in women would occur more rapidly if a unified, cross disciplinary approach to disorders of the pelvic support was developed.

Wall & DeLancey (1991) mentioned only the different medical professions as part of a multidisciplinary team. In this book we will argue that physical therapists (PTs), having assessment and treatment of the musculoskeletal system in general as their speciality, should be core professionals in a multidisciplinary approach to pelvic floor dysfunction.

PHYSICAL THERAPY FOR THE PELVIC FLOOR

The nature of physical therapy

In May 1999, at the 14th General Meeting of The World Confederation for Physical Therapy (WCPT), a position statement describing the nature and process of physical therapy/physical therapy was approved by all member nations (1999). This description will be used as a foundation and framework to give an overview of physical therapy/physical therapy in the area of pelvic floor dysfunction. The term 'physical therapy' will be used throughout this book, in accordance with the guidelines of the WCPT Europe.

According to the WCPT, physical therapy is 'providing services to people and populations to develop, maintain and restore maximum movements and functional ability throughout the lifespan'.

The main area of practice for PT is musculoskeletal pain and dysfunction. However, many PTs also specialize in other areas such as the cardiorespiratory field, neurology, and coronary disease. In all areas PTs aim to improve functional capacity and improve the patients' ability to maintain or increase physical activity level.

The PFM are not responsible for gross motor movements alone, but work in synergy with other trunk muscles. Therefore, pelvic floor dysfunction may lead to symptoms during movement and perceived restriction in the ability to stay physically active (Bø et al 1989, Nygaard et al 1990). Several studies have shown that, for example, urinary incontinence may lead to a change in movement patterns during physical activities (Bø et al 1989, Nygaard et al 1990), withdrawal from regular fitness activities and bother when being active (Brown & Miller 2001, Nygaard et al 1990).

Lifelong participation in regular moderate physical activity is important in the prevention of several dis-

eases, and is an independent factor in the prevention of osteoporosis, obesity, diabetes mellitus, high blood pressure, coronary heart disease, breast and colon cancer, depression and anxiety (Bouchard et al 1993).

In addition, limitations in the ability to move or conduct activities of daily living either due to age or injuries may also lead to other problems, such as secondary incontinence.

Physical therapy for pelvic floor dysfunction may therefore also include physical activities for increasing general function and fitness level.

'Physical therapy includes the provision of services in circumstances where movement and function are threatened by the process of aging or that of injury or disease'

WCPT

Hippocrates (5th–4th centuries BC) claimed that 'all parts of the body which have a function, if used in moderation and exercised in labors in which each is accustomed, become thereby healthy, well-developed and age more slowly, but if unused and left idle they become liable to disease, defective in growth, and age quickly'.

The PFM are subject to continuous strain throughout the lifespan. In particular, the pelvic floor of women is subject to tremendous strain during pregnancy and childbirth (Mørkved 2003). In addition, hormonal changes may influence the pelvic floor and pelvic organs and a decline in muscle strength may occur due to aging. Hence, the PFM may need regular training to stay healthy throughout life.

'Physical therapy is concerned with identifying and maximizing movement potential, within the spheres of health promotion, prevention, treatment, and rehabilitation'

WCPT

Physical therapists may promote PFM training (PFMT) by writing about the issue in newspapers and women's magazines, informing all their regular patients about PFMT, including PFMT in regular exercise classes and in particular in antenatal and postnatal training, as well as before and after pelvic surgery in men and women. Physical therapists who treat pelvic floor dysfunction should be fully trained in this specialty or should refer to colleagues who have the thorough knowledge to treat patients according to the principles of evidence based physical therapy.

'Physical therapy is an essential part of the health services delivery system'

WCPT

'PTs practice independently of other health care providers and also within interdisciplinary rehabilitation/habilitation programs for the restoration of optimal function and quality of life in individuals with loss and disorders of movement'

WCPT

In most countries physical therapy work is by referral from medical practitioners. However, during recent decades this has changed in some countries such as Australia and New Zealand. In 2006 Dutch PTs have also become primary contact practitioners. Both systems require good collaboration between the medical and physical therapy professions.

The referral system implies that the medical practitioner is aware of what the PT can offer, and also has PTs available to send referrals to. One of the weaknesses of this system is that medical practitioners who are not motivated or who have insufficient knowledge about the evidence for different physical therapy interventions will not send suitable patients to physical therapy. The patients will more likely be offered traditional medical treatment options such as medication or surgery. These treatments may have adverse effects and are more expensive than exercise therapy (Black & Downs 1996, Smith et al 2002). In addition, the referral system is expensive because it involves an extra consultation.

The argument against PTs as primary contact practitioners has been that PTs do not have enough education to make differential diagnoses, and may therefore not detect more serious diseases such as cancer or neurological disease underlying the symptoms.

The editors of this book do not take a stand for either system of physical therapy service. We believe that prevention and treatment of pelvic floor dysfunction needs a multidisciplinary approach and would encourage collaboration between physicians and PTs at all levels of assessment and treatment.

'Physical therapy involves ". . . using knowledge and skills unique to physical therapists and, is the service ONLY (author's emphasis) provided by, or under the direction and supervision of a physical therapist"'

WCPT

The educational standard of PTs differs between countries throughout the world. In the US, physical therapy is at master's degree level (although this is based on an undergraduate degree other than physical therapy), whereas in most countries in Europe, Asia, Africa, it is a 3-year bachelor degree and in Australia and New Zealand it is a 4-year bachelor degree with the possibility to continue with a master's degree and PhD.

Physical therapy schools are within the university in many countries, but in other countries physical therapy is taught in polytechnic schools or colleges below university level.

There can be different educational requirements for entry into undergraduate programmes within one country and from country to country. In most countries, however, physical therapy is a professional education and the entry level for physical therapy undergraduate studies is very high, in some countries being at the same level as medicine. In the area of pelvic floor dysfunction, several PTs are professors and many PTs throughout the world have master's and PhDs.

The emphasis on pelvic floor dysfunction in undergraduate physical therapy curricula varies between countries at both undergraduate and postgraduate physical therapy level. The broad knowledge of anatomy and physiology, medical science, clinical assessment and treatment modalities learnt by all PTs can be applied to the pelvic floor. Several countries also have postgraduate education programmes for PTs specializing either in women's health or pelvic or pelvic floor physical therapy with education level and content varying between countries.

'The physical therapy process includes assessment, diagnosis, planning, intervention, and evaluation'

WCPT

Assessment

'Assessment includes both the examination of individuals or groups with actual or potential impairments, functional limitations, disabilities, or other conditions of health by history taking, screening and the use of specific tests and measures, and evaluation of the results of examination through analysis and synthesis within a process of clinical reasoning'

WCPT

In patients with pelvic floor dysfunction, after thorough history taking, the PT will assess the function of the pelvic floor by visual observation, vaginal palpation and/or measurement of muscle activity (measurement of vaginal or urethral squeeze pressure, electromyography [EMG], ultrasound) (Bø & Sherburn 2005).

Diagnosis

'In carrying out the diagnostic process, physical therapists may need to obtain additional information from other professionals'

WCPT

Most PTs in private practice obtain referrals of patients from general practitioners. These medical practitioners themselves seldom have access to urodynamics, EMG, magnetic resonance imaging (MRI) or ultrasound.

According to the Report from the Standardization Subcommittee of the International Continence Society (Abrams et al 2002) a diagnosis of stress or urge incontinence or pelvic pain syndrome cannot be based on history taking alone. Therefore, interdisciplinary collaborations with other professionals are highly recommended. In real life most PTs in private practice treat patients who have not undergone a thorough diagnostic investigation.

DeLancey (1996) has suggested that the cure and improvement rates of PFMT would be higher for stress urinary incontinence (SUI) if more detailed knowledge about the pathophysiology of each patient was available.

Planning

'A plan of intervention includes measurable outcome goals negotiated in collaboration with the patient/client, family or care giver. Alternatively it may lead to referral to another agency in cases which are inappropriate for physical therapy'

                                                    WCPT

It is extremely important that the patient decides the final goal of the treatment. For example, not all women need to be totally dry during jumping because they may never perform this activity.

One goal for an elderly woman might be to be able to lift her grandchild without leaking or feeling heaviness from a pelvic organ prolapse. If she is able to contract the PFM with a certain degree of strength this may be quite easy to accomplish with proper instruction of pre-contraction of the PFM before and during lifting.

Another woman may have the goal of being totally dry or having good organ support while playing tennis (Bø et al 2004a). To achieve this she may need much more intensive PFM training because she needs to build up muscle volume and stiffness of the pelvic floor and gain an automatic PFM action during an increase in abdominal pressure or a high ground reaction force (Bø 2004b).

Because most PTs treat patients with pelvic floor dysfunction without a full diagnosis it is of utmost importance that they communicate with other medical professions if they discover discrepancies between expected outcomes, or suspect other underlying conditions to be the cause of the patient's complaints. For example, urgency and urge incontinence may be the first signs of multiple sclerosis.

Intervention

'In general physical therapy intervention is implemented and modified in order to reach agreed goals and may include: manual handling; movement enhancing; physical, electro-therapeutic and mechanical agents; functional training (muscle strength and endurance, coordination, motor control, body-awareness, flexibility, relaxation, cardiorespiratory fitness); provision of aids and appliances; patient/client related instruction and counseling; documentation and coordination, and communication'

                                                    WCPT

In treating pelvic floor dysfunction the mainstay of physical therapy is education about the dysfunction, in-formation regarding lifestyle interventions, manual techniques and PFMT.

PFMT can be taught with or without the use of biofeedback or other adjunctive therapies, such as electrical stimulation or mechanical agents. It includes teaching of the correct contraction, muscle and body awareness, coordination and motor control, muscle strength and endurance, and relaxation.

The PT will choose different treatment programmes for different conditions and different patients. In some cases the PT will also provide preventive devices to the patients, and teach them how to use them.

Interventions may also be aimed at preventing impairments, functional limitations, disability and injury and include the promotion and maintenance of health, quality of life, and fitness in all ages and populations.

To prevent urinary incontinence, teaching pelvic floor exercises in pregnancy and after childbirth is essential.

The choice of interventions should always be based on the highest level of evidence available.

Ideally, the PT will choose the protocol from a randomized controlled trial (RCT) where the intervention has been shown to be effective and adjust this to the patient's needs and practical requirements.

In the area of SUI there is sufficient knowledge from RCTs to choose an effective training protocol. However, in other conditions that may be caused by pelvic floor dysfunction such knowledge is not yet available. The PT then has to develop a programme on the basis of clinical experience (his or her own or other experts), small experimental studies or theories. It is essential that such experience or theories are quickly developed into research hypotheses and tested in RCTs by trained researchers to see if there is a clinically worthwhile effect.

Collaboration between experienced clinicians and researchers is extremely important in planning clinical research. Experienced clinicians should not jump at new theories and ideas or change their practice based on theories and small experimental studies alone. Ideally, the only information that should lead to a drastic change of clinical practice are results (positive or negative) from RCTs.

When undertaking research and deciding on a PT intervention, the PT must be aware that the 'quality of the intervention', particularly the intensity of the physical therapy intervention, will affect the outcome. Ineffective (low dose) or even harmful treatments can be in a RCT that has high-quality methodology. These research challenges are the same when conducting RCTs that include both surgery and PFMT, and the methodological quality of studies of both surgery and PFMT has been variable (Hay-Smith et al 2001, Smith et al 2002).

When participating in research led by other professionals it is important that the physical therapy intervention meets quality standards. No drug company would dream of conducting a study with a non-optimal dosage of the drug. In published RCTs, there are several PFMT programmes with low dosage showing little or no effect (Hay-Smith et al 2001).

Evaluation

'Evaluation necessitates re-examination for the purpose of evaluating outcomes'

WCPT

Using the same outcome measures before and after treatment is mandatory for the purpose of evaluating outcomes in clinical practice.

In treating symptoms of pelvic floor dysfunction the PT uses different forms of PFMT (**independent variable** in experimental research) to change the condition (named **dependent variable** in experimental research e.g. stage of pelvic organ prolapse, pelvic pain or SUI).

It is mandatory that PTs use the concept of the International Classification of Impairment, Disability and Handicap (ICIDH) (1997), later changed to International Classification of Function (ICF) (2002) to evaluate efficacy of the intervention. The ICF is a World Health Organization (WHO)-approved system designed to classify health and health related states. According to this system (see Ch. 5.1) different health components are related to specific diseases and conditions:

- body functions: physiological and psychological functions of body systems (e.g. delayed motor latency of the nerves to the PFM);
- body structures: anatomical parts (e.g. rupture or atrophy of the PFM);
- impairments: problems in body function or structure such as significant deviation or loss (e.g. weak or non-coordinated PFM);

- activity: execution of a task or action by an individual (e.g. to stay continent during increase in abdominal pressure);
- participation: involvement in a life situation (being able to participate in social situations such as playing tennis or aerobic dancing without fear or embarrassment of leaking);
- environment (e.g. easy access to the bathroom).

Physical therapy aims to improve factors involving all these components. Therefore we need to select different outcome measures for different components. For example, PFMT may improve timing of the co-contraction during cough (ICF: body functions; neurophysiology). This may be measured by wire or needle EMG.

One of the aims for PFMT in treating pelvic organ prolapse (POP) is to alter the length/stiffness of the PFM so they sit at a higher anatomical location inside the pelvis (ICF: body structure, anatomy). This may be measured using MRI or ultrasound.

Impairment of the PFM can result from inability to produce optimal strength (force). Muscle strength can be measured by manometers or dynamometers during attempts of maximal contraction.

Ambulatory urodynamics of urethral pressure during physical activities may be developed as a future measure of automatic co-contraction during activity.

Urinary leakage could be classified as disability in the ICIDH and as activity in the new ICF system. The actual leakage can be measured by number of leakage episodes (self report) or pad tests.

Physical therapy also aims at, for example, reducing urinary leakage to a point where this is no longer restricting the patient from participation in social activities (ICF: participation). This can be measured by quality of life questionnaires. PTs can also work politically to improve the environment such as advocating for easy access to toilets in public buildings.

Ideally, PTs should assess the effect of the physical therapy intervention in all these components using outcome measures with high responsiveness (measurement tools that can detect small differences), reliability (intra- and inter-tester reproducibility), and validity (to what degree the measurement tool measures what it is meant to measure).

PTs should 'use terminology that is widely understood and adequately defined' and 'recognize internationally accepted models and definitions'

WCPT

In the area of pelvic floor dysfunction we are fortunate to have international committees working on standardization and terminology. The International Continence Society (ICS) constantly revises its standardization of terminology (Abrams et al 2002), and the Clinical Assessment Group within the same society has also delivered a standardization document (www.icsoffice.com).

Physical therapists must refer to definitions and terminology from the WHO, the WCPT and for definitions and standards developed in exercise science and motor learning and control to be able to communicate effectively with other professions.

Linking research and practice

'Emphasise the need for practice to be evidence-based whenever possible' and *'appreciate the interdependence of practice, research and education within the profession'*

WCPT

Sackett et al (2000) has defined evidence-based medicine as 'the conscientious, explicit and judicious use of current best evidence in making decisions about care of individual patients'. Neither the best available external clinical evidence (RCTs) nor clinical expertise alone is good enough for decision making in clinical practice. Without clinical experience, 'evidence' can ignore the individual's needs and circumstances, and without evidence, 'experience' can become old fashioned/out of date.

Evidence-based (PT) practice has a theoretical body of knowledge, uses the best available scientific evidence in clinical decision making and uses standardized outcome measures to evaluate the care provided (Herbert et al 2005).

Herbert et al (2005) have stated that research conducted as part of routine clinical practice can be prone to bias because there is often a lack of comparison of outcomes with outcomes of randomized controls. In such studies it may be difficult to distinguish between effects of intervention and natural recovery or statistical regression. In addition, self-reported outcomes may be biased because patients may feel obliged to the therapist. There may be no record or follow-up of dropouts, outcome measures may be distorted by assessors' expectations of intervention, adherence to the training protocol is seldom reported and long-term results are often not available. The best evidence of effects of intervention comes from randomized trials with adequate follow-up and blinding of assessors and, where possible, blinding of patients too.

Our understanding of the mechanisms of therapies is often incomplete, and it is unknown whether the effects of some PT interventions are large enough to be worthwhile (effect size).

Only high-quality clinical research (RCTs) potentially provides unbiased estimates of the effect size (Herbert 2000a, b). This provides several challenges in clinical practice.

To increase their level of knowledge in clinical practice PTs need to:

- stay updated in pathophysiology;
- use interventions for which we have evidence-based knowledge of dose–response issues;
- if possible: use interventions/protocols based on results/protocols from high quality RCTS with positive results (clinically relevant effect-size);
- use pre- and post-treatment tests that are responsive, reliable, and valid;
- measure adherence and adverse effects!

ROLE OF THE PHYSICAL THERAPIST IN PELVIC FLOOR DYSFUNCTION

- Work in a team with other professions in medicine (e.g. general practitioner, urologist, gynecologist, radiologist).

- Evaluate the degree of pelvic floor dysfunction symptoms and complaints and overall condition by covering all components of the ICF.

- Fully evaluate PFM performance, including ability to contract and strength.

- Set individual treatment goals and plan treatment programmes in collaboration with the patient.

- Treat the condition individually and/or conduct PFM exercise classes.

- Teach preventive PFM exercise individually or in classes during pregnancy and postnatally.

- Clinicians without a research background can participate in high-standard research as deliverers of high-quality physical therapy and conduct evaluation of the intervention. They should, however, refuse to be involved in studies with low-quality methodology and/or low-quality intervention (e.g. inadequate dosage).

- Research PTs should:
  - conduct basic research on tissue adaptation to different treatment modalities;
  - participate in the development of responsive, reliable and valid tools to assess PFM function and strength and outcome measures;
  - conduct high-quality methodological and interventional RCTs to evaluate effect of different physical therapy interventions.

REFERENCES

Abrams P, Cardozo L, Fall M et al 2002 The standardization of terminology of lower urinary tract function: report from the standardization sub-committee of the International Continence Society. Neurourology and Urodynamics 21:167–178

Black N A, Downs S H 1996 The effectiveness of surgery for stress urinary incontinence in women: a systematic review. British Journal of Urology 78:487–510

Bø K 2004a Urinary incontinence, pelvic floor dysfunction, exercise and sport. Sports Medicine 34(7):451–464

Bø K 2004b Pelvic floor muscle training is effective in treatment of stress urinary incontinence, but how does it work? International Urogynecology Journal and Pelvic Floor Dysfunction 15:76–84

Bø K, Mæhlum S, Oseid S, Larsen S 1989 Prevalence of stress urinary incontinence among physically active and sedentary female students. Scandinavian Journal of Sports Sciences 11(3):113–116

Bø K, Sherburn M 2005 Evaluation of female pelvic-floor muscle function and strength. Physical Therapy 85(3):269–282

Bouchard C, Shephard R J, Stephens T 1993 Physical activity, fitness, and health. Consensus Statement. Human Kinetics Publishers, Champaign IL

Brown W, Miller Y 2001 Too wet to exercise? Leaking urine as a barrier to physical activity in women. Journal of Science and Medicine in Sport 4(4):373–378

Bump R C, Norton P A 1998 Epidemiology and natural history of pelvic floor dysfunction. Obstetrics and Gynecology Clinics of North America 25(4):723–746

DeLancey J O L 1993 Anatomy and biomechanics of genital prolapse. Clinical Obstetrics and Gynecology 36(4):897–909

DeLancey J 1996 Stress urinary incontinence: where are we now, where should we go? American Journal of Obstetrics and Gynecology 175:311–319

Description of Physical Therapy 1999 14th General Meeting, Yokohama, World Confederation of Physical Therapy

Hay-Smith E, Bø K, Berghmans L et al 2001 Pelvic floor muscle training for urinary incontinence in women (Cochrane review). [3] The Cochrane Library, Oxford

Herbert R D 2000a Critical appraisal of clinical trials. I: estimating the magnitude of treatment effects when outcomes are measured on a continuous scale. Australian Journal of Physiotherapy 46:229–235

Herbert R D 2000b Critical appraisal of clinical trials. II: estimating the magnitude of treatment effects when outcomes are measured on a dichotomous scale. Australian Journal of Physiotherapy 46:309–313

Herbert R D, Jamtvedt G, Mead J et al 2005 Practical evidence-based physiotherapy. Elsevier, Oxford

International Classification of Impairment, Disability, and Handicap (ICIDH) 1997 WHO, Zeist

International Classification of Functioning, Disability and Health (ICF) 2002 WHO, Marketing and Dissemination, Geneva

Mørkved S 2003 Urinary incontinence during pregnancy and after childbirth. Effect of pelvic floor muscle training in prevention and treatment. Doctoral thesis. NTNU, Trondheim, Norway

Nygaard I, DeLancey J O L, Arnsdorf L et al 1990 Exercise and incontinence. Obstetrics and Gynecology 75:848–851

Norton P 1993 Pelvic floor disorders: the role of fascia and ligaments. Clinical Obstetrics and Gynecology 36(4):926–938

Sackett D, Straus S, Richardson W et al 2000 Evidence based medicine. How to practice and teach EBM, 2nd edn. Churchill Livingstone, London

Smith T, Daneshgari F, Dmochowski R et al 2002 Surgical treatment of incontinence in women. In: Abrams P, Cardozo L, Khoury S et al (eds) Incontinence, 2nd edn. Plymbridge Distributors, Plymouth, UK, p 823–863

Wall L, DeLancey J 1991 The politics of prolapse: a revisionist approach to disorders of the pelvic floor in women. Perspectives of Biological Medicine 34(4):486–496

Chapter 2

Critical appraisal of randomized trials and systematic reviews of the effects of physical therapy interventions for the pelvic floor

Rob Herbert

In the preceding chapter, Kari Bø described her vision of physical therapy for the pelvic floor. A core part of that vision is that practice should be guided by evidence in the form of high-quality clinical research. This chapter develops that theme by considering one specific sort of evidence: evidence about the effects of interventions. The chapter begins by identifying the sorts of evidence that tell us about the effects of intervention. It then explores how readers of the research literature can differentiate between high- and low-quality evidence. The chapter concludes by briefly considering how high-quality evidence of the effects of intervention can be used to assist clinical decisions.

RANDOMIZED TRIALS AND SYSTEMATIC REVIEWS

Randomized trials

Randomized trials (also called randomized **controlled** trials or randomized **clinical** trials [RCTs]) provide a mechanism for estimating the effects of interventions. They involve samples of people (trial 'subjects' or 'participants') drawn from clinical populations who either have a health disorder (in studies of treatment) or are at risk of a health disorder (in studies of prevention).

Each participant in the trial is randomly allocated to receive the intervention of interest or not. The group of participants that does not receive the intervention of interest is often called the 'control group'. Subsequently the experimenter compares the outcomes of participants in the intervention and control groups.

There are a number of variations on this broad approach (Herbert et al 2005). In the simplest version, participants are allocated to groups that receive intervention or a group that receives no intervention. Alternatively, participants in both groups could receive standard care but participants in one group could receive, in addition, the intervention of interest. Or one group could receive an intervention and the other group could receive a different intervention. If participants are randomized to groups all of these variations can be called randomized trials.

Two features differentiate randomized trials from other studies of the effects of intervention: there is comparison between outcomes of groups that do and do not receive a particular intervention, and participants are allocated to conditions using a random procedure. These features make it possible to separate out the effects of intervention from other factors that influence clinical outcomes, such as the natural history of a condition, or statistical phenomena such as statistical regression. The logic is as follows: randomization generates groups that are likely to be very similar, especially in large trials. So when we give the intervention of interest to one group and not the other, differences in the outcomes of the two groups are attributable to the intervention. A complication is that, because randomization produces similar but not identical groups, differences in outcomes could be due to small differences between groups at baseline. Statistical methods can be used to assess whether this is plausible or not. This means that the difference between the outcomes of the two groups in a randomized trial provides an estimate of the effect of intervention.

Importantly, randomization is the **only** way to generate two groups that we can know are comparable. No other method can assure a 'fair comparison' between intervention and control groups. (Some empirical evidence suggests well-conducted non-randomized trials often produce similar results to randomized trials [Benson & Hartz 2000, Concato et al 2000; but see Kunz & Oxman 1998], but there is no reason why we should **expect** that to be so.) For this reason randomized trials can claim to be the only method that can be expected to generate unbiased estimates of the effects of interventions.

Systematic reviews

Many physical therapy practices, including several interventions for the pelvic floor, have been subjected to multiple randomized trials. Where more than one trial has examined the effects of the same intervention we can potentially learn more from a careful examination of the totality of evidence provided by all relevant randomized trials than from any individual trial. Potentially we can get more information about the effects of an intervention from literature reviews rather than from individual studies.

Until a couple of decades ago, reviews of the literature were conducted in an unsystematic way. Authors of reviews would find what they considered to be relevant trials, read them carefully, and write about the findings of those trials. The authors of the best reviews were able to differentiate between high- and low-quality trials to bring together a balanced synthesis that fairly reflected what existing trials said about the effects of the intervention.

Nonetheless, traditional (narrative) reviews have always had one important shortcoming: their methods are inscrutable. It is hard for readers of narrative reviews to know if the review was carried out optimally. Readers cannot determine, without specific knowledge of the literature under review, whether the reviewer identified all of the relevant trials or properly weighted the findings of high-quality and low-quality studies. Also, readers usually cannot know how the reviewer went about drawing together the findings of the relevant trials to synthesize the review's conclusions. There must always be some concern that the evidence provided in narrative reviews is biased by selective reporting of studies, unbalanced assessment of trial quality, or partial interpretations of what the best trials mean.

The method of **systematic** reviews was developed in the late 1970s to overcome some of the shortcomings of narrative reviews (Egger et al 2001, Glass et al 1981). The most important characteristic of systematic reviews is that they explicitly describe the methods used to conduct the review; typically systematic reviews have a methods section that describes how the search was conducted, how trials were selected, how data were extracted, and how the data were used to synthesize the findings of the review. Thus, in systematic reviews, the methods are transparent. This means the reader can make judgments about how well the review was conducted.

A principle that underlies the design of most systematic reviews is that the methods should minimize bias by attempting to find all relevant trials, or at least a representative subset of the relevant trials. Also, predetermined criteria are used to assess the quality of trials, and to draw together the findings of individual trials to generate an overall conclusion.

To summarize, systematic reviews generally provide a better source of information about the effects of an intervention than narrative reviews because they employ transparent methods designed to minimize bias (Box 2.1).

What can't randomized trials and systematic reviews tell us?

Theoretically, randomized trials could provide us with estimates of the effects of every physical therapy intervention and every component of every physical therapy intervention. In practice, we are a long way from that position, and it is likely we will never get there.

Randomized trials are cumbersome instruments. They are able to provide unbiased estimates of the effects of interventions, but do so at a cost. Many trials enroll hundreds or even thousands of participants and follow them for months or years. The magnitude of this undertaking means that it is not possible to conduct trials to examine the effects of every permutation of every component of every intervention for every patient group.

In practice the best that randomized trials can provide us with is indicative estimates of effects of typical interventions administered in a small subset of reasonable ways to typical populations, even though we know that when the intervention is applied in clinical settings its effects will vary depending on precisely how the intervention is administered and precisely who the intervention is administered to.

Randomized trials can suggest treatment approaches, but the fine detail of how interventions are implemented will always have to be supplemented by clinical experience, by our understandings of how the intervention works, and by common sense.

Randomized trials and systematic reviews of randomized trials are suited to answering questions about the effects of interventions, but are not able to answer other sorts of questions. Different sorts of designs are required to answer questions about the prognosis of a particular condition or about the interpretation of a diagnostic test (Herbert et al 2005).

A major limitation of randomized trials is that the methods developed for analysing randomized trials can only be applied to quantitative measures of outcomes. But it is not possible to quantify the full complexity of people's thoughts and feelings with quantitative measures (Herbert & Higgs 2004). If we want to understand how people experience an intervention we need to consult studies that employ qualitative methods, such as focus groups or in-depth interviews, rather than randomized trials. In general, qualitative methods cannot tell us about the effects of intervention but, because they can tell us about people's experiences of intervention, they can inform decisions about whether or not to intervene in a particular way.

How can the evidence be located, and how much evidence is there?

Several databases can be used to locate randomized trials and systematic reviews of the effects of intervention.

PubMed indexes the general health literature and can be accessed free of charge at http://www.pubmed.gov.

CENTRAL, part of the Cochrane Library (http://www.mrw.interscience.wiley.com/cochrane/), specifically indexes randomized trials and is free in many countries. (To see a list of countries from which CENTRAL can be accessed free of charge, follow the link to 'Do you already have access?').

The only database that specifically indexes randomized trials and systematic reviews of physical therapy interventions is PEDro. It is freely available at www.pedro.fhs.usyd.edu.au. In May 2005, a quick search of the PEDro database for records indexed as relevant to the 'pelvic floor or genitourinary system' yielded 183 randomized trials and 40 systematic reviews. The quality of these trials will be discussed in the next section.

Dimensions of quality of randomized trials and systematic reviews

Randomized trials and systematic reviews vary greatly in quality. There are high-quality studies that have been carefully designed, meticulously conducted and rigorously analysed, and there are low-quality studies that have not!

Physical therapists must be able to differentiate between high- and low-quality studies if they are to be able to discern the real effects of intervention.

A key characteristic of high-quality randomized trials and systematic reviews is that they are relatively **unbiased**. That is, they do not systematically underestimate or overestimate effects of intervention.

And of course high-quality trials and reviews must also be **relevant** to clinical practice. That is, they must tell us about the effects of interventions when administered well to appropriate patients, and about the effects of the intervention on outcomes that are important. Finally, high-quality trials and reviews provide us with **precise estimates** of the size of treatment effects. The precision of the estimates is primarily a function of the sample size (the number of subjects in a trial or the number of subjects in all studies in the review). Thus the highest quality trials and reviews, those that best support clinical decision making, are large, unbiased and relevant.

The following sections consider how readers of trials and reviews can assess these aspects of quality.

SEPARATING THE WHEAT FROM THE CHAFF: DETECTING BIAS IN TRIALS AND REVIEWS

Detecting bias in randomized trials

When we read reports of randomized trials we would like to know if the trials are biased or not. Another way of saying this is that we need to assess the validity (or 'internal validity') of the trials.

One way to assess internal validity is to see how well the trial has been designed. Over the past 50 years methodologists have refined the methods used to conduct randomized trials to the extent that there is now consensus, at least with regards to the main features of trial design, about what constitutes best practice in the design of clinical trials (Moher et al 2001, Pocock 1984). This suggests we could assess internal validity of individual trials by examining how well their methods correspond to what is thought to be best practice in trial design.

Alternatively, we could base judgments about the validity of trials on empirical evidence of bias. Several studies have shown that, all else being equal, certain design features are associated with smaller estimates of the effects of intervention (e.g. Chalmers et al 1983, Colditz et al 1989, Moher et al 1998, Schulz et al 1995). This has been interpreted as indicating that these design features are markers of bias.

Potentially we could use either of these approaches: we could base decisions about the validity of trials either on expert opinion or empirical evidence. There is much debate about which is the best way to assess validity. But fortunately both approaches suggest that trial validity should be assessed by looking for the presence of similar features of trial design (Box 2.2).

Random allocation

Most methodologists believe that true random allocation reduces the possibilities for bias, and some empirical evidence supports this position (Kunz & Oxman 1998). To ensure that allocation is truly randomized it is important to ensure that the person who recruits patients into the trial is unaware, at the time he or she makes

> **Box 2.2:** Key features conferring validity to clinical trials
>
> - True (concealed) random allocation of participants to groups
> - Blinding of participants and assessors
> - Adequate follow-up

decisions about whether or not to admit a patient into the trial which group the patient would subsequently be allocated to. Similarly, it is important that patients do not know which group they would be allocated to. This is referred to as **concealment** of the allocation schedule.

Failure to conceal allocation potentially distorts randomization because experimenters might be reluctant to let patients with the most serious symptoms into the trial if they know the patient is to be allocated to the control group, and patients may be less likely to choose to participate in the trial if they know they will subsequently be allocated to the control group. This would generate groups that are not comparable at baseline with regard to disease severity, so it introduces potential for serious bias. For this reason concealment is thought to protect against bias in randomized trials. Indeed, empirical evidence suggests failure to conceal allocation may be one of the most important indicators of bias (Chalmers et al 1983, Schulz et al 1995).

Of the trials of physical therapy for the pelvic floor listed on the PEDro database, only 27% explicitly conceal the allocation schedule.

Blinding

A second key design feature is blinding. Blinding implies that a person (such as a trial participant or a person assessing trial outcomes) is unaware of whether the trial participant is in the intervention group or the control group.

Blinding of the **participants** in a trial is achieved by giving a sham intervention to subjects in the control group. Sham interventions are interventions that resemble the intervention of interest, but are thought to have no specific therapeutic effect. (An example of an attempt to use a sham condition in a trial of an intervention for the pelvic floor is the trial by Sand et al (1995) which compared the effects of active transvaginal electrical stimulation with sham stimulation.)

By providing a sham intervention all trial participants can appear to receive intervention, but only the intervention group receives active intervention. Consequently trial participants can be 'kept in the dark' about whether they are receiving the intervention or control condition.

The usual justification for blinding trial participants is that this makes it possible to determine if an intervention has more of an effect than just a placebo effect. In so far as placebo effects occur, they are expected to occur to an equal degree in intervention and sham-intervention groups, so in sham-controlled trials the estimated effect of intervention – the difference between group outcomes – is not influenced by placebo effects.

An additional and perhaps more important justification is that, in trials with self-reported outcomes, blinding of participants removes the possibility of bias created by patients misreporting their outcomes. In unblinded trials, patients in the intervention group could exaggerate improvements in their outcomes and patients in the control group could understate improvements in their outcomes, perhaps because they think this is what assessors want to hear. When participants are blinded (when they do not know if they received the intervention or control conditions) there should be no difference in reporting tendencies of the two groups, so estimates of the effect of intervention (the difference between groups) cannot be biased by differential reporting.

In most trials of physical therapy interventions for the pelvic floor it is difficult to administer a sham intervention that is both credible and inactive. For example, it is difficult to conceive of a sham intervention for training pelvic floor muscles. In that case the best alternative may be to deliver an inactive intervention to the control group, even if the inactive intervention does not exactly resemble the active intervention. An example is the trial by Dumoulin et al (2004) that compared pelvic floor rehabilitation (electrical stimulation of pelvic floor muscles plus pelvic floor muscle exercises) with biofeedback. These authors gave the control group relaxation massage to the back and extremities in the belief that this would control, to some degree, the effects of placebo and misreporting of outcomes. Such trials provide some control, but perhaps not complete control, of the confounding effects of placebo and misreporting of outcomes.

The difficulties of providing an adequate sham intervention preclude participant blinding in most trials of physical therapy interventions for the pelvic floor. Only 6% of these trials truly blind participants.

It is also desirable that the **person assessing trial outcomes** is blinded. Blinding of assessors ensures that assessments are not biased by the assessor's expectations of the effects of intervention. When objective outcome measures are used, blinding of assessors is easily achieved by using assessors who are not otherwise involved in the study and are not told about which patients are in the intervention and control groups.

However, blinding of assessors is more difficult when trial outcomes are self-reported (as, for example, in studies which ask women whether they 'leak'). In that case the assessor is really the participant, and the assessor is only blind if the participant is blind.

Follow-up

A third feature of trial design that is likely to determine a trial's validity is the level of follow-up.

In most trials participants are randomized to groups, but for various reasons outcome measures are not subsequently obtained from all participants. Such 'loss to follow-up' occurs, for example, when subjects become too ill to be measured, or they die, go on holiday, or have major surgery, or because the researchers lose contact with the participant. Loss to follow-up potentially 'unrandomizes' allocation, and can produce systematic differences in the characteristics of the two groups, so it potentially biases estimates of the effects of intervention.

How much loss to follow-up is acceptable in a randomized trial? When is loss to follow-up so extreme that it potentially causes serious bias? There is no simple and universally applicable answer to these questions. However methodologists have applied threshold losses to follow-up of between about 10 and 20%. Losses to follow-up of less than 10% of randomized subjects are usually considered unlikely to produce serious bias, and losses to follow-up of greater than 20% are thought be a potential source of serious bias.

Fortunately most trials of physical therapy interventions for the pelvic floor have adequate follow-up: 67% of the relevant trials have loss to follow-up of less than 15%.

A related but more technical issue concerns problems with deviations from the trial protocol. Protocol deviations occur when, for example, people do not receive the intervention as allocated (e.g. if participants in an exercise group do not do their exercise), or if outcome measures are not measured at the allocated times. This presents a dilemma for the person analysing the data: should data from these subjects be excluded? Should data from subjects who did not receive the intervention be analysed as if those subjects had been allocated to the control group? The answer to both questions is no!

Most methodologists believe that the best way to deal with protocol violations is to analyse the data as if the protocol violation did not occur. In this approach, called 'analysis by intention to treat' (Hollis & Campbell 1999), all subjects' data are analysed, regardless of whether they received the intervention as allocated or not, and their data are analysed in the group to which they were allocated.

Analysis by intention to treat is thought to be the least biased way to analyse trial data in the presence of protocol violations. Of the relevant trials on PEDro 24% explicitly analyse by intention to treat.

Detecting bias in systematic reviews

The search strategy

Systematic reviewers attempt to provide an unbiased summary of the findings of relevant trials. Ideally systematic reviews summarize the findings of all relevant trials that had ever been conducted. That would achieve two ends: it would ensure that the reviewer had taken full advantage of all of the information available from all extant trials, and it would mean that the summary of the findings of the trials was not biased by selective reporting of only those trials with atypical estimates of the effects of the intervention.

Unfortunately it is usually not possible to find complete reports of all relevant trials: reports of some trials are published in obscure journals, others are published in obscure languages, many are published only in abstract format, and some are not published at all. Consequently even the most diligent reviewers will fail to find some trial reports.

Given that it is usually not possible to find reports of all relevant trials the next best thing is for reviewers to obtain reports of **nearly all** trials. We can use reviews that summarize nearly all relevant trial reports to tell nearly all of what is known about the effectiveness of the intervention.

Incomplete retrieval of trial reports raises another problem. If reviewers do not identify all trial reports then there is the possibility that they have retrieved a particular subset of trials with exceptionally optimistic or pessimistic estimates of the effect of the intervention. We would like to be reassured when reading a systematic review that the reviewer has located a representative subset of all trials. That is, we would like to know that the reviewer has not selectively reported on trials that provide overly optimistic or pessimistic estimates of the effects of intervention. Even if we cannot expect reviewers to find reports of all trials we can require that they find an **unbiased subset of nearly all trials**.

To this end, most reviewers conduct quite thorough literature searches. For a Cochrane systematic review of pelvic floor muscle training (PFMT), for urinary incontinence in women, Hay-Smith et al (2000) searched the Cochrane Incontinence Group trials register, Medline, Embase, the database of the Dutch National Institute of Allied Health Professions, CENTRAL, Physical Therapy Index and the reference lists of relevant articles. They also searched the proceed-

ings of the International Continence Society page by page. Some reviewers include trials published only as abstract form, whereas others include only full papers on the grounds that most abstracts have not been peer reviewed and often contain too little information to be useful.

Occasionally systematic reviewers conduct limited searches, for example by searching only Medline. This is potentially problematic: although Medline is the largest database of the medical literature such searches are likely to miss much of the relevant literature. It has been estimated that Medline only indexes between 17 and 82% of all relevant trials (Dickersin et al 1994).

When reading a systematic review it is important to check that the literature search in the review is reasonably recent. If a report of a systematic review is more than a few years old it is likely several trials will have been conducted since the search was conducted, and the review may provide an out-of-date summary of the literature.

Assessment of trial quality

Systematic reviewers may find a number of trials that investigate the effects of a particular intervention, and often the quality of the trials is varied. Obviously it is not appropriate to weight the findings of all trials without regard to trial quality. Particular attention should be paid to the highest quality trials because these trials are likely to be least biased; the poorest quality trials should be ignored. Systematic reviews should assess the quality of the trials in the review, and quality assessments should be taken into account when drawing conclusions from the review.

A range of methods have been used to assess the quality of trials in systematic reviews. The most common approach is to use a quality scale to assess quality, and then to ignore the findings of trials with low-quality scores. Commonly used scales include the Maastricht scale (Verhagen et al 1998) and the PEDro scale (Maher et al 2003); a copy of the PEDro scale is shown in Box 2.3. These scales assess quality based on the presence or absence of design features thought to influence validity, including true concealed randomization, blinding of participants and assessors, adequate follow-up and intention to treat analysis.

This approach sounds sensible, but there are some reasons to think that it may discriminate inappropriately between trials. The available evidence suggests there is only moderate agreement between the ratings of different quality scales (Colle et al 2002). Nonetheless, it is not known how better to assess trial quality, so these rudimentary procedures must suffice for now. For the time being we should expect systematic reviews to take

Box 2.3: The PEDro scale

(More details on this scale are available from http://www.pedro.fhs.usyd.edu.au/scale_item.html.)

1. Eligibility criteria were specified
2. Subjects were randomly allocated to groups (in a crossover study, subjects were randomly allocated an order in which treatments were received)
3. Allocation was concealed
4. The groups were similar at baseline regarding the most important prognostic indicators
5. There was blinding of all subjects
6. There was blinding of all therapists who administered the therapy
7. There was blinding of all assessors who measured at least one key outcome
8. Measures of at least one key outcome were obtained from more than 85% of the subjects initially allocated to groups
9. All subjects for whom outcome measures were available received the treatment or control condition as allocated or, where this was not the case, data for at least one key outcome was analysed by 'intention to treat'
10. The results of between-group statistical comparisons are reported for at least one key outcome
11. The study provides both point measures and measures of variability for at least one key outcome

Box 2.4: Key features conferring validity to systematic reviews

- An adequate search strategy (that finds an unbiased subset of nearly all relevant trials)
- The review considers trial quality when drawing conclusions about the effects of intervention

into account the quality of trials, but we cannot be too discerning about how quality is assessed (Box 2.4).

ASSESSING RELEVANCE OF TRIALS AND SYSTEMATIC REVIEWS

Not all valid trials are useful trials. Some provide valid tests of poorly administered interventions, others provide valid tests of the effects of intervention on inappropriate samples of patients, and yet others provide valid tests of the effect of intervention on meaningless outcomes.

The following sections consider how the quality of the intervention, the selection of patients, and outcomes can influence the **relevance** of randomized trials and systematic reviews.

Quality of intervention

Randomized trials are most easily applied to pharmacological interventions. In one sense pharmacological interventions are relatively simple: they involve the delivery of a drug to a patient. Because pharmacological interventions are quite simple they tend to be administered in quite similar ways in all trials. (One possible exception is the dose of the drug, but toxicity studies, pharmacokinetic studies and dose-finding studies often constrain the range of doses before definitive trials are carried out, so even this parameter is often fairly consistent across studies.) In contrast, many physical therapy interventions are complex. In trials of physical therapy interventions the intervention is often tailored to the individual patient based on specific examination findings, and sometimes the intervention consists of multiple components, perhaps administered in a range of settings by a range of health professionals. Consequently a single intervention (such as PFMT) may be administered in quite different ways across trials.

Wherever there is the possibility of administering the intervention in a range of ways we need to consider whether, in a particular trial, the intervention was administered well (Herbert & Bø 2005). It is reasonable to be suspicious of the findings of trials where the intervention was administered in a way that would appear to be suboptimal.

Criticisms have been leveled against trials because the interventions were administered by unskilled therapists (Brock et al 2002) or because the intervention was administered in a way that was contrary to the way in which the intervention is generally administered (Clare et al 2004), or because the intervention was not sufficiently intense to be effective (Ada 2002, Herbert & Bø 2005). Such criticisms are sometimes reasonable and sometimes not.

Of course it is impossible to know with any certainty how an intervention should be administered before first knowing how effective the intervention is. Trials must necessarily be conducted before good information is available about how to administer the intervention. Consequently a degree of latitude ought to be offered to clinical trialists: we should be prepared to trust the findings of trials that test interventions that are applied in ways other than the ways we might choose to apply the intervention, as long as the application of the intervention in the trial was not obviously suboptimal.

Patients

Trials of a particular intervention may be carried out on quite different patient groups. Readers need to be satisfied that the trial was applied to an appropriate group of patients. It could be reasonable to ignore the findings of a trial if the intervention was administered to a group of patients for whom the intervention was generally considered inappropriate. An example might be the application of pelvic floor exercises to reverse prolapse in women who already have complete prolapse of the internal organs. Most therapists would agree that once prolapse is complete conservative intervention is no longer appropriate and surgical intervention is necessary.

The same caveat applies here: it is impossible to know with certainty, at the time a trial is conducted, who an intervention will be most effective for. Again we must be prepared to give trialists some latitude: we should be prepared to trust the findings of trials that test interventions on patients other than the patients we might choose to apply the intervention to, as long as the patient group was not obviously inappropriate.

Outcomes

The last important dimension of the relevance of a clinical trial concerns the outcomes that are measured. Ultimately, if an intervention for the pelvic floor is to be useful, it must improve quality of life. Arguably there is little value in an intervention that increases the strength of pelvic floor muscles if it does not also increase quality of life.

Studies of variables such as muscle strength can help us understand the mechanisms by which interventions work, but they cannot tell us if the intervention is worth doing. The trials that best help us to decide whether or not to apply an intervention are those that determine the effect of intervention on quality of life.

Many trials do not measure quality of life directly, but instead they measure variables that are thought to be closely related to quality of life. For example, Bø et al (2000) determined the effect of PFMT for women with stress urinary incontinence (SUI) on the risk of incontinence-related problems with social life, sex life, and physical activity. It would appear reasonable to expect that problems with social life, sex life and physical activity directly influence quality of life, so this trial provides useful information with which to make decisions about PFMT for women with SUI.

In general trials can help us make decisions about intervention in so far as they measure outcomes that are related to quality of life.

USING ESTIMATES OF EFFECTS OF INTERVENTION TO MAKE DECISIONS ABOUT INTERVENTION

The most useful piece of information a clinical trial can give us is an estimate of the size of the effects of the intervention. We can use estimates of the effect of intervention to help us decide if an intervention does enough good to make it worth its expense, risks and inconvenience (Herbert 2000a, 2000b).

Obtaining estimates of the effects of intervention from randomized trials and systematic reviews

Most people experience an improvement in their condition over the course of any intervention. But the magnitude of the improvement only partly reflects the effects of intervention. People get better, often partly because of intervention, but usually also because the natural course of the condition is one of gradual improvement or because apparently random fluctuations in the severity of the condition tend to occur in the direction of an improvement in the condition. (The latter is called statistical regression; for an explanation see Herbert et al 2005.) In addition, part of the recovery may be due to placebo effects or to patients politely overstating the magnitude of the improvements in their condition.

As several factors contribute to the improvements that people experience over time, the improvement in the condition of treated patients cannot provide a measure of the effect of intervention.

A far better way to estimate the effects of intervention is to look at the magnitude of the difference in outcomes of the intervention and control groups. This is most straightforward when outcomes are measured on a continuous scale. Examples of continuous outcome measurements are pad test weights, measures of global perceived effect of intervention, or duration of labour. These variables are continuous because it is possible to measure the amount of the variable on each subject.

An estimate of the mean effects of intervention on continuous variables is obtained simply by taking the difference between the mean outcomes of the intervention and control groups. For example, a study by Bø et al (1999) compared pelvic floor exercises with a no-exercise control condition for women with SUI. The primary outcome was urine leakage measured using a stress pad test. Over the 6-month intervention period women in the control group experienced a mean reduction in leakage of 13 g whereas women in the PFMT group experienced a mean reduction of 30 g. Thus the mean effect of exercise, compared to controls, was to reduce leaking by about 17 g (or about 50% of the initial leakage).

Other outcomes are dichotomous. Dichotomous outcomes cannot be quantified on a scale; they are events that either happen or not. An example comes from the trial by Chiarelli & Cockburn (2002) of a programme of interventions designed to prevent post-partum incontinence. Three months postpartum, women were classified as being continent or incontinent. This outcome (incontinent/continent) is dichotomous, because it can have only one of two values.

When outcomes are measured on a dichotomous scale we can no longer talk meaningfully about the mean outcome. Instead we talk about the risk (or probability) of the outcome; our interest is in how much intervention changes the risk of the outcome.

Chiarelli and colleagues found that 125 of the 328 women in the control group were still incontinent at 3 months, and 108 of 348 women in the intervention group were still incontinent at 3 months. Thus the risk of being incontinent at 3 months was 125/328 (38.1%) for women in the control group, but this risk was reduced to 108/348 (31%) in the intervention group. So

the effect of the 3-month intervention was to reduce the risk of incontinence at 3 months postpartum by 7.1% (i.e. 38.1 – 31.0%). This figure, the difference in risks, is sometimes called the absolute risk reduction. An absolute risk reduction of 7.1% is equivalent to preventing incontinence in one in every 14 women treated with the intervention.

Using estimates of the effects of intervention

Estimates of the effects of intervention can be used to inform the single most important clinical decision: whether or not to apply a particular intervention for a particular patient.

Decisions about whether to apply an intervention need to weigh the potential benefits of intervention against all negative consequences of intervention. So, for example, when deciding whether or not to undertake a programme of PFMT, a woman with SUI has to decide if the effects of intervention (including an expected reduction in leakage of about one-half) warrants the inconvenience of daily exercise. And when deciding whether to embark on a programme to prevent postpartum incontinence a woman needs to decide whether she is prepared to undertake the programme for a 1 in 14 chance of being continent when she otherwise would not be.

REFERENCES

Ada L 2002 Commentary on Green J, Forster A, Bogle S et al 2002 Physiotherapy for patients with mobility problems more than 1 year after stroke: a randomized controlled trial [Lancet 359:199–203]. Australian Journal of Physiotherapy 48:318

Benson K, Hartz A J 2000 A comparison of observational studies and randomized, controlled trials. New England Journal of Medicine 342:1878–1886

Bø K, Talseth T, Holme I 1999 Single blind, randomized controlled trial of pelvic floor exercises, electrical stimulation, vaginal cones, and no treatment in management of genuine stress incontinence in women. BMJ 318:487–493

Bø K, Talseth T, Vinsnes A 2000 Randomized controlled trial on the effect of pelvic floor muscle training on quality of life and sexual problems in genuine stress incontinent women. Acta Obstetricia Gynecologica Scandinavica 79:598–603

Brock K, Jennings K, Stevens J, Picard S 2002 The Bobath concept has changed [Comment on Critically Appraised Paper, Australian Journal of Physiotherapy 48:59]. Australian Journal of Physiotherapy 48:156

Chalmers T C, Celano P, Sacks H S et al 1983 Bias in treatment assignment in controlled clinical trials. New England Journal of Medicine 309:1358–1361

Chiarelli P, Cockburn J 2002 Promoting urinary continence in women after delivery: randomized controlled trial. BMJ 324:1241

Clare H A, Adams R, Maher C G 2004 A systematic review of efficacy of McKenzie therapy for spinal pain. Australian Journal of Physiotherapy 50:209–216

Colditz G A, Miller J N, Mosteller F 1989 How study design affects outcomes in comparisons of therapy. I: Medical. Statistics in Medicine 8:441–454

Colle F, Rannou F, Revel M et al 2002 Impact of quality scales on levels of evidence inferred from a systematic review of exercise therapy and low back pain. Archives of Physical Medicine and Rehabilitation 83:1745–1752

Concato J, Shah N, Horwitz R I 2000 Randomized controlled trials, observational studies, and the hierarchy of research designs. New England Journal of Medicine 342:1887–1892

Dickersin K, Scherer R, Lefebvre C 1994 Systematic reviews: identifying relevant studies for systematic reviews. BMJ 309:1286–1291

Dumoulin C, Gravel D, Bourbonnais D et al 2004 Reliability of dynamometric measurements of the pelvic floor musculature. Neurology and Urodynamics 23(2):134–142

Egger M, Davey Smith G, Altman D G (eds) 2001 Systematic reviews in health care. Meta-analysis in context. BMJ Books, London

Glass G V, McGaw B, Smith M L 1981 Meta-analysis in social research. Sage, Beverly Hills

Hay-Smith E J C, Bø K, Berghmans L C M et al 2000 Pelvic floor muscle training for urinary incontinence in women. The Cochrane Database of Systematic Reviews

Herbert R D 2000a Critical appraisal of clinical trials. I: estimating the magnitude of treatment effects when outcomes are measured on a continuous scale. Australian Journal of Physiotherapy 46:229–235

Herbert R D 2000b Critical appraisal of clinical trials. II: estimating the magnitude of treatment effects when outcomes are measured on a dichotomous scale. Australian Journal of Physiotherapy 46:309–313

Herbert R D, Bø K 2005 Analysing effects of quality of interventions in systematic reviews. BMJ 331(7515):507–509

Herbert R D, Higgs J 2004 Complementary research paradigms. Australian Journal of Physiotherapy 50:63–64

Herbert R D, Jamtvedt G, Mead J et al 2005 Practical evidence-based physiotherapy. Elsevier, Oxford

Hollis S, Campbell F 1999 What is meant by intention to treat analysis? Survey of published randomized trials. BMJ 319:670–674

Kunz R, Oxman A D 1998 The unpredictability paradox: review of empirical comparisons of randomized and non-randomized clinical trials. BMJ 317:1185–1190

Maher C G, Sherrington C, Herbert R D et al 2003 Reliability of the PEDro scale for rating quality of randomized controlled trials. Physical Therapy 83:713–721

Moher D, Pham B, Cook D et al 1998 Does quality of reports of randomized trials affect estimates of intervention efficacy reported in meta-analyses? Lancet 352:609–613

Moher D, Schulz K F, Altman D G 2001 The CONSORT statement: revised recommendations for improving the quality of reports of parallel group randomized trials. BMC Medical Research Methodology 1:2

Pocock S J 1984 Clinical trials: a practical approach. Wiley, New York

Sand P K, Richardson D A, Staskin D R et al 1995 Pelvic floor electrical stimulation in the treatment of genuine stress incontinence: a multicenter, placebo-controlled trial. American Journal of Obstetrics and Gynecology 173:72–79

Schulz K, Chalmers I, Hayes R et al 1995 Empirical evidence of bias: dimensions of methodological quality associated with estimates of treatment effects in controlled trials. Journal of the American Medical Association 273:408–412

Verhagen A P, de Vet H C, de Bie R A et al 1998 Balneotherapy and quality assessment: interobserver reliability of the Maastricht criteria list and the need for blinded quality assessment. Journal of Clinical Epidemiology 51:335–341

Chapter 3

Functional anatomy of the female pelvic floor

James A Ashton-Miller and John O L DeLancey

SUMMARY

The anatomic structures that prevent incontinence and a prolapse during elevations in abdominal pressure include sphincteric and supportive systems. In the urethra, for example, the action of the vesical neck and urethral sphincteric mechanisms at rest constrict the urethral lumen and keep urethral closure pressure higher than bladder pressure. The striated urogenital sphincter, the smooth muscle sphincter in the vesical neck, and the circular and longitudinal smooth muscle of the urethra all contribute to closure pressure. The mucosal and vascular tissues that surround the lumen provide a hermetic seal via coaptation, aided by the connective tissues in the urethral wall. Decreases in the number of striated muscle sphincter fibres occur with age and parity, but changes in the other tissues are not well understood.

The supportive hammock under the urethra and vesical neck provides a firm backstop against which the urethra is compressed during increases in abdominal pressure to maintain urethral closure pressures above the rapidly increasing bladder pressure. This supporting layer consists of the anterior vaginal wall and the connective tissue that attaches it to the pelvic bones through the pubovaginal portion of the levator ani muscle and the uterosacral and cardinal ligaments comprising the tendinous arch of the pelvic fascia.

At rest the levator ani act to maintain the urogenital hiatus closed in the face of hydrostatic pressure due to gravity and slight abdominal pressure. During the dynamic activities of daily living they are additionally recruited to maintain hiatal closure in the face of inertial loads related to visceral accelerations as well as abdominal pressure resulting from activation of the abdominal wall musculature and diaphragm.

Urinary incontinence is a common condition in women, with prevalence ranging from 8.5 to 38% depending on age, parity, and definition (Herzog et al 1990, Thomas et al 1980). Most women with incontinence have stress urinary incontinence (SUI) (Diokno et al 1987), which is treated using conservative therapy or surgery. Despite its common occurrence, there have been few advances in our understanding of its cause in the past 40 years. Most of the many surgical procedures for alleviating SUI involve the principle of improving bladder neck support (Bergman & Elia 1995, Colombo et al 1994). Treatment selection based on specific anatomic abnormalities has awaited identification, in each case, of the muscular, neural, and/or connective tissues involved.

Understanding how the pelvic floor structure/function relationships provide bladder neck support can help guide treatment selection and effect. For example if, while giving vaginal birth, a woman sustains a partial tear of a portion of her pelvic muscles that influence her continence, then pelvic muscle exercises may be effective.

On the other hand, if portions of those muscles are irretrievably lost, for example due to complete and permanent denervation, then no amount of exercising will restore them; pelvic muscle exercises may well lead to agonist muscle hypertrophy, but whether or not this will restore continence will depend upon whether the agonist muscles can compensate for the lost muscle function.

This chapter reviews the functional anatomy of the pelvic floor structures and the effects of age on urethral support and the urethral sphincter, and attempts to clarify what is known about the different structures that influence stress continence. This mechanistic approach should help guide research into pathophysiology, treatment selection, and prevention of SUI. In addition, we also review the structures that resist genital prolapse because vaginal delivery confers a 4–11-fold increase in risk of developing pelvic organ prolapse (Mant et al 1997).

HOW IS URINARY CONTINENCE MAINTAINED?

Urethral closure pressure must be greater than bladder pressure, both at rest and during increases in abdominal pressure to retain urine in the bladder. The resting tone of the urethral muscles maintains a favourable pressure relative to the bladder when urethral pressure exceeds bladder pressure.

During activities such as coughing, when bladder pressure increases several times higher than urethral pressure, a dynamic process increases urethral closure pressure to enhance urethral closure and maintain continence (Enhörning 1961). Both the magnitude of the resting pressure in the urethra and the increase in pressure generated during a cough determine the pressure at which leakage of urine occurs (Kim et al 1997).

Although analysis of the degree of resting closure pressure and pressure transmission provides useful theoretical insights, it does not show how specific injuries to individual component structures affect the passive or active aspects of urethral closure. A detailed examination of the sphincteric closure and the urethral support subsystems (Fig. 3.1) is required to understand these relationships.

The dominant element in the urethral sphincter is the striated urogenital sphincter muscle, which contains a striated muscle in a circular configuration in the middle of the urethra and strap-like muscles distally. In its sphincteric portion, the urogenital sphincter muscle surrounds two orthogonally-arranged smooth muscle layers and a vascular plexus that helps to maintain closure of the urethral lumen.

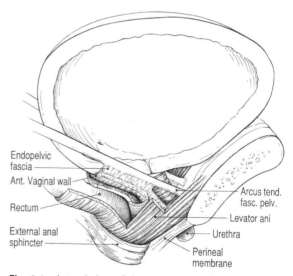

Fig. 3.1 Lateral view of the components of the urethral support system. Note how the levator ani muscles support the rectum, vagina, and urethrovesical neck. Also note how the endopelvic fascia beside the urethra attaches to the levator ani muscle; contraction of the levator muscle leads to elevation of the urethrovesical neck. Puborectalis muscle is removed for clarity. (Redrawn from DeLancey 1994, with permission of C V Mosby Company, St Louis. © DeLancey 2005.)

THE URINARY SPHINCTERIC CLOSURE SYSTEM

Sphincteric closure of the urethra is normally provided by the urethral striated muscles, the urethral smooth muscle, and the vascular elements within the submucosa (Figs 3.2 and 3.3) (Strohbehn et al 1996, Strohbehn & DeLancey 1997). Each is believed to contribute equally to resting urethral closure pressure (Rud et al 1980).

Anatomically, the urethra can be divided longitudinally into percentiles, with the internal urethral meatus representing point 0 and the external meatus representing the 100th percentile (Table 3.1). The urethra passes through the wall of the bladder at the level of the vesical neck where the detrusor muscle fibres extend below the internal urethra meatus to as far as the 15th percentile.

The striated urethral sphincter muscle begins at the termination of the detrusor fibres and extends to the 64th percentile. It is circular in configuration and completely surrounds the smooth muscle of the urethral wall.

Starting at the 54th percentile, the striated muscles of the urogenital diaphragm, the compressor urethrae, and the urethrovaginal sphincter can be seen. They are continuous with the striated urethral sphincter and extend to the 76th percentile. Their fibre direction is no longer circular. The fibres of the compressor urethrae pass over the urethra to insert into the urogenital diaphragm near the pubic ramus.

The urethrovaginal sphincter surrounds both the urethra and the vagina (Fig. 3.4). The distal terminus of the urethra runs adjacent to, but does not connect with, the bulbocavernosus muscles (DeLancey 1986).

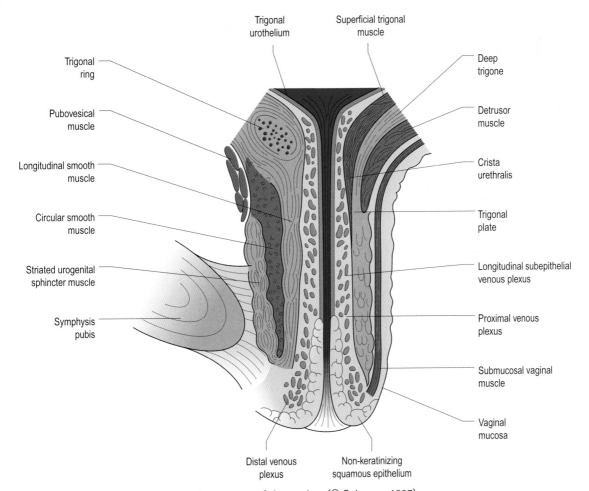

Fig. 3.2 Midsagittal section showing the anatomy of the urethra. (© DeLancey 1997)

Functionally, the urethral muscles maintain continence in various ways. The U-shaped loop of the detrusor smooth muscle surrounds the proximal urethra, favouring its closure by constricting the lumen.

The striated urethral sphincter is composed mainly of type 1 (slow twitch) fibres, which are well suited to maintaining constant tone as well as allowing voluntary increases in tone to provide additional continence protection (Gosling et al 1981). Distally, the recruitment of the striated muscle of the urethrovaginal sphincter and the compressor urethrae compress the lumen.

The smooth muscle of the urethra may also play a role in determining stress continence. The lumen is surrounded by a prominent vascular plexus that is believed to contribute to continence by forming a watertight seal via coaptation of the mucosal surfaces. Surrounding this plexus is the inner longitudinal smooth muscle layer. This in turn is surrounded by a circular layer, which itself lies inside the outer layer of striated muscle.

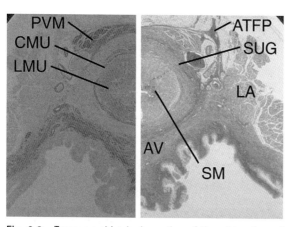

Fig. 3.3 Transverse histologic section of the midurethra of a 21-year-old woman. On the left structures are visualized using a sigma-actin smooth muscle stain, which shows the pubovesical muscle (PVM), the circumferential smooth muscle (CMU) layer, and the longitudinal smooth muscle (LMU) layer. On the right, the contralateral side is stained with Masson's trichrome to show the arcus tendineus fascia pelvis (ATFP), the striated urogenital sphincter (SUG), the levator ani (LA), the anterior vaginal wall (AV), and the submucosa of the urethra (SM). (From Strohbehn et al 1996, with permission of Lippincott Williams Wilkins, Baltimore, MD.)

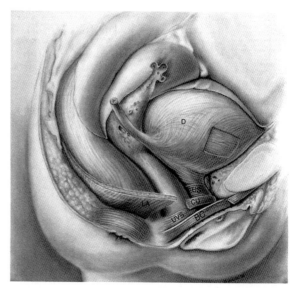

Fig. 3.4 Lateral view of urethral and pelvic floor muscular anatomy. BC, bulbocavernosus; CU, compressor urethrae; D, detrusor; LA, levator ani; US, urethral sphincter; UVS, urethrovaginal sphincter. Puborectalis muscle is removed for clarity. (© DeLancey 2004.)

Table 3.1 Urethral topography and urethral and paraurethral structures

Percentile of urethral length	Location–Region of the urethra	Structures
0–20	Intramural	Internal urethral meatus Detrusor loop
20–60	Mid-urethra	Striated urethral sphincter muscle Smooth muscle
60–80	Urogenital diaphragm	Compressor urethrae muscle Urethrovaginal sphincter Smooth muscle
80–100	Distal urethra	Bulbocavernosus muscle

The smooth muscle layers are present throughout the upper four-fifths of the urethra. The circular configuration of the smooth muscle and outer striated muscle layers suggests that the contraction of these layers has a role in constricting the lumen. The mechanical role of the inner longitudinal smooth muscle layer is presently unresolved. Contraction of this longitudinal layer may help to open the lumen to initiate micturition rather than to constrict it.

CLINICAL CORRELATES OF URETHRAL ANATOMY AND EFFECTS OF AGEING

There are several important clinical correlates of urethral muscular anatomy. Perhaps the most important is that SUI is caused by problems with the urethral sphincter mechanism as well as with urethral support. Although this is a relatively new concept, the supporting scientific evidence is strong.

The usual argument for urethral support playing an important role in SUI is that urethral support operations cure SUI without changing urethral function. Unfortunately, this logic is just as flawed as suggesting that obesity is caused by an enlarged stomach because gastric stapling surgery, which makes the stomach smaller, is effective in alleviating obesity. The fact that urethral support operations cure SUI does not implicate urethral hypermobility as the cause of SUI.

Most studies have shown not only that there is substantial variation in resting urethral closure pressures in normal women compared with those with SUI, but also that the severity of SUI correlates quite well with resting urethral closure pressure.

Loss of urethral closure pressure probably results from age-related deterioration of the urethral musculature as well as from neurologic injury (Hilton & Stanton 1983, Smith et al 1989a, b, Snooks et al 1986). For example, the total number of striated muscle fibres within the ventral wall of the urethra has been found to decrease seven-fold as women progress from 15 to 80 years of age, with an average loss of 2% per year (Fig. 3.5) (Perucchini et al 2002a).

Because the mean fibre diameter does not change significantly with age, the cross-sectional area of striated muscle in the ventral wall decreases significantly with age; however, nulliparous women seemed relatively protected (Perucchini et al 2002b). This 65% age-related loss in the number of striated muscle fibres found in vitro is consistent with the 54% age-related loss in closure pressure found in vivo by Rud et al 1980, suggesting that it may be a contributing factor. However, prospective studies are needed to directly correlate the loss in the number of striated muscle fibres with a loss in closure pressure in vivo.

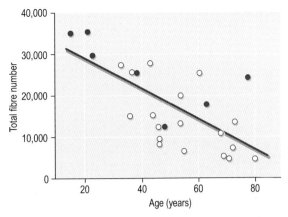

Fig. 3.5 Decrease in total number of striated muscle fibres in the ventral wall with age. The closed circles denote data from nulliparous women, and the open circles denote data from parous women. (From Perruchini et al 2002a, with permission of Lippincott Williams Wilkins, Baltimore, MD.)

It is noteworthy that in our in-vitro study, thinning of the striated muscle layers was particularly evident in the proximal vesical neck and along the dorsal wall of the urethra in older women (Perucchini et al 2002b). The concomitant seven-fold age-related loss of nerve fibres in these same striated urogenital sphincters (Fig. 3.6) directly correlated with the loss in striated muscle fibres (Fig. 3.7) in the same tissues (Pandit et al 2000); and the correlation supports the hypothesis of a neurogenic source for SUI and helps to explain why faulty innervation could affect continence.

We believe that the ability of pelvic floor exercise to compensate for this age-related loss in sphincter striated muscle may be limited under certain situations. Healthy striated muscle can increase its strength by about 30% after an intensive 8–12 week progressive resistance training intervention (e.g. Skelton et al 1995). For example suppose an older woman had a maximum resting urethral closure pressure of 100 cmH$_2$O when she was young but it is now 30 cmH$_2$O due to loss of striated sphincter muscle fibres. If she successfully increases her urethral striated muscle strength by 30% through an exercise intervention and there is a one-to-one correspondence between urethral muscle strength and resting closure pressure, she will only be able to increase her resting closure pressure by 30%, from 30 cmH$_2$O to 39 cmH$_2$O, an increment less than one-tenth of the 100 cmH$_2$O increase in intravesical pressure that occurs during a hard cough. It remains to be determined whether pelvic floor muscle exercise is as effective in alleviating SUI in women with low resting

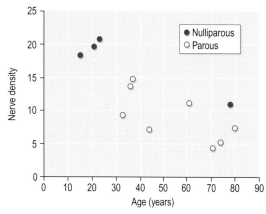

Fig. 3.6 Decreasing nerve density (number per mm²) in the ventral wall of the urethra with age. This is a subgroup of the data in Fig. 3.5 (Perucchini et al 2002a). The closed circles denote data from nulliparous women, and the open circles denote data from parous women. (From Pandit et al 2000, with permission of Lippincott Williams & Wilkins, Baltimore, MD.)

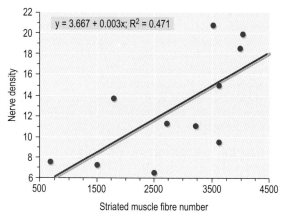

Fig. 3.7 Correlation between nerve density (number per mm²) and total fibre number in the ventral wall of the urethra. No distinction is made between nulliparous and parous women (Perucchini et al 2002a). In the equation given for the regression line, Y denotes the ordinate, X the abscissa, and R^2 the coefficient of variation. (From Pandit et al 2000, with permission of Lippincott Williams & Wilkins, Baltimore, MD.)

urethral pressures as it can be in women with higher resting pressures, especially for women participating in activities with large transient increases in abdominal pressure.

URETHRAL (AND ANTERIOR VAGINAL WALL) SUPPORT SYSTEM

Support of the urethra and vesical neck is determined by the endopelvic fascia of the anterior vaginal wall through their fascial connections to the arcus tendineus fascia pelvis and connection to the medial portion of the levator ani muscle.

It is our working hypothesis that both urethral constriction and urethral support contribute to continence. Active constriction of the urethral sphincter maintains urine in the bladder at rest. During increases in abdominal pressure, the vesical neck and urethra are compressed to a closed position when the raised abdominal pressure surrounding much of the urethra exceeds the fluid pressure within the urethral lumen (see Fig. 3.1). The stiffness of the supportive layer under the vesical neck provides a backstop against which abdominal pressure compresses the urethra. This anatomic division mirrors the two aspects of pelvic floor function relevant to SUI: urethral closure pressure at rest and the increase in urethral closure caused by the effect of abdominal pressure.

Support of the urethra and distal vaginal wall are inextricably linked. For much of its length, the urethra is fused with the vaginal wall, and the structures that determine urethral position and distal anterior vaginal wall position are the same.

The anterior vaginal wall and urethral support system consists of all structures extrinsic to the urethra that provide a supportive layer on which the proximal urethra and midurethra rest (DeLancey 1994). The major components of this supportive structure are the vaginal wall, the endopelvic fascia, the arcus tendineus fasciae pelvis, and the levator ani muscles (see Fig. 3.1).

The endopelvic fascia is a dense, fibrous connective tissue layer that surrounds the vagina and attaches it to each arcus tendineus fascia pelvis laterally. Each arcus tendineus fascia pelvis in turn is attached to the pubic bone ventrally and to the ischial spine dorsally.

The arcus tendineus fasciae pelvis are tensile structures located bilaterally on either side of the urethra and vagina. They act like the catenary-shaped cables of a suspension bridge and provide the support needed to suspend the urethra on the anterior vaginal wall. Although it is well defined as a fibrous band near its origin at the pubic bone, the arcus tendineus fascia pelvis becomes a broad aponeurotic structure as it passes dorsally to insert into the ischial spine. It therefore appears as a sheet of fascia as it fuses with the endopelvic fascia, where it merges with the levator ani muscles (see Fig. 3.1).

Levator ani muscles

The levator ani muscles also play a critical role in supporting the pelvic organs (Berglas & Rubin 1953, Halban & Tandler 1907, Porges et al 1960). Not only has evidence of this been seen in magnetic resonance scans (Kirschner-Hermanns et al 1993, Tunn et al 1998) but histological evidence of muscle damage has been found (Koelbl et al 1998) and linked to operative failure (Hanzal et al 1993).

There are three basic regions of the levator ani muscle (Kearney et al 2004) (Figs 3.8 and 3.9):

- the first region is the iliococcygeal portion, which forms a relatively flat, horizontal shelf spanning the potential gap from one pelvic sidewall to the other;
- the second portion is the pubovisceral muscle, which arises from the pubic bone on either side and attaches to the walls of the pelvic organs and perineal body;

- the third region, the puborectal muscle, forms a sling around and behind the rectum just cephalad to the external anal sphincter.

The connective tissue covering on both superior and inferior surfaces are called the superior and inferior fasciae of the levator ani. When these muscles and their associated fasciae are considered together, the combined structures make up the pelvic diaphragm.

The opening within the levator ani muscle through which the urethra and vagina pass (and through which prolapse occurs), is called the urogenital hiatus of the levator ani. The rectum also passes through this opening, but because the levator ani muscle attaches directly to the anus it is not included in the name of the hiatus. The hiatus, therefore, is supported ventrally (anteriorly) by the pubic bones and the levator ani muscles, and dorsally (posteriorly) by the perineal body and external anal sphincter.

The normal baseline activity of the levator ani muscle keeps the urogenital hiatus closed by compressing the vagina, urethra and rectum against the pubic bone, the pelvic floor and organs in a cephalic direction (Taverner 1959). This constant activity of the levator ani muscle is analogous to that in the postural muscles of the spine. This continuous contraction is also similar to the

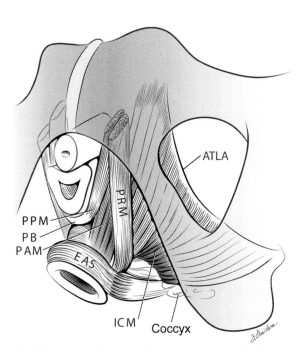

Fig. 3.8 Schematic view of the levator ani muscles from below after the vulvar structures and perineal membrane have been removed showing the arcus tendineus levator ani (ATLA); external anal sphincter (EAS); puboanal muscle (PAM); perineal body (PB) uniting the two ends of the puboperineal muscle (PPM); iliococcygeal muscle (ICM); puborectal muscle (PRM). Note that the urethra and vagina have been transected just above the hymenal ring. (© DeLancey 2003.)

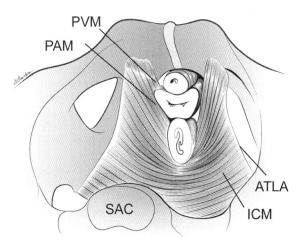

Fig. 3.9 The levator ani muscle seen from above looking over the sacral promontory (SAC) showing the pubovaginal muscle (PVM). The urethra, vagina, and rectum have been transected just above the pelvic floor. PAM, puboanal muscle; ATLA, arcus tendineus levator ani; ICM, iliococcygeal muscle. (The internal obturator muscles have been removed to clarify levator muscle origins.) (From Kearney et al 2004, with permission of Elsevier North Holland, New York, © DeLancey 2003.)

continuous activity of the external anal sphincter muscle, and closes the lumen of the vagina in a manner similar to that by which the anal sphincter closes the anus. This constant action eliminates any opening within the pelvic floor through which prolapse could occur.

A maximal voluntary contraction of the levator ani muscles causes the pubovisceral muscles and the puborectalis muscles to further compress the mid-urethra, distal vagina and rectum against the pubic bone distally and against abdominal hydrostatic pressure more proximally. It is this compressive force and pressure that one feels if one palpates a pelvic floor muscle contraction intravaginally. Contraction of the bulbocavernosus and the ventral fibres of the iliococcygeus will only marginally augment this compression force developed by the pubovisceral and puborectalis muscles because the former develops little force and the latter is located too far dorsally to have much effect intravaginally.

Finally, maximal contraction of the mid and dorsal iliococcygeus muscles elevates the central region of the posterior pelvic floor, but likely contributes little to a vaginal measurement of levator strength or pressure because they do not act circumvaginally.

Interactions between the pelvic floor muscles and the endopelvic fasciae

The levator ani muscles play an important role in protecting the pelvic connective tissues from excess load. Any connective tissue within the body may be stretched by subjecting it to a tensile force. Skin expanders used in plastic surgery stretch the dense and resistant dermis to extraordinary degrees, and flexibility exercises practiced by dancers and athletes elongate leg ligaments. Both these observations underscore the adaptive nature of connective tissue when subjected to repeated tension over time.

If the ligaments and fasciae within the pelvis were subjected to continuous stress imposed on the pelvic floor by the great force of abdominal pressure, they would stretch. This stretching does not occur because the constant tonic activity of the pelvic floor muscles (Parks et al 1962) closes the urogenital hiatus and carries the weight of the abdominal and pelvic organs, preventing constant strain on the ligaments and fasciae within the pelvis.

The interaction between the pelvic floor muscles and the supportive ligaments is critical to pelvic organ support. As long as the levator ani muscles function to properly maintain closure of the genital hiatus, the ligaments and fascial structures supporting the pelvic organs are under minimal tension. The fasciae simply act to stabilize the organs in their position above the levator ani muscles.

When the pelvic floor muscles relax or are damaged, the pelvic floor opens and the vagina lies between the zones of high abdominal pressure and low atmospheric pressure outside the body. In this situation it must be held in place by the suspensory ligaments. Although the ligaments can sustain these loads for short periods of time, if the pelvic floor muscles do not close the pelvic floor then the connective tissue will eventually fail, resulting in pelvic organ prolapse.

The support of the uterus has been likened to a ship in its berth floating on the water attached by ropes on either side to a dock (Paramore 1918). The ship is analogous to the uterus, the ropes to the ligaments, and the water to the supportive layer formed by the pelvic floor muscles. The ropes function to hold the ship (uterus) in the center of its berth as it rests on the water (pelvic floor muscles). If, however, the water level falls far enough that the ropes are required to hold the ship without supporting water, the ropes would break.

The analogous situation in the pelvic floor involves the pelvic floor muscles supporting the uterus and vagina, which are stabilized in position by the ligaments and fasciae. Once the pelvic floor musculature becomes damaged and no longer holds the organs in place, the supportive connective tissue is placed under stretch until it fails.

The attachment of the levator ani muscles into the perineal body is important and damage to this part of the levator ani muscle during delivery is one of the irreparable injuries to pelvic floor. Recent magnetic resonance imaging (MRI) has vividly depicted these defects and it has been shown that up to 20% of primiparous women have a visible defect in the levator ani muscle on MRI (DeLancey et al 2003).

It is likely that this muscular damage is an important factor associated with recurrence of pelvic organ prolapse after initial surgical repair. Moreover, these defects were found to occur more frequently in those individuals complaining of SUI (DeLancey et al 2003). An individual with muscles that do not function properly has a problem that is not surgically correctable.

PELVIC FLOOR FUNCTION RELEVANT TO STRESS URINARY INCONTINENCE

Functionally, the levator ani muscle and the endopelvic fascia play an interactive role in maintaining continence and pelvic support. Impairments usually become evident when the system is stressed.

One such stressor is a hard cough that, driven by a powerful contraction of the diaphragm and abdominal muscles, can cause a transient increase of 150 cmH$_2$O, or more, in abdominal pressure. This transient pressure increase causes the proximal urethra to undergo a downward (caudodorsal) displacement of about 10 mm in the midsagittal plane that can be viewed on ultrasonography (Howard et al 2000a). This displacement is evidence that the inferior abdominal contents are forced to move caudally during a cough.

Because the abdominal contents are essentially incompressible, the pelvic floor and/or the abdominal wall must stretch slightly under the transient increase in abdominal hydrostatic pressure, depending on the level of neural recruitment. The ventrocaudal motion of the bladder neck that is visible on ultrasonography indicates that it and the surrounding passive tissues have acquired momentum in that direction. The pelvic floor then needs to decelerate the momentum acquired by this mass of abdominal tissue.

The resulting inertial force causes a caudal-to-cranial pressure gradient in the abdominal contents, with the greatest pressure arising nearest the pelvic floor. While the downward momentum of the abdominal contents is being slowed by the resistance to stretch of the pelvic floor, the increased pressure compresses the proximal intra-abdominal portion of the urethra against the underlying supportive layer of the endopelvic fasciae, the vagina, and the levator ani muscles.

We can estimate the approximate resistance of the urethral support layer to this displacement. The ratio of the displacement of a structure in a given direction to a given applied pressure increase is known as the compliance of the structure.

If we divide 12.5 mm of downward displacement of the bladder neck (measured on ultrasonography) during a cough by the transient 150 cmH$_2$O increase in abdominal pressure that causes it, the resulting ratio (12.5 mm divided by 150 cmH$_2$O) yields an average compliance of 0.083 mm/cmH$_2$O in healthy nullipara (Howard et al 2000a). In other words, the cough displaces the healthy intact pelvic floor 1 mm for every 12 cmH$_2$O increase in abdominal pressure. (Actually, soft tissue mechanics teaches us to expect ever smaller displacements as the abdominal pressure increments towards the maximum value).

The increase in abdominal pressure acts transversely across the urethra, altering the stresses in the walls of the urethra so that the anterior wall is deformed toward the posterior wall, and the lateral walls are deformed towards one another, thereby helping to close the urethral lumen and prevent leakage due to the concomitant increase in intravesical pressure.

If pelvic floor exercises lead to pelvic floor muscle hypertrophy, then the resistance of the striated components of the urethral support layer can be expected to also increase. This is because the longitudinal stiffness and damping of an active muscle are linearly proportional to the tension developed in the muscle (e.g. Blandpied & Smidt 1993); this is partly because, for the same muscle tone, the hypertrophied muscle contains more cross-bridges in the strongly-bound state (across the cross-sectional area of the muscle) and these provide greater resistance to stretch of the active muscle.

If there are breaks in the continuity of the endopelvic fascia (Richardson et al 1981) or if the levator ani muscle is damaged, the supportive layer under the urethra will be more compliant and will require a smaller pressure increment to displace a given distance.

Howard et al 2000a showed that compliance increased by nearly 50% in healthy primipara to 0.167 mm/cmH$_2$O and increased even further in stress-incontinent primipara by an additional 40% to 0.263 mm/cmH$_2$O. Thus, the supportive layer is considerably more compliant in these incontinent patients than in healthy women; it provides reduced resistance to deformation during transient increases in abdominal pressure so that closure of the urethral lumen cannot be ensured and SUI becomes possible.

An analogy that we have used previously is attempting to halt the flow of water through a garden hose by stepping on it (DeLancey 1990). If the hose was lying on a noncompliant trampoline, stepping on it would change the stress in the wall of the hose pipe, leading to a deformation and flattening of the hose cross-sectional area, closure of the lumen, and cessation of water flow, with little indentation or deflection of the trampoline.

If, instead, the hose was resting on a very compliant trampoline, stepping on the hose would tend to accelerate the hose and underlying trampoline downward because the resistance to motion (or reaction force) is at first negligible, so little flattening of the hose occurs as the trampoline begins to stretch. While the hose and trampoline move downward together, water would flow unabated in the hose. As the resistance of the trampoline to downward movement increasingly decelerates the downward movement of the foot and hose, flow will begin to cease. Thus, an increase in compliance of the supporting tissues essentially delays the effect of abdominal pressure on the transverse closure of the urethral lumen, allowing leakage of urine during the delay.

Additionally, the constant tone maintained by the pelvic muscles relieves the tension placed on the endopelvic fascia. If the nerves to the levator ani muscle are damaged (such as during childbirth) (Allen et al 1990), the denervated muscles would atrophy and leave the responsibility of pelvic organ support to the endopelvic fascia alone. Over time, these ligaments gradually stretch under the constant load and this viscoelastic behaviour leads to the development of prolapse.

There are several direct clinical applications for this information. The first concerns the types of damage that can occur to the urethral support system. An example is the paravaginal defect, which causes separation in the endopelvic fascia connecting the vagina to the pelvic sidewall and thereby increases the compliance of the fascial layer supporting the urethra. When this occurs, increases in abdominal pressure can no longer effectively compress the urethra against the supporting endopelvic fascia to close it during increases in abdominal pressure. When present, this paravaginal defect can be repaired surgically and normal anatomy can thus be restored.

Normal function of the urethral support system requires contraction of the levator ani muscle, which supports the urethra through the endopelvic fascia. During a cough, the levator ani muscle contracts simultaneously with the diaphragm and abdominal wall muscles to build abdominal pressure. This levator ani contraction helps to tense the suburethral fascial layer, as evidenced by decreased vesical neck motion on ultrasonographic evaluation (Miller et al 2001), thereby enhancing urethral compression. It also protects the connective tissue from undue stresses. Using an instrumented speculum (Ashton-Miller et al 2002), the strength of the levator ani muscle has recently been quantified under isometric conditions (Sampselle et al 1998), and racial differences have also been found in the levator muscle contractile properties (Howard et al 2000b).

Striated muscle takes 35% longer to develop the same force in the elderly as in young adults, and its maximum force is also diminished by about 35% (Thelen et al 1996a). These changes are due not to alterations in neural recruitment patterns, but rather to age-related changes in striated muscle contractility (Thelen et al 1996b). Furthermore, if the striated muscle of the levator ani becomes damaged or if its innervation is impaired, the muscle contraction will take even longer to develop the same force. This decrease in levator ani strength, in turn, is associated with decreased stiffness, because striated muscle strength and stiffness are directly and linearly correlated (Sinkjaer et al 1988).

Alternatively, if the connection between the muscle and the fascia is broken (Klutke et al 1990), then the normal mechanical function of the levator ani during a cough is lost. This phenomenon has important implications for clinical management. Recent evidence from MRI scans, reviewed in a blinded manner, shows the levator ani can be damaged unilaterally or bilaterally in certain patients (DeLancey et al 2003).

URETHROVESICAL PRESSURE DYNAMICS

The anatomical separation of sphincteric elements and supportive structures is mirrored in the functional separation of urethral closure pressure and pressure transmission. The relationship between resting urethral pressure, pressure transmission, and the pressure needed to cause leakage of urine are central to understanding urinary continence. These relationships have been described in what we have called the 'pressuregram' (Kim et al 1997). The constrictive effect of the urethral

Table 3.2 Effects of changes in cough pressure and pressure transmission ratio on urethral closure pressure and the potential leakage of urine

Example	Pves$_R$	Pura$_R$	UCP$_R$ (Pura − Pves)	Cough	PTR (%)	ΔPura$_c$	Pves$_c$	Pura$_c$	UCPc	Status
1	10	60	+50	200	100	200	210	260	+50	C
2	10	60	+50	200	70	140	210	200	−10	I
3	10	30	+20	100	70	70	110	100	−10	I
4	10	60	+50	100	70	70	110	130	+20	C
5	10	30	+20	50	70	35	60	55	−5	I

Primary variables shown in bold from which other pressures are derived.
Parameters that have been varied are italicized to show how changes in specific parameters can change continence status.
All pressures are expressed as cmH$_2$O.
C, continent; ΔPura, change in urethral pressure; I, incontinent; PTR, pressure transmission ratio; Pura$_c$, urethral pressure during cough; Pura$_R$, urethral pressure at rest; Pves$_c$, bladder pressure during cough; Pves$_R$, vesical pressure at rest; UCP$_c$, urethral closure pressure during cough; UCP$_R$, urethral closure pressure at rest.

sphincter deforms the wall of the urethra so as to main-tain urethral pressure above bladder pressure, and this pressure differential keeps urine in the bladder at rest. For example, if bladder pressure is 10 cmH_2O while urethral pressure is 60 cmH_2O, a closure pressure of 50 cmH_2O prevents urine from moving from the bladder through the urethra (Table 3.2, example 1).

Bladder pressure often increases by 200 cmH_2O or more during a cough, and leakage of urine would occur unless urethral pressure also increases. The efficiency of this pressure transmission is expressed as a percentage. A pressure transmission of 100% means, for example, that during a 200 cmH_2O increase in bladder pressure (from 10 cmH_2O to 210 cmH_2O), the urethral pressure would also increase by 200 cmH_2O (from 60 to 260 cmH_2O) (see Table 3.2, example 1).

The pressure transmission is less than 100% for incontinent women. For example, abdominal pressure may increase by 200 cmH_2O while urethral pressure may only increase by 140 cmH_2O, for a pressure trans-mission of 70% (see Table 3.2, example 2).

If a woman starts with a urethral pressure of 30 cmH_2O, resting bladder pressure of 10 cmH_2O and her pressure transmission is 70%, then with a cough pressure of 100 cmH_2O her bladder pressure would increase to 110 cmH_2O while urethral pressure would increase to just 100 cmH_2O and leakage of urine would occur (see Table 3.2, example 3).

In Table 3.2, example 4 shows the same elements, but with a higher urethral closure pressure; and similarly example 5 shows what happens with a weaker cough.

According to this conceptual framework, resting pressure and pressure transmission are the two key con-tinence variables. What factors determine these two phenomena? How are they altered to cause inconti-nence? Although the pressuregram concept is useful for understanding the role of resting pressure and pressure transmission, it has not been possible to reliably make these measurements because of the rapid movement of the urethra relative to the urodynamic transducer during a cough.

CLINICAL IMPLICATIONS OF LEVATOR FUNCTIONAL ANATOMY

Pelvic muscle exercise has been shown to be effective in alleviating SUI in many, but not all, women (Bø & Talseth 1996). Having a patient cough with a full bladder and measuring the amount of urine leakage is quite simple (Miller et al 1998a). If the muscle is normally innervated and is sufficiently attached to the endopelvic fascia, and if by contracting her pelvic muscles before and during a cough a woman is able to decrease that leakage (Fig. 3.10) (Miller et al 1998b), then simply learn-ing when and how to use her pelvic muscles may be an

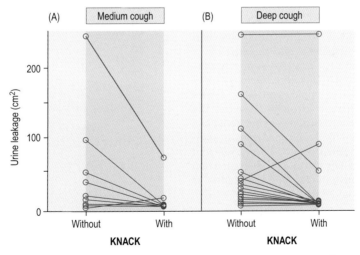

Fig. 3.10   The effect of learning the 'knack' (precontracting the pelvic muscles before a cough) on reducing the total amount of urine leaked during three separate medium-intensity coughs (left panel) and during three separate deep coughs (right panel) measured 1 week after the women had learned the skill. Each line joins the wet area on one trifold paper towel for each of the 27 women observed coughing without the knack (denoted by 'without knack') with that observed on a second paper towel when the same women used the knack (denoted 'with knack') (Miller et al 1998b). With regard to the units on the ordinate, a calibration test showed that every cm^2 of wetted area was caused by 0.039 mL urine leakage. (From Miller et al 1998b, with permission of Blackwell Science, Malden, Massachusetts.)

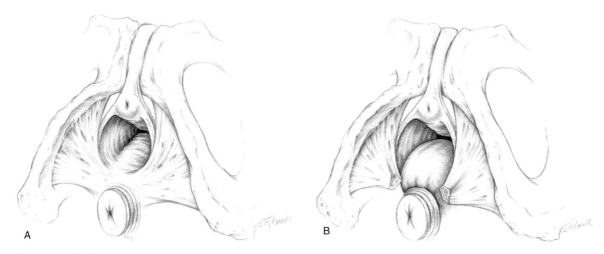

A   B

Fig. 3.11 (A) The perineal membrane spans the arch between the ischiopubic rami with each side attached to the other through their connection in the perineal body. (B) Note that separation of the fibres in this area leaves the rectum unsupported and results in a low posterior prolapse. (© DeLancey 1999.)

effective therapy. If this is the case, then the challenge is for the subject to remember to use this skill during activities that transiently increase abdominal pressure.

If the pelvic floor muscle is denervated as a result of substantial nerve injury, then it may not be possible to rehabilitate the muscle sufficiently to make pelvic muscle exercise an effective strategy. In order to use the remaining innervated muscle, women need to be told **when** to contract the muscles to prevent leakage, and they need to learn to strengthen pelvic muscles.

A stronger muscle that is not activated during the time of a cough cannot prevent SUI. Therefore, teaching proper timing of pelvic floor muscles would seem logical as part of a behavioural intervention involving exercise. The efficacy of this intervention is currently being tested in a number of ongoing randomized controlled trials. In addition, if the muscle is completely detached from the fascial tissues, then despite its ability to contract, the contraction may no longer be effective in elevating the urethra or maintaining its position under stress.

ANATOMY OF THE POSTERIOR VAGINAL WALL SUPPORT AS IT APPLIES TO RECTOCELE

The posterior vaginal wall is supported by connections between the vagina, the bony pelvis and the levator ani muscles (Smith et al 1989b). The lower one-third of the vagina is fused with the perineal body (Fig. 3.11), which is the attachment between the perineal membranes on

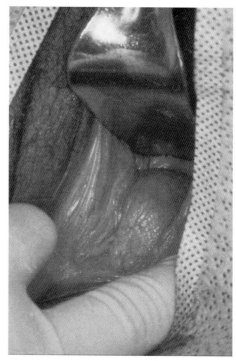

Fig. 3.12 Posterior prolapse due to separation of the perineal body. Note the end of the hymenal ring, which lies laterally on the side of the vagina, no longer united with its companion on the other side. (© DeLancey 2004.)

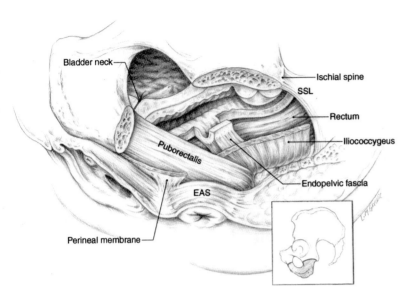

Fig. 3.13 Lateral view of the pelvis showing the relationships of the puborectalis, iliococcygeus and pelvic floor structures after removal of the ischium below the spine and sacrospinous ligament (SSL) (EAS, external anal sphincter). The bladder and vagina have been cut in the midline, yet the rectum left intact. Note how the endopelvic fascial 'pillars' hold the vaginal wall dorsally, preventing its downward protrusion. (© DeLancey 1999.)

either side. This connection prevents downward descent of the rectum in this region.

If the fibres that connect one side with the other rupture then the bowel may protrude downward resulting in a posterior vaginal wall prolapse (Fig. 3.12).

The midposterior vaginal wall is connected to the inside of the levator ani muscles by sheets of endopelvic fascia (Fig. 3.13). These connections prevent ventral movement of the vagina during increases in abdominal pressure. The medial most aspect of these paired sheets is referred to as the rectal pillars.

In the upper one-third of the vagina, the vaginal wall is connected laterally by the paracolpium. In this region there is a single attachment to the vagina, and a separate system for the anterior and posterior vaginal walls does not exist. Therefore when abdominal pressure forces the vaginal wall downward towards the introitus, attachments between the posterior vagina and the levator muscles prevent this downward movement.

The uppermost area of the posterior vagina is suspended, and descent of this area is usually associated with the clinical problem of uterine and/or apical prolapse. The lateral connections of the midvagina hold this portion of the vagina in place and prevent a midvaginal posterior prolapse (Fig. 3.14). The multiple connections of the perineal body to the levator muscles and the pelvic sidewall (Figs 3.15 and 3.16) prevent a low posterior prolapse from descending downward through the opening of the vagina (the urogenital hiatus and the levator ani muscles). Defects in the support at the level of the perineal body most frequently occur during vaginal delivery and are the most common type of posterior vaginal wall support problem.

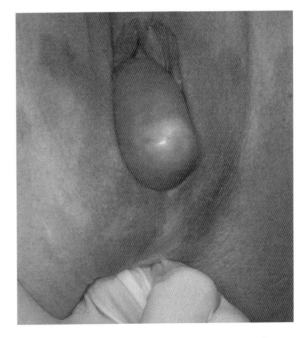

Fig. 3.14 Midvaginal posterior prolapse that protrudes through the introitus despite a normally supported perineal body. (© DeLancey 2004.)

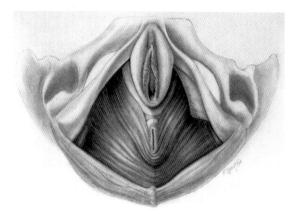

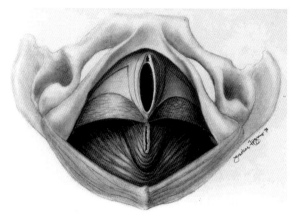

Fig. 3.15 Levator ani muscles seen from below the edge of the perineal membrane (urogenital diaphragm) can be seen on the left of the specimen. (© DeLancey 1999.)

Fig. 3.16 Position of the perineal membrane and its associated components of the striated urogenital sphincter, the compressor urethrae and the urethrovaginal sphincter. (© DeLancey 1999.)

REFERENCES

Allen R E, Hosker G L, Smith A R B et al 1990 Pelvic floor damage and childbirth: a neurophysiological study. British Journal of Obstetrics and Gynaecology 97(9):770–779

Ashton-Miller J A, DeLancey J O L, Warwick D N 2002 Method and apparatus for measuring properties of the pelvic floor muscles. US Patent # 6,468,232 B1

Berglas B, Rubin I C 1953 Study of the supportive structures of the uterus by levator myography. Surgery, Gynecology and Obstetrics 97:677–692

Bergman A, Elia G 1995 Three surgical procedures for genuine stress incontinence: five-year follow-up of a prospective randomized study. American Journal of Obstetrics and Gynecology 173(1):66–71

Blandpied P, Smidt G L 1993 The difference in stiffness of the active plantarflexors between young and elderly human females. Journals of Gerontology 48(2):M58–M63

Bø K, Talseth T 1996 Long-term effect of pelvic floor muscle exercise 5 years after cessation of organized training. Obstetrics and Gynecology 87(2):261–265

Colombo M, Scalambrino S, Maggioni A et al 1994 Burch colposuspension versus modified Marshal–Marchetti–Krantz urethropexy for primary genuine stress urinary incontinence: a prospective, randomized clinical trial. American Journal of Obstetrics and Gynecology 171(6):1573–1579

DeLancey J O L 1986 Correlative study of paraurethral anatomy. Obstetrics and Gynecology 68(1):91–97

DeLancey J O L 1990 Anatomy and physiology of urinary continence. Clinical Obstetrics and Gynecology 33(2):298–307

DeLancey J O L 1994 Structural support of the urethra as it relates to stress urinary incontinence: the hammock hypothesis. American Journal of Obstetrics and Gynecology 170(6):1713–1723

DeLancey J O L 1999 Structural anatomy of the posterior pelvic compartment as it relates to rectocele [Comment]. American Journal of Obstetrics and Gynecology, 180(4):815–823

DeLancey J O L, Kearney R, Chou Q et al 2003 The appearance of levator ani muscle abnormalities in magnetic resonance images after vaginal delivery. Obstetrics and Gynecology 101(1):46–53

Diokno A C, Wells T J, Brink C A 1987 Urinary incontinence in elderly women: urodynamic evaluation. Journal of the American Geriatrics Society 35(10):940–946

Enhörning G 1961 Simultaneous recording of intravesical and intra-urethral pressure. Acta Chirurgica Scandinavica 276(suppl):1–68

Gosling J A, Dixon J S, Critchley H O D et al 1981 A comparative study of the human external sphincter and periurethral levator ani muscles. British Journal of Urology 53(1):35–41

Halban J, Tandler I 1907 Anatomie und aetiologie der genitalprolapse beim weibe. Vienna

Hanzal E, Berger E, Koelbl H 1993 Levator ani muscle morphology and recurrent genuine stress incontinence. Obstetrics and Gynecology 81(3):426–429

Herzog A R, Diokno A C, Brown M B et al 1990 Two-year incidence, remission, and change patterns of urinary incontinence in noninstitutionalized older adults. Journal of Gerontology 45(2):M67–M74

Hilton P, Stanton S L 1983 Urethral pressure measurement by micro-transducer: the results in symptom-free women and in those with genuine stress incontinence. British Journal of Obstetrics and Gynaecology 90(10):919–933

Howard D, Miller J M, DeLancey J O L et al 2000a Differential effects of cough, valsalva, and continence status on vesical neck movement. Obstetrics and Gynecology 95(4):535–540

Howard D, DeLancey J O L, Tunn R et al 2000b Racial differences in the structure and function of the stress urinary continence mechanism in women. Obstetrics and Gynecology 95(5):713–717

Kearney R, Sawhney R, DeLancey J O L 2004 Levator ani muscle anatomy evaluated by origin–insertion pairs. Obstetrics and Gynecology 104(1):168–173

Kim K-J, Ashton-Miller J A, Strohbehn K et al 1997 The vesico-urethral pressuregram analysis of urethral function under stress. Journal of Biomechanics 30(1):19–25

Kirschner-Hermanns R, Wein B, Niehaus S et al 1993 The contribution of magnetic resonance imaging of the pelvic floor to the understanding of urinary incontinence. British Journal of Urology 72(5 Pt 2):715–718

Klutke G C, Golomb J, Barbaric Z et al 1990 The anatomy of stress incontinence: magnetic resonance imaging of the female bladder neck and urethra. Journal of Urology 43(3):563–566

Koelbl H, Saz V, Doerfler D et al 1998 Transurethral injection of silicone microimplants for intrinsic urethral sphincter deficiency. Obstetrics and Gynecology 92(3):332–336

Mant J, Painter R, Vessey M 1997 Epidemiology of genital prolapse: observations from the Oxford Planning Association Study. British Journal of Obstetrics and Gynaecology 104(5):579–585

Miller J M, Ashton-Miller J A, DeLancey J O L 1998a Quantification of cough-related urine loss using the paper towel test. Obstetrics and Gynecology 91(5 Pt 1):705–709

Miller J M, Ashton-Miller J A, DeLancey J O L 1998b A pelvic muscle precontraction can reduce cough-related urine loss in selected women with mild SUI. Journal of the American Geriatrics Society 46(7):870–874

Miller J M, Perucchini D, Carchidi L T et al 2001 Pelvic floor muscle contraction during a cough and decreased vesical neck mobility. Obstetrics and Gynecology, 97(2):255–260

Pandit M, DeLancey J O L, Ashton-Miller JA et al 2000 Quantification of intramuscular nerves within the female striated urogenital sphincter muscle. Obstetrics and Gynecology 95(6 Pt 1):797–800

Paramore R H 1918 The uterus as a floating organ. In: The statics of the female pelvic viscera. HK Lewis and Company, London, p 12

Parks A G, Porter N H, Melzak J 1962, Experimental study of the reflex mechanism controlling muscles of floor. Diseases of the Colon and Rectum 5:407–414

Perucchini D, DeLancey J O L, Ashton-Miller J A et al 2002a Age effects on urethral striated muscle: I. changes in number and diameter of striated muscle fibers in the ventral urethra. American Journal of Obstetrics and Gynecology 186(3):351–355

Perucchini D, DeLancey J O L, Ashton-Miller J A et al 2002b Age effects on urethral striated muscle: II. Anatomic location of muscle loss. American Journal of Obstetrics and Gynecology 186(3):356–360

Porges R F, Porges J C, Blinick G 1960 Mechanisms of uterine support and the pathogenesis of uterine prolapse. Obstetrics and Gynecology 15:711–726

Richardson A C, Edmonds P B, Williams N L 1981 Treatment of stress urinary incontinence due to paravaginal fascial defect. Obstetrics and Gynecology 57(3):357–362

Rud T, Andersson K E, Asmussen M et al 1980 Factors maintaining the intraurethral pressure in women. Investigative Urology 17(4):343–347

Sampselle C M, Miller J M, Mims B et al 1998 Effect of pelvic muscle exercise on transient incontinence during pregnancy and after birth. Obstetrics and Gynecology 91(3):406–412

Sinkjaer T, Toft E, Andreassen S et al 1988 Muscle stiffness in human ankle dorsiflexors: intrinsic and reflex components. Journal of Neurophysiology 60(3):1110–1121

Skelton D A, Young A, Greig C A et al 1995 Effects of resistance training on strength, power, and selected functional abilities of women aged 75 and older. Journal of the American Geriatrics Society 43(10):1081–1087

Smith A R B, Hosker G L, Warrell D W 1989a The role of partial denervation of the pelvic floor in the aetiology of genitourinary prolapse and stress incontinence of urine: a neurophysiological study. British Journal of Obstetrics and Gynaecology 96(1):24–28

Smith A R B, Hosker G L, Warrell D W 1989b The role of pudendal nerve damage in the aetiology of genuine stress incontinence in women. British Journal of Obstetrics and Gynaecology 96(1):29–32

Snooks S J, Swash M, Henry M M et al 1986 Risk factors in childbirth causing damage to the pelvic floor innervation. International Journal of Colorectal Disease 1(1):20–24

Strohbehn K, DeLancey J O L 1997 The anatomy of stress incontinence. Operative Techniques in Gynecological Surgery 2:15–16

Strohbehn K, Quint L E, Prince M R et al 1996 Magnetic resonance imaging anatomy of the female urethra: a direct histologic comparison. Obstetrics and Gynecology 88(5):750–756

Taverner D 1959 An electromyographic study of the normal function of the external anal sphincter and pelvic diaphragm. Diseases of the Colon and Rectum 2:153–160

Thelen D G, Ashton-Miller J A, Schultz A B et al 1996a Do neural factors underlie age differences in rapid ankle torque development? Journal of the American Geriatric Society 44(7):804–808

Thelen D G, Schultz A B, Alexander N B et al 1996b Effects of age on rapid ankle torque development. Journals of Gerontology. Series A, Biological Sciences and Medical Sciences 51(5):M226–M232

Thomas T M, Plymat K R, Blannin J et al 1980 Prevalence of urinary incontinence. British Medical Journal 281(6250):1243–1245

Tunn R, Paris S, Fischer W et al 1998 Static magnetic resonance imaging of the pelvic floor muscle morphology in women with stress urinary incontinence and pelvic prolapse. Neurourology and Urodynamics 17(6):579–589

ACKNOWLEDGEMENT

Supported by Public Health Service grants R01 DK 47516 and 51405, and P30 AG 08808.

Chapter 4

Neuroanatomy and neurophysiology of pelvic floor muscles

David B Vodušek

INTRODUCTION

Pelvic floor muscles (PFM) support pelvic organs, they are actively involved in their function, and probably the main culprits in some dysfunctions. A good example is stress urinary incontinence (SUI), which may develop due to weakness and/or activation and coordination disturbances of PFM. All activity of PFM is mediated (controlled) by the nervous system.

INNERVATION OF PELVIC FLOOR MUSCLES

Somatic motor pathways

The motor neurons that innervate the striated muscle of the external urethral and anal sphincters originate from a localized column of cells in the sacral spinal cord called Onuf's nucleus (Mannen et al 1982), expanding in humans from the second to third sacral segment (S2–S3) and occasionally into S1 (Schroder 1985). Within Onuf's nucleus there is some spatial separation between motor neurons concerned with the control of the urethral and anal sphincters. Spinal motor neurons for the levator ani group of muscles seem to originate from S3–S5 segments and show some overlap (Barber et al 2002).

Sphincter motor neurons are uniform in size and smaller than the other alpha motor neurons. They also differ with respect to their high concentrations of amino acid, neuropeptide, noradrenaline (norepinephrine), serotonin and dopamine-containing terminals, which represent the substrate for the distinctive neuropharmacological responses of these neurons, and differ from those of limb muscles, the bladder and the PFM.

The somatic motor fibres leave the spinal cord in the anterior roots and fuse with the posterior roots to constitute the spinal nerve. After passing through the intravertebral foramen the spinal nerve divides into a posterior and an anterior ramus (Bannister 1995). Somatic fibres from the anterior rami (also called the sacral plexus) form the pudendal nerve.

Traditionally the pudendal nerve is described as being derived from the S2–S4 anterior rami, but there may be some contribution from S1, and possibly little or no contribution from S4 (Marani et al 1993).

The pudendal nerve continues through the greater sciatic foramen and enters in a lateral direction through the lesser sciatic foramen into the ischiorectal fossa (Alcock's canal). In the posterior part of Alcock's canal the pudendal nerve gives off the inferior rectal nerve; then it branches into the perineal nerve, and the dorsal nerve of the penis/clitoris.

Although still controversial, it is generally accepted that the pudendal nerve supplies not only the anal but also the urinary sphincter. On the other hand it is mostly agreed that the main innervation for the PFM is through direct branches from the sacral plexus ('from above') rather than predominantly by branches of the pudendal nerve ('from below') (Fig. 4.1).

Significant variability of normal human neuroanatomy is probably the source of remaining controversies originating from anatomical studies of peripheral innervation of pelvis, which have so far been performed in only a small number of cases.

Higher nervous system regions control spinal cord motor nuclei by descending pathways; these inputs to

PFM motor neurons are manifold, and mostly 'indirect' (through several interneurons). More direct connections to Onuf's nucleus are from some nuclei in the brainstem (raphe, ambiguous) and from paraventricular hypothalamus.

Functional brain imaging is a powerful new tool to demonstrate functional anatomy of the human brain, and has already increased our knowledge in the realm of neural control of the lower urinary tract (LUT). Functional brain imaging techniques are based in particular on registering – directly or indirectly – the blood flow in the living human brain. Those brain areas, which during a particular manoeuvre (e.g. pelvic floor contraction) are controlling that particular activity, are more metabolically active than other 'nonactive' brain areas. The increase in metabolism is accompanied by an increase in blood flow through the particular area, and this can be recorded.

The established way of recording the 'amount' of blood flow in parenchymatous organs is by nuclear medicine techniques, by making the blood flow 'visible' by a radioisotope injected into the blood. Positron emission tomography (PET) relies on this principle and is able to render enough anatomical detail to be useful also for functional anatomical studies.

Using a different recording principle (but based on similar physiological principles), functional magnetic resonance tomography (fMR) is even better for providing detailed functional anatomical data. (These techniques can also demonstrate brain areas with 'less activity' as in the 'resting state', thus indicating inhibition of certain brain areas during execution of some manoeuvres.)

PET studies have revealed activation of the (right) ventral pontine tegmentum (in the brainstem) during holding of urine in human subjects (Blok et al 1997). This finding is consistent with the location of the 'L region' in cats, proposed to control PFM nuclei. The connections serve the coordinated inclusion of PFM into 'sacral' (LUT; anorectal, and sexual) functions. Individual PFM and sphincters need not only be neurally coordinated 'within' a particular function (e.g. with bladder activity), but the single functions need to be neurally coordinated with each other (e.g. voiding and defecation, voiding and erection).

Sacral function control system is proposed to be a part of the 'emotional motor system' derived from brain or brainstem structures belonging to the limbic system. It consists of the medial and a lateral component (Holstege 1998). The medial component represents diffuse pathways originating in the caudal brainstem and terminating on (almost all) spinal grey matter, using serotonin in particular as its neurotransmitter. This system is proposed to 'set the threshold' for overall

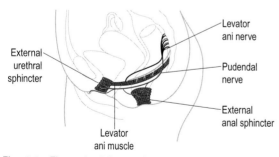

Fig. 4.1 The pudendal nerve is derived from the anterior rami of roots S1–S4. It continues through the greater sciatic foramen and enters in a lateral direction into the ischiorectal fossa. Its muscular branches innervate the external anal sphincter and the external urethral sphincter. There may be muscular branches for the levator ani, which is as a rule innervated by direct branches from the sacral plexus (from above) – the levator ani nerve.

changes in muscle activity, such as for instance in muscle tone under different physiological conditions (e.g. sleeping).

The lateral component of the emotional motor system consists of discrete areas in the hemispheres and the brainstem responsible for specific motor activities such as micturition and mating. The pathways belonging to the lateral system use spinal premotor interneurons to influence motor neurons in somatic and autonomic spinal nuclei, thus allowing for confluent interactions of various inputs to modify the motor neuron activity.

PFM nuclei also receive descending corticospinal input from the cerebral cortex. PET studies have revealed activation of the superomedial precentral gyrus during voluntary PFM contraction, and of the right anterior cingulate gyrus during sustained PFM straining (Blok et al 1997). Not surprisingly, PFM contraction can be obtained by electrical or magnetic transcranial stimulation of the motor cortex in man (Brostrom 2003, Vodušek 1996).

Afferent pathways

Because PFM function is intimately connected to pelvic organ function, it is proposed that all sensory information from the pelvic region is relevant for PFM neural control.

The sensory neurons are bipolar. Their cell bodies are in spinal ganglia. They send a long process to the periphery and a central process into the spinal cord where it terminates segmentally or – after branching for reflex connections – ascends in some cases as far as the brainstem (Bannister 1995).

The afferent pathways from the anogenital region and pelvic region are divided into somatic and visceral. Somatic afferents derive from touch, pain and thermal receptors in skin and mucosa and from proprioceptors in muscles and tendons. (Proprioceptive afferents arise particularly from muscle spindles and Golgi tendon organs.) The visceral afferents accompany both parasympathetic and sympathetic efferent fibres. The somatic afferents accompany the pudendal nerves, the levator ani nerve and direct somatic branches of the sacral plexus. The different groups of afferent fibres have different reflex connections, and transmit at least to some extent different afferent information.

The terminals of pudendal nerve afferents in the dorsal horn of the spinal cord are found ipsilaterally, but also bilaterally, with ipsilateral predominance (Ueyama et al 1984).

The proprioceptive afferents form synaptic contacts in the spinal cord and have collaterals ('primary afferent collaterals'), which run ipsilaterally in the dorsal spinal columns to synapse in the gracilis (dorsal column) nuclei in the brainstem. This pathway transmits information about innocuous sensations from the PFM.

The lateral columns of the spinal cord transmit information concerning pain sensations from perineal skin, as well as sexual sensations. In humans this pathway is situated superficially just ventral to the equator of the cord and is probably the spinothalamic tract (Torrens & Morrison 1987).

The spinal pathways that transmit sensory information from the visceral afferent terminations in the spinal cord to more rostral structures can be found in the dorsal, lateral, and ventral spinal cord columns.

NEURAL CONTROL OF SACRAL FUNCTIONS

Neural control of continence

At rest continence is assured by a competent sphincter mechanism, including not only the striated and smooth muscle sphincter but also the PFM and an adequate bladder storage function.

Normal kinesiological sphincter EMG recordings show continuous activity of motor units at rest (as defined by continuous firing of motor unit potentials), which as a rule increase with increasing bladder fullness. Reflexes mediating excitatory outflow to the sphincters are organized at the spinal level (the guarding reflex).

The L region in the brainstem has also been called the 'storage centre' (Blok et al 1997). This area was active in PET studies of those volunteers, who could not void, but contracted their PFM. The L region is thought to exert a continuous exciting effect on the Onuf's nucleus and thereby on the striated urinary sphincter during the storage phase; in humans it is probably part of a complex set of 'nerve impulse pattern generators' for different coordinated motor activities such as breathing, coughing, straining, etc.

During physical stress (e.g. coughing, sneezing) the urethral and anal sphincters may not be sufficient to passively withhold the pressures arising in the abdominal cavity, and hence within the bladder and lower rectum. Activation of the PFM is mandatory, and may be perceived as occurring in two steps by two different activation processes.

Coughing and sneezing are thought to be generated by individual pattern generators within the brainstem, and thus activation of PFM is a preset coactivation – and not primarily a 'reflex' reaction to increased intra-abdominal pressure. But, in addition, there may be an additional reflex PFM response to increased abdominal pressure due to distension of muscle spindles within PFM.

The PFM can of course also be voluntarily activated anticipating an increase in abdominal pressure. Such timed voluntary activity may be learned (the 'knack procedure') (Miller et al 1998).

Neural control of micturition

Centres in the pons (brainstem) coordinate micturition as such, but areas rostral to the pons (the hypothalamus and other parts of the brain including the frontal cortex) are responsible for the timing of the start of micturition. The pontine micturition centre (PMC) coordinates the activity of motor neurons of the urinary bladder and the urethral sphincter (both nuclei located in the sacral spinal cord), receiving afferent input via the periaqueductal grey matter. The central control of LUT function is organized as an on–off switching circuit (or a set of circuits, rather) that maintains a reciprocal relationship between the urinary bladder and urethral outlet.

Without the PMC and its spinal connections coordinated bladder/sphincter activity is not possible, thus patients with lesions of the PMC and its spinal connections demonstrate bladder sphincter discoordination (dyssynergia). Patients with lesions above the pons do not show detrusor–sphincter dyssynergia, but have urge incontinence (due to bladder overactivity) and demonstrate noninhibited sphincter relaxation and an inability to delay voiding to an appropriate place and time.

Voluntary micturition is a behaviour pattern that starts with relaxation of the striated urethral sphincter and PFM. Voluntary PFM contraction during voiding can lead to a stop of micturition, probably because of collateral connections to detrusor control nuclei. Descending inhibitory pathways for the detrusor have been demonstrated (de Groat et al 2001). Bladder contractions are also inhibited by reflexes, activated by afferent input from the PFM, perineal skin, and anorectum (Sato et al 2000).

Neural control of anorectal function

Faeces stored in the colon are transported past the rectosigmoid 'physiological sphincter' into the normally empty rectum, which can store up to 300 mL of contents. Rectal distension causes regular contractions of the rectal wall, which is effected by the intrinsic nervous (myenteric) plexus, and prompts the desire to defecate (Bartolo & Macdonald 2002).

Stool entering the rectum is also detected by stretch receptors in the rectal wall and PFM; their discharge leads to the urge to defecate. It starts as an intermittent sensation, which becomes more and more constant. Contraction of the PFM may interrupt the process, probably by concomitant inhibitory influences to the defecatory neural 'pattern generator', but also by 'mechanical' insistence on sphincter contraction and the propelling of faeces back to the sigmoid colon (Bartolo & Macdonald 2002).

The PFM are intimately involved in anorectal function. Apart from the 'sensory' role of the PFM and the external anal sphincter function, the puborectalis muscle is thought to maintain the 'anorectal' angle, which facilitates continence, and has to be relaxed to allow defecation. Current concepts suggest that defecation requires increased rectal pressure coordinated with relaxation of the anal sphincters and PFM.

Pelvic floor relaxation allows opening of the anorectal angle and perineal descent, facilitating fecal expulsion. Puborectalis and external anal sphincter activity during evacuation is generally inhibited. However, observations by EMG and defecography suggest that the puborectalis may not always relax during defecation in healthy subjects (Fucini et al 2001).

Neural control of the sexual response

The PFM are actively involved in the sexual response. Their activation has been mostly explored in males during ejaculation, where their repetitive activation during a several seconds interval is responsible for the expulsion of semen from the urethra, particularly by the bulbocavernosus muscles (Petersen et al 1955). Little is known on PFM activity patterns during other parts of the human sexual response cycle.

It is assumed that apart from general changes in muscle tone set by the emotional motor system, the sacral reflex circuitry governs much of the PFM activity during the sexual response cycle. The bulbocavernosus reflex behaviour, as known from studies (Vodušek 2002a) would allow for reflex activation of the PFM during genital stimulation. Tonic stimulation of the reflex is postulated to hinder venous outflow from penis/clitoris, thus helping erection. Reflex contraction of the PFM should conceivably contribute to the achievement of the 'orgasmic platform' (contraction of the levator ani and – in the female – the circumvaginal muscles). Climax in humans (in both sexes, and in experimental animals) elicits rhythmic contractions of the PFM/perineal muscles, which in the male drives the ejaculate from the urethra (assisted by a coordinated bladder neck closure).

NEUROPHYSIOLOGY OF PELVIC FLOOR MUSCLES

Muscle activity is thoroughly dependent on neural control. 'Denervated' muscle atrophies and turns into fibrotic tissue. Muscle – like every tissue – consists of cells (muscle fibres). But the functional unit within striated muscle is not a single muscle cell, but a motor unit. A motor unit consists of one alpha (or 'lower') motor neuron (from the motor nuclei in spinal cord), and all the muscle cells this motor neuron innervates. The motor unit – in other words – is the basic functional unit of the somatic motor system; control of a muscle means control of its motor units. Thus, in discussing neural control of muscle, we really only need to consider the motor neurons in the spinal cord and all the influences they are exposed to.

The function of pelvic floor and sphincter lower motor neurons is organized quite differently from other groups of motor neurons. In contrast to the reciprocal innervation that is common in limb muscles, the neurons innervating each side of the PFM have to work in harmony and synchronously. Indeed, sphincters may be morphologically considered to constitute 'one' muscle – which is innervated by two nerves (left and right)!

By concomitant activity the PFM act as the 'closure unit' of the excretory tracts, the 'support unit' for pelvic viscera, and an 'effector unit' in the sexual response. In general, muscles involved in these functions from both sides of the body act in a strictly unified fashion as 'one muscle': this has been demonstrated for the pubococcygei muscles, but has not really been documented for the whole group of PFM and sphincters (Deindl et al 1993). However, as each muscle in the pelvis has its own unilateral peripheral innervation, dissociated activation patterns are possible and have been reported between the two pubococcygei (Deindl et al 1994) and between levator ani and the urethral sphincter (Kenton & Brubaker 2002).

The differences in evolutionary origin of the sphincter muscles and levator ani furthermore imply that unilateral activation may be less of an impossibility for the PFM than for sphincters. It can be postulated that the neural mechanisms controlling the different muscles involved in sphincter mechanisms and pelvic organ support may not be as uniform as has been assumed. How much variability there is in normal activation patterns of PFM is not yet clarified. It is clear, however, that the coordination between individual PFM can definitively be impaired by disease or trauma.

Tonic and phasic pelvic floor muscle activity

The normal striated sphincter muscles demonstrate some continuous motor unit activity at rest as revealed by kinesiological EMG (Fig. 4.2). This differs between individuals and continues also after subjects fall asleep during the examination (Chantraine 1973). This physiological spontaneous activity may be called tonic, and depends on prolonged activation of certain tonic motor units (Vodušek 1982).

The 'amount' of tonic motor unit activity can in principle be assessed counting the number of active motor unit potentials or analysing the interference pattern by EMG; this has so far not been much studied. Thus, little is known about the variability and the normal range of tonic activity in normal subjects, and the reproducibility of findings; this makes it difficult to assess the validity of results from the few studies reporting activity changes accompanying LUT, anorectal or sexual dysfunction.

As a rule tonic motor unit activity increases with bladder filling, at the same time depending on the rate of filling. Any reflex or voluntary activation is mirrored first in an increase of the firing frequency of these motor units. On the contrary, inhibition of firing is apparent on initiation of voiding.

With any stronger activation manoeuvre (e.g. contraction, coughing), and only for a limited length of time, new motor units are recruited (see Fig. 4.2). These may be called 'phasic' motor units. As a rule, they have potentials of higher amplitudes and their discharge rates are higher and irregular. A small percentage of motor units with an 'intermediate' activation pattern

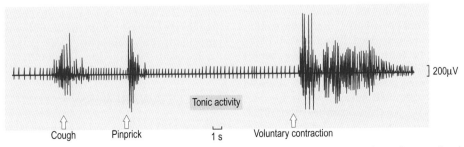

Fig. 4.2 Kinesiological EMG recordings from urethral sphincter muscle. Concentric needle electrode recording in a 53-year-old continent woman: recruitment of motor units on reflex manoeuvres and on command to contract. (From Vodušek 1994, with kind permission of Springer Science and Business Media.)

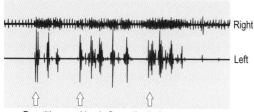

Repetitive coughing (reflex activation)

Fig. 4.3 Patterns of activation of pubococcygei muscles in a normal continent nulliparous woman – the tonic (above) and the phasic (below) pattern at two discrete recording sites within the right and left muscle. (From Deindl et al 1993, with permission.)

can also be encountered (Vodušek 1982). It has to be stressed that this typing of motor units is electrophysiological, and no direct correlation to histochemical typing of muscle fibres has so far been achieved.

With regard to tonic activity, sphincters differ from some perineal muscles; tonic activity is encountered in many but not all detection sites for the levator ani muscle (Deindl et al 1993, Vodušek 1982) (Fig. 4.3) and is practically never seen in the bulbocavernosus muscle (Vodušek 1982). In the pubococcygeus of the normal female there is some increase of activity during bladder filling, and reflex increases in activity during any activation manoeuvre performed by the subject (e.g. talking, deep breathing, coughing).

On voiding, inhibition of the tonic activity of the external urethral sphincter – and also the PFM – leads to relaxation. This can be detected as a disappearance of all EMG activity, which precedes detrusor contraction. Similarly, the striated anal sphincter relaxes with defecation and also micturition (Read 1990).

Reflex activity of pelvic floor muscles

The human urethral and anal striated sphincters seem to have no muscle spindles; their reflex reactivity is thus intrinsically different from the levator ani muscle complex, in which muscle spindles and Golgi tendon organs have been demonstrated (Borghi et al 1991). Thus, PFM have the intrinsic proprioceptive 'servomechanism' for adjusting muscle length and tension, whereas the sphincter muscles depend on afferents from skin and mucosa. Both muscle groups are integrated in reflex activity, which incorporates pelvic organ function.

The reflex activity of PFM is clinically and electrophysiologically evaluated by eliciting the bulbocavernosus and anal reflex. The bulbocavernosus reflex is evoked on nonpainful stimulation of the glans (or – electrically – the dorsal penile/clitoral nerve). As recorded electromyographically, it is a complex response: its first component thought to be an oligosynaptic and the later component a polysynaptic reflex (Vodušek & Janko 1990). The polysynaptic anal reflex is elicited by painful (pinprick) stimulation in the perianal region.

The constant tonic activity of sphincter muscles is thought to result from the characteristics of their 'low-threshold' motor neurons and the constant 'inputs' (either of reflex segmental or suprasegmental origin). It is supported by cutaneous stimuli, by pelvic organ distension, and by intra-abdominal pressure changes.

Sudden increases in intra-abdominal pressure as a rule lead to brisk PFM (reflex) activity, which has been called the 'guarding reflex'; it is organized at the spinal level. It needs to be considered that 'sudden increases in intra-abdominal pressure', if caused by an intrinsically driven manoeuvre (i.e. coughing) include feed forward activation of the PFM as part of the complex muscle activation pattern. The observed PFM activation in the normal subject (e.g. during coughing) is thus a compound 'feed-forward' and 'reflex' muscle activation.

Another common stimulus leading to an increase in PFM activity is pain. The typical phasic reflex response to a nociceptive stimulus is the anal reflex. It is commonly assumed that prolonged pain in pelvic organs is accompanied by an increase in 'reflex' PFM activity, which would indeed be manifested as 'an increased tonic motor unit activity'. This has so far not been much formally studied. Whether such chronic PFM overactivity might itself generate a chronic pain state and even other dysfunctions may be a tempting hypothesis, but has not been well demonstrated so far.

To correspond to their functional (effector) role as pelvic organ supporters (e.g. during coughing, sneezing), sphincters for the LUT and anorectum, and as an effector in the sexual arousal response, orgasm and ejaculation, PFM have also to be involved in very complex involuntary ('reflex') activity, which coordinates the behaviour of pelvic organs (smooth muscle) and several different groups of striated muscles. This activity is to be understood as originating from so called 'pattern generators' within the central nervous system, particularly the brainstem. These pattern generators ('reflex centres') are genetically inbuilt.

MUSCLE AWARENESS

The sense of position and movement of one's body is referred to as 'proprioception', and is particularly important for sensing limb position (stationary proprioception) and limb movement (kinaesthetic proprioception).

Proprioception relies on special mechanoreceptors in muscle tendons and joint capsules. In muscles there are specialized stretch receptors (muscle spindles) and in tendons there are Golgi tendon organs, which sense the contractile force. In addition, stretch sensitive receptors signalling postural information are in the skin. This cutaneous proprioception is particularly important for controlling movements of muscles without bony attachment (lips, anal sphincter). By these means of afferent input the functional status of a striated muscle (or rather: a certain movement) is represented in the brain. Indeed, muscle awareness reflects the amount of sensory input from various sites. Typically, feedback to awareness on limb muscle function (acting at joints) is derived not only from their input from muscle spindles, and receptors in tendons, but also from the skin, and from visual input, etc. The concept of the 'awareness' thus in fact overlaps with the ability to voluntarily change the state of a muscle (see below).

In contrast to limb muscles, the PFM (and sphincters) lack several of the above mentioned sensory input mechanisms and therefore the brain is not 'well informed' on their status. Additionally, there may be a gender difference, inasmuch as pelvic floor muscle awareness in females seems to be in general less compared to males. (The author concludes this on the basis of long personal experience with PFM EMGs in both genders; there seems to be no formal study on PFM activation patterns in man apart from ejaculation.)

Healthy males have no difficulties in voluntarily contracting the pelvic floor, but up to 30% of healthy women cannot do it readily on command. The need for 'squeezing out' the urethra at the end of voiding and the close relationship of penile erection and ejaculation to PFM contractions may be the origin of this gender difference. The primarily weak awareness of PFM in women seems to be further jeopardized by vaginal delivery.

Voluntary activity of pelvic floor muscles

Skilled movement of distal limb muscles requires individual motor units to be activated in a highly focused manner by the primary motor cortex. By contrast, activation of axial muscles (necessary to maintain posture etc.) – while also under voluntary control – depends particularly on vestibular nuclei and reticular formation to create predetermined 'motor patterns'.

The PFM are not, strictly speaking, axial muscles, but several similarities to axial muscles can be proposed as regards their neural control. In any case, PFM are under voluntary control (i.e. it is possible to voluntarily activate or inhibit the firing of their motor units). EMG studies have shown that the activity of motor units in

the urethral sphincter can be extinguished at both low and high bladder volumes even without initiating micturition (Sundin & Petersen 1975, Vodušek 1994).

To voluntarily activate a striated muscle we have to have the appropriate brain 'conceptualization' of that particular movement, which acts as a rule within a particular complex 'movement pattern'. This evolves particularly through repeatedly executed commands and represents a certain 'behaviour'.

Proprioceptive information is crucial for striated muscle motor control both in the 'learning' phase of a certain movement and for later execution of overlearnt motor behaviours. It is passed to the spinal cord by fast-conducting large-diameter myelinated afferent fibres and is influenced not only by the current state of the muscle, but also by the efferent discharge the muscle spindles receive from the nervous system via gamma efferents. To work out the state of the muscle, the brain must take into account these efferent discharges and make comparisons between the signals it sends out to the muscle spindles along the gamma efferents and the afferent signals it receives from the primary afferents.

Essentially, brain compares the signal from the muscle spindles with the copy of its motor command (the 'corollary discharge' or 'efferents copy') which was sent to the muscle spindle intrafusal muscle fibres by the CNS via gamma efferents. The differences between the two signals are used in deciding on the state of the muscle. The experiments were carried out in limb muscles (McCloskey 1981), but it has been suggested (Morrison 1987) that similar principles rule in bladder neurocontrol.

NEUROMUSCULAR INJURY TO THE PELVIC FLOOR DUE TO VAGINAL DELIVERY

Many studies using different techniques have demonstrated neurogenic and structural damage to the PFM and sphincter muscles as a consequence of vaginal delivery (Vodušek 2002b). Other lesion mechanisms, such as muscle ischaemia, may also be operative during childbirth. As a consequence, the PFM would become weak; such weakness has indeed been demonstrated (Verelst & Leivseth 2004). The sphincter mechanisms and pelvic organ support become functionally impaired, with SUI and prolapse being a logical consequence.

Although muscle weakness may be a common consequence of childbirth injury, there seem to be further pathophysiological possibilities for deficient PFM function; it is not only the strength of muscle contraction that defines its functional integrity.

Normal neural control of muscle activity leads to coordinated and timely responses to ensure appropriate

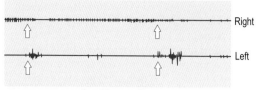

Right

Left

Repetitive coughing

Fig. 4.4 Patterns of activation of pubococcygei muscles in a parous woman with stress incontinence. A paradoxical inhibition of firing of motor units occurs during coughing in one of the pubococcygei. (From Deindl et al 1994, with permission)

muscle function as required. Muscular 'behavioural' patterns have been studied by kinesiological EMG recording (Deindl et al 1993). Changes in muscular behaviour may originate from minor and repairable neuromuscular pelvic floor injury (Dendl et al 1994).

In nulliparous healthy women two types of behavioural patterns named as tonic and phasic pattern, respectively, can be found (see Fig. 4.3):

- the tonic pattern consists of a crescendo–decrescendo type of activity (probably derived from grouping of slow motor units) that may be the expression of constant ('tonic') reflex input parallel to the breathing pattern;

- the phasic pattern, probably related to fast-twitch motor unit activation, is motor unit activity seen only during activation manoeuvres, either voluntary contraction or coughing.

With respect to these muscle activation patterns parous women with SUI are subject to a number of possible changes (Dendl et al 1994), such as a significant reduction of duration of motor unit recruitment, unilateral recruitment of reflex response in the pubococcygeal muscle, and paradoxical inhibition of continuous firing of motor units (Fig. 4.4) in PFM activation on coughing.

The reasons for such persisting abnormalities are not clear and are difficult to explain by muscle denervation (which has been amply studied) alone.

Although not proven in studies, it is reasonable to assume that motor denervation is accompanied also by sensory denervation of the PFM. In addition to denervation injury there may be some further temporary 'inhibitors' of PFM activity, such as periods of pain and discomfort after childbirth (e.g. perineal tears, episiotomy), increased by attempted PFM contraction.

All above mentioned factors may lead to a temporary disturbance of PFM neural control after childbirth. This, in combination with a particularly vulnerable pelvic floor neural control (which only evolved in its complexity phylogenetically after the attainment of the upright stance), might become persistent, even if the factors originally leading to the problem disappear.

CONCLUSION

The PFM are a deep muscle group that have some similarities in their neural control as axial muscles. They are under prominent reflex and relatively weak voluntary control, with few and poor sensory data contributing to awareness of the muscles. Furthermore their neural control mechanism is fragile due to its relative phylogenetic recency, and is exposed to trauma and disease due to its expansive anatomy (from frontal cortex to the 'tail').

Vaginal delivery may lead to structural and denervation changes in the PFM, but also to secondary changes in their activation patterns. Dysfunctional neural control induced by trauma, disease, or purely functional causes may manifest itself by over- or underactivity, and/or by discoordination of PFM activity. Often these disturbances are not 'hard-wired' into the nervous system, but only a problem of neural control 'software' (which can be 're-programmed'). Therefore, physical therapy should in many patients provide an appropriate, and even best available treatment.

REFERENCES

Bannister L H (ed) 1995 Gray's anatomy. The anatomical basis of medicine and surgery, 38th edn. Churchill Livingstone, New York

Barber M D, Bremer R E, Thor K B et al 2002 Innervation of the female levator ani muscles. American Journal of Obstetrics and Gynecology 187:64–71

Bartolo D C C, Macdonald A D H 2002 Fecal continence and defecation. In: Pemberton J H, Swash M, Henry M M (eds) The pelvic floor. Its function and disorders. W B Saunders, London, p 77–83

Blok B F M, Sturms L M, Holstege G 1997 A PET study on cortical and subcortical control of pelvic floor musculature in women. Journal of Comparative Neurology 389:535–544

Borghi F, Di Molfetta L, Garavoglia M et al 1991 Questions about the uncertain presence of muscle spindles in the human external anal sphincter. Panminerva Medica 33: 170–172

Brostrom S 2003 Motor evoked potentials from the pelvic floor. Neurourology and Urodynamics 22:620–637

Bump R, Mclish D 1992 Cigarette smoking and urinary incontinence in women. American Journal of Obstetrics and Gynaecology 167:1213

Chantraine A 1973 Examination of the anal and urethral sphincters. In: Desmedt J E (ed) New developments in electromyography and clinical neurophysiology, vol. 2. Karger, Basel, p 421–432

de Groat W C, Fraser M O, Yoshiyama M et al 2001 Neural control of the urethra. Scandinavian Journal of Urology and Nephrology. Supplementum 207:35–43, discussion 106–125

Deindl F M, Vodušek D B, Hesse U et al 1993 Activity patterns of pubococcygeal muscles in nulliparous continent women. British Journal of Urology 72:46–51

Deindl F M, Vodušek D B, Hesse U et al 1994 Pelvic floor activity patterns: comparison of nulliparous continent and parous urinary stress incontinent women. A kinesiological EMG study. British Journal of Urology 73:413–417

Fucini C, Ronchi O, Elbetti C 2001 Electromyography of the pelvic floor musculature in the assessment of obstructed defecation symptoms. Diseases of the Colon and Rectum 44:1168–1175

Holstege G 1998 The emotional motor system in relation to the supraspinal control of micturition and mating behavior. Behavioural Brain Research 92:103–109

Kenton K, Brubaker L 2002 Relationship between levator ani contraction and motor unit activation in the urethral sphincter. American Journal of Obstetrics and Gynecology 187:403–406

Mannen T, Iwata M, Toyokura Y et al 1982 The Onuf's nucleus and the external anal sphincter muscles in amyotrophic lateral sclerosis and Shy–Drager syndrome. Acta Neuropathologica 58:255–260

Marani E, Pijl M E, Kraan M C et al 1993 Interconnections of the upper ventral rami of the human sacral plexus: a reappraisal for dorsal rhizotomy in neurostimulation operations. Neurourology and Urodynamics 12:585–598

McCloskey D I 1981 Corollary changes: motor commands and perception. In: Brookhart J M, Mountcastle V B (eds) Handbook of physiology, Section I, The nervous system, vol. 2 (part 2). American Physiological Society, Bethesda, MD, p 1415–1447

Miller J M, Ashton-Miller J A, DeLancey J O 1998 A pelvic muscle precontraction can reduce cough-related urine loss in selected women with mild SUI. Journal of the American Geriatrics Society 46:870–874

Morrison J F B 1987 Reflex control of the lower urinary tract. In: Torrens M, Morrison JF (eds) The physiology of the lower urinary tract. Springer–Verlag, London, p 193–235

Petersen I, Franksson C, Danielson C O 1955 Electromyographic study of the muscles of the pelvic floor and urethra in normal

females. Acta Obstetricia et Gynecologica Scandinavica 34: 273–285

Read N W 1990 Functional assessment of the anorectum in faecal incontinence. Neurobiology of incontinence (Ciba Foundation Symposium 151). John Wiley, Chichester, p 119–138

Sato A, Sato Y, Schmidt R F 2000 Reflex bladder activity induced by electrical stimulation of hind limb somatic afferents in the cat. Journal of the Autonomic Nervous System 1:229–241

Schroder H D 1985 Anatomical and pathoanatomical studies on the spinal efferent systems innervating pelvic structures. 1. Organization of spinal nuclei in animals. 2. The nucleus X-pelvic motor system in man. Journal of the Autonomic Nervous System 14:23–48

Sundin T, Petersen I 1975 Cystometry and simultaneous electromyography from the striated urethral and anal sphincters and from levator ani. Investigative Urology 13:40–46

Swash M 2002 Electrophysiological investigation of the posterior pelvic floor musculature. In: Pemberton J H, Swash M, Henry M M (eds) The pelvic floor. Its functions and disorders. Saunders, London, p 213–236

Torrens M, Morrison J F B (eds) 1987 The physiology of the lower urinary tract. Springer–Verlag, London

Ueyama T, Mizuno N, Nomura S et al 1984 Central distribution of afferent and efferent components of the pudendal nerve in cat. Journal of Comparative Neurology 222:38–46

Verelst M, Leivseth G 2004 Are fatigue and disturbances in pre-programmed activity of pelvic floor muscles associated with female stress urinary incontinence? Neurourology and Urodynamics 23:143–147

Vodušek D B 1994 Electrophysiology. In: Schuessler B, Laycock J, Norton P et al (eds) Pelvic floor re-education, principles and practice. Springer–Verlag, London, p 83–97

Vodušek D B 1996 Evoked potential testing. Urologic Clinics of North America 23:427–446

Vodušek D B 1982 Neurophysiological study of sacral reflexes in man (in Slovene). Institute of Clinical Neurophysiology. University E Kardelj in Ljubljana, Ljubljana, p 55

Vodušek D B 2002a Sacral reflexes. In: Pemberton JH, Swash M, Henry MM, eds. Pelvic floor. Its functions and disorders. Saunders, London, p 237–247

Vodušek D B 2002b The role of electrophysiology in the evaluation of incontinence and prolapse. Current Opinion in Obstetrics and Gynecology 14:509–514

Vodušek D B, Janko M 1990 The bulbocavernosus reflex. A single motor neuron study. Brain 113(Pt 3):813–820

Chapter 5

Measurement of pelvic floor muscle function and strength and pelvic organ prolapse

Introduction

Kari Bø and Margaret Sherburn

The International Classification of Impairments, Disabilities and Handicaps (ICIDH) (1997), lately changed to International Classification of Functioning, Disability, and Health (ICF) (2002), is a World Health Organization (WHO)-approved system for classification of health and health-related states in rehabilitation science. According to this system, the causes of a non-optimally functioning pelvic floor (e.g. muscle and nerve damage after vaginal birth) can be classified as the **pathophysiological** component. Nonfunctioning pelvic floor muscles (PFM) (reduced force generation, incorrect timing or coordination) are the **impairment** component, and the symptom of pelvic floor dysfunction (e.g. urinary leakage, fecal incontinence, or pelvic organ prolapse) is a **disability**. How the symptoms and conditions affect the women's quality of life and participation in fitness activities is an **activity** or **participation** component.

Physiotherapists working to prevent or treat pelvic floor dysfunction aim to improve disability and activity/participation components by improving PFM function and strength. Hence, it is important to measure all ICF components. In this chapter we deal only with the pathophysiological and impairment component with a focus on assessment of ability to contract the PFM and measurement of PFM strength.

The main reasons for physical therapists to conduct high-quality assessment of ability to contract the PFM and PFM strength are as follows.

1. Without proper instruction, many women are unable to volitionally contract PFM on demand. This may be because they are situated at the floor of the pelvis and are not visible from the outside. In addition the muscles are seldom used consciously. Several studies have shown that more than 30% of women do not contract their PFM correctly at their first consultation, even after thorough individual instruction (Benvenuti et al 1987, Bump et al 1991, Bø et al 1988, Kegel 1948). The most common errors are to contract the gluteal, hip adductor, or abdominal muscles instead of the PFM (Bø et al 1988). Some women also stop breathing or try to exaggerate inspiration instead of contracting the PFM. Some studies have demonstrated that many women strain, causing PFM descent, instead of actively squeezing and lifting the PFM upward (Bump et al 1991, Bø et al 1990). For proper contraction of the PFM, it is mandatory that women receive precise training with appropriate monitoring and feedback. Hay-Smith et al (2001) found that in the reports of only 15 of 43 RCTs they reviewed did the authors state that a correct PFM contraction was checked before training began.

2. In intervention studies evaluating the effect of PFM training, the training is the independent variable meant to cause a change in the dependent variable (e.g. stress urinary incontinence [SUI] or pelvic organ prolapse; Thomas & Nelson 1996). Thus, measurement of PFM function and strength before and after training is important to determine whether the intervention has made significant changes. Even in the presence of tissue pathology (e.g. neuropathy), if there is no change in PFM function or strength after a training programme commensurate with that pathology, the training programme has been of insufficient dosage (intensity, frequency or duration of the training period) or the participants have had inadequate adherence (Bouchard et al 1994). It is likely that such programmes have not followed muscle training recommendations.

In this chapter we describe different measurement tools such as clinical observation, vaginal palpation, electromyography (EMG), vaginal squeeze pressure measurement (manometry), urethral pressure measurement (stationary and ambulatory), dynamometry, ultrasonography and magnetic resonance imaging (MRI) in use for assessment of the PFM. This can be either assessment of unconscious co-contraction of the PFM during an increase in abdominal pressure or ability to volitionally perform a correct contraction. A correct voluntary contraction is described as an elevation and squeeze around the pelvic openings (Kegel 1948).

Muscle strength has been defined as 'the maximum force that can be exerted against an immovable object (static or isometric strength), the heaviest weight which can be lifted or lowered (dynamic strength), or the maximal torque which can be developed against a pre-set rate-limiting device (isokinetic strength)' (Frontera & Meredith 1989). Maximum strength is often referred to as the maximum weight the individual can lift once. This is named the one repetition maximum or 1RM (Wilmore & Costill 1999).

Maximum strength is measured through a **maximum voluntary contraction**. Maximum voluntary contraction refers to a condition in which a person attempts to recruit as many fibers in a muscle as possible for the purpose of developing force (Knuttgen & Kraemer 1987). The force generated is dependent on the cross-sectional area of the muscle and the neural components (e.g. number of activated motor units and frequency of excitation; Wilmore & Costill 1999). Hence, PFM strength is a surrogate for underlying factors that will change with regular strength training.

Muscle power is the explosive aspect of strength and is the product of strength and speed of movement [power = (force × distance)/time] (Wilmore & Costill 1999). Muscle force is reduced with speed of the contraction. Power is the key component of functional application of strength. Speed, however, changes little with training, thus power is changed almost exclusively through gains in strength (Wilmore & Costill 1999).

Muscular endurance can be classified as:

1. ability to sustain near maximal or maximal force, assessed by the time one is able to maintain a maximum static or isometric contraction;
2. ability to repeatedly develop near maximal or maximal force determined by assessing the maximum number of repetitions one can perform at a given percentage of 1RM (Wilmore & Costill 1999).

Muscle strength measurement may be considered an indirect measure of PFM function in real-life activities. Women with no leakage do not contract voluntarily before coughing or jumping. Their PFM contraction is considered to be an automatic co-contraction occurring as a quick and effective activation of an intact neural system.

Other important factors for a quick and effective contraction are the location of the pelvic floor within the pelvis, the muscle bulk, stiffness/elasticity of the pelvic floor and intact connective tissue.

A stretched and weak pelvic floor may be positioned lower within the pelvis compared with a well-trained or non-injured pelvic floor (Bø 2004). The time for stretched muscles to reach an optimal contraction may be too slow to be effective in preventing descent against increased abdominal pressure (e.g. sneeze), thereby allowing leakage to occur.

In general, when measuring muscle strength it can be difficult to isolate the muscles to be tested, and many test subjects need adequate time and instruction in how to perform the test. In addition, the test situation may not reflect the whole function of the muscles, and the generalizability from the test situation to real-world activity (external validity) has to be established (Thomas & Nelson 1996). Therefore, when reporting results from muscle testing, it is important to specify the equipment used, position during testing, testing procedure, instruction and motivation given, and what parameters are tested (e.g. ability to contract, maximum strength, endurance). When testing the PFM, additional challenges are present because muscle action and location are not easily observable.

Whether a measurement tool should be used in clinical practice or in research depends on its responsiveness, reliability and validity. These terms are used slightly different in different research areas and have somewhat different definitions in different textbooks of research methodology. The definitions given below are the ones we have chosen to use in this textbook.

- **Responsiveness**: the degree or amount of variation that the device is capable of measuring; the ability of a tool to detect small differences or small changes (Currier 1990).

- **Reliability**: consistency or repeatability of a measure. The most common way to establish stability of a test is to perform a test–retest. **Intratest** reliability is conducted by one researcher measuring the same procedure in the same subjects twice. **Inter-test** reliability is conducted when two or more clinicians or researchers are conducting measurement of the same subjects (Currier 1990).

- **Validity**: degree to which a test or instrument measures what it is supposed to measure.

- **Logical (face) validity**: condition that is claimed when the measure obviously involves the performance being measured (e.g. squeeze and elevation of the PFM can be felt by vaginal palpation).

- **Content validity**: condition that is claimed when a test adequately samples what it should cover (few methods measure both squeeze pressure and elevation of the PFM).

- **Criterion validity**: the degree to which the scores on a test are related to some recognized standard, or criterion (e.g. clinical observation of inward movement of the perineum during attempts to contract the PFM compared with ultrasonography).

- **Concurrent validity**: involves a measuring instrument being correlated with some criterion administered at the same time or concurrently (e.g. simultaneous observation of inward movement during measurement of PFM strength with manometers and dynamometers).

- **Predictive validity**: degree to which scores of predictor variables can accurately predict criterion scores.
- **Diagnostic validity**: ability of a measure to detect differences between those having a diagnosis/problem/condition/symptom with those not.
- **Sensitivity**: the proportion of positives that are correctly identified by the test.
- **Specificity**: the proportion of negatives that are correctly identified by the test (Altman 1997, Currier 1990, Thomas & Nelson 1996).

It is important for physiotherapists (PTs) who treat patients with pelvic floor dysfunction to understand the qualities and limitations of the measurement tools they use (Bø & Sherburn 2005). This chapter will provide the information needed for PTs to understand the application of each tool to the measurement of the PFM. In many instances the PT may need thorough supervised instruction from other professionals before starting to use new equipment. In most cases, when available, receiving results from assessment of PFM activity from other professionals (e.g. radiologists) provides the best results.

REFERENCES

Altman D G 1997 Practical statistics for medical research, 9th edn. Chapman & Hall, London

Benvenuti F, Caputo G M, Bandinelli S et al 1987 Reeducative treatment of female genuine stress incontinence. American Journal of Physical Medicine 66:155–168

Bø K 2004 Pelvic floor muscle training is effective in treatment of stress urinary incontinence, but how does it work? International Journal of Urogynecology and Pelvic Floor Dysfunction 15:76–84

Bø K, Kvarstein B, Hagen R et al 1990 Pelvic floor muscle exercise for the treatment of female stress urinary incontinence, II: validity of vaginal pressure measurements of pelvic floor muscle strength and the necessity of supplementary methods for control of correct contraction. Neurourology and Urodynamics 9:479–487

Bø K, Larsen S, Oseid S, et al 1988 Knowledge about and ability to correct pelvic floor muscle exercises in women with urinary stress incontinence. Neurourology and Urodynamics 7:261–262

Bø K, Sherburn M 2005 Evaluation of female pelvic floor muscle function and strength. Physiotherapy 85(3):269–282

Bouchard C, Shephard R J, Stephens T 1994 Physical activity, fitness, and health: international proceedings and consensus statement. Human Kinetics, Champaign, IL

Bump R, Hurt W G, Fantl J A et al 1991 Assessment of Kegel exercise performance after brief verbal instruction. American Journal of Obstetrics and Gynecology 165:322–329

Currier D P 1990 Elements of research in physiotherapy, 3rd edn. Williams &Wilkins, Baltimore

Frontera W R, Meredith C N 1989 Strength training in the elderly. In: Harris R, Harris S Physical activity, aging and sport, Vol 1, Scientific and medical research. Center for the Study of Aging, Albany NY, p 319–331

Hay-Smith E, Bø K, Berghmans L et al 2001 Pelvic floor muscle training for urinary incontinence in women. The Cochrane Library, Oxford, p 3

International Classification of Impairments, Disabilities, and Handicaps (ICIDH) 1997. ICIDH-2 Beta-1 Draft. World Health Organization, Zeist

International Classification of Functioning, Disability, and Health (ICF) 2002. World Health Organization, Geneva

Kegel A H 1948 Progressive resistance exercise in the functional restoration of the perineal muscles. American Journal of Obstetrics and Gynecology 56:238–249

Knuttgen H G, Kraemer W J 1987 Terminology and measurement of exercise performance. Journal of Applied Sports Science Research 1(1):1–10

Thomas J R, Nelson J K 1996 Research methods in physical activity, 3rd edn. Human Kinetics, Champaign, IL

Wilmore J, Costill D 1999 Physiology of sport and exercise, 2nd edn. Human Kinetics, Champaign, IL

Visual observation and palpation

Kari Bø and Margaret Sherburn

VISUAL OBSERVATION

A correct contraction can be observed clinically (Kegel 1948), by ultrasound (Beco et al 1987, Dietz et al 2002, Petri et al 1999) or with dynamic magnetic resonance imaging (MRI) (Bø et al 2001, Stoker et al 2001).

In 1948, Kegel described a correct PFM contraction as squeeze around the urethral, vaginal and anal openings, and an inward lift that could be observed at the perineum (Kegel 1948, Kegel 1952). He estimated the inward movement in the lying position to be 3–4 cm (Kegel 1952). However, newer research visualizing lifting distance inside the body with MRI and ultrasound has not supported his estimation, which was based on visual observation. Bø et al (2001) demonstrated a mean inward lift during PFM contraction to be 10.8 mm (SD 6.0) in 16 women using dynamic MRI in a sitting position. This corresponded with an inward lift of 11.2 mm (95% CI: 7.2–15.3) measured with suprapubic ultrasound in a supine position (Bø et al 2003).

Most physiotherapists (PTs) would use visual observation of the PFM contraction as a starting point for measurement of ability to contract. In spite of this, there is a paucity of research on responsiveness, reliability and validity of this method.

Bø et al (1990) used observation of movement of a vaginal catheter, vaginal palpation, and vaginal squeeze pressure to measure PFM function and strength. They registered the ability to contract from visual observation as:

- correct (inward movement of the catheter);
- no contraction (no movement);
- straining (outward movement).

There was 100% agreement between observation and the vaginal palpation test in women who either contracted correctly or were not able to contract according to the palpation test. The observation classified six who were straining and were not detected on the palpation test. Hence observation of movement may be more sensitive to straining and Valsalva manoeuvre than palpation.

Responsiveness

No studies have been found evaluating the responsiveness of visual observation.

Intra- and inter-rater reliability

Devreese et al (2004) developed an inspection scale for the PFM and abdominal muscles to be used in crook lying, sitting and standing position. Contractions were inspected during both voluntary contraction and reflex contraction during coughing. They classified the contraction of the PFM as either 'coordinated' (inward movement of 1 cm of the perineum and a visible contraction of the deep abdominal muscle) or 'not coordinated' (downward movement of the pelvic floor and/or an outward movement of the abdominal wall. The results of inter-tester reliability showed kappa coefficients between 0.94 and 0.97.

Validity

Shull et al (2002) stated that by visual observation one is generally observing superficial perineal muscles. From this observation researchers assume that the levator ani is responding similarly. It may, however, not be the case.

Observing the inward movement of a correct PFM contraction is the starting point for measurement of PFM function, and has the advantage of being a simple, noninvasive method. However, the inward lift may be created by contraction of superficial muscle layers only, and have no influence on urethral closure mechanism. Conversely, there may be palpable PFM contraction with no visible outside movement. A correct lift can be difficult to observe from the outside, particularly in obese women. Also it is questionable whether it is possible to grade cm of inward movement from the outside of the body. In the future ultrasound may take over the role of visual observation, and would also serve as a biofeedback and teaching tool.

Whether the muscle action observed by visual observation or ultrasound is sufficiently strong to increase urethral closure pressure can only be measured by urodynamic assessment in the urethra and bladder. Interestingly Bump et al (1991) found that, although contracting correctly, only 50% of a population of continent and incontinent women were able to voluntarily contract the PFM with enough force to increase urethral pressure.

Sensitivity and specificity

Devreese et al (2004) used observation scores of coordinated contractions during PFM contraction and coughing, and compared continent and incontinent women with blinded investigators. The results showed that continent women exhibited significantly better coordination between the pelvic floor and lower abdominal muscles during coughing in all three positions (crook lying sitting and standing).

Conclusion

Visual observation can be used in clinical practice to give a first impression about ability to contract. Further estimation about the amount of the inward movement is not recommended. Visual observation should not be used for scientific purposes because MRI and ultrasound are more responsive, reliable and valid methods to assess movement during contraction, straining and physical exertion.

CLINICAL RECOMMENDATIONS

PFM assessment using observation

- Inform and explain the procedure to the patient.

- Teach the patient how to contract the PFM by use of models, anatomical drawings and imagery.

- After the patient has undressed, ask the patient to lie down on the bench with hips and knees bent and shoulder width apart (crook lying). Cover pelvic area with a towel. Support legs of patient (one leg against the wall, the other leg support with one hand).

- Allow some time for patient to practice before observing the contraction.

- Ask the patient to breathe normally and then lift the perineum inwards and squeeze around the openings without any movement of the pelvis or visible co-contraction of the gluteal or hip-adductor muscles. A small drawing in of the lower abdomen by transversus abdominis with the PFM contraction is accepted.

Observe the patient's attempt to contract and register how the contraction was performed (correct, no contraction, inconclusive, straining).

- If there is an observable contraction, give positive feedback and explain that you will palpate to register action of the deeper muscles, and coordination and strength of the contraction. If you are not able to observe inward movement, explain that this is common at the first attempt, and that it is not always easy to assess from the outside, and that you need to conduct a vaginal palpation to be sure whether there is a contraction or not.

VAGINAL PALPATION

Vaginal palpation (Fig. 5.1) is used to:

1. assess the ability of the patient to contract and relax the PFM correctly;

2. measure PFM muscle strength via a maximal occlusive and lifting force (assessing the person's attempt to conduct a maximum voluntary contraction), ability to sustain a contraction (endurance) or perform a number of repeated contractions (endurance);

3. assess other elements of PFM, such as resting tone, the ability to fully relax after a contraction, coordination with lower abdominal muscles, symmetry of right and left PFM contraction, scarring and adhe-

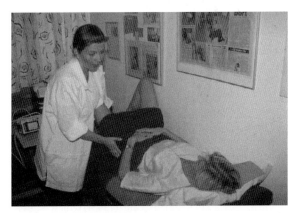

Fig. 5.1 During vaginal palpation the physiotherapist (PT) instructs the patient about how to perform a contraction correctly (squeeze around my finger and try to lift the finger inwards) and tells her how well she is able to do it and also about coordination skills and strength. With encouragement most patients are able to contract harder.

sions and the presence of pain, speed and sequence of recruitment of levator ani with the perineal muscles, and transverse and anteroposterior diameters of the urogenital hiatus.

As there is yet no evidence for the responsiveness or reliability of measurement of these other elements of muscle parameters, they will not be discussed further in this chapter.

The ICS Clinical Assessment Group (see www.icsoffice.org) has proposed qualitative scales of measurement for some of these parameters (absent, partial, full), but there has been a lack of psychometric testing of these scales or development of more responsive scales. This is an area needing further research.

Kegel described vaginal palpation as a method to evaluate the ability to perform a correct contraction (Kegel 1948, Kegel 1952). He placed one finger in the distal one-third of the vagina and asked the woman to lift inwards and squeeze around the finger. Kegel did not use this method to measure PFM strength. He classified the contraction qualitatively as correct or not. In addition, he developed the 'perineometer', a pressure manometer, to measure PFM strength through vaginal squeeze pressure (Kegel 1948).

Van Kampen et al (1996) reported that after Kegel first described vaginal palpation as a method to evaluate PFM function, more than 25 different palpation methods have been developed. Some examiners use one, and others two fingers.

Worth et al (1986) and Brink et al (1989) have evaluated pressure, duration, muscle 'ribbing', and displacement of the examiner's finger in a specific scoring system. This system has mainly been used by American nurses. There has been no systematic research to determine the best method of palpation to assess ability to contract, or any of the parameters of muscle strength, endurance, or power.

Laycock has developed the modified Oxford grading system (Box 5.1) to measure PFM strength (British Medical Research Council 1943, Laycock 1994), and this seems to be the system mostly used by PTs to assess PFM strength in clinical practice.

Responsiveness

The Oxford grading system has been modified from the Medical Research Council scale (1943) which suffers from poor responsiveness and non-linearity (Beasley 1961).

One of the difficulties of measurement using the modified Oxford scale is that it produces one value for two elements (occlusion and lift) in the one scale. The palpating fingers may not be sensitive enough to dif-

---

Box 5.1: The modified Oxford grading scale

The modified Oxford grading scale is a six-point scale where half numbers of + and − can be added when a contraction is considered to fall between two full grades, so it expands to a 15-point scale when both + and − are used:
- 0 = no contraction
- 1 = flicker
- 2 = weak
- 3 = moderate (with lift)
- 4 = good (with lift)
- 5 = strong (with lift)

---

ferentiate the proportions of occlusion versus lift. To separate these two elements, manometers or dynamometers can be used to evaluate occlusion, and ultrasound to measure the lift component. When the responsiveness of this scale is tested against vaginal squeeze pressure, it should be recognized that only one element, occlusion, is being compared.

Bø & Finckenhagen (2001) questioned the responsiveness of the original scale (without + and −) because they did not find that the scale could separate between weak, moderate, good, or strong when comparing measurement of vaginal squeeze pressure. This was supported by Morin et al (2004) comparing vaginal palpation and dynamometry in continent and incontinent women. They found that important overlaps were observed between each category of vaginal palpation. Mean force values differed significantly only between nonadjacent levels in palpation assessment (e.g. between 1 and 3, 1 and 4, 1 and 5, 2 and 4, and 2 and 5 [p < 0.05]).

Frawley et al (2006) found that the Oxford grading scale using + and − had lower kappa values in intratest reliability testing and recommended using the original six-point scale in research.

Intra- and inter-rater reliability

The results from studies evaluating intra- and inter-rater reliability of vaginal palpation for strength measurement are conflicting (Bø & Finckenhagen 2001, Frawley et al 2006, Hahn et al 1996, Isherwood & Rane 2000, Jeyaseelan et al 2001, Laycock & Jerwood 2001, McKey & Dougherty 1986).

Isherwood & Rane (2000) found high inter-rater reliability whereas Jeyaseelan et al (2001) concluded that inter-tester reliability should not be assumed, and needs to be established when two or more clinicians are involved in pre- and post-treatment assessment.

Bø & Finckenhagen (2001) using the six-point scale and Laycock & Jerwood (2001) using the 15-point scale found agreement between testers in only 45% and 45% of the tested cases, respectively.

Frawley et al (2005) found 79% complete agreement in both crook lying and supine using the six-point scale but this dropped to 53 and 58%, respectively, using the 15-point scale. They tested intratester reliability of vaginal digital assessment and found good to very good kappa values of 0.69, 0.69, 0.86, and 0.79 for crook lying, supine, sitting, and standing positions, respectively. In addition, they compared vaginal palpation with vaginal squeeze pressure measurement with the Peritron perineometer and found that the Peritron was more reliable than vaginal palpation (Frawley et al 2006).

Devreese et al (2004) developed a new vaginal palpation system assessing muscle tone, endurance, speed of contraction, strength, lift (inward movement) and coordination, and evaluated both superficial and deep PFM. They found high agreement in interobserver reliability in tone (95–100% agreement) and reliability coefficients between 0.75 and 1.00 for measurements of the other parameters above. The scoring system developed is qualitative and open to personal interpretation, but is a first step towards standardizing a measurement system for observation and palpation.

Muscle 'tone' requires a universally acceptable definition to establish a reliable measurement system, and to differentiate 'tone' from 'stiffness', 'contracture' and 'spasm'. Simons & Mense (1998) have proposed that muscle tone specific to a muscle rather than generalized tone be defined as 'the elastic and viscoelastic stiffness of a muscle in the absence of motor unit activity'. The elastic component or 'elastic stiffness' is measured qualitatively by pressing or squeezing a muscle. However, measurement of the viscoelastic component is more complex and is dependent on the speed at which the muscle is moved using pendular, oscillatory and resonant frequency measurements (Simons & Mense 1998). These viscoelastic measurements are not possible for the PFM because the PFM do not pass over a joint to allow elongation then shortening. If the PFM are elongated using vaginal palpation to stretch the muscle fibres, the muscle belly is actually being compressed by the examining digit and elastic stiffness is again being measured.

One can also discuss how one can assess that there is no motor unit activity. At least for the PFM, there is always electromyographic (EMG) activity except before and during voiding (Fowler et al 2002).

Validity

Several investigators have studied criterion validity of vaginal palpation comparing vaginal palpation and vaginal squeeze pressure (Bø & Finckenhagen 2001, Hahn et al 1996, Isherwood & Rane 2000, Jarvis et al 2001, Kerschan-Schindel et al 2002, McKey & Dougherty 1986).

Isherwood & Rane (2000) compared vaginal palpation using the Oxford Grading System and compared it with an arbitrary scale on a perineometer from 1 to 12. They found a high kappa of 0.73. In contrast, Bø and Finckenhagen (2001) found a kappa of 0.37 comparing the Oxford grading system with vaginal squeeze pressure. Heitner (2000) concluded that lift was most reliably tested with palpation, and that all other measures of muscle function were better tested with EMG.

Hahn et al (1996) found that there was a better correlation of vaginal palpation and pressure measurement in continent than in incontinent women ($r = 0.86$ and 0.75, respectively). This was supported by Morin et al (2004) comparing vaginal palpation with dynamometry, finding $r = 0.73$ in continent and $r = 0.45$ in incontinent women, respectively.

Lying, sitting or standing?

PFM function and strength is often measured in a supine position, despite the fact that urinary leakage is more common in the upright position with gravity acting on the PFM. Very few studies have addressed measurement in different positions.

Devreese et al (2004) investigated inter-rater reliability of clinical observation and vaginal palpation in crook lying, sitting, and standing positions. They found high inter-tester reliability in all positions, but did not report whether there were differences in measurement values in the different positions.

Frawley et al (2005) found that vaginal palpation of PFM contraction had moderate to high intratest reliability in crook lying, supine, sitting and standing position.

Both Bø & Finckenhagen (2003) and Frawley et al (2006) found that PTs and patients preferred testing using vaginal palpation and vaginal squeeze pressure in lying positions.

Bø & Finckenhagen (2003) found that the testing procedure was easiest to standardize when the patient was supine, and therefore recommend this in clinical practice.

For scientific purposes the position of the patient should be chosen according to the research question.

One or two fingers?

There is a discussion whether one or two fingers should be used for vaginal palpation (Bø et al 2005, Shull et al 2002) and this may depend on factors such as whether the patient is nulliparous and has a narrow vaginal introitus and urogenital hiatus, or whether there is introital discomfort or pain.

Hoyte et al (2001) reported increased diameters from nonsymptomatic parous women, to parous women with pelvic organ prolapse (POP). In parous women, vaginal birth may have stretched the PFM and its investing fascia. However, time and PFM training may normalize this in many women.

When palpating, the anterior and posterior vaginal walls are always in apposition and in contact with the finger. The lateral vaginal walls expand in the upper vagina at the level of the fornices and above the level of the levator ani. At the PFM level, the lateral diameter of the urogenital hiatus marks the medial borders of the levator ani and these borders may be palpated through the intervening vaginal mucosa.

Ghetti et al (2005) stated that intra- and inter-rater reliability of vaginal palpation to assess the diameter of the hiatus needs to be done. In addition, criterion validity between magnetic resonance imaging (MRI)/ultrasound and vaginal palpation of the hiatus has to be established.

Putting a muscle on stretch makes it more difficult to perform a maximal contraction (Frontera & Meredith 1989). Therefore the aim of palpation should be to gain maximum sensation for the palpation with no stretch. This must not be confused with the fact that a quick stretch can be used to facilitate the stretch reflex. Quick stretch is one technique used by PTs to facilitate a correct PFM contraction if the patients are unable to contract (Brown 2001).

Sensitivity and specificity

There are few studies comparing measurement of PFM function and strength in continent and incontinent women using vaginal palpation.

Hahn et al (1996) compared 30 continent and 30 incontinent women using vaginal palpation and found that the group of incontinent women had lower scores on palpation test (1.0 ± 0.1) compared to the group of continent women (1.9 ± 0.1) ($p < 0.001$).

Devreese et al (2004) found a significant difference in favour of continent women in speed of contraction, maximum strength and coordination of both superficial and deep PFM, and inward movement of the superficial, but not the deep PFM, assessed with vaginal palpation.

Conclusion

Today most PTs use vaginal palpation to evaluate PFM function because both squeeze pressure and lift can be registered, though with poor discrimination. It is a low-cost method, and is relatively easy to conduct.

Vaginal palpation of PFM contraction is recommended as a good technique for use by PTs to understand, teach, and give feedback to patients about correctness of the contraction. Position of the patient, instruction given, and the use of one or two fingers have to be standardized and reported. However, whether palpation is robust enough to be used for scientific purposes to measure muscle strength is questionable. Palpation as a method to detect morphological abnormalities also needs to be tested before being used in clinical assessment and research.

CLINICAL RECOMMENDATIONS

Following perineal observation, with patient in crook lying position

- Explain the palpation procedure to patient and obtain consent.

- Prepare examination gloves, gel and tissues, and check with the patient for latex and gel allergy. Use vinyl gloves for preference.

- Wash hands, put on gloves and apply a little gel on the palpating gloved finger(s).

- Gently part the labia and insert one finger in the outer one-third of the vagina.

- Ask the patient whether she feels comfortable.

- If appropriate, insert the second finger.

- Ask the patient to lift in and squeeze around the finger(s) and observe or control the action so that the pelvis is not moving or the hip adductor or gluteal muscles are not contracted.

- Give feedback of correctness, performance and strength.

- Record whether PFM contraction is:
  - Correct;
  - only possible with visible co-contraction of other muscles;
  - not present;
  - in the opposite direction (straining or Valsalva).

- To record the maximum voluntary contraction (MVC) request a 3–5 s maximum effort PFM contraction after one or two submaximal 'practice' contractions.

If you do not have a sensitive, reliable and valid tool to measure strength, use the Oxford grading scale to record the MVC. Separately record the lift component as absent, partial or complete.

- Note the voluntary relaxation after these contractions and record this as absent, partial or full.

- If no further vaginal measurements are to be made, discard the examination gloves into the appropriate waste disposal and allow the patient privacy for dressing.

REFERENCES

Beasley W C 1961 Quantitative muscle testing: principles and applications to research and clinical services. Archives of Physical Medicine Rehabilitation 42:398–425

Beco J, Sulu M, Schaaps JP et al 1987 A new approach to urinary continence disorders in women: urodynamic ultrasonic examination by the vaginal route [French]. Journal de Gynécologie, Obstétrique et Biologie de la Reproduction 16:987–998

Bø K, Finckenhagen H B 2001 Vaginal palpation of pelvic floor muscle strength: inter-test reproducibility and the comparison between palpation and vaginal squeeze pressure. Acta Obstetricia et Gynecologica Scandinavica 80:883–887

Bø K, Finckenhagen H B 2003 Is there any difference in measurement of pelvic floor muscle strength in supine and standing position? Acta Obstetricia Gynecologica Scandinavica 82:1120–1124

Bø K, Kvarstein B, Hagen R et al 1990 Pelvic floor muscle exercise for the treatment of female stress urinary incontinence: II. Validity of vaginal pressure measurements of pelvic floor muscle strength and the necessity of supplementary methods for control of correct contraction. Neurourology and Urodynamics 9: 479–487

Bø K, Lilleås F, Talseth T et al 2001 Dynamic MRI of pelvic floor muscles in an upright sitting position. Neurourology and Urodynamics 20:167–174

Bø K, Raastad R, Finckenhagen H B 2005 Does the size of the vaginal probe affect measurement of pelvic floor muscle strength? Acta Obstetricia Gynecologica Scandinavica 84:129–133

Bø K, Sherburn M, Allen T 2003 Transabdominal ultrasound measurement of pelvic floor muscle activity when activated directly or via transversus abdominis muscle contraction. Neurourology and Urodynamics 22:582–588

Brink C, Sampselle C M, Wells T et al 1989 A digital test for pelvic muscle strength in older women with urinary incontinence. Nursing Research 38(4):196–199

Brown C 2001 Pelvic floor re-education: a practical approach. In: Corcos J, Schick E (eds) The urinary sphincter. Marcel Dekker, New York, p 459–473

British Medical Research Council 1943 Aid to the investigation of peripheral nerve injuries. War Memorandum, Her Majesty's Stationery Office, London, p 11–46

Bump R, Hurt W G, Fantl J A et al 1991 Assessment of Kegel exercise performance after brief verbal instruction. American Journal of Obstetrics and Gynecology 165:322–329

Devreese A, Staes F, De Weerdt W et al 2004 Clinical evaluation of pelvic floor muscle function in continent and incontinent women. Neurourology and Urodynamics 23:190–197

Dietz H, Jarvis S, Vancaillie T 2002 The assessment of levator muscle strength: a validation of three ultrasound techniques. International Urogynecological Journal 13:156–159

Fowler C J, Benson J T, Craggs M D et al 2002 Clinical neurophysiology. In: Abrams P, Cardozo L, Khourhy S et al. Incontinence, 2nd edn. Plymbridge Distributors, Plymouth, UK, p 389–424

Frawley H C, Galea M P, Philips B A et al 2006 Reliability of pelvic floor muscle strength assessment using different test positions and tools. Neurourology and Urodynamics

Frontera W, Meredith C 1989 Strength training in the elderly. In: Harris R, Harris S (eds) Physical activity, aging and sports, Vol 1, Scientific and medical research. Center for the Study of Aging, Albany, NY, p 319–331

Ghetti C, Gregory W T, Edwards S R et al 2005 Severity of pelvic organ prolapse associated with measurements of pelvic floor function. International Urogynecology Journal and Pelvic Floor Dysfunction 16(6):432–436

Hahn I, Milsom I, Ohlson BL et al 1996 Comparative assessment of pelvic floor function using vaginal cones, vaginal digital palpation and vaginal pressure measurement. Gynecological and Obstetric Investigation 41:269–274

Heitner C 2000 Valideringsonderzoek naar palpatie en myofeedback bij vrouwen met symptomen van stress urine-incontinentie. Master Thesis. University of Maastricht, The Netherlands

Hoyte L, Schierlitz L, Zou K et al 2001 Two- and 3-dimensional MRI comparison of levator ani structure, volume, and integrity in women with stress incontinence and prolapse. American Journal of Obstetrics and Gynecology 185(1):11–19

Isherwood P, Rane A 2000 Comparative assessment of pelvic floor strength using a perineometer and digital examination. British Journal of Obstetrics and Gynaecology 107:1007–1011

Jarvis S, Dietz H, Vancaillie T 2001 A comparison between vaginal palpation, perineometry and ultrasound in the assessment of levator function. International Urogynecolgy Journal and Pelvic Floor Dysfunction 12(suppl 3):31

Jeyaseelan S, Haslam J, Winstanley J et al 2001 Digital vaginal assessment. An inter-tester reliability study. Physiotherapy 87(5):243–250

Kegel A H 1948 Progressive resistance exercise in the functional restoration of the perineal muscles. American Journal of Obstetrics and Gynecology 56:238–249

Kegel A H 1952 Stress incontinence and genital relaxation. Ciba Clinical Symposia 2:35–51

Kerschan-Schindel K, Uher E, Wiesinger G et al 2002 Reliability of pelvic floor muscle strength measurement in elderly incontinent women. Neurourology and Urodynamics 21:42–47

Laycock J 1994 Clinical evaluation of the pelvic floor. In: Schussler B, Laycock J, Norton P et al (eds) Pelvic floor re-education. Springer–Verlag, London, p 42–48

Laycock J, Jerwood D 2001 Pelvic floor muscle assessment: The PERFECT scheme. Physiotherapy 87(12):631–642

McKey P L, Dougherty M C 1986 The circumvaginal musculature: correlation between pressure and physical assessment. Nursing Research 35(5):307–309

Morin M, Dumoulin C, Bourbonnais D et al 2004 Pelvic floor maximal strength using vaginal digital assessment compared to dynamometric measurements. Neurourology and Urodynamics 23:336–341

Petri E, Koelbl H, Schaer G 1999 What is the place of ultrasound in urogynecology? A written panel. International Urogynecology Journal and Pelvic Floor Dysfunction 10:262–273

Shull B, Hurt G, Laycock J et al 2002 Physical examination. In: Abrams P, Cardozo L, Khoury S et al (eds) Incontinence. Plymbridge Distributors, Plymouth, UK, p 373–388

Simons D G, Mense S 1998 Understanding and measurement of muscle tone as related to clinical muscle pain. Pain 75:1–17

Stoker J, Halligan S, Bartram C 2001 Pelvic floor imaging. Radiology 218:621–641

Van Kampen M, De Weerdt W, Feys H et al 1996 Reliability and validity of a digital test for pelvic muscle strength in women. Neurourology and Urodynamics 15:338–339

Worth A, Dougherty M, McKey P 1986 Development and testing of the circumvaginal muscles rating scale. Nursing Research 35(3):166–168

Electromyography

David B Vodušek

INTRODUCTION

Electromyography (EMG) is the extracellular recording of bioelectrical activity generated by muscle fibres. The term indeed stands for at least two different clinically used methods, which are quite distinct and as a rule performed in different settings (laboratories), for different purposes. On the one hand EMG can reveal the 'behaviour' (i.e. patterns of activity) of a particular muscle, or it can also be used to demonstrate whether a muscle is normal, myopathic or denervated/reinnervated. The former can be called 'kinesiological EMG' and the latter 'motor unit' EMG, but usually this division is not specified and both types of examination are just called 'EMG', which can confuse the uninitiated.

In clinical neurophysiology, EMG techniques are combined with conduction studies to assess involvement of the neuromuscular system by trauma or disease (Aminoff 2005).

MUSCLE FIBRE, MOTOR UNIT, MUSCLE

A single muscle fibre (cell) does not contract on its own, but rather in concert with other muscle fibres that are part of the same motor unit (i.e. innervated by the same motor neuron). Its axon reaches the muscle via a motor nerve. Within the muscle the motor axon tapers and then branches to innervate muscle fibres, which are scattered throughout the muscle. Fibres that are part of the same motor unit are not adjacent to one another. Bioelectrical activity generated by the concomitant activation of muscle fibres from one motor unit is 'summated' by the recording electrode as a 'motor unit action potential'

(MUP). As many motor units are active within a contracting muscle and the recording surface of the EMG electrode is adjacent to muscle fibres from several motor units, several MUPs are recorded by the recording electrode. This produces an 'interference pattern' of MUPs in a given time interval of recording. If the activation of a normal muscle is strong, most motor units are activated and the interference pattern is 'full' (Podnar & Vodušek 2005, Vodušek & Fowler 2004).

KINESIOLOGICAL EMG

Prolonged recording of bioelectrical activity of a muscle provides a qualitative and quantitative description of its activity over time, thus characterising its 'behaviour' during particular manoeuvres (see Ch. 4, Fig. 4.2). It should be borne in mind that kinesiological EMG does not provide information on the 'state' of the muscle (i.e. whether its motor units have been changed due to neuropathy or myopathy). A special analysis of the EMG signal is necessary to provide that information. Meaningful kinesiologic EMG can, of course, only be obtained from innervated muscle.

When we are interested in the pattern of activity of an individual muscle, the EMG should ideally provide a selective recording, uncontaminated by neighbouring muscles on one hand, and a faithful detection of any activity within the source muscle on the other hand. Both objectives are difficult to achieve simultaneously. Overall detection from the bulk of a muscle can only be achieved with non-selective electrodes, selective recordings from small muscles can only be made with intramuscular electrodes with small detection surfaces. Non-selective recordings carry the risk of contamination with activity from other muscles; selective recordings may fail to detect activity in all parts of the source muscle. Meaningful recordings from deep muscles can only be accomplished by invasive techniques.

Considering the above, truly selective recording from sphincter muscles can probably only be obtained by intramuscular electrodes. In clinical routine the concentric needle electrode is used as a rule. Needle electrodes, however, may produce some pain on movement, and can be dislodged. Instead, two thin isolated/bare tip wires (with a hook at the end) can be introduced into the muscle with a cannula, which is then withdrawn, and the wires stay in place (Deindl et al 1993). The advantage of this type of recording is good positional stability and painlessness once the wires are inserted, though their position cannot be much adjusted.

To make EMG recording less invasive various surface-type electrodes have been devised – also for special use in the perineum. Small skin-surface electrodes can be applied to the perineal skin. Other special intravaginal, intrarectal or catheter-mounted recording devices have been described. Recordings with surface electrodes are more artefact prone and furthermore the artefacts may be less easily identified.

Critical online assessment of the 'quality of the EMG signal' is mandatory in kinesiological EMG, and this requires either auditory or oscilloscope monitoring of the raw signal. Integration of high-quality EMG signals by the software of modern recording systems may help in quantification of results. It should be borne in mind that kinesiological EMG needs some concomitant event markers to make it a valid indicator of muscle activity correlated with specific manoeuvres or other physiologic events (e.g. detrusor pressure).

EMG METHODS TO DIFFERENTIATE NORMAL FROM PATHOLOGICAL MUSCLE

EMG may help to differentiate between normal, denervated and reinnervated and myopathic muscle. In pelvic floor muscles (PFM) and sphincter muscles, 'neurogenic' changes are sought as a rule because only patients with suspected denervation injury are routinely referred for assessment. One or several muscles may be examined, according to the clinical problem in the individual patient. The levator ani, anal and urethral sphincter, and bulbocavernosus are the muscles routinely examined, but if a rather equal involvement of PFM is suspected, examination of the external anal sphincter (on one or both sides) suffices (Podnar et al 1999).

Concentric needle EMG

Single-use disposable concentric needle EMG (CN EMG) electrodes are used as a rule to diagnose striated muscle denervation/reinnervation. The CN EMG electrode records spike (or 'near') activity from about 20 muscle fibres in the vicinity of its active recording surface at the bevelled tip (Vodušek & Fowler 2004). The number of motor units recorded depends both upon the local arrangement of muscle fibres within the motor unit and the level of contraction of the muscle.

CN EMG can provide information on insertion activity, abnormal spontaneous activity, MUPs, and interference pattern (Podnar & Vodušek 2005).

In healthy skeletal muscle initial placement of the needle (and any movement of the tip) elicits a short burst of 'insertion activity' due to mechanical stimulation of excitable membranes. Absence of insertion activity with an appropriately placed needle electrode usually means a complete denervation atrophy of the examined muscle (Podnar & Vodušek 2005). At rest, tonic MUPs are the only normal bioelectrical activity recorded.

In partially denervated sphincter muscle there is – by definition – a loss of motor units, but this is difficult to estimate. Normally, MUPs should intermingle to produce an 'interference' pattern on the oscilloscope during strong muscle contraction, and during a strong cough. The number of continuously active MUPs during relaxation can be estimated by counting the number of continuously firing low-threshold MUPs (Podnar et al 2002a).

In patients with lesions of peripheral innervation, fewer MUPs fire continuously during relaxation. In addition to continuously firing low threshold ('tonic') motor units, new motor units ('phasic') are recruited voluntarily and reflexly. It has been shown that the two motor unit populations differ in their characteristics: reflexly or voluntarily activated 'high-threshold' MUPs being larger than continuously active 'low-threshold' MUPs (Podnar & Vodušek 1999).

Using the standard recording facilities available on all modern EMG machines, individual MUPs can be captured and their characteristics determined (Fig. 5.2). Typically MUP amplitude and duration are measured.

To allow identification of MUPs and to be certain the 'late' MUP components of complex potentials are not due to superimposition of several MUPs, it is necessary to capture the same potential repeatedly. MUPs are mostly below 1 mV and certainly below 2 mV in the normal urethral and anal sphincter; most are less than 7 ms in duration, and few (less than 15%) are above 10 ms; most are bi- and triphasic, but up to 15–33% may be polyphasic. Normal MUPs are stable – their shape on

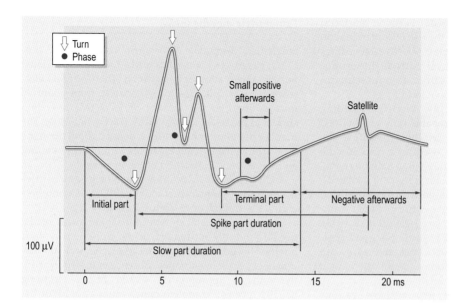

Fig. 5.2 Schematic representation of the motor unit potential (MUP) to demonstrate different components, and parameters analysed. (Modified from Podnar et al 2002a, b)

repetitive recording does not change (Fowler et al 1984, Rodi et al 1996, Vodušek & Light 1983) (Fig. 5.3).

There are indeed two approaches to analysing quantitatively the bioelectrical activity of motor units: either individual MUPs are analysed (Podnar et al 2002a, b), or the overall activity of intermingled MUPs (the 'interference pattern' – IP) is analysed (see Fig. 5.3) (Aanestad et al 1989, Podnar et al 2002a, b).

Generally three techniques of MUP analysis ('manual-MUP', 'single-MUP' and 'multi-MUP') and one technique of IP analysis (turn/amplitude – T/A) are available on advanced EMG systems. By either method a relevant sample of EMG activity needs to be analysed for the test to be valid.

In the small half of the sphincter muscle collecting ten different MUPs has been accepted as the minimal requirement for using single-MUP analysis. Using manual-MUP and multi-MUP techniques sampling of 20 MUPs (standard number in limb muscles) from each EAS poses no difficulty in healthy controls and most of patients (Podnar et al 2000, Podnar et al 2002b). Normative data obtained from the external anal sphincter (EAS) muscle by standardized EMG technique using all three MUP analysis techniques (multi-MUP, manual-MUP, single-MUP) have been published (Podnar et al 2002b). There are several technical differences in the methods. The template based multi-MUP analysis of MUP is fast, easy to apply, and allows little examiner bias (see Fig. 5.3).

Use of quantitative MUP and IP analyses of the EAS is facilitated by the availability of normative values (Podnar et al 2002b) that can be introduced into the EMG system software. It has been shown that normative data are not significantly affected by age, gender (Podnar et al 2002a), number of uncomplicated vaginal deliveries (Podnar et al 2000), mild chronic constipation (Podnar & Vodušek 2000), and the part of the external anal sphincter muscle (i.e. subcutaneous or deeper) examined (Podnar et al 2002a, b). This makes quantitative analysis much simpler and results from different laboratories easily comparable.

Similar in-depth analysed normative data by standardized technique for other pelvic floor and perineal muscles are not yet available, but individual laboratories use their own normative data.

CN EMG findings due to denervation and reinnervation

In PFM and perineal muscles, complete or partial denervation may be observed after lesions to its nerves. The changes occurring in striated muscles after denervation are in principle similar. After complete denervation all motor unit activity ceases and there may be electrical silence for several days; 10–20 days after a denervating injury, 'insertion activity' becomes more prolonged and abnormal spontaneous activity in the form of short biphasic spikes, 'fibrillation potentials', biphasic potentials with prominent positive deflections, and 'positive sharp waves' appear. With successful axonal reinnervation MUPs appear again; first short bi- and triphasic, soon becoming polyphasic, serrated and of prolonged duration (Podnar & Vodušek 2005, Vodušek & Fowler 2004). In partially denervated muscle some MUPs remain and mingle eventually with abnormal

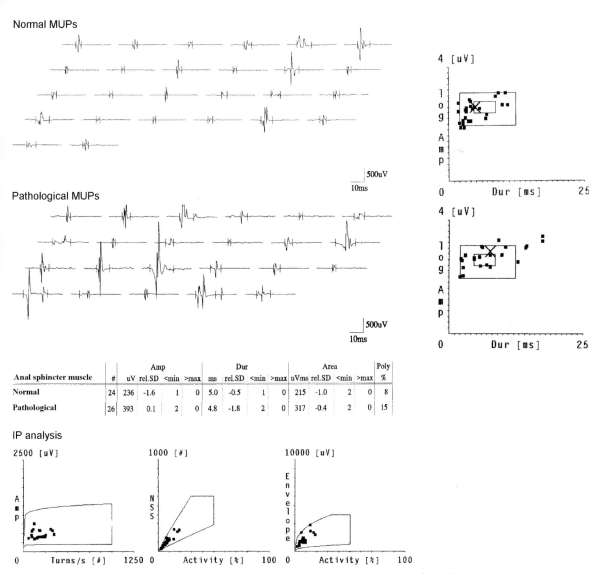

Fig. 5.3 Comparison of normal (above) and pathological (below) motor unit potentials (MUPs) sampled by multi-MUP analysis from the right halves of the subcutaneous parts of the external anal sphincter (EAS) muscles. On the right, logarithm amplitude vs duration plots of the MUPs are shown; the inner rectangle presents the normative range for mean values, and the outer rectangle for outliers. Below the MUP samples values are tabulated. Three plots on the bottom were obtained by turn/amplitude analysis of the interference pattern (IP) in a patient with a cauda equina lesion. Delineated areas (clouds) present the normative range, and dots individual IP samples. The normal subject was a 45-year-old woman. Results of MUP and IP analysis were normal. The pathological sample was obtained from a 36-year old man with cauda equina lesion caused by central herniation of the intervertebral disc 13 months before the examination, with perianal sensory loss. Mean values for MUP amplitude and area are above the normative range, and polyphasicity is increased. In addition, for all MUP parameters shown, individual values of more than 2 MUPs are above the outlier limits. Note that IP analysis in the patient is within the normative range despite marked MUP abnormalities.

spontaneous activity. In longstanding partially denervated muscle a peculiar abnormal insertion activity appears, so-called 'repetitive discharges'. This activity may be found in the striated urethral sphincter without any other evidence of neuromuscular disease (Podnar & Vodušek 2005).

In partially denervated muscle, collateral reinnervation takes place. Surviving motor axons will sprout and grow out to reinnervate denervated muscle fibres. This will result in a change in the arrangement of muscle fibres within the motor unit. Following reinnervation several muscle fibres belonging to the same motor unit come to be adjacent to one another; this is reflected in changes of MUPs (increased duration and amplitude).

In the late stage, after reinnervation has been completed, CN EMG as a rule finds a reduced number of remaining motor units (i.e. the IP of MUPs is reduced). The MUPs are of higher amplitudes, and longer duration, and the percentage of polyphasic MUPs is increased. Such a finding may be taken as proof of previous denervation and successful reinnervation. The function of the reinnervated muscle will depend on the number (and size) of remaining motor units. The relative amount of remaining motor units can only be estimated (Podnar et al 2002a, b, Vodušek & Fowler 2004).

Single fibre electromyography

The single fibre electromyography (SFEMG) electrode has similar external proportions to a CN EMG electrode, but instead of having the recording surface at the tip, it is on the side above the tip and its recording surface is much smaller. Because of the arrangement of muscle fibres in a normal motor unit, a SFEMG needle will record only 1–3 single muscle fibres from the same motor unit.

The SFEMG parameter that reflects motor unit morphology is fibre density (FD), which is the mean number of muscle fibres belonging to an individual motor unit per detection site. To measure FD, recordings from 20 different detection sites within the examined muscle are necessary and the number of component potentials to each motor unit recorded and averaged. The normal fibre density for the anal sphincter is less than 2.0 (Neill & Swash 1980, Vodušek & Janko 1981).

Due to its technical characteristics a SFEMG electrode is able to record changes that occur in motor units due to reinnervation, but is less suitable to detect changes due to denervation itself (i.e. abnormal insertion and spontaneous activity). The SFEMG electrode is also suitable for recording instability of motor unit potentials, the 'jitter' (Stalberg & Trontelj 1994). This parameter has not been much used in PFM.

SFEMG has been used in research but is not widely used, even for diagnostics in general clinical neurophysiological laboratories. The recording needles are very expensive, and disposable needles are not available.

USEFULNESS OF EMG IN CLINICAL PRACTICE AND RESEARCH

The validity, reliability, responsiveness and sensitivity/specificity of EMG have to be discussed separately for the particular physiological information sought from EMG, and for various EMG techniques, types of recording, and applications. EMG is often falsely understood as 'one method', and as a method precisely measuring muscle 'function'. Muscle function is, however, complex and different EMG techniques address different aspects of it, but never really cover all of it. Indeed, motor unit EMG techniques, for instance, are more useful in diagnosing denervation and reinnervation (i.e. helping in diagnosing a neurological lesion) than in diagnosing the functional deficit (i.e. quantifying the number of motor units and thus providing data that would be directly functionally relevant).

It has to be distinguished whether EMG is used to detect the pattern of muscle activity, or rather to detect muscle denervation/reinnervation. EMG methods are reasonably reliable, reproducible, sensitive and specific to diagnose muscle denervation/reinnervation – but this is mostly 'expert opinion' relying on long-term correlation of clinical and EMG findings in conditions affecting musculature in general. Correlation of EMG findings to muscle function (strength, power and endurance) is – in the individual – insecure (excluding instances of minor or severe/complete denervation).

Validity of the EMG signal

(Kinesiological) EMG has good logical validity (i.e. it measures the presence/absence of striated muscle activity), but technical expertise is required. EMG recording has to be differentiated from artefacts, which is very straightforward for intramuscular recordings (particularly if also amplified as an acoustic signal). In surface recordings, the artefacts are much more difficult to sort out. With surface electrodes there may be a problem of changing contact quality, particularly with prolonged recordings, creating a variability of recording quality. For detection with surface EMG there are studies claiming sound reliability and clinical predictive validity for intra-anal electrodes (Glazer et al 1999).

Content validity of kinesiological EMG recording implies a continuous recording from the same defined source; needle electrodes may become dislodged, therefore intramuscular wire electrodes are much more intrinsically reliable for long-term recordings. The content validity of recordings with surface-type electrodes depends on the type of electrode, and the possibility of their movement (displacement). A particular problem is content validity of repeated EMG recordings, which should sample the same source; this is intrinsically better for surface recordings, which are less selective. On the other hand, content validity of surface recordings may be questioned if the source of EMG activity is claimed to be only one of several muscles in the vicinity of the electrodes. With surface-type electrodes the overall anatomical source of the EMG signal in the pelvic region is often uncertain – is the EMG really derived only from the muscle which is claimed as the source? The other relevant issue is the question of representativeness – is the EMG signal really representative for the muscle or muscle group for which it is being claimed to be representative of? In other words, for all electrode types, content validity needs to be established for the physiological relevance of the particular source recording. Thus, for example, anal sphincter recording may not be conclusive for urethral sphincter behaviour.

The kinesiological EMG (as obtained during polygraphic urodynamic recording) has accepted diagnostic validity to detect detrusor/striated sphincter dyssynergia, but this has not been formally researched much and probably holds true particularly for intramuscular recordings for the urethral sphincter. Indeed, the test has not yet been standardized. Its sensitivity and specificity are not known, but are far from ideal.

The logical and content validity of CN EMG to diagnose muscle reinnervation is good, but is usually not discussed in these terms. The diagnostic validity of CN EMG to detect striated muscle denervation and reinnervation is generally accepted. CN EMG sensitivity and specificity to detect moderate to severe denervation and reinnervation is accepted as good. These statements are supported by a large body of experience with nerve and muscle lesions as defined clinically, electrophysiologically and histopathologically (see Aminoff 2005). The sensitivity and specificity to diagnose changes of reinnervation may vary for different types of CN EMG signal analysis (Podnar et al 2002b).

SFEMG has good logical and content validity, and good diagnostic validity to detect changes due to reinnervation, but does not seem to be used clinically for PFM.

Responsiveness

A technically good EMG recording is capable of demonstrating absence of electrical activity in a non-active muscle ('electrical silence') and a graded response to increasing muscle activation. There is no difficulty in detecting even small differences in EMG activity from a given source with a good (technically reliable) technique.

Reliability

The consistency and reproducibility (Engstrom & Olney 1992) of results of diagnostic EMG (quantitative techniques using concentric and single fibre needle electrodes) is accepted as good if performed by experienced testers (see Aminoff 2005). Extensive experience is needed for either method, possibly even more for CN EMG.

Straightforward parameters from surface EMG recordings (presence/absence of muscle activation) are much easier to interpret than CN EMG, and the consistency and reproducibility of such recordings (if technical issues are solved) are good. The overall consistency and reproducibility of results of the kinesiological EMG as a tool to investigate physiology lies more with the reproducibility of the 'physiology' that is being assessed (i.e. reproducibility of muscle 'behaviour').

USE OF KINESIOLOGICAL EMG AND CN EMG IN PARTICULAR PATIENT GROUPS

Kinesiological EMG recordings of sphincter and PFM are used in research, and diagnostically in selected patients with voiding dysfunction to ascertain striated muscle behaviour during bladder filling and voiding, and in selected patients with anorectal dysfunction. The method is not standardized.

The demonstration of voluntary and reflex activation of PFM is indirect proof of the integrity of respective (central and peripheral) neural pathways. The demonstration of a normal PFM behaviour pattern (i.e. striated sphincter non-activity during voiding) is indirect proof of integrity of the relevant central nervous system centres for lower urinary tract neural control.

Kinesiological EMG as a tool (if a sound technique is used) is not controversial, but there is little knowledge on behavioural patterns of PFM in health and disease. Therefore, short intervals of EMG in a particular patient may be misinterpreted as indicating significant pathology, whereas it only may represent normal variability of muscle behaviour or some non-specific muscle response to the experimental setting. Kinesiological EMG is also used as a therapeutic tool in biofeedback.

CN EMG is performed particularly in neurological, neurosurgical and orthopaedic patients with (suspected) lesions to the conus, cauda equina, the sacral plexus or the pudendal nerve, and only rarely in urological, uro-gynecological and proctological patients with suspected 'neurogenic' uro-ano-genital dysfunction.

Pelvic floor muscle denervation has been implicated in the pathophysiology of genuine stress incontinence (Snooks et al 1984) and genitourinary prolapse (Smith et al 1989); different EMG techniques have been used in research to identify sphincter injury after childbirth. The usefulness of CN EMG in routine investigation of women after vaginal delivery and/or with urinary incontinence is, however, minimal and seems to be restricted in practice to the rare cases of severe sacral plexus involvement (Vodušek 2002).

Isolated urinary retention in young women was tra-ditionally thought to be due either to multiple sclerosis or psychogenic factors (Siroky & Krane 1991). Profuse complex repetitive discharges and 'decelerating burst activity' in the urethral sphincter muscle have been, however, described by CN EMG in such patients (Fowler et al 1988). It was proposed that this pathological spon-taneous activity leads to sphincter contraction, which endures during micturition and causes obstruction to flow (Deindl et al 1994). The syndrome was associated with polycystic ovaries (Fowler & Kirby 1986) and is now referred to as Fowler's syndrome. Because CN EMG will detect both changes of denervation and rein-nervation that occur with a cauda equina lesion, as well as abnormal spontaneous activity, it has been argued that this test is mandatory in women with urinary reten-tion (Fowler et al 1988). The specificity of CN EMG pathological changes in women in retention has, however, been questioned.

The CN EMG electrode can be employed at the same diagnostic session for recording motor evoked responses and/or reflex responses for a more comprehensive eval-uation of the nervous system (Podnar & Vodušek 2005; Vodušek & Fowler 2004).

In conclusion, both 'kinesiological' and 'motor unit' EMG have contributed significantly to our understand-ing of pelvic floor, lower urinary tract, anorectal and sexual function in health and disease, but there is still much research to be done.

EMG is helpful in diagnosing selected patients with suspected neurogenic PFM dysfunction, either to dem-onstrate dysfunction of detrusor–sphincter coordination (kinesiological EMG) or to prove denervation/reinner-vation in striated PFM and sphincters. In the case of mild to moderate partial denervation EMG is very limited in providing data on muscle strength (which is logically impaired due to denervation).

CLINICAL RECOMMENDATIONS

- Any EMG method should be, as a rule, used by prop-erly trained examiners. Even surface EMG record-ings – noninvasive and apparently easy to use – need training and experience. There are many technical pitfalls, and not all are apparent to the unsuspicious and uninformed untrained examiner. Close collabo-ration of physiotherapists with neurologists and clinical neurophysiologists is recommended.

- At present, the only widely accepted diagnostic use of kinesiological EMG is to diagnose detrusor–stri-ated sphincter dyssynergia. Any other use of kinesio-logical EMG recordings should follow a protocol, after determining the validity and reliability of the recordings, and minutely describing all aspects of the technique in publications. Standardization of the method in different settings should be strived for.

- CN EMG is the electrophysiologic method of choice in the routine examination of skeletal muscle sus-pected to be denervated/reinnervated. CN EMG of PFM and sphincter muscles is an optional method in incontinent patients with suspected peripheral nervous system involvement. Extrapolation from EMG data to muscle strength, power and endurance should be undertaken cautiously.

- CN EMG should be performed only by properly trained examiners who are licensed by the relevant national authority.

REFERENCES

Aanestad O, Flink R, Norlen B J 1989 Interference pattern in perineal muscles: I. A quantitative electromyographic study in normal subjects. Neurourology and Urodynamics 8:1–9

Aminoff M J 2005 Clinical electromyography. In: Aminoff M J (ed) Electrodiagnosis in clinical neurology, 5th edn. Churchill Livingstone, Philadelphia, p 233–259

Deindl F M, Vodušek D B, Hesse U et al 1993 Activity patterns of pubococcygeal muscles in nulliparous continent women. British Journal of Urology 72(1):46–51

Deindl F M, Vodušek D B, Hesse U et al 1994 Pelvic floor activity patterns: comparison of nulliparous continent and parous urinary stress incontinent women. A kinesiological EMG study. British Journal of Urology 73(4):413–417

Engstrom J W, Olney R K 1992 Quantitative motor unit analysis: the effect of sample size. Muscle & Nerve 15:277–281

Fowler C J, Christmas T J, Chapple C R et al 1988 Abnormal electromyographic activity of the urethral sphincter, voiding dysfunction, and polycystic ovaries: a new syndrome? British Medical Journal 297(6661):1436–1438

Fowler C J, Kirby R S 1986 Electromyography of urethral sphincter in women with urinary retention. Lancet 1(8496):1455–1457

Fowler C J, Kirby R S, Harrison M J et al 1984 Individual motor unit analysis in the diagnosis of disorders of urethral sphincter innervation. Journal of Neurology, Neurosurgery, and Psychiatry 47(6):637–641

Glazer H I, Romanzi L, Polaneczky M 1999 Pelvic floor muscle surface electromyography; Reliability and clinical predictive validity. The Journal of Reproductive Medicine 44:779–782

Neill M E, Swash M 1980 Increased motor unit fibre density in the external anal sphincter muscle in ano-rectal incontinence: a single fibre EMG study. Journal of Neurology, Neurosurgery, and Psychiatry 43(4):343–347

Podnar S, Lukanovic A, Vodušek D B 2000 Anal sphincter electromyography after vaginal delivery: neuropathic insufficiency or normal wear and tear? Neurourology and Urodynamics 19(3):249–257

Podnar S, Mrkaic M, Vodušek D B 2002a Standardization of anal sphincter electromyography: quantification of continuous activity during relaxation. Neurourology and Urodynamics 21(6):540–545

Podnar S, Rodi Z, Lukanovic A et al 1999 Standardization of anal sphincter EMG: technique of needle examination. Muscle & Nerve 22(3):400–403

Podnar S, Vodušek D B 1999 Standardisation of anal sphincter EMG: high and low threshold motor units. Clinical Neurophysiology 110(8):1488–1491

Podnar S, Vodušek D B 2000 Standardization of anal sphincter electromyography: effect of chronic constipation. Muscle & Nerve 23(11):1748–1751

Podnar S, Vodušek D B 2005 Electrophysiologic evaluation of sacral function. In: Aminoff M J (ed) Electrodiagnosis in clinical neurology, 5th edn. Churchill Livingstone, Philadelphia, p 649–670

Podnar S, Vodušek D B, Stalberg E 2000 Standardization of anal sphincter electromyography: normative data. Clinical Neurophysiology 111(12):2200–2207

Podnar S, Vodušek D B, Stalberg E 2002b Comparison of quantitative techniques in anal sphincter electromyography. Muscle & Nerve 25(1):83–92

Rodi Z, Vodušek D B et al 1996 Clinical uro-neurophysiological investigation in multiple sclerosis. European Journal of Neurology 3:574–580

Siroky M B, Krane R J 1991 Functional voiding disorders in women. In: Krane R, Siroky M B (eds) Clinical neuro-urology. Little Brown & Company, Boston, p 445–457

Smith A R, Hosker G L, Warrell D W 1989 The role of pudendal nerve damage in the aetiology of genuine stress incontinence in women. British Journal of Obstetrics and Gynaecology 96(1):29–32

Snooks S J, Barnes P R, Swash M 1984 Damage to the innervation of the voluntary anal and periurethral sphincter musculature in incontinence: an electrophysiological study. Journal of Neurology, Neurosurgery, and Psychiatry 47(12): 1269–1273

Stalberg E, Trontelj J V 1994 Single fiber electromyography: studies in healthy and diseased muscle, 2nd edn. Raven Press, New York

Vodušek D B 2002 The role of electrophysiology in the evaluation of incontinence and prolapse. Current Opinion in Obstetrics & Gynecology 14(5):509–514

Vodušek D B, Fowler C J 2004 Pelvic floor clinical neurophysiology. In: Binnie C, Cooper R, Mauguiere F et al (eds) Clinical neurophysiology vol. 1, EMG, nerve conduction and evoked potentials. Elsevier, Amsterdam, p 281–307

Vodušek D B, Janko M 1981 SFEMG in striated sphincter muscles [abstract]. Muscle & Nerve 4:252

Vodušek D B, Light J K 1983 The motor nerve supply of the external urethral sphincter muscles. Neurourology and Urodynamics 2:193–200

Vaginal squeeze pressure measurement

Kari Bø and Margaret Sherburn

Measurement of squeeze pressure is the most commonly used method to measure pelvic floor muscle (PFM) maximum strength and endurance. The patient is asked to contract the PFM either as hard as possible (maximum strength), to sustain a contraction (endurance), or repeat as many contractions as possible (endurance). The measurement can be done either in the urethra, vagina or rectum.

Kegel (1948) developed a vaginal pressure device connected to a manometer (named the perineometer) showing the pressure in millimetres of mercury as a measure of PFM strength. He did not report any data about responsiveness, reliability or validity for his method. The term 'perineometer' is somewhat misleading because the pressure-sensitive region of the probe of the manometer is not placed at the perineum, but in the vagina at the level of the levator ani. Currently several types of vaginal pressure devices are available to measure vaginal squeeze pressure, all with different device sizes and technical parameters (Bø et al 1990a, Dougherty et al 1986, Laycock & Jerwood 1994) (Figs 5.4–5.6). The tools measure pressure in either mmHg or cmH_2O.

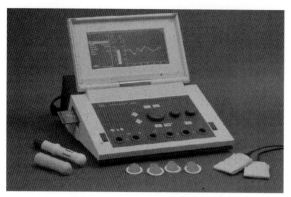

Fig. 5.4 Apparatus with multiple functions: measurement of pelvic floor muscle function with surface EMG and vaginal and rectal squeeze pressure (Enraf Nonius International, 2600 AV Delft, The Netherlands).

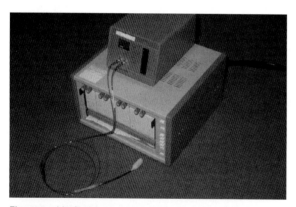

Fig. 5.5 Vaginal squeeze pressure measured with a vaginal balloon connected to a microtip pressure transducer (Camtech AS, Sandvika, Norway).

RESPONSIVENESS

In most studies describing measurement tools, data on responsiveness are not reported. However, in a newer type of apparatus, a specialized balloon catheter connected to a fibreoptic microtip and strain gauge pressure transducer has shown high responsiveness (Abrams et al 1986, Bø et al 1990a, Dougherty et al 1986, Kvarstein et al 1983, Svenningsen & Jensen 1986). In the apparatus of Bø et al (1990a) (Camtech AS, Sandvika, Norway), the transducer's measurement range is 0–400 cmH$_2$O, with linearity of 0.5–1%, hysteresis less than 0.5%, thermal baseline drift less than 0.5% (typically 0.2 cmH$_2$O per °C), and thermal sensitivity drift less than 0.1% per °C (Kvarstein et al 1983, Svenningsen & Jensen 1986).

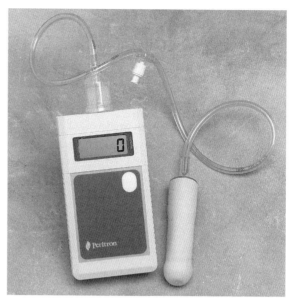

Fig. 5.6 One commonly used perineometer – Peritron with vaginal probe (Cardio Design Pty Ltd, Oakleigh VIC 3166, Australia).

INTRA- AND INTER-TESTER RELIABILITY

Several authors (Bø et al 1990a, Dougherty et al 1986, Frawley et al 2006, McKey & Dougherty 1986, Wilson et al 1991) have shown that vaginal squeeze pressure can be measured with satisfactory reliability. However, Dougherty et al (1991) reported a within-subjects mean of 15.5 mmHg (SD 3.9) and a between-subjects mean of 132.4 mmHg (SD 11.5) in healthy subjects age range from 19 to 61 years. A significant variation was confirmed by Bø et al (1990a) who also showed that at the first attempt some women needed some time to find and recruit motor units, whereas other women fatigued, causing the strength to drop considerably after only a few attempts. However, comparing the results of the whole group of women on two different occasions 14 days apart, reproducible results were found. Wilson et al (1991) also found a significant difference between first and last contractions. They did not find a significant difference between measurements obtained with a full or empty bladder or during the menstrual cycle. Dougherty et al (1991) did not find a significant difference when muscle strength was measured on different days, at different times of the day, or during stress.

Kerschan-Schindl et al (2002) tested intratester reliability of the Peritron perineometer and found that the absolute difference in maximal contraction force and mean contraction force within 5 s was less than 5.3 mmHg and 4.5 mmHg, respectively. Frawley et al (2006) tested intratester reliability of the Peritron perineometer, and found ICC values for squeeze pressure readings to be 0.95, 0.91, 0.96, and 0.92 for crook lying, supine, sitting and standing positions, respectively. The ICC values for endurance testing in the same positions were much lower: 0.05, 0.42, 0.13, and 0.35. ICC values for resting pressure were 0.74, 0.77, 0.47 and 0.29. They concluded that there were high values of reliability of maximal voluntary contraction measured by the Peritron. However, endurance testing was unreliable, and so also was resting pressure in sitting and standing position.

VALIDITY

Of the three pelvic canals, measurement within the urethra has the best face and content validity for measuring urethral closure pressure caused by the force of muscle contraction. This is where the increased pressure created by the PFM contraction is required to prevent urinary leakage. However, because of the risk of infection and the lack of availability of equipment in most physical therapy clinics, this method has mostly been used for research purposes (Benvenuti et al 1987, Lose 1992). Rectal pressure may not be a valid measure of the PFM in relation to urinary incontinence because it also includes contraction of the anal sphincter muscle. However, in men rectal pressure is the only practical option. In contrast to men, most women would have little sense of where the urethra is located, and most women probably would have the optimal sense of PFM contraction in the vagina. Therefore, vaginal squeeze pressure is the most commonly used method clinically.

PLACEMENT OF THE DEVICE

Size of the vaginal probe differs between devices. Some devices cover the full length of the vagina and placement of the probe is therefore not a problem. Using smaller devices (Bø et al 1990a, Dougherty et al 1986), location of the probe in the vagina creates both a reliability and validity problem because the balloon may be located outside the anatomical location of the PFM. The balloon or transducer has to be placed at the same anatomical level and at the level where the PFM are located. Kegel (1948, 1952) suggested that the PFM were located in the distal one-third of the vagina, and Bø (1992) found that most women had the highest pressure rise when the balloon was placed with the middle of the balloon

3.5 cm inside the introitus. However, individual differences were found.

SIZE AND SHAPES OF THE DEVICE

Results reported from different squeeze pressure and electromyography (EMG) apparatus can not be compared due to differences in the diameter of the vaginal devices. There is discussion regarding the optimum diameter of vaginal devices (Schull et al 2002). It is unknown whether a wide-diameter vaginal device stretches the PFM, inhibiting its activity or, conversely, increasing activity by providing firm proprioceptive feedback. In a study by Bø et al (2005), measurement of PFM maximum strength was compared using two commonly used apparatus with different size of the vaginal probe. Significant differences were found, and it was concluded that measurements obtained with different methods cannot be compared.

INFLUENCE FROM INCREASED ABDOMINAL PRESSURE

Squeeze pressure measurements obtained from all three canals can be invalid because an increase in abdominal pressure will increase the measured pressures. The PFM form one wall of the abdominopelvic cavity, and all rises in abdominal pressure will increase the pressure measured in the urethra, vagina and rectum.

Both Bø et al (1988) and Bump et al (1991) have shown that straining is a common error when women attempt to contract their PFM, and therefore an erroneous measurement can be registered. However, because a correct contraction involves an observable inward movement of the perineum or the instrument, and straining creates a downward movement, some authors (Bø et al 1990b, Bump et al 1996) have suggested that a valid measurement can be ensured by simultaneous observation of inward movement of the perineum.

Some researchers (Cammu & Van Nylen 1998) have tried to avoid co-contraction of the abdominal muscles interfering with measurement of PFM strength by use of surface EMG on the rectus abdominis muscle to train subjects to relax their abdominal muscles or by simultaneous abdominal pressure measurement. Performance of a near-maximal PFM contraction is important to achieve the best training effect (Komi 1992, Wilmore & Costill 1999). Several researchers (Bø et al 1990b, Dougherty et al 1991, Neumann & Gill 2002, Sapsford et al 2001), however, have shown that there is a co-contraction of the deep abdominal muscles (lower transversus abdominis and internal oblique) during attempts at a correct, maximal contraction. Neumann & Gill (2002) also reported that during a maximum PFM contraction the mean abdominal pressure was 9 mmHg (range 2–19). The abdominal pressure rose to a mean of 27 mmHg (range 11–34) with a head and leg lift from supine while performing a PFM contraction, and 36 mmHg (range 33–52 during forced expiration and PFM contraction when supine, two activities which require diaphragmatic and outer abdominal muscles (external oblique and rectus abdominis) activity. A normal co-contraction of the lower abdominal wall, therefore, can be allowed because abdominal pressure rise is small with this co-contraction.

Dougherty et al (1991) allowed an increase in abdominal pressure of 5 mmHg only, to ensure the least abdominal pressure interference with the measurement results. Bø et al (1990b) standardized the testing by not allowing any movement of the pelvis during measurement. Further investigation is required to assess how subtle changes in postural activity might affect vaginal pressure measurements.

Contraction of other muscles such as the hip adductor and external rotator muscles and gluteals, also alters intravaginal pressure measurement (Bø et al 1990b, Peschers et al 2001). Bø & Stien (1994) showed with concentric needle EMG in women without urinary incontinence that contraction of these other muscles increased muscle activity in both the striated urethral wall muscle and the PFM. However, when analysing the whole group of women, contraction of the other pelvic muscles did not give a higher pressure response than contraction of the PFM alone. Caution has to be taken though because for some individuals this may occur. Because the gross motor pattern of gluteal and adductor activity is not part of the normal neuromuscular action of the PFM and lower transversus abdominis synergy, co-contractions of the outer pelvic muscles are discouraged when measuring PFM action and strength.

SENSITIVITY AND SPECIFICITY

Several case–control studies comparing PFM strength with vaginal squeeze pressure in continent and incontinent women have demonstrated that continent women have better strength than incontinent women (Hahn et al 1996, Mørkved et al 2004), and that there is an association between improvement in muscle function or strength and reduction in urinary incontinence (Bø 2003). However, some studies have not found an association between increase in muscle strength and improvement in incontinence (Elser et al 1999), which may be explained by the fact that there was no improvement in muscle strength following the low-dosage exercise protocol.

CONCLUSION

Because all increases in abdominal pressure will affect urethral, vaginal, and rectal pressures, squeeze pressure cannot be used alone. With simultaneous observation of inward movement of the perineum, it is likely that a correct contraction is measured. Cautious teaching of the patient, standardization of instruction and motivation, and standardization of the patient's position and performance are mandatory. If the aim is to measure the ability to close the urethra, urethral pressure should be measured. If overall PFM strength is the aim of the investigation, vaginal squeeze pressure (pressure manometry or dynamometric force) is preferred because this is the least invasive method with a low risk of infection in women.

CLINICAL RECOMMENDATIONS

Measurement of vaginal squeeze pressure is difficult, and clinical skills and experience are important factors in achieving reliable and valid results. The method has to be used with caution. However, when used in accordance with knowledge from research in this area, measurement of PFM contraction can give important information and feedback to both the patient and therapist (Fig. 5.7).

• Fully inform the patient about the test procedure and gain consent.
• Give the patient privacy to undress and a drape to place over her on the examination couch.
• Always start the instruction with observation and palpation of PFM contraction.
• If the patient is unable to contract, strains or uses other muscles instead of the PFM, pressure measurement is not possible.
• Patient can be supine, crook lying, sitting or standing. Use the same position for each assessment for that patient.
• The physiotherapist must be in a position to be able to observe the perineum.
• Prepare the measuring device before washing hands and putting on examination gloves.
• Follow local infection control guidelines with regard to covering the probe or use a single-use apparatus.
• Gently insert the probe or ask the patient to do it.
• Once the probe is comfortably in place, instruct the patient to relax and breathe normally before the PFM contraction.

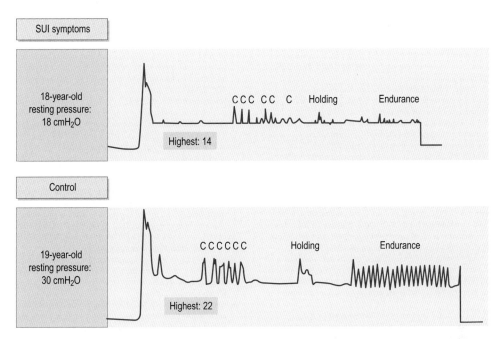

Fig. 5.7 Measurement of resting pressure, pelvic floor muscle maximal strength, attempts of holding, and repeated contractions at first time consultation in two nulliparous female sports students. Both were able to contract the PFM as assessed by vaginal palpation. The first had proven urodynamic stress urinary incontinence (SUI) with 43 g of leakage on ambulatory urodynamics. The second had no symptoms of pelvic floor dysfunction.

- Support the device to keep it in the same intravaginal position.
- Instruct the patient to contract the PFM as hard as possible with no visible co-contraction of hip adductor, gluteal or rectus abdominis muscles (pelvic tilt) and then to relax without pressing the perineum downwards.
- A small indrawing or 'hollowing' using internal abdominals (transversus abdominis and internal oblique) with maximum contraction and no tilting of the pelvis is allowed.
- Resting pressure, holding time and repeated contractions can also be registered depending on the device parameters.
- Only contractions with simultaneous visible inward movement of the perineum or the measurement device can be considered valid measurements of PFM strength.
- Register at least three contractions and use the maximum or mean of the three contractions.
- Other aspects of muscle performance, such as holding time and number of repeated contractions (endurance), onset of contraction, slope and area under the curve, and resting pressure (relaxation) can be measured if the equipment used provides for this.
- Gently remove the probe, and either dispose of the intravaginal component or wash it according to local guidelines before sterilization.
- Allow the patient privacy to dress before discussing the results.

REFERENCES

Abrams R, Batich C, Dougherty M et al 1986 Custom-made vaginal balloons for strengthening circumvaginal musculature. Biomaterials, Medical Devices, and Artificial Organs 14(3–4): 239–248

Benvenuti F, Caputo G M, Bandinelli S et al 1987 Reeducative treatment of female genuine stress incontinence. American Journal of Physical Medicine 66:155–168

Bø K 1992 Pressure measurements during pelvic floor muscle contractions: the effect of different positions of the vaginal measuring device. Neurourology and Urodynamics 11:107–113

Bø K 2003 Pelvic floor muscle strength and response to pelvic floor muscle training for stress urinary incontinence. Neurourology and Urodynamics 22:654–658

Bø K, Larsen S, Oseid S et al 1988 Knowledge about and ability to correct pelvic floor muscle exercises in women with urinary stress incontinence. Neurourology and Urodynamics 7:261–262

Bø K, Kvarstein B, Hagen R et al 1990a Pelvic floor muscle exercise for the treatment of female stress urinary incontinence, I: reliability of vaginal pressure measurements of pelvic floor muscle strength. Neurourology and Urodynamics 9:471–477

Bø K, Kvarstein B, Hagen R et al 1990b Pelvic floor muscle exercise for the treatment of female stress urinary incontinence, II: validity of vaginal pressure measurements of pelvic floor muscle strength and the necessity of supplementary methods for control of correct contraction. Neurourology and Urodynamics 9:479–487

Bø K, Raastad R, Finckenhagen HB 2005 Does the size of the vaginal probe affect measurement of pelvic floor muscle strength? Acta Obstetricia et Gynecologica Scandinavica 84:129–133

Bø K, Stien R 1994 Needle EMG registration of striated urethral wall and pelvic floor muscle activity patterns during cough, Valsalva, abdominal, hip adductor, and gluteal muscle contractions in nulliparous healthy females. Neurourology and Urodynamics 13:35–41

Bump R, Hurt W G, Fantl J A et al 1991. Assessment of Kegel exercise performance after brief verbal instruction. American Journal of Obstetrics and Gynecology 165:322–329

Bump R, Mattiasson A, Bø K et al 1996 The standardization of terminology of female pelvic organ prolapse and pelvic floor dysfunction. American Journal of Obstetrics and Gynecology 175:10–17

Cammu H, Van Nylen M 1998 Pelvic floor exercises versus vaginal weight cones in genuine stress incontinence. European Journal of Obstetrical and Gynecological Reproductive Biology 77:89–93

Dougherty M C, Abrams R, McKey P L 1986 An instrument to assess the dynamic characteristics of the circumvaginal musculature. Nursing Research 35:202–206

Dougherty M, Bishop K, Mooney R et al 1991 Variation in intravaginal pressure measurement. Nursing Research 40:282–285

Elser D, Wyman J, McClish D et al 1999 The effect of bladder training, pelvic floor muscle training, or combination training on urodynamic parameters in women with urinary incontinence. Neurourology and Urodynamics 18:427–436

Frawley H C, Galea M P, Phillips B A et al 2006 Reliability of pelvic floor muscle strength assessment using different test positions and tools. Neurourology and Urodynamics 25(3):236–242

Hahn I, Milsom I, Ohlson B L et al 1996 Comparative assessment of pelvic floor function using vaginal cones, vaginal digital palpation and vaginal pressure measurement. Gynecological and Obstetrical Investigation 41:269–274

Kegel A H 1948 Progressive resistance exercise in the functional restoration of the perineal muscles. American Journal of Obstetrics and Gynecology 56:238–249

Kegel A H 1952 Stress incontinence and genital relaxation; a nonsurgical method of increasing the tone of sphincters and their supporting structures. Ciba Clinical Symposia 4(2):35–51

Kerschan–Schindl K, Uher E, Wiesinger G et al 2002 Reliability of pelvic floor muscle strength measurement in elderly incontinent women. Neurourology and Urodynamics 21:42–47

Komi P V 1992 Strength and power in sport. The encyclopaedia of sports medicine. An IOC Medical Commission Publication in collaboration with the International Federation of Sports Medicine. Blackwell Science, Oxford

Kvarstein B, Aase O, Hansen T et al 1983 A new method with fiberoptic transducers used for simultaneous recording of intravesical and urethral pressure during physiological filling and voiding phases. Journal of Urology 130:504–506

Laycock J, Jerwood D 1994 Development of the Bradford perineometer. Physiotherapy 80:139–142

Lose G 1992 Simultaneous recording of pressure and cross-sectional area in the female urethra: a study of urethral closure function in healthy and stress incontinent women. Neurourology and Urodynamics 11:54–89

McKey PL, Dougherty MC 1986 The circumvaginal musculature: correlation between pressure and physical assessment. Nursing Research 35:307–309

Mørkved S, Salvesen K Å, Bø K et al 2004 Pelvic floor muscle strength and thickness in continent and incontinent nulliparous pregnant women. International Urogynecology Journal and Pelvic Floor Dysfunction 15:384–390

Neumann P, Gill V 2002 Pelvic floor and abdominal muscle interaction: EMG activity and intra–abdominal pressure. International Urogynecology Journal and Pelvic Floor Dysfunction 13:125–132

Peschers U, Gingelmaier A, Jundt K et al 2001 Evaluation of pelvic floor muscle strength using four different techniques. International Urogynecology Journal and Pelvic Floor Dysfunction 12:27–30

Sapsford R, Hodges P, Richardson C et al 2001 Co-activation of the abdominal and pelvic floor muscles during voluntary exercises. Neurourology and Urodynamics 20:31–42

Schull B, Hurt G, Laycock J et al 2002 Physical examination. In: Abrams P, Cardozo L, Khoury S et al (eds). Incontinence. Plymbridge Distributors Ltd, Plymouth UK, p 373–388

Svenningsen L, Jensen Ø 1986 Application of fiberoptics to the clinical measurement of intra-uterine pressure in labour. Acta Obstetricia et Gynecologica Scandinavica 65:551–555

Wilmore J, Costill D 1999 Physiology of sport and exercise, 2nd edn. Human Kinetics, Champaign, IL

Wilson P, Herbison G, Heer K 1991 Reproducibility of perineometry measurements. Neurourology and Urodynamics 10:399–400

Urethral pressure measurements

Mohammed Belal and Paul Abrams

Continence depends on the intramural and extramural forces that maintain urethral closure while the bladder is filling. Stress leakage may occur if the urethral resistance is overcome by abdominal forces, therefore resulting in a vesical pressure that is higher than urethral pressure (Barnes 1961). An understanding of urethral function is vital in incontinence.

Urethral pressure measurements are a common method of measuring urethral function. They assess the ability of the urethra to prevent urinary incontinence. They can be measured at single points in the urethra or most commonly over the entire length of the urethra (urethral pressure profile). We begin with the definitions of urethral pressure parameters, followed by the different methods and techniques used to obtain urethral pressures. The advantages and disadvantages of the different methods and techniques will be discussed.

DEFINITIONS

Urethral pressure is defined as **the fluid pressure needed to just open a closed (collapsed) urethra** (Griffiths 1985). This definition implies that the urethral pressure is similar to an ordinary fluid pressure (i.e. is a scalar [does not have a direction] quantity with a single value at each point along the length of the urethra; Lose et al 2002).

From the definition, it is apparent that the introduction of catheters changes the properties of the closed urethra but the effect on the urethral pressure measurement was considered to be small (Griffiths 1985). Urethral pressure measures the intra and extramural forces that cause apposition of the urethral walls and associated definitions are as follows (Fig. 5.8).

- **Urethral pressure profile (UPP)** is a graph indicating the intraluminal pressure along the length of the urethra.
- **Urethral closure pressure profile** is given by the subtraction of intravesical pressure from urethral pressure.

- **Maximum urethral pressure (MUP)** is the maximum pressure of the measured profile.
- **Maximum urethral closure pressure (MUCP)** is the maximum difference between the urethral pressure and the intravesical pressure. This is the reserve pressure of the urethra to prevent leakage. The calculation of MUCP (p_{ucp}) requires the simultaneous recording of both intraurethral (p_{ura}) and intravesical (p_{ves}) pressure. The calculation is as follows: $p_{ucp} = p_{ura} - p_{ves}$.
- **Functional urethral length (FUL)** is the length of the urethra along which the urethral pressure exceeds intravesical pressure in women.

METHODS OF MEASURING URETHRAL PRESSURE PROFILOMETRY

There are currently three methods of measuring urethral pressure profilometry:

- fluid perfusion technique or the Brown Wickham technique (Brown & Wickham 1969);
- microtip/fibreoptic catheters;
- balloon catheters.

A summary of the advantages and disadvantages of the different methods is shown in Table 5.1.

Fluid perfusion technique

The fluid perfusion technique measures the pressure needed to perfuse the catheter, which is withdrawn at a constant speed, at a constant rate. The constant rate of infusion is usually provided by a syringe driver. The measured quantity can be very close to the local urethral pressure, provided that the urethra is highly distensible (Griffiths 1980). Several factors affect the technique, as discussed below.

Catheter size

Catheter sizes from 4- to 10-French gauge are satisfactory to use in the fluid perfusion technique (Harrison

Table 5.1 Advantages and disadvantages of the different methods of measuring urethral pressures

	Fluid perfusion technique	Microtip/fibreoptic catheters	Balloon catheters
Advantages	Less prone to movement artefacts Cheap	Measure rapid pressure changes	No orientation dependence
Disadvantages	Slow response to pressure changes	Influenced by transducer shape and orientation Stiffness of the catheter can lead to further artefacts, so a flexible catheter is required Expensive and fragile	Dilating effect on urethra Expensive

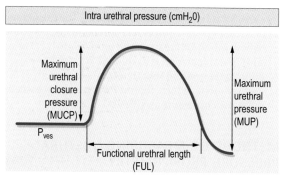

Fig. 5.8 The measurement of urethral pressure parameters.

1976). Large-sized catheters give a falsely higher reading because they record urethral elasticity as well as the urethral closure pressure (Lose 1992).

Catheter eyeholes

Two opposing side holes 5 cm from the tip of the catheter are satisfactory (Abrams et al 1978). A larger number of holes does not improve accuracy. The orientation is not important.

Perfusion rate

A perfusion rate of 2–10 mL/min will give an accurate measurement of closure pressure (Abrams et al 1978). A syringe driver is preferable to a peristaltic pump.

Catheter withdrawal speed

The catheter should preferably be withdrawn continuously with the optimal withdrawal speed of less than

7 mm/s (Hilton 1982). The usual rate of withdrawal is between 1 and 5 mm/s.

Response time

Response time is dependent on the rate of perfusion and the rate of catheter withdrawal. The perfusion method is able to record a maximum rate of change between 34 and 50 cmH$_2$O/s.

Microtip/fibreoptic catheters

The microtransducer catheters have the ability to measure rapid changes in pressure. However they appear to have several disadvantages. First there is a significant degree of positional dependence (Hilton & Stanton 1983a). For example if the catheter microtransducer is facing anteriorly, then the MUP is greater and FUL shorter than posteriorly (Abrams et al 1978). Secondly bending in urethral wall tissue may lead to a superimposition of local urethral tissue and transducer interactions on the urethral pressure: this requires the catheters to be very flexible. If used it is recommended that the transducer faces laterally (Anderson et al 1983).

Balloon catheters

The advantages of balloon catheters in measuring urethral pressures are that they avoid orientation dependence. However, in the past technical problems meant that the balloons were too large, causing a dilatation effect on the urethra. This results in an overestimation of the urethral pressure. Additionally the length of the balloon is also important. If the balloon is too long this averages out the pressure variations along the length of the urethra. Recent balloon catheters have overcome these difficulties (Pollak et al 2004).

FACTORS AFFECTING MAXIMUM URETHRAL CLOSURE PRESSURES

Urethral pressure measurement can be carried out at different bladder volumes and in different subject positions at rest, during coughing or straining and during voiding.

Bladder volume

Urethral closure pressure measurement in women depends on bladder volume. In continent women the urethral closure pressure increases with increasing volume. However, in women with stress incontinence it tends to decrease with increasing volume (Awad et al 1978).

Patient position

Position also has an effect on urethral closure pressure: continent women showing an increase in urethral closure pressure on standing whereas women with stress incontinence show a decrease in pressure on standing (Henriksson et al 1977; Hendriksson et al 1979). However, there is poor reproducibility of the urethral closure pressure in the standing position, thus limiting clinical use (Dorflinger et al 2002).

Pelvic floor activity

Pelvic floor muscle (PFM) activity is always active except before and during voiding. However, a failure of relaxation of the voluntary pelvic floor contraction increases urethral closure pressure. This can usually be overcome by repeating the urethral pressure profilometry twice more or until a reproducible pattern is obtained, and if need be, over a longer period of time. Conversely, the effect of pelvic floor activity on the urethra can be assessed during measurement of urethral pressure. The catheter is placed at the point of MUP and the patient is asked to contract the pelvic floor voluntarily as if trying to stop themselves from passing urine. In normal women an increment above the MUCP is seen. A value of less than 10 cmH$_2$O above the MUCP denotes a poor pelvic floor squeeze in the fluid perfusion technique (Table 5.2).

The variation of urethral closure pressures depends on the method used and the position, and to facilitate reliable recordings, recommendations on the standardization of urethral pressure measurements have been made. Below are some of the recommendations of the International Continence Society (ICS) sub-committee on the standardization of urethral pressure measurements (Lose et al 2002).

Table 5.2 Comparison of clinical PFM strength assessment by experienced clinicians and urethral pressure assessment (fluid perfusion technique)

PFM strength as assessed by urologist/ urogynaecologist	Normal	Reduced	Absent
Number of patients	2757	3399	485
Urethral pressure assessment (cmH$_2$O) (SD)	18.1 (15.5)	8.8 (11.1)	3.6 (7.5)

A large series from the Bristol Urological Institute over a period of 15 years.
PFM, pelvic floor muscle.

STANDARDIZATION OF URETHRAL PRESSURE MEASUREMENTS

The investigator is asked to specify:

1. type of measurement (point – profilometry – ambulatory);
2. period of time over which the measurement was recorded;
3. constant (given by the probe) or variable cross-sectional area of the urethra (i.e. inflation of a balloon);
4. patient position;
5. bladder volume;
6. manoeuvres (coughing, Valsalva, other);
7. withdrawal speed (for profilometry);
8. infusion medium and rate of infusion (for fluid-perfused catheters);
9. type of catheter;
10. size of catheter;
11. catheter material – flexibility;
12. orientation of a directional sensor;
13. sensor position fixation (for point pressures or during coughing/straining);
14. zeroing of pressure sensors:
    - external transducers (and fluid-filled catheters)
    - superior edge of the symphysis pubis (piezometric) for pressure reference height; to correct for viscous pressure losses within the catheter zero of pressure should be set as the reading in

air when the fluid is flowing. (zero reference point is atmospheric pressure)
- microtip transducers calibrated to atmospheric pressure, but no pressure reference height is needed for catheter-mounted transducers; when calculating closure pressure using multisensor microtips, any difference in vertical height between the 'bladder' transducer and urethral transducer(s) should be taken into account

15. recording apparatus:
    - describe type of recording apparatus – the frequency response of the total system should be stated; equipment with a sampling rate of 18 Hz can satisfactorily record cough-produced pressure changes in the urethra (Thind et al 1994).

NORMAL URETHRAL PRESSURE PROFILES

There are sex differences between men and women in the range of normal urethral pressure values. In men, MUP does not significantly decrease with age (Abrams 1997), whereas in women, after the menopause, MUP decreases. Prostatic length tends to increase with age in men; however urethral length tends to decrease in women. A rough guide to MUP in women is a value of 92 – age (cmH$_2$O) using values obtained from the fluid perfusion technique (Edwards & Malvern 1974).

Urethral pressure profile shape

Men

Certain features are seen in the male UPP; there are two peaks – the presphincter peak followed by the prostatic plateau and then the sphincter peak (Fig. 5.9). Abnormalities in the presphincteric prostatic plateau can be

due to bladder neck hypertrophy or prostatic enlargement. The sphincter peak in men can be too high, as seen in some neurogenic patients, or too low in male patients with iatrogenic causes of stress incontinence, such as after prostate surgery.

Women

The female urethral pressure profile tends to symmetrical in shape as seen in Fig. 5.8.

Normal and abnormal urethral pressure profiles are shown in Figs 5.10 and 5.11, respectively. Women can also have low or high urethral pressures. A high urethral pressure sometimes denotes Fowler's syndrome, a condition in which idiopathic sphincter overactivity causes voiding difficulties (Fowler et al 1988). A low urethral pressure may denote intrinsic sphincter deficiency, which usually results from childbirth and may lead to stress urinary incontinence (SUI).

The measurement of resting UPPs has several uses.

- In post-prostatectomy incontinence; there is a close association between sphincter damage and a reduction in the MUCP (Hammerer & Huland 1997).

- There is some evidence that a low MUCP is associated with a poor outcome with surgery in women for SUI (Hilton & Stanton 1983b).

- Urethral pressure measurements may provide an answer to unexplained incontinence in women.

- When considering patients for urinary diversion surgery the MUCP gives an indication as to whether an artificial sphincter is necessary. An MUCP greater than 50 cmH$_2$O would not require a sphincter if a good-volume, low-pressure reservoir is created (Abrams 1997).

Urethral pressure profile and incontinence surgery

Several studies have suggested that female patients with a low urethral closure pressure and urethral length have a worst outcome after incontinence surgery (Bhatia & Ostergard 1982; Hilton 1989; Hilton & Stanton 1983b). Some have not shown any difference (Sand et al 2000).

RESTING URETHRAL PRESSURE PROFILES

Responsiveness

The microtip catheters have a high frequency response of over 2000 Hz, which is more than adequate to record physiological events in the lower urinary tract. The fluid

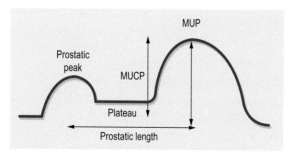

Fig. 5.9 The male urethral pressure profile measurements, demonstrating the prostatic peak, plateau and length. MUP, maximum urethral pressure; MUCP, maximum urethral closure pressure (MUCP).

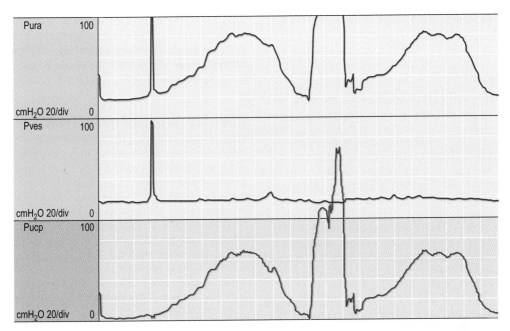

Fig. 5.10 Normal urethral pressures in women: the diagram shows two urethral pressure profiles (UPPs) with the shorter higher peak being the artefact recorded when the catheter is passed though the sphincter area to perform the second UPP seen on the right. (p_{ucp}, urethral closure pressure, p_{ura}, intraurethral pressure, p_{ves}, intravesical pressure.)

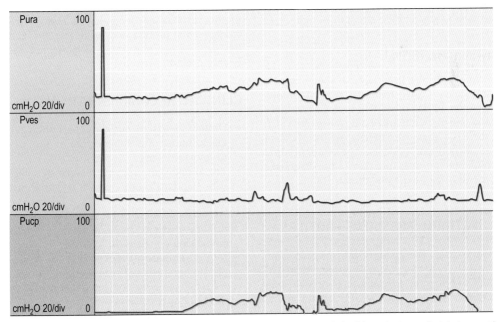

Fig. 5.11 Reduced urethral pressures: two urethral pressure profiles are recorded with a short artefact between them (see Fig. 5.10). ($Pucp_c$, urethral closure pressure, Pura, intraurethral pressure, Pves, intravesical pressure.)

perfusion technique has a reduced responsiveness in comparison.

Reliability

The reproducibility and repeatability of the fluid perfusion technique and the microtip catheter have been shown to be reasonable (Abrams et al 1978; Hilton 1982; Wang & Chen 2002). The standard deviation of measurements made in a single occasion of the fluid perfusion technique and the microtip catheter is shown to be approximately 5 and 3 cmH$_2$O, respectively (Abrams et al 1978; Hilton & Stanton 1983a). The inter-test measurements showing a standard deviation of 3.5–5 cmH$_2$O depending on menstrual status (van Geelen et al 1981; Hilton 1982). Recently balloon catheters have shown reasonable correlations with microtip catheters (Pollak et al 2004).

Validity

The validity of the measurements of resting urethral pressure profilometry depends on the technique used The measured quantity can be very close to the local urethral pressure, provided that the urethra is highly distensible (Griffiths 1980) in the case of the fluid perfusion technique.

Microtip catheters measure the stress of the urethral wall, not the pressure. The validity of urethral pressure measurements in assessing PFM strength is high.

Sensitivity and specificity

Female patients with SUI generally have significantly lower mean values of MUP than in continent women (Hilton & Stanton 1983a). The MUP is lowest in those women (and men) with increasingly severe SUI. However, there is a large overlap between the MUPs of normal and incontinent patients. Therefore urethral pressure profilometry does not have the diagnostic accuracy for SUI to be used alone (Versi 1990).

STRESS URETHRAL PRESSURE PROFILES

This method assesses the pressure transmission from the abdominal cavity to the proximal urethra. Decreased conductance of abdominal pressure is associated with stress incontinence. Essentially a UPP is performed, preferably with a microtip catheter with the patient coughing. If the urethral closure pressures become negative on coughing, then leakage is likely and represents a positive test. Ideally the stress UPP should be carried out in the erect position with a full bladder. This poses practical issues. A lack of specificity with the test has limited its use (Versi 1990). Stress UPPs are no longer used regularly in clinical practice.

NEW METHODS OF MEASURING URETHRAL PRESSURES

A recent technique devised called the retrograde urethral pressure has been described for women. This is the pressure required to achieve and keep the urethral sphincter open. The mean retrograde urethral pressure was shown to be lower in continent women (Slack et al 2004b). There appears to be some association with MUP and severity of incontinence (Slack et al 2004a). However further work is required to test its clinical diagnostic value in diagnosing SUI and the technique has been criticised as being incompletely validated (Abrams & Cardozo 2004).

CONCLUSION

Resting urethral pressure measurements can be made using several techniques and the results are influenced by the technique used and biological factors. Urethral pressure measurements are static measurements that do not reflect the forces exerted on the urethra at leakage. Increases in abdominal pressure compress the urethra and result in reflex activation of the periurethral muscles, which are not assessed by resting urethral pressures.

CLINICAL RECOMMENDATIONS

- Urethral pressure measurements should be undertaken under the supervision of the urologist or urogynaecologist.
- The urologist or urogynaecologist should refer to the ICS standardization report on urethral pressure measurements.
- An understanding of the limitations of the different urethral pressure measurements is required before embarking on research.
- Multidisciplinary collaboration is required when physiotherapists perform research in this area with the urologist or urogynaecologist providing the urethral pressure measurements.
- Urethral pressure measurements, if done correctly, are good valid measurements for assessing PFM strength.

REFERENCES

Abrams P 1997 Urodynamics, 2nd edn. Springer, London

Abrams P, Cardozo L 2004 Technique of urethral retro-resistance pressure measurement. Neurourology and Urodynamics 23(4):385

Abrams P H, Martin S, Griffiths D J 1978 The measurement and interpretation of urethral pressures obtained by the method of Brown and Wickham. British Journal of Urology 50(1):33–38

Anderson R S, Shepherd A M, Feneley R C 1983 Microtransducer urethral profile methodology: variations caused by transducer orientation. The Journal of Urology 130(4):727–728

Awad S A, Bryniak S R, Lowe P J et al 1978 Urethral pressure profile in female stress incontinence. The Journal of Urology 120(4):475–479

Barnes A 1961 The method of evaluating the stress of urinary incontinence. Obstetrics and Gynecology 81:108

Bhatia N N, Ostergard D R 1982 Urodynamics in women with stress urinary incontinence. Obstetrics and Gynecology 60(5):552–559

Brown M, Wickham J E 1969 The urethral pressure profile. British Journal of Urology 41(2):211–217

Dorflinger A, Gorton E, Stanton S et al 2002 Urethral pressure profile: is it affected by position? Neurourology and Urodynamics 21(6):553–557

Edwards L, Malvern J 1974 The urethral pressure profile: theoretical considerations and clinical application. British Journal of Urology 46(3):325–335

Fowler C J, Christmas T J, Chapple C R et al 1988 Abnormal electromyographic activity of the urethral sphincter, voiding dysfunction, and polycystic ovaries: a new syndrome? BMJ 297(6661):1436–1438

Griffiths D S 1980 Urodynamics. Adam Hilger, Bristol

Griffiths D 1985 The pressure within a collapsed tube, with special reference to urethral pressure. Physics in Medicine and Biology 30(9):951–963

Hammerer P, Huland H 1997 Urodynamic evaluation of changes in urinary control after radical retropubic prostatectomy. The Journal of Urology 157(1):233–236

Harrison N W 1976 The urethral pressure profile. Urological Research 4(3):95–100

Hendriksson L, Andersson KE, Ulmsten U 1979 The urethral pressure profiles in continent and stress-incontinent women. Scandinavian Journal of Urology and Nephrology 13(1):5–10

Henriksson L, Ulmsten U, Andersson K E 1977 The effect of changes of posture on the urethral closure pressure in healthy women. Scandinavian Journal of Urology and Nephrology 11(3):201–206

Hilton P 1982 Urethral pressure measurements at rest: an analysis of variance. Neurourology and Urodynamics 1:303

Hilton P 1989 A clinical and urodynamic study comparing the Stamey bladder neck suspension and suburethral sling

procedures in the treatment of genuine stress incontinence. British Journal of Obstetrics and Gynaecology 96(2):213–220

Hilton P, Stanton S L 1983a Urethral pressure measurement by microtransducer: the results in symptom-free women and in those with genuine stress incontinence. British Journal of Obstetrics and Gynaecology 90(10):919–933

Hilton P, Stanton S L 1983b A clinical and urodynamic assessment of the Burch colposuspension for genuine stress incontinence. British Journal of Obstetrics and Gynaecology 90(10):934–939

Lose G 1992 Simultaneous recording of pressure and cross sectional area in the female urethra: a study of urethral closure function in healthy and stress incontinent women. Neurourology and Urodynamics 11:55

Lose G, Griffiths D, Hosker G et al 2002 Standardisation of urethral pressure measurement: report from the Standardisation Sub-Committee of the International Continence Society. Neurourology and Urodynamics 21(3):258–260

Pollak J T, Neimark M, Connor J T et al 2004. Air-charged and microtransducer urodynamic catheters in the evaluation of urethral function. International Urogynecology Journal and Pelvic Floor Dysfunction 15(2):124–128

Sand P K, Winkler H, Blackhurst D W et al 2000 A prospective randomized study comparing modified Burch retropubic urethropexy and suburethral sling for treatment of genuine stress incontinence with low-pressure urethra. American Journal of Obstetrics and Gynecology 182(1 Pt 1):30–34

Slack M, Culligan P, Tracey M et al 2004a Relationship of urethral retro-resistance pressure to urodynamic measurements and incontinence severity. Neurourology and Urodynamics 23(2):109–114

Slack M, Tracey M, Hunsicker K et al 2004b Urethral retro-resistance pressure: a new clinical measure of urethral function. Neurourology and Urodynamics 23(7):656–661

Thind P, Bagi P, Lose G et al 1994 Characterization of pressure changes in the lower urinary tract during coughing with special reference to the demands on the pressure recording equipment. Neurourology and Urodynamics 13(3):219–225

van Geelen J M, Doesburg W H, Thomas C M et al 1981 Urodynamic studies in the normal menstrual cycle: the relationship between hormonal changes during the menstrual cycle and the urethral pressure profile. American Journal of Obstetrics and Gynecology 141(4):384–392

Versi E 1990 Discriminant analysis of urethral pressure profilometry data for the diagnosis of genuine stress incontinence. British Journal of Obstetrics and Gynaecology 97(3):251–259

Wang A C, Chen M C 2002 A comparison of urethral pressure profilometry using microtip and double-lumen perfusion catheters in women with genuine stress incontinence. BJOG 109(3):322–326

Pelvic floor dynamometry

Chantale Dumoulin and Mélanie Morin

INTRODUCTION

Precise, quantitative measurements of strength are critical for determining the clinical progression of neuromuscular weakness and assessing the response to an intervention aimed at increasing strength. Dynamometers accurately measure forces produced during a muscle contraction independently of the evaluator's judgement. Although these instruments have been widely use by physiotherapists for the evaluation of trunk, upper and lower extremity muscles for more than 40 years (Bohanon 1990), pelvic floor dynamometers are fairly new. Caufriez (1993, 1998) and Rowe (1995) were the first to report the development of dynamometers for measuring the PFM function. However, only in non-peer reviewed manuscripts (Caufriez 1998, 1993) and in one brief conference abstract (Rowe 1995). Sampselle et al (1998) and Howard et al (2000) were the first to mention the use of a pelvic floor dynamometer in clinical trials. In a patent document published in 2002, Ashton-Miller described the strain gage device used in those trials (Ashton-Miller et al 2002). However, no report on the reliability and validity of this apparatus has been published so far.

Four years ago, our research team designed and developed an original dynamometric speculum for measuring isometric dorsoventral pelvic floor muscle (PFM) forces (Dumoulin et al 2003). This new PFM dynamometer comprises a dynamometric speculum and a computerized central unit (Dumoulin et al 2003) consisting of a laptop computer and a PCMCIA data acquisition card. The dynamometric speculum (Fig. 5.12) consists of two aluminium branches. The upper branch of the speculum is fixed while an adjustable screw can slowly open the lower one. The distance between the two branches can be adjusted from 5 mm (minimum) to 40 mm. Once the aperture is determined, a second screw fixes the moveable branch of the speculum. PFM forces are measured using two pairs of strain gauges glued on each side of the dynamometer lower branch.

For the evaluation of the PFM function, which refers to PFM parameters such as strength, endurance, speed of contraction and passive forces, the patient adopts a supine position, with hips and knees flexed and feet flat, on a conventional gynaecologist's table. The evaluator prepares the instrument by covering each branch with a latex condom and lubricating it with a hypoallergenic gel. The dynamometer is then inserted into the vagina to a depth of 5 cm, which allows the forces exerted by the pelvic floor musculature to be measured. PFM contraction results in lengthening or shortening of a strain gauge causing its electrical resistance to change, which in turn, is measured as a voltage variation. Voltage values from the strain gauge are amplified then digitized and converted into units of force (N). Then, a computer program (Numeri) presents the PFM force measurements in written and graphic form. Fig. 5.13 presents a typical recording of a pelvic floor strength measurement in a female subject (Dumoulin et al 2003).

More recently, Verelst & Leivseth (2004a, 2004b) developed a PFM dynamometer. The originality of this instrument is that it measures PFM forces in the transverse direction of the urogenital hiatus. Verelst and Leivseth's dynamometer consists of two semi-round parallel branches, one of which is spliced with a metal plate on which a strain gauge is glued. During PFM contraction, the metal plate is deformed and the various forces can be measured. Both branches can be opened to permit measurement from 30 mm to 50 mm of mediolateral opening. The sensor is connected to a signal processing system.

IN-VITRO CALIBRATION STUDIES

Only three investigators have reported conducting in vitro calibration studies for their PFM dynamometers (Rowe, Dumoulin, Verelst). Rowe reported that his device exhibited good linearity with a quantification accuracy of 0.07 N, a maximum experimental error of 0.3 N and minimum hysteresis for the range of forces from −5 N to +5 N. Output was found to drift by less than 0.14 N in 2 hours of continuous service and to be repeatable within and between days and at both room and body temperature (Rowe 1995).

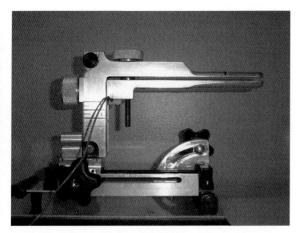

Fig. 5.12   Dynamometric speculum.

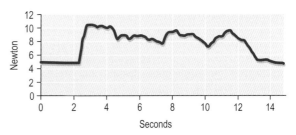

Fig. 5.13   Recording of a maximal PFM strength measurement.

Dumoulin's dynamometer was assessed for linearity, repeatability, ability to measure the resultant force independently of its point of application on the branch of the speculum, and hysteresis (Dumoulin et al 2003). The linearity proved excellent for a range of forces from 0 to 15 N, with regression coefficients close to unity ($R^2 = 0.999$). To evaluate the repeatability, the dynamometer was loaded twice with the same loading technique. The slopes and intercepts of the regression lines were not significantly different between loading trials, indicating the high reliability of these in-vitro measurements.

To verify that the force was measured independently of its exact site of application to the lower branch of the speculum, successive loading using the same loading technique was done at distances of 2.5 cm, 3.5 cm and 4.5 cm from the tip of the lower branch of the speculum. The slopes and intercepts of the regression lines in the three loading trials were not significantly different, confirming that the force measurement was independent of the force application site. Finally, the hysteresis was computed by dividing the maximum difference in voltage output between two loading conditions by the maximum scale output recorded with the highest load. The device exhibited minimal hysteresis of 0.000 06%. Furthermore, the output of the strain gauges was found to drift by less than 0.003 N in 1 hour of continuous service.

Verelst & Leivseth (2004b) reported very good linearity to 60 N with quantification of non-linearity of ±2% of rate output at temperatures ranging between 15 and 50°C, and resolution of 0.06 N. No further details regarding calibration techniques were given in either Rowe's or Verelst's paper.

TEST–RETEST RELIABILITY STUDIES

Only two investigators (Verelst and Dumoulin) have reported on test–retest reliability. With regard to Dumoulin's dynamometer, two studies were undertaken to evaluate the intra-rater test–retest reliability of the dynamometric strength, speed and endurance measurements of the PFM among women with persistent postpartum stress urinary incontinence (SUI) (Dumoulin et al 2004, Morin et al 2004a).

In the Dumoulin et al study, there were 29 female participants, primipara and multipara, aged between 23 and 42 years, presenting different severity levels of SUI (Dumoulin et al 2004). Of these, 17 reported episodes of urinary incontinence when coughing or sneezing or during physical exertion or effort but did not demonstrate any involuntary leakage in the provocative stress test. The others (n = 12) reported the same symptoms but had involuntary leakage in the provocative stress test. Strength, speed and endurance evaluations using the new PFM dynamometer were repeated in three successive sessions by the same evaluator.

For the strength measurements, participants were instructed to contract their PFM as hard as they could for 10 s. Standard verbal encouragement was given throughout the effort (Dumoulin et al 2004). Maximal strength values were recorded at three dynamometer openings (0.5 cm, 1.0 cm and 1.5 cm between the two dynamometer branches).

The endurance measurement consisted of a 1-min maximum contraction with standardized verbal encouragement. The participants were instructed to contract as hard and as fast as possible while breathing in and out for 60 s. The maximal rate of force development (MRFD) or rapidity of PFM contraction and the percentage of strength lost after 10 s and 60 s were computed from the endurance trial (Dumoulin et al 2004).

The generalizability theory (Shavelson 1988) was applied to estimate the reliability of the PFM measurements. The reliability was quantified by the index of dependability (Φ) and the corresponding standard error of measurement (SEM) for the mean of three trials performed in one session for the strength measurements and one trial completed in one session for the endurance and speed measurements. Results are presented in Tables 5.3 and 5.4.

For the maximal strength measurements, the largest coefficient of dependability, with a value of 0.88, was obtained at the 1.0-cm opening. The corresponding SEM reached 1.49 N. Regarding the endurance measurements, the reliability of the MRFD was also very good, with a coefficient of 0.86 and an SEM of 0.056 N/s.

Table 5.3 Dependability index (Φ) and standard error of measurement (SEM) for the strength measurements at different dynamometer openings

Strength measurement	Dynamometer opening (cm)		
	0.5	1.0	1.5
Φ	0.71	0.88	0.76
SEM (N)	1.22	1.49	2.11

Table 5.4 Dependability index (Φ) and standard error of measurement (SEM) for the endurance measurements

	Endurance measurement		
	MRFD	Loss of strength % after 10 s	Loss of strength % after 60 s
Φ	0.86	0.38	0.10
SEM	0.056 N/s	15.71%	20.75%

MRFD, maximal rate of force development.

However, the strength loss measurements at 10 s and 60 s were unreliable, with coefficient values of only 0.38 and 0.10 respectively (Dumoulin et al 2004).

In the study by Morin et al 19 women with SUI, six of them primipara and 13 multipara, aged between 23 and 41 years, were recruited at Ste-Justine Hospital in Montreal (Morin 2004a). Stress incontinence was confirmed by the 20-min pad test with standardized bladder volume (Abrams 1988, Sand 1992) and the absence of detrusor overactivity was verified by cystometry. Two sessions to assess the speed of contraction and endurance by different techniques to those used in the study of Dumoulin et al (2004) were conducted at 8-week intervals by a single evaluator. In the endurance test, the maximum sustained contraction was prolonged to 90 s (Morin 2004a) and the normalized area under the force curve was taken as the endurance parameter: (area under the curve/maximal strength) × 100. For the speed measurements, the women were instructed to contract maximally and relax as fast as possible for 15 s (Morin 2004a). The speed of contraction was quantified by the MRFD of the first contraction and the number of full contractions performed during the 15-s period. The maximum strength during the speed test was also extracted from the curves (Morin 2004a). The reliability of the data was evaluated using the generalizability theory (Shavelson 1988). These estimates are reported for one measurement session involving one trial (Table 5.5).

The normalized area under the force curve showed good reliability with a coefficient of 0.81 and an SEM of 298%. For the speed measurements, the range of observed coefficients of dependability from 0.79 to 0.92 indicates a good to very good test–retest reliability. The associated SEM for the rate of force development, number of contractions and maximum strength were 1.39 N/s, 1.4 contractions and 1.00 N respectively.

The results of these two studies show that the test–retest reliability of the PFM parameters (maximum strength, speed and endurance measurements) was high enough for future investigations into pelvic floor reha-

Table 5.5 Dependability index (Φ) and standard error of measurement (SEM) for the speed and endurance measurements

	Speed measurement		Endurance measurement	
	MRFD	Number of contractions	Maximal strength	Normalized area under the curve
Φ	0.92	0.79	0.79	0.81
SEM	1.39 N/s	1.4	1.0 N	298%

MRFD, maximal rate of force development.

bilitation programmes (Dumoulin et al 2004, Morin et al 2004a).

Verelst & Leivseth (2004b) completed an intra-rater test–retest reliability study of dynamometric strength measurements of the PFM in the transverse direction of the urogenital hiatus. Twenty healthy parous women volunteers with no history of urinary incontinence participated in the study. Dynamometric measurements were taken with a consecutively increasing diameter in the transverse plane at 30, 35, 40, 45 and 50 mm. The procedure was repeated with 2- to 4-day intervals. Within-subject day-to-day variability at all dynamometer openings tested was non-significant, indicating that the measurements were reliable, the 40-mm dynamometer opening being the most favourable (Verelst & Leivseth 2004b).

Although the intra-rater reliability of dynamometric measurements has been studied quite extensively for different PFM functional tests and in different populations, the inter-rater reliability of dynamometric measurements remains to be investigated.

Acceptance

Dumoulin et al assessed women's acceptance of the dynamometric measuring procedure during the course of their test–retest reliability study. The subjects' unanimous appreciation when asked to comment on the measurement procedure implied that the instrument was acceptable and that the measuring procedure was not painful (Dumoulin et al 2004).

VALIDITY STUDIES

Only one investigator team, Morin et al, has reported on the validity of the dynamometer developed by Dumoulin.

Validity criterion: To date, there is no recognized gold standard for evaluating PFM function so it is impossible to evaluate the dynamometric instrument's validity criterion. Consequently, validation of the PFM dynamometer has to rely on the construct validity, which Dunn (1989) has defined as the extent to which a test can be proven to measure a hypothetical construct (the PFM function, in this case). Various studies need to be performed to support the construct validity, namely correlation with another instrument and the Known Groups Method (Nunnally & Bernstein 1994, Portney & Watkins 2000).

Convergent validity: A study was carried out to compare the new dynamometer with the digital assessment for evaluating pelvic floor maximum strength (Morin et al 2004b). The focus of this approach is convergent validity, one of several components of construct validity (Nunnally & Bernstein 1994, Portney & Watkins 2000). Digital assessment was chosen over other tools because it is the approach currently used by most physiotherapists to evaluate pelvic floor function. Thirty continent women and 59 women with SUI, aged between 21 and 44 years, participated in the study. Spearman's rho coefficients were calculated to assess the correlation between the dynamometric and the modified Oxford grading system (Laycock 1992). Significant correlations were found between the two measurements with coefficients of $r = 0.727$, $r = 0.450$ and $r = 0.564$ for continent, incontinent and all women, respectively ($p < 0.01$). According to the standards proposed by Portney & Watkins (2000), these correlations can be defined as moderate to good.

In conclusion, the significant relations observed between digital and dynamometric assessments support some of the various aspects of construct validity of the dynamometric speculum.

Sensitivity and specificity

Known groups method: This type of construct validity focuses on the ability of the new instrument to discriminate between groups that are known to be different (Dunn 1989, Portney & Watkins 2000). In other words, if the new dynamometer proved capable of differentiating between the PFM function of continent women and women with SUI, this would support its validity (Morin et al 2004c).

Thirty continent women and 59 women with SUI, aged between 21 and 44 and parous, were recruited. A 20-min pad test was performed to confirm continence in the asymptomatic women and to appreciate the severity of incontinence in the women who had reported leakage. A conventional urodynamic examination was also carried out on the incontinent women to exclude those experiencing uninhibited detrusor contractions.

The new dynamometer was used to assess the following static parameters of the PFM: (1) passive force, (2) maximal strength in a self-paced effort, (3) rate of force development and number of contractions during a protocol of rapidly repeated 15-s contractions and, lastly, (4) absolute endurance recorded over a 90-s period during a sustained maximal contraction.

Analyses of covariance were used to control the confounding variables of age and parity when comparing the PFM function in the continent and incontinent women. The incontinent women demonstrated a lower passive force and absolute endurance than the continent women ($p \leq 0.001$). In the protocol of rapidly repeated contractions, the rate of force development and number of contractions were both lower among the SUI subjects ($p \leq 0.01$).

In conclusion, the capacity of the dynamometer to discriminate between women with SUI and continent postpartum women confirms further aspects of construct validity.

CONCLUSION

Although the new dynamometer seems a highly promising tool for assessing PFM function, it is not yet available commercially. Psychometric evaluation is still in progress and further inter-rater reliability and validation studies are required. The effect of intra-abdominal pressure on dynamometric measurements needs to be investigated. During coughing or straining, an increase in force is recorded by the dynamometer. This is probably caused by a reflex contraction in the PFM during effort and tension coming from vaginal tissues. Thus intra-abdominal pressure might influence the force recording. Whether this systematic bias is important and can be compensated for needs to be studied in more depth.

CLINICAL RECOMMENDATIONS

- Inform and explain the procedure to the patient.
- After the patient has undressed, ask her to adopt a supine lying position, with hips and knees flexed and supported, and feet flat on a treatment table.
- Before insertion of the dynamometer, give detailed instructions about contracting the PFM using anatomical models, drawings or vaginal palpation.
- Prepare the dynamometer by covering each branch of the speculum with a condom and lubricating it with a hypoallergenic gel.
- Bring the two branches of the measuring device to minimum opening and insert the dynamometer gently into the vaginal cavity in an anteroposterior axis to a depth of 5 cm.
- Separate the two branches with the screw to obtain the appropriate opening.
- Allow some time for the woman to get used to the unit inside the vagina and time for practice before recording a PFM contraction.
- Ask the patient to breathe normally and then to squeeze and lift the pelvic floor musculature as if preventing the escape of flatus and urine while recording.
- Give positive feedback throughout measurement of strength, endurance and coordination.
- After the evaluation session, discard the condoms and disinfect the dynamometer.

REFERENCES

Abrams P, Blaivas J G, Stanton S L et al 1988 The standardisation of terminology of lower urinary tract function. The International Continence Society Committee on Standardisation of Terminology. Scandinavian Journal of Urology Nephrology Supplementum 114:5–19

Ashton-Miller J A, DeLancey J O L, Warwick D N 2002 Method and apparatus for measuring the properties of the pelvic floor muscles. U.S. Patent No. 6,468,232 B1. Oct. 22, 2002

Bohanon R W 1990 Testing isometric limb muscle strength with dynamometers. Physical Therapy 2(2):75–86

Caufriez M 1993 Post-partum: rééducation urodynamique. Tome 3. Maïte Collection, Brussels, Belgium

Caufriez M 1998 Thérapies manuelles et instrumentales en urogynécologie. Brussels, Belgium

Dumoulin C, Bourbonnais D, Lemieux M C 2003 Development of a dynamometer for measuring the isometric force of the pelvic floor musculature. Neurourology and Urodynamics 22(7):648–653

Dumoulin C, Gravel D, Bourbonnais D et al 2004 Reliability of dynamometric measurements of the pelvic floor musculature. Neurourology and Urodynamics 23(2):134–142

Dunn W 1989 Reliability and validity. In: Miller L J (ed) Developing norm–referenced standardized tests. Haworth Press, New York, p 149–168

Howard D, DeLancey J O, Tynn R et al 2000 Racial differences in the structure and function of the stress urinary incontinence mechanism. Obstetrics and Gynecology 95:713–717

Laycock J 1992 Assessment and treatment of pelvic floor dysfunction [Doctoral thesis]. Bradford University

Morin M, Dumoulin C, Gravel D et al 2004a Test-retest reliability of speed of contraction and endurance parameters of the pelvic floor muscles using an instrumented speculum [Abstract #40]. Progrès en Urologie 3(3)

Morin M, Dumoulin C, Bourbonnais D et al 2004b Pelvic floor maximal strength using vaginal digital assessment compared to dynamometric measurements. Neurourology and Urodynamics 23(4):336–341

Morin M, Bourbonnais D, Gravel D et al 2004c Pelvic floor muscle function in continent and stress urinary incontinent women using dynamometric measurements. Neurourology and Urodynamics 23(7):668–674

Nunnally J C, Bernstein I H 1994 Psychometric Theory. 3rd edn. McGraw-Hill, p 83–113

Portney L G, Watkins M P 2000 Foundations of clinical research. Applications to practice. Prentice Hall, Boston, p 79–110

Rowe P 1995 A new system for the measurement of pelvic floor muscle strength in urinary incontinence. In: 12th International Congress of the World Confederation for Physical Therapy Abstract book: 1193

Sand P K 1992 The evaluation of incontinent females. Current Problems in Obstetrics, Gynecology and Fertility 15:107–151

Sampselle C, Miller J, Mims B et al 1998 Effect of pelvic muscle exercise on transient incontinence during pregnancy and after birth. Obstetrics and Gynecology 91:406–412

Shavelson R 1988 Generalizability theory: a primer. Sage Publications, California

Verelst M, Leivseth G 2004a Are fatigue and disturbances in pre–programmed activity of pelvic floor muscles associated with female stress urinary incontinence? Neurourology and Urodynamics 23(2):143–147

Verelst M, Leivseth G 2004b Force–length relationship in the pelvic floor muscles under transverse vaginal distension: a method study in healthy women. Neurourology and Urodynamics 23(7):662–667

Ultrasound in the assessment of pelvic floor muscle and pelvic organ descent

Hans Peter Dietz

INTRODUCTION

Ultrasound is increasingly used for the morphological and functional assessment of the muscles of the pelvic floor. Recent developments have greatly simplified the direct demonstration of the inferior parts of the levator ani (i.e. the pubovisceral muscle complex [puborectalis and pubococcygeus]) by ultrasound.

The advent of 3D ultrasound has given us access to the axial plane. 4D ultrasound now allows realtime imaging of the effect of maneouvres such as cough, Valsalva manoeuvre and pelvic floor muscle (PFM) contraction in any arbitrarily defined plane (Dietz 2004b). Most recently, volume contrast and speckle reduction algorithms as well as multislice or tomographic ultrasound imaging have enabled us to reach resolutions equivalent to magnetic resonance imaging (MRI) in all three dimensions, while delivering temporal resolution far above anything possible on MRI today.

This discussion will be limited to translabial or transperineal ultrasound, the only sonographic imaging modality to allow direct assessment of levator structure and function. Although transabdominal ultrasound has been used to describe levator activity (Thompson & O'Sullivan 2003), such an assessment is necessarily indirect and very limited.

TECHNIQUE

Translabial or perineal ultrasound (Dietz 2004c, Koelbl & Hanzal 1995, Schaer 1997) is performed by placing a transducer (usually a 3.5–5, 4–8 or 6–9 MHz curved array) on the perineum, after covering the instrument with a glove or thin plastic wrap for hygienic reasons. Powdered gloves can markedly impair imaging quality due to reverberations and should be avoided. Imaging can be performed in the dorsal lithotomy position, with the hips flexed and slightly abducted, or in the standing position. Bladder filling should be specified; for some applications prior voiding is preferable. The presence of a full rectum may impair diagnostic accuracy and sometimes necessitates a repeat assessment after bowel emptying. Parting of the labia may improve image quality.

The transducer can generally be placed quite firmly against the symphysis pubis without causing significant discomfort, unless there is marked atrophy. The resulting image includes the symphysis anteriorly, the urethra and bladder neck, the vagina, cervix, rectum and anal canal (Fig. 5.14). Posterior to the anorectal junction a hyperechogenic area indicates the central portion of the levator plate (i.e. the puborectalis/pubococcygeus or pubovisceral muscle). The cul de sac may also be seen, filled with a small amount of fluid, echogenic fat or peristalsing small bowel. Parasagittal or transverse views may yield additional information (e.g. enabling assessment of the puborectalis muscle and its insertion on the arcus tendineus of the levator ani [ATLA]).

BLADDER NECK POSITION AND MOBILITY

Bladder neck position and mobility can be determined with a high degree of reliability. Intra- and interobserver

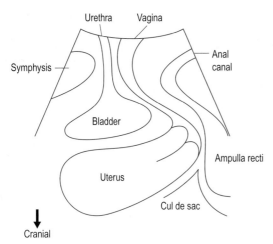

Fig. 5.14 Field of vision for translabial/perineal ultrasound, midsagittal plane. (From Dietz 2004c. © International Society of Ultrasound in Obstetrics and Gynecology. Reproduced with permission from John Wiley & Sons Ltd on behalf of the ISUOG.)

variability have been published, with a test–retest series on 50 young nulliparous women seen after a minimum interval of 4 weeks showing an intraclass correlation of 0.77 (Dietz et al 2005). This was confirmed in another series where an intraclass correlation of 0.79 was obtained in 47 women seen by two trained observers within 30 minutes (Dietz 2003).

It is essential, however, to ensure an adequate Valsalva manoeuvre. This means that the patient has to be coached to breathe in, hold her breath, and 'push as if you had to push a baby out' or 'push as if you had to pass a hard motion' to achieve adequate abdominal pressures. At the same time, one should ensure that the patient does not produce a concomitant levator contraction, which will result in artificially low values for pelvic organ descent. This is most common in young women with good PFM function and is evident as a reduction in the anteroposterior diameter of the levator hiatus, and as a posterior displacement of the prepubic fat pad, seen inferior or caudal to the inferior surface of the symphysis pubis, due to contraction of the superficial perineal muscles. Pressure on the transducer has to be reduced during a Valsalva manoeuvre to allow full descent of pelvic organs.

Points of reference are the central axis of the symphysis pubis (Schaer 1997) or its inferoposterior margin (Dietz 2004c). The former may be more accurate because measurements are independent of transducer position or movement; however, due to calcification of the inter-

pubic disc the central axis is often difficult to obtain in older women, reducing accuracy. There have been no comparative studies on repeatability of measurements to date.

Measurements of bladder neck position are generally performed at rest and on maximal Valsalva manoeuvre. The difference yields a numerical value for bladder neck descent (Fig. 5.15). On Valsalva manoeuvre, the proximal urethra may be seen to rotate in a posteroinferior direction. The extent of rotation can be measured by comparing the angle of inclination between the proximal urethra and any other fixed axis (see Fig. 5.15).

Fig. 5.16 illustrates how pelvic floor ultrasound can be used to quantify descent not just of the bladder neck and urethra, but also of the most dependent part of a cystocele, an enterocele or a rectocele.

There is no definition of 'normal' for bladder neck descent although cut-offs of 20 and 25 mm have been proposed to define hypermobility. Average measurements in women with stress incontinence are consistently around 30 mm (own unpublished data). Fig. 5.17 shows a relatively immobile bladder neck before a first delivery (left), and a marked increase in bladder neck mobility after childbirth (right). Bladder filling, patient position and catheterization have been shown to influence measurements, and it can occasionally be quite difficult to obtain an effective Valsalva manoeuvre, especially in nulliparous women (Dietz 2004c).

The aetiology of increased bladder neck descent is likely to be multifactorial. The wide range of values obtained in young nulliparous women suggests a congenital component, and a recently published twin study has confirmed a high degree of heritability for anterior vaginal wall mobility (Dietz et al 2005). Vaginal childbirth (Dietz & Bennett 2003, Meyer et al 1998, Peschers et al 1996) is probably the most significant environmental factor (see Fig. 5.17), with a long second stage of labour and vaginal operative delivery being associated with increased postpartum descent (Dietz & Bennett 2003). This association between increased bladder descent and vaginal parity is also evident in older women with symptoms of pelvic floor dysfunction (Dietz et al 2002a). Although the pelvic floor is undoubtedly affected by pregnancy and childbirth, labour and delivery are in turn affected by pelvic floor characteristics: anterior vaginal wall mobility on Valsalva manoeuvre has been found to be a potential predictor of delivery mode (Balmforth et al 2003, Dietz et al 2003).

LEVATOR ACTIVITY

Perineal ultrasound has been used for the quantification of PFM activity, both in women with stress incontinence

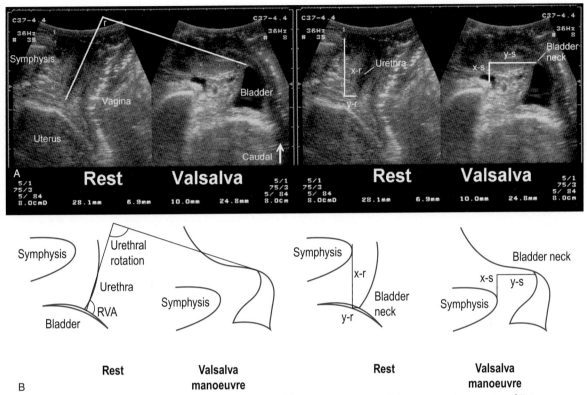

Fig. 5.15 Perineal ultrasound image (A) and line drawing (B), illustrating some of the measured parameters (distance between bladder neck and symphysis pubis [at rest: x-r and y-r, on Valsalva: x-s and y-s], urethral inclination and retrovesical angle [RVA]). (From Dietz 2004c. © International Society of Ultrasound in Obstetrics and Gynecology. Reproduced with permission from John Wiley & Sons Ltd on behalf of the ISUOG.)

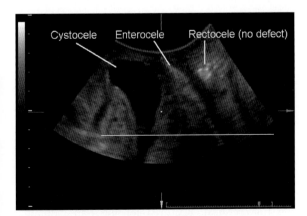

Fig. 5.16 Three-compartment prolapse as seen on translabial ultrasound. A line of reference is placed through the inferior margin of the symphysis pubis to enable quantification of prolapse. There is a cystocele with intact retrovesical angle, an enterocele and a 'false' rectocele due to perineal hypermobility. (© Dietz 2006.)

and in continent controls (Wijma et al 1991), as well as before and after childbirth (Dietz 2004a, Peschers et al 1997a). A cranioventral shift of pelvic organs imaged in a sagittal midline orientation is taken as evidence of a levator contraction (Dietz 2004c). The resulting displacement of the internal urethral meatus is measured relative to the infero-posterior symphyseal margin (Fig. 5.18). In this way pelvic floor activity is assessed at the bladder neck. Another means of quantifying levator activity is to measure reduction of the levator hiatus in the midsagittal plane, or the change in the main hiatal plane relative to the central symphyseal axis.

Ultrasound can also be used for PFM exercise teaching by providing visual biofeedback (Dietz et al 2001). The technique has helped validate the concept of 'the knack' (i.e. of a reflex levator contraction immediately before increases in intra-abdominal pressure such as those resulting from coughing; Miller et al 1996).

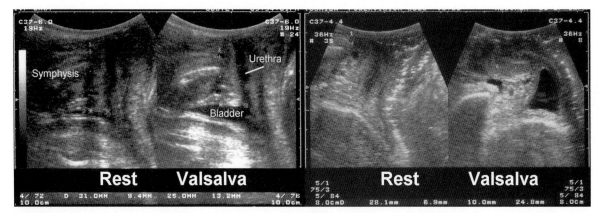

Fig. 5.17 Immobile bladder neck (bladder neck descent [BND] 6 mm) before first delivery (left pair of images), and a marked increase in bladder neck mobility (BND 38.1 mm) after childbirth (right pair of images). (From Dietz & Bennett 2003, with permission.)

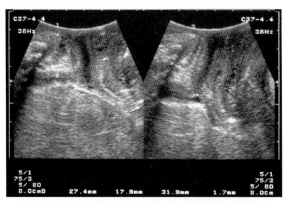

Fig. 5.18 Quantification of levator contraction: cranioventral displacement of the bladder neck is measured relative to the inferoposterior symphyseal margin. The measurements indicate 4.5 (31.9–27.4) mm of cranial displacement and 16.2 (17.9–1.7) mm of ventral displacement of the bladder neck. (From Dietz 2004c, with permission. © International Society of Ultrasound in Obstetrics and Gynecology. Reproduced with permission from John Wiley & Sons Ltd on behalf of the ISUOG.)

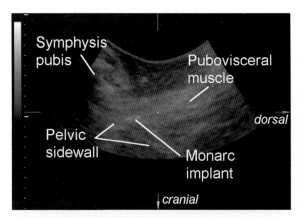

Fig. 5.19 Demonstration of the pubococcygeus/ puborectalis complex by oblique parasagittal imaging. In this case, there is a transobturator tape (Monarc) perforating the most inferomedial aspects of the muscle close to its insertion on the arcus tendineus of the levator ani. This orientation can be used to directly observe shortening of the pubovisceral muscle complex on contraction. (© Dietz 2006.)

Correlations between cranioventral shift of the bladder neck on the one hand and palpation/perineometry on the other have been shown to be good (Dietz et al 2002b). A recent study comparing transabdominal and transperineal ultrasound for the visualization of PFM activity showed good repeatability of both techniques (intra-class correlation coefficient [ICC] 0.91 for the transperineal, ICC 0.93 for the transabdominal approach) (Thompson et al 2005).

Finally, direct visualization of a levator contraction and shortening of fibres is possible on 2D ultrasound using an oblique parasagittal plane (Fig. 5.19), although there are no published reports on this technique.

PROLAPSE QUANTIFICATION

Translabial ultrasound can demonstrate uterovaginal prolapse (Dietz et al 2001). The inferior margin of the symphysis pubis serves as a line of reference against which the maximal descent of bladder, uterus, cul de sac and rectal ampulla on Valsalva manoeuvre can be measured (see Fig. 5.16). Findings have been validated against clinical staging and the results of a standardized assessment according to criteria developed by the International Continence Society, with good correlations shown for the anterior and central compartments (Dietz et al 2001). Although there may be poorer correlation between posterior compartment clinical assessment and ultrasound, it is possible to distinguish between 'true' and 'false' rectocele (i.e. a true fascial defect of the rectovaginal septum, and perineal hypermobility without fascial defects; Steensma & Dietz 2004a, b). Hopefully the ability to differentiate between different forms of posterior compartment descent will allow better surgical management in the future, not least because enterocele (see Fig. 5.16) can easily be distinguished from rectocele. Most recently, it appears that colorectal surgeons are starting to use the technique to complement or replace defecography (Beer-Gabel 2002), and perineal ultrasound can also be used for exoanal imaging of the anal sphincter (Peschers et al 1997b).

Disadvantages of the method include incomplete imaging of bladder neck, cervix and vault with large rectoceles and the possible underestimation of severe prolapse due to transducer pressure. Procidentia or complete vaginal eversion preclude translabial imaging. Occasionally, apparent anterior vaginal wall prolapse will turn out to be due to a urethral diverticulum, a vaginal cyst such as a Gartner duct cyst (cystic remnant of the mesonephric or Wolffian ducts), a cyst due to epithelial inversion after repair surgery, or even a vaginal fibroma.

3D PELVIC FLOOR IMAGING

3D and 4D pelvic floor ultrasound is currently performed using systems that have evolved around transducers that allow motorized acquisition. The first such motorized probe was developed in 1974, and by 1987 transducers for clinical use were becoming commercially available (Gritzky & Brandl 1998). The first system platform, the Kretz Voluson, was developed around such a 'fan scan' probe. With these types of transducer, automatic image acquisition is achieved by rapid oscillation of a group of elements, as with the abdominal and endovaginal probes used in systems such as the GE Kretz Voluson 730/730 expert series, Medison SA 8000–

9900 and Accuvix systems, Phillips IU 22 and HD 11 or Siemens sonoline G50/G60 systems. The results have been the abdominal and endovaginal probes used in systems such as the GE Kretz Voluson 730 series, the Philips HDI 4000 and the Medison SA 8000–9000 series. The widespread acceptance of 3D ultrasound in obstetrics and gynaecology was helped considerably by the development of such transducers because they do not require any movement relative to the investigated tissue during acquisition. A single volume obtained at rest with an acquisition angle of 70° or higher will include the entire levator hiatus with symphysis pubis, urethra, paravaginal tissues, the vagina, anorectum and pubovisceral muscle from the pelvic sidewall in the area of the ATLA to the posterior aspect of the anorectal junction (see Figs 5.20–5.25).

There has been some controversy as to whether to include the rectum in the levator hiatus (DeLancey 1993, Tunn et al 1999), but for practical purposes the levator hiatus as seen on translabial 3D/4D ultrasound or MRI is the plane of minimal dimensions between the symphysis pubis/pubic rami anteriorly and the pubovisceral muscle laterally and posteriorly. It is understood that this plane, strictly speaking, is not linear in all directions but very likely somewhat warped, especially anteriorly. For measurement purposes it appears most appropriate to select minimal anteroposterior hiatal dimensions in the midsagittal plane and then rotate to the axial plane at this level, an approach that is highly reproducible (Dietz et al 2005c, Majida et al 2006, Shek et al 2004, Yang et al 2006).

Depending on the dimensions of the hiatus and pubovisceral muscle, the field of vision may also include the anal canal and even the external sphincter. Of course

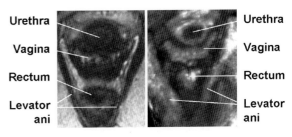

Fig. 5.20   The axial plane on magnetic resonance (MR) imaging (left) and ultrasound (US, freehand 3D, right). Although these images were obtained in different patients, all significant structures can be identified by both methods. (MRI image courtesy of Dr Ben Adekamni, Plymouth UK. From Dietz 2004b. © International Society of Ultrasound in Obstetrics and Gynecology. Reproduced with permission from John Wiley & Sons Ltd on behalf of the ISUOG.)

this also holds true for volumes acquired on levator contraction because this shortens the levator hiatus in the anteroposterior direction without altering its lateral dimensions significantly. A Valsalva manoeuvre however may result in lateral or posterior parts of the pubovisceral muscle being pushed outside the field of vision, especially in women with significant prolapse and hiatal areas over 40 cm^2 on Valsalva manoeuvre (see below). The currently offered abdominal 8–4 MHz volume transducer for Voluson 730 expert systems allows acquisition angles of up to 85°, ensuring that the levator hiatus can be imaged in its entirety even in women with significant enlargement ('ballooning') of the hiatus on Valsalva manoeuvre.

The main advantage of volume ultrasound for pelvic floor imaging is that the method gives access to the plane of the levator hiatus (i.e. the axial or transverse plane). Up until recently, pelvic floor ultrasound was limited to the midsagittal plane. Parasagittal (see Fig. 5.19) and coronal plane imaging (see Fig. 5.21, top right, for an example) have not been reported, which may be because there are no obvious points of reference, as opposed to the convenient reference point of the symphysis pubis on midsagittal views. The axial plane was accessible only on MRI (DeLancey et al 1999) (see Fig. 5.20 for an axial view of the levator hiatus on MRI and 3D ultrasound).

Imaging planes on 3D ultrasound can be varied in a completely arbitrary fashion to enhance the visibility of a given anatomical structure, either at the time of acquisition or offline at a later time. The levator ani usually requires an axial plane that is tilted in a cranioventral to dorsocaudal direction, and this is also true for imaging of the hiatus itself. The three orthogonal images (i.e. three planes at right angles to each other – sagittal, transverse and axial) are complemented by a 'rendered image' (i.e. a semitransparent representation of all volume pixels [voxels] in an arbitrarily definable 'box'). The bottom right hand image in Fig. 5.21 shows a standard surface rendered image of the levator hiatus, with the rendering direction set from caudally to cranially, which seems to be most convenient for imaging of the pubovisceral muscle. Midsagittal, axial and coronal views of the levator hiatus are given in the 'orthogonal' images in the top row and bottom left.

4D IMAGING

4D imaging implies the realtime acquisition of volume ultrasound data, which can then be represented in orthogonal planes or rendered volumes. Recently, it has become possible to save cine loops of volumes, which is of major importance in pelvic floor imaging because it

allows enhanced documentation of functional anatomy. Avulsion of the pubovisceral muscle from the ATLA is often more evident on Valsalva manoeuvre or levator contraction, and most significant pelvic organ prolapse is not visible at rest in the supine position. Fascial defects such as those defining a true rectocele (Dietz 2004b) usually only become visible on Valsalva manoeuvre.

The ability to perform a realtime 3D (or 4D) assessment of pelvic floor structures makes the technology potentially superior to MR imaging because the absence of realtime observation of manoeuvres means that patient compliance with instructions during MRI acquisition is impossible to ensure. Therefore, ultrasound has potential advantages when it comes to describing prolapse, especially when associated with fascial or muscular defects, and in terms of defining functional levator anatomy.

VOLUME CONTRAST IMAGING

Latest technical developments have focused mainly on the use of software algorithms as a means of improving resolutions and enhancing clinical applications. Different manufacturers use different proprietary terms such as 'volume contrast imaging (VCI)' and 'speckle reduction imaging (SRI)' to describe rendering algorithms employed to reduce speckle artefact (random noise) (Ruano et al 2004). Such algorithms may result in very

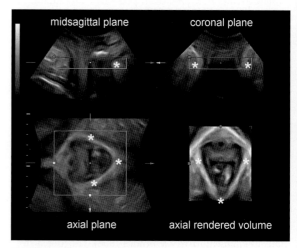

Fig. 5.21 The levator hiatus in three orthogonal planes (midsagittal on top right, coronal on top left, axial on bottom left) and as a rendered volume (bottom right). This case illustrates normal anatomy at rest. The pubovisceral muscle is marked with a star wherever it is visible in the different planes. (© Dietz 2006.)

significant gains in resolution, especially in the axial plane (see Figs 5.25 and 5.26). Tomographic or 'multi-slice' imaging or 'sonoCT' allow the representation of volume data in a series of slices of predetermined thickness and spacing, analogous to other cross-sectional imaging methods. Tomographic ultrasound is particularly useful in pelvic floor imaging as shown in Fig. 5.25. As a result of these developments, pelvic floor ultrasound has become more 'user-friendly' and has reached spatial resolutions very close to, if not similar to MR, while temporal resolutions are higher by several orders of magnitude.

CLINICAL RESEARCH USING 3D/4D PELVIC FLOOR ULTRASOUND

To date, there are few published data on imaging of the levator ani by 3D/4D ultrasound, and most of it has been accumulated over the last 3 years. We do know, however, what a normal, healthy pelvic floor in a nulligravid young woman looks like. In a series of 52 women aged 18–24 years, no significant asymmetry of the levator was observed, supporting the hypothesis that significant morphological abnormalities of the levator are likely to be evidence of delivery-related trauma (Dietz et al 2005c). Contrary to MRI data, there was no significant side difference, neither for thickness nor for area (Fielding et al 2000).

A number of biometric parameters of the puborectalis/pubococcygeus complex itself and of the levator hiatus were defined in this series (Dietz et al 2005c) and have recently been confirmed by others (Kruger et al 2000b, Majida et al 2006, Yang et al 2006). Results agreed with MRI data obtained in small numbers of nulliparous women for dimensions of the levator hiatus (Fielding et al 2000) and levator thickness (Tunn et al 1999). In a test–retest series, it became evident that diameter and area measurements of the pubococcygeus/puborectalis complex are less reproducible than measures of the levator hiatus. Possibly as a consequence, measures of muscle mass did not correlate with levator function as determined by displacement of the bladder neck on levator contraction.

Hiatal depth, width and area measurements (see Fig. 5.22) seem highly reproducible (ICC of 0.70–0.82) compared to muscle diameter (axial ICC 0.52, coronal 0.54) and cross-sectional area (axial ICC 0.44, coronal 0.45) (Dietz et al 2005c). Depth, width and area of the hiatus correlate strongly with pelvic organ descent, both at rest and on Valsalva manoeuvre (Dietz et al 2005c, Dietz & Steensma 2006). Although this is not surprising for the correlation between hiatal area on Valsalva manoeuvre and descent (because downwards displacement of

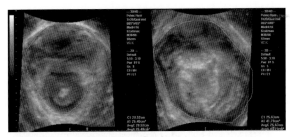

Fig. 5.22 Quantification of hiatal dimensions in a patient with a wide hiatus at rest (area 26.4 cm^2) and marked asymmetrical levator ballooning (to 41.8 cm^2) on Valsalva manoeuvre. Clinically, there was a recurrent large enterocele (which is visible as a large echogenic mass within the hiatus) and voiding dysfunction. (© Dietz 2006.)

organs may push the levator laterally), it is much more interesting that hiatal area at rest is associated with pelvic organ descent on Valsalva manoeuvre. These data constitute the first real evidence for the hypothesis that the state of the levator ani is important for pelvic organ support (DeLancey 2001), even in the absence of levator trauma.

The typical form of levator trauma, a unilateral avulsion of the pubovisceral muscle off the pelvic sidewall, is clearly related to childbirth (see Figs 5.23–5.25 and 5.27) and is palpable as an asymmetrical loss of substance in the anteromedial portion of the muscle. In the author's and others' experience (DeLancey, personal communication), digital evaluation for morphological abnormalities is not easy and requires significant operator experience (Dietz et al 2006b, Kearney et al 2006b). Bilateral defects (see Fig. 5.24) are even more difficult to palpate and much less common. In a recently completed study the author found that over one-third of women delivering vaginally suffered such injuries (Dietz & Lanzarone 2005), an incidence that is unexpectedly high compared to observations in older symptomatic women (Steensma & Dietz 2004b).

The clinical significance of such defects, however, remains in doubt. Own data suggest that levator avulsion is common (about 15% in parous women) which agrees approximately with comparable MRI data (DeLancey et al 2003). Defects were associated with anterior and central compartment prolapse, but not with urodynamic findings or symptoms of bladder dysfunction in a series of over 300 primary urogynaecological assessments (Dietz & Steensma 2006). Cross-sectional studies of levator anatomy in asymptomatic and symptomatic older women are needed to determine whether such abnormalities are associated with clinical symptoms or conditions in the general population. Another interesting question is whether major morphological

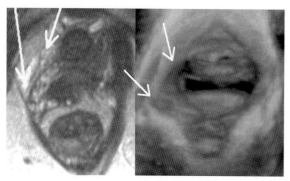

Fig. 5.23 Levator avulsion (arrows) on magnetic resonance imaging (MRI; left) and 3D ultrasound (right). Although these images were obtained in different patients, the appearances are typical in that a levator avulsion frequently seems to occur on the patient's right (left side of the images). (MRI image courtesy of Dr Ben Adekamni, Plymouth UK. From Dietz 2004b. © International Society of Ultrasound in Obstetrics and Gynecology. Reproduced with permission from John Wiley & Sons Ltd on behalf of the ISUOG.)

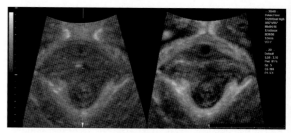

Fig. 5.24 Axial plane translabial imaging at rest, illustrating both a severe case of delivery-related pelvic floor trauma and the impact of the most recent technological developments in pelvic floor ultrasound. The left image shows a bilateral avulsion and complete loss of tenting bilaterally on conventional axial plane 3D ultrasound. The right image shows the same plane in the same volume dataset using volume contrast imaging (VCI). The patient has severe stress incontinence and prolapse 3 years after a rotational forceps delivery. (© Dietz 2006.)

abnormalities of the levator ani affect surgical outcomes. From experience to date, it appears to the author that major levator trauma (i.e. avulsion of the pubovisceral muscle from the pelvic sidewall) seems to be associated with early presentation and recurrent prolapse after surgical repair.

It is highly likely that levator avulsion injury is the missing link – or a large part of the missing link – between vaginal childbirth and female pelvic organ prolapse, with a relative risk of 6.6 recently defined by DeLancey's group (Margulies et al 2006). Not just the presence of defects, but defect width and depth are determinants of both objective prolapse and symptoms of prolapse (Dietz 2006). Neuropathic damage to the levator ani muscle probably exists, but we seem to have massively overestimated its importance relative to direct muscle trauma.

Of major interest is the recent observation of an almost linear relationship between maternal age at first delivery and levator trauma (Dietz & Lanzarone 2005, Dietz & Lekskulchai 2006, Kearney et al 2006), suggesting that the biomechanical properties of the muscle-bone interface may be of paramount importance. Every year of delayed childbearing increases the risk of levator injury by more than 10%. This implies that this risk triples or quadruples during the reproductive years, from below 15% shortly after menarche to over 50% at age 40. Vaginal operative delivery is a clear risk factor, almost doubling the injury rate at a given age (Dietz & Lekskulchai 2006).

OUTLOOK

The ready availability of axial plane imaging is likely to have a significant impact on conservative and surgical treatment paradigms for pelvic floor disorders. Since the 19th century, gynaecologists and surgeons have attempted to cure prolapse and incontinence by pushing organs cranially using a vaginal approach. Since the middle of the 20th century, pulling those organs up by means of sutures and/or mesh has become popular, and so far those methods seem to give the best long-term results in curing prolapse. Since the mid-seventies, the defect-specific approach blames all prolapse on distinct fascial defects and sets out to repair these discrete defects. Neither concept is entirely satisfactory, as evidenced by the large and growing number of techniques on offer.

Now largely forgotten, Bob Zacharin of Melbourne, Australia, developed a rather different approach in the 1960s and 70s. He appreciated the central role of the levator ani in pelvic organ support long before the advent of modern cross-sectional imaging and proposed focussing on levatorplasty as the primary means of curing pelvic organ descent (Zacharin 1980). Levatorplasty is rather unpopular at present, but it appears likely that an increased awareness of the importance of levator biomechanics and function may change this. It seems blatantly obvious to the observer of severe levator ballooning on Valsalva manoeuvre that poor levator resting tone and marked distensibility will not be cured by a Burch colposuspension or an abdominal vault suspension. Such women are destined for recur-

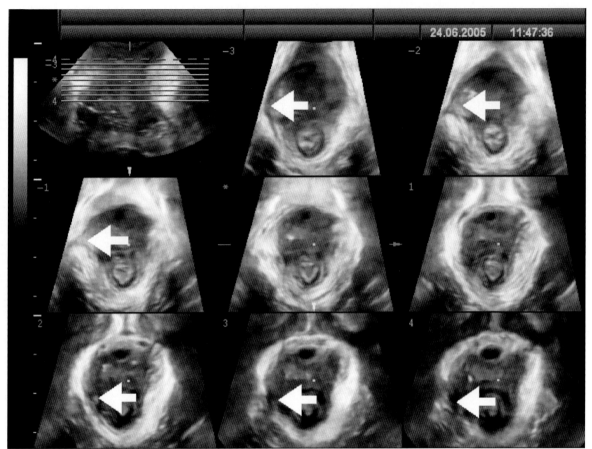

Fig. 5.25 Tomographic ultrasound imaging of a complex right-sided levator injury, imaged from 7.5 mm below to 10 mm above the plane of minimal dimensions. The slices are obtained at 2.5 mm intervals. There is a defect of the right pubovisceral muscle (arrows), involving both the lower three and the top three slices, with the central two slices appearing relatively normal, though the muscle is clearly thinner on the right. (© Dietz 2006.)

rence of prolapse, often in another location, but recurrence all the same. They undergo a vaginal hysterectomy with repairs, come back with incontinence, have a Burch colposuspension, come back with a rectoenterocele, have a sacrocolpopexy or sacrospinous fixation, and then come back with a large high cystocele or anterior enterocele, get an anterior mesh repair, which then erodes, until either they give up on us or we give up on them.

A focus on (and understanding of) functional levator anatomy may change all that. Clearly, in some women the pubovisceral muscle has to be the target of our therapeutic efforts, at least in an adjunctive sense. This may not have to involve the morbidity and technical difficulty of the original Zacharin procedure. Prediction of levator trauma appears feasible and prevention trials are already in progress, focusing either on elective caesarean section in high-risk women or on modification of biomechanical properties of the muscle-bone interface. Pelvic floor physiotherapy will have to play a major part in this regard. Secondary prevention has become at least theoretically feasible with the observation that major levator trauma can sometimes be diagnosed in the labour ward, provided it is not occult but overt due to a large vaginal tear (see Fig. 5.27).

Conventional suturing techniques are unlikely to be successful, but it would be rather premature to assume that the peculiar nature of this trauma should preclude successful surgical management. Conventional trauma management strategies require identification of trauma and early intervention, potentially opening up new indications for pelvic floor physiotherapy.

Conservative treatment may also be enhanced by an improved understanding of levator functional anatomy.

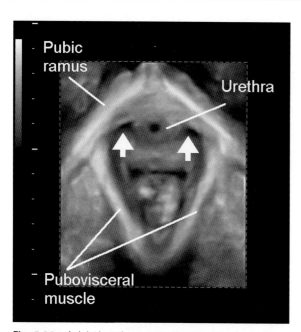

Fig. 5.26 Axial plane image representing the plane of minimal dimensions, showing the levator urethra gaps (arrows). These gaps are the key to palpating levator trauma. (© Dietz 2006.)

Our goal should be to increase resting tone and bulk of the pubovisceral muscle, reducing downwards displacement of pelvic organs and improving pressure transmission to the urethra – and there may be other ways of doing this than with conventional physical therapy. An increase in resting tone or stiffness and a reduction in hiatal dimensions may in theory be achievable by direct electrophysiological, pharmacological or surgical means. Axial plane imaging will hopefully deliver the means of optimizing treatment regimens to achieve these goals.

Some women suffer significant pelvic floor damage in labour, be it due to overdistension, avulsion or denervation of the pubovisceral muscle. In the future, we may be able to identify those women most at risk of such injury and intervene to prevent such damage from occurring in the first instance. In the meantime however, it appears that demographic trends, especially delayed childbearing and the obesity epidemic, are likely to further increase the incidence of such trauma.

CONCLUSIONS

Ultrasound imaging, and in particular translabial or transperineal ultrasound, has become an important research tool for assessing the levator ani. Although much information can be obtained easily and cheaply using 2D ultrasound systems, direct demonstration of the inferior aspects of the levator is much simplified by axial plane imaging (i.e. 3D/4D ultrasound). The availability of this technology is rapidly increasing, with tens

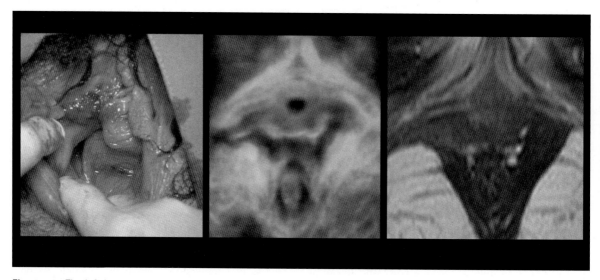

Fig. 5.27 The left image shows a major levator avulsion injury with concomitant large vaginal tear as diagnosed immediately after normal vaginal delivery. The defect is clearly evident 3 months postpartum, as shown on translabial 4D ultrasound (middle) and MR (right).

of thousands of such systems now installed worldwide. Most tertiary obstetrics and gynaecology units in the developed world (and increasingly in the developing world) have access to 3D capable systems, enabling them to obtain a functional and morphological assessment of the PFM with minimal discomfort to the patient and at little cost. Physiotherapists, urologists and gynaecologists are in the process of discovering the usefulness of such systems for their field. Undoubtedly, pelvic floor imaging by ultrasound provides a superior tool for research and clinical assessment. It will alter our perception of pelvic floor morbidity and hopefully enhance our means of treating it.

There is currently no evidence to prove that the use of modern imaging techniques improves patient outcomes in pelvic floor medicine. However, this limitation is true for many diagnostic modalities in clinical medicine. Due to methodological problems, the situation is unlikely to improve soon. In the meantime, it has to be recognized that any diagnostic method is only as good as the operator behind the machine, and diagnostic ultrasound is well known for its operator-dependent nature. Teaching is therefore of paramount importance to ensure that imaging techniques are used appropriately and effectively.

CLINICAL RECOMMENDATIONS

Pelvic floor imaging is unlikely to become a routine intervention in the hands of each and every clinical practitioner providing pelvic floor re-education, but it already is a very useful tool for research and the most convenient imaging method currently available. Below is a list of recommendations for the clinical use of 2D ultrasound equipment in assessing pelvic floor function via the translabial route. Recommendations for 3D/4D applications are available from the author on request.

Equipment

- Realtime B-mode capable diagnostic ultrasound system
- Cine loop function
- 3.5–6 Mhz curved array transducers with a footprint of at least 6 cm
- Black and white videoprinter, VHS recorder
- Nonpowdered gloves
- Ultrasound gel
- Alcoholic wipes for disinfection of probes between patients.

Examination

- Position patient supine (lithotomy position), with feet close to buttocks, and lower abdomen and legs covered with sheet for privacy.
- Examine after voiding (and defaecation if possible).
- Cover contact surface of transducer with gel, and then with glove/transducer cover while avoiding bubbles between the transducer and cover.
- Place the transducer in the midsagittal plane after parting the labia (if necessary).
- Ask the patient to cough to clear bubbles/detritus.
- Perform at least three manoeuvres (Valsalva manoeuvre, PFM contraction [PFMC]) each and watch for incorrect manoeuvres such as levator activation with Valsalva manoeuvre and vice versa.
- Observe presence/absence of 'the knack' (i.e. dorso-caudal movement of the prepubic fat pad and ventral movement of the posterior aspect of the pubovisceral muscle on coughing, which implies a reflex activation of the external perineal muscles and the levator ani).
- Provide biofeedback teaching – make the contraction look stronger on the monitor!
- Compare images and measurements at rest and on manoeuvre.

Documentation for assessment of PFMC

- Position of bladder neck at rest and on PFMC.
- Need for teaching/biofeedback, and success of teaching.
- Presence of reflex contraction on coughing ('the knack').

REFERENCES

Balmforth J, Toosz-Hobson P, Cardozo L 2003 Ask not what childbirth can do to your pelvic floor but what your pelvic floor can do in childbirth. Neurourology and Urodynamics 22(5): 540–542

Beer-Gabel M M D 2002 Dynamic transperineal ultrasound in the diagnosis of pelvic floor disorders: pilot study. Diseases of the Colon and Rectum 45(2):239–248

DeLancey J O 1993 Anatomy and biomechanics of genital prolapse. Clinical Obstetrics and Gynecology 36(4):897–909

DeLancey J O 2001 Anatomy. In: Cardozo L, Staskin D (eds) Textbook of female urology and urogynaecology. Isis Medical Media, London, p 112–124

DeLancey J O, Kearney R, Chou Q et al 2003 The appearance of levator ani muscle abnormalities in magnetic resonance images after vaginal delivery. Obstetrics and Gynecology 101(1):46–53

DeLancey J O, Speights S E, Tunn R et al 1999 Localized levator ani muscle abnormalities seen in MR images: site, size and side of occurrence. International Urogynecology Journal and Pelvic Floor Dysfunction 10(S1):S20–S21

Dietz H 2003 The female lower urinary tract and pelvic floor in pregnancy and puerperium. PhD, University of New South Wales

Dietz H 2004a Levator function before and after childbirth. The Australian & New Zealand Journal of Obstetrics & Gynaecology 44(1):19–23

Dietz H 2004b Ultrasound imaging of the pelvic floor: 3D aspects. Ultrasound in Obstetrics & Gynecology 23(6):615–625

Dietz H P 2004c Ultrasound imaging of the pelvic floor. Part I: two-dimensional aspects [Review]. Ultrasound in Obstetrics & Gynecology 23(1):80–92

Dietz H 2006 Classifying major delivery-related pelvic floor trauma. International Urogynecology Journal 17(S2):S124–S125

Dietz H P, Bennett M J 2003 The effect of childbirth on pelvic organ mobility [comment]. Obstetrics and Gynecology 102(2):223–228

Dietz H P, Clarke B, Vancaillie T G 2002a Vaginal childbirth and bladder neck mobility. The Australian & New Zealand Journal of Obstetrics & Gynaecology 42(5):522–525

Dietz H P, Hansell N, Grace M et al 2005a Bladder neck mobility is a heritable trait. British Journal of Obstetrics and Gynaecology 112:334–339

Dietz H P, Haylen B T, Broome J 2001 Ultrasound in the quantification of female pelvic organ prolapse. Ultrasound in Obstetrics & Gynecology 18(5):511–514

Dietz H P, Hay-Smith J, Hyland G 2006a Vaginal palpation and 3D pelvic floor ultrasound in the diagnosis of avulsion defects of the levator ani. Neurourology and Urodynamics. Accepted June 2006

Dietz H P, Hyland G, Hay-Smith J 2006b The assessment of levator trauma: A comparison between palpation and 4D pelvic floor ultrasound. Neurourology and Urodynamics 25(5):424–427

Dietz H P, Jarvis S K, Vancaillie T G 2002b The assessment of levator muscle strength: a validation of three ultrasound techniques. International Urogynecology Journal and Pelvic Floor Dysfunction 13(3):156–159

Dietz H P, Lanzarone V 2005b Levator trauma after vaginal delivery. Obstetrics and Gynecology 106:707–712

Dietz H, Lekskulchai O 2006 Does delayed childbearing increase the risk of levator injury in labour? Neurourology and Urodynamics 25:509–510

Dietz H P, Moore K H, Steensma A B 2003 Antenatal pelvic organ mobility is associated with delivery mode. Australian & New Zealamics Journal of Obstetrics & Gynaecology 43(1):70–74

Dietz H, Shek K, Clarke B 2005c Biometry of the pubovisceral muscle and levator hiatus by three-dimensional pelvic floor ultrasound. Ultrasound Obstetrics and Gynaecology 25:580–585

Dietz H P, Steensma A 2006 The prevalence and clinical significance of major morphological abnormalities of the levator ani. BJOG 113:225–30

Dietz H P, Wilson P D, Clarke B 2001 The use of perineal ultrasound to quantify levator activity and teach pelvic floor muscle exercises. International Urogynecology Journal and Pelvic Floor Dysfunction 12(3):166–168, discussion 168–169

Fielding J R, Dumanli H, Schreyer A G et al 2000 MR-based three-dimensional modeling of the normal pelvic floor in women: quantification of muscle mass. American Journal of Roentgenology 174(3):657–660

Gritzky A, Brandl H 1998 The Voluson (Kretz) technique. In: Merz E (ed) 3-D ultrasound in obstetrics and gynecology. Lippincott Williams and Wilkins Healthcare, Philadelphia, p 9–15

Kearney R, Miller J, Ashton-Miller et al 2006a Obstetric factors associated with levator ani muscle injury after vaginal birth. Obstetrics and Gynaecology 107(1):144–149

Kearney R, Miller J M, DeLancey J 2006b Interrater reliability and physical examination of the pubovisceral portion of the levator ani muscle, validity comparisons using MR imaging. Neurourology and Urodynamics 25(1):50–54

Koelbl H, Hanzal E 1995 Imaging of the lower urinary tract. Current Opinion in Obstetrics & Gynecology 7(5):382–385

Kruger J, Dietz H P 2006 A comparison of pelvic floor function in nulliparous elite athletes and nulliparous controls. ICS Annual General Meeting, Christchurch, New Zealand

Majida M, Hoff Braekken I et al 2006 3D and 4D ultrasound of the pelvic floor. An interobserver reliability study. International Urogynecology Journal 17(S2):S136–S137

Margulies R, Huebner et al 2006 Levator ani muscle defects: what origina and insertion points are affected? International Urogynecology Journal 17(S2):S110–S119

Meyer S, Schreyer A, De Grandi P et al 1998 The effects of birth on urinary continence mechanisms and other pelvic-floor characteristics. Obstetrics and Gynecology 92(4 Pt 1):613–618

Miller J, Ashton-Miller J O 1996 The knack: Use of precisely timed pelvic floor muscle contraction can reduce leakage in SUI. Neurourology and Urodynamics 15(4):392–393

Peschers U M, DeLancey J O, Schaer G N et al 1997b Exoanal ultrasound of the anal sphincter: normal anatomy and sphincter defects. British Journal of Obstetrics and Gynaecology 104(9):999–1003

Peschers U M, Schaer G N, DeLancey J O et al 1997a Levator ani function before and after childbirth. British Journal of Obstetrics and Gynaecology 104(9):1004–1008

Peschers U, Schaer G, Anthuber C et al 1996 Changes in vesical neck mobility following vaginal delivery. Obstetrics and Gynecology 88(6):1001–1006

Ruano R, Benachi A, Aubry M et al 2004 Volume contrast imaging: A new approach to identify fetal thoracic structures. Journal of Ultrasound in Medicine 23:403–408

Schaer G N 1997 Ultrasonography of the lower urinary tract. Current Opinion in Obstetrics & Gynecology 9:313–316

Shek K, Dietz H, Clarke B 2004 Biometry of the puborectalis muscle and levator hiatus by 3D pelvic floor ultrasound. Neurourology and Urodynamics 23:577–578

Steensma A B, Dietz H 2004a 3D pelvic floor ultrasound in the assessment of the levator ani muscle complex. Ultrasound in Obstetrics & Gynecology 24:258

Steensma A B, Dietz H 2004b The prevalence of defects of the rectovaginal septum. Ultrasound in Obstetrics & Gynecology 24:259

Thompson J A, O'Sullivan P B 2003 Levator plate movement during voluntary pelvic floor muscle contraction in subjects with incontinence and prolapse: a cross-sectional study and review. International Urogynecology Journal and Pelvic Floor Dysfunction 14(2):84–88

Thompson J, O'Sullivan P B, Briffa K et al 2005 Assessment of pelvic floor movement using transabdominal and transperineal ultrasound. International Urogynecology Journal and Pelvic Floor Dysfunction 16(4):285–292

Tunn R, DeLancey J O, Howard D et al 1999 MR imaging of levator ani muscle recovery following vaginal delivery. International Urogynecology Journal and Pelvic Floor Dysfunction 10(5):300–307

Wijma J, Tinga D J, Visser G H 1991 Perineal ultrasonography in women with stress incontinence and controls: the role of the pelvic floor muscles. Gynecologic and Obstetric Investigation 32(3):176–179

Yang J, Yang S, Huang W C 2006 Biometry of the pubovisceral muscle and levator hiatus in nulliparous Chinese women. Ultrasound in Obstetrics and Gynecology 26:710–716

Zacharin R F 1980 Pulsion enterocele: review of functional anatomy of the pelvic floor. Obstetrics and Gynecology 55(2):135–140

MRI of intact and injured female pelvic floor muscles

John O L DeLancey and James A Ashton-Miller

INTRODUCTION

Pelvic striated muscle activity is critical to normal continence and pelvic organ support. Three portions of the levator ani muscle support the pelvic organs and influence continence as described in Ch. 4. These muscles must constantly adjust to the widely varying stresses placed on the pelvic floor during daily activities that may range from sitting and reading, to jumping on a trampoline, to forcefully sneezing. This chapter will focus on the levator ani muscle damage seen after vaginal delivery and the implications of this damage for muscle rehabilitation.

Each muscle in the body has its own specific action. Knowing the functional loss that occurs when a muscle is injured is important to understanding the dysfunction that arises from muscle injury. When one of the levator ani muscle elements is damaged knowing how pelvic muscle training is influenced by muscle injury type has relevance to clinical therapy. If one muscle in the shoulder, for example, is damaged, there is a characteristic impairment that results. Damage to the pectoral muscle for example, would limit forward motion of the arm, while not limiting its backward movement. Now that MRI can show us evidence of localized muscle injury in an individual it will be possible to better understand the relationship between injury to a specific part of the muscle and specific female pelvic floor problems.

The mechanism of injury to a muscle may also influence its rehabilitation. If a muscle is weak it can be strengthened. If a portion of the muscle is partially denervated then the remaining muscle parts can be recruited to compensate for its muscle loss. If, on the other hand, an entire muscle is lost through avulsion from its attachment and subsequent atrophy or is lost through complete denervation, then it may not be possible to improve the function of the missing muscle. In the past, knowing how a given type of pelvic floor muscle injury would respond to treatment has not been possible because it has not been possible to visualize and locate the injury. Now, with the advent of modern imaging, we can directly see the pelvic floor muscles and their injuries. There is the very real possibility that failure rates with muscle training will decline as patients are more appropriately selected for treatment based on each individual's specific situation.

MRI ANATOMY OF THE NORMAL LEVATOR ANI MUSCLE STRUCTURE

The levator ani muscle consists of several parts. Each has its own origin and insertion. The suggested terms for these components, along with their origin/insertion and function, are listed in Table 5.6 based on a review of anatomical descriptions available in the literature (Kearney et al 2004). These are shown in Figs 5.28 and 5.29. Although these parts are simple and are described consistently by authors that have personally studied the muscle, a profusion of conflicting terms that have historically applied to this region makes it somewhat complicated to interpret the literature, as described in Kearney et al (2004).

The iliococcygeal muscle is a thin sheet of muscle that spans the pelvic canal from the tendinous arch of the pelvic fascia to the midline iliococcygeal raphe where it interdigitates with the muscle of the other side and connects with the superior surface of the sacrum and coccyx.

Arising from the pubic bone and passing beside the pelvic organs is the pubovisceral muscle. This muscle has previously been called the pubococcygeal muscle, but we favour Lawson's term 'pubovisceral' (Lawson 1974) because it describes the origin and insertion accurately, whereas the older term is based on evolutionary considerations rather than human anatomy. Within the pubovisceral muscle are parts that attach to the perineal body (puboperinealis), and a part that inserts into the anal canal and skin (puboanal). The vaginal wall is attached to this mass of muscle and those fibres to which the vaginal wall is attached belong to the pubovaginal portion of the pubovisceral muscle. Arising near the

Table 5.6   Overview of the nomenclature and functional anatomy of the levator ani

Terminologia Anatomica	Origin	Insertion	Function
Pubococcygeal (we favour 'puboviseral')			
Puboperineal	Pubis	Perineal body	Tonic activity pulls perineal body ventrally toward pubis
Pubovaginal	Pubis	Vaginal wall at the level of the mid-urethra	Elevates vagina in region of mid-urethra
Puboanal	Pubis	Intersphincteric groove between internal and external anal sphincter to end in the anal skin	Inserts into the intersphincteric groove to elevate the anus and its attached anoderm
Puborectal	Pubis	Sling behind rectum	Forms sling behind the rectum forming the anorectal angle and closing the pelvic floor
Iliococcygeal	Tendinous arch of the levator ani	Two sides fuse in the iliococcygeal raphe	The two sides form a supportive diaphragm that spans the pelvic canal

perineal membrane and coursing lateral to the remainder of the levator ani muscle is the puborectal muscle. It forms a sling behind the rectum and is distinct from the puboviseral muscle. While the puborectal muscle creates an angulation in the rectum, the puboviseral muscle elevates the anus, perineal body and vagina. (Lawson includes this muscle within the puboviseral muscle complex, but we prefer a separate designation because it has a very different muscle fibre direction.)

Each of these different origin/insertion pairs has its unique mechanical action. Injury to one component may have different mechanical effects than damage to another. For example, loss of the pubovaginal muscle would prevent elevation of the anterior vaginal wall (and urethra), while loss of the puborectal muscle would prevent kinking of the rectum in the post-anal angle. Therefore knowing their subdivisions will make a difference.

Magnetic resonance imaging (MRI) is a new and exciting investigative tool that provides anatomical detail in the pelvic floor. It has, for the first time, allowed the detailed anatomy and integrity of the levator ani muscles to be examined. Not only has this technique revealed important insights about normal anatomy, but it also allows investigators to study muscle damage while providing permanent records of muscle morphology that can be evaluated by researchers blinded to the

subject's clinical status, minimizing potential observer bias. Systematic studies concerning repeatability of these techniques, their validity and their responsiveness to change are yet to be carried out. However, the detailed anatomical information that can be gained from these techniques has already established their use in research, and data concerning the performance of these measures are certain to be forthcoming.

MRI APPEARANCE OF THE LEVATOR ANI MUSCLES

Damage to the levator ani muscle has been described in cadavers with pelvic organ prolapse for 100 years (Halban & Tandler 1907). Matched cross-sections of a cadaver pelvis and MR images clarified the anatomy of the levator ani muscles in cross-sectional imaging (Strohbehn et al 1996). Recent advances in MRI have allowed the muscles to be examined and demonstrated the anatomy of the muscles in 2D images (Fig. 5.30) and in 3D reconstructions (Fig. 5.31) (Hoyte et al 2001, Kirschner-Hermanns et al 1993). These scans show considerable variation in the normal thickness and configuration of the muscle from one individual to another (Tunn et al 2003) (Fig. 5.32). As is true in other parts of the body this variation in muscle bulk is likely attribut-

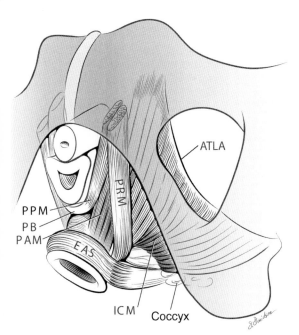

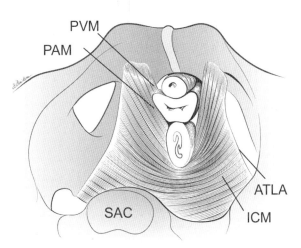

Fig. 5.28 Schematic view of the levator ani muscles from below after the vulvar structures and perineal membrane have been removed showing the arcus tendineus levator ani (ATLA); external anal sphincter (EAS); puboanal muscle (PAM); perineal body (PB) uniting the two ends of the puboperineal muscle (PPM); iliococcygeal muscle (ICM); puborectal muscle (PRM). Note that the urethra and vagina have been transected just above the hymenal ring. (From Kearney et al 2004. © DeLancey 2003.)

Fig. 5.29 The levator ani muscle seen from above looking over the sacral promontory (SAC) showing the pubovaginal muscle (PVM). The urethra, vagina, and rectum have been transected just above the pelvic floor. PAM, puboanal muscle; ATLA, arcus tendineus levator ani, ICM, iliococcygeal muscle. (The internal obturator muscles have been removed to clarify levator muscle origins.) (From Kearney et al 2004. © DeLancey 2003.)

able to a combination of genetic factors, daily demands and exercise. The amount of muscle that an individual has should have implications for pelvic floor function and injury. A woman with a naturally bulky set of muscles may lose half of her muscle bulk due to injury or atrophy and still have the same amount of muscle as a woman with naturally delicate muscles. The consequences of these variations and damage remain to be determined.

BIRTH IS A MAJOR EVENT CAUSING PELVIC FLOOR DYSFUNCTION

Vaginal birth increases the likelihood that a woman will have pelvic floor dysfunction (Mant et al 1997, Rortveit et al 2003) and vaginal birth has been identified as a cause of damage to the muscle (DeLancey et al 2003). The levator ani muscles and pelvic floor undergo

remarkable changes during the second stage of labour to dilate sufficiently for the fetal head to be delivered. Understanding how injury can occur and how recovery does or does not proceed are central to understanding the role of rehabilitation.

Recovery after vaginal birth

Pelvic muscle training is a mainstay of recovery after vaginal birth, decreasing incontinence and improving muscle function more rapidly than occurs without regular exercise (Mørkved et al 2003, Sampselle et al 1998). Imaging has allowed us to study the process of normal recovery and has given insight into changes the muscle must undergo to return to its normal healthy state.

Soon after delivery the pelvic floor sags and the urogenital hiatus is wider than normal (Fig. 5.33) (Tunn et al 1999). Muscle recovery results in resumption of the near-normal position in most women over the course of the first 6 months, the time when normal pelvic muscle strength also returns to normal (Sampselle et al 1998). Chemical changes in the muscle where there is increased fluid from edema in certain muscle parts early in the recovery reveal the changes in muscular tissue during the normal healing process (Fig. 5.34).

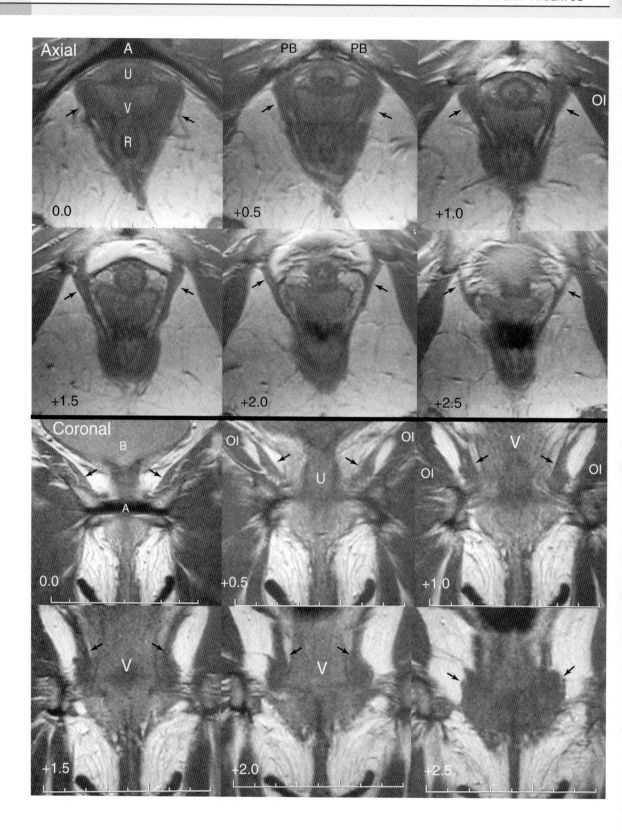

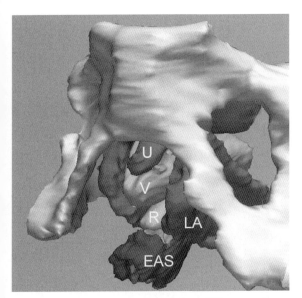

Fig. 5.31 View of 3D model made from MRI scans of a 34-year-old woman with normal anatomy showing the urethra (U), vagina (V), anal sphincter (AS), rectum (R), and levator ani (LA). (© DeLancey 2005.)

Injury from vaginal birth

In a study of primiparous women 32 of 160 primiparous women (20%) had damage to the levator ani muscles (DeLancey et al 2003). A nulliparous control group of 80 women was also studied, and none of these women had injuries; identifying birth as a cause of the type of levator ani muscle injury seen in women with pelvic floor dysfunction (Hoyte et al 2001). Twenty-nine of these visible injuries occurred in the pubovisceral muscle and only three of these were in the iliococcygeal portion of the muscle (Fig. 5.35). This was a study originally designed to study stress incontinence: equal numbers of women that had developed de-novo stress incontinence and women that remained continent after their first birth

Fig. 5.30 Axial and coronal images from a 45-year-old nulliparous woman. The urethra (U), vagina (V), rectum (R), arcuate pubic ligament (A), pubic bones (PB), and bladder (B) are shown. The arcuate pubic ligament is designated as zero for reference, and the distance from this reference plane is indicated in the lower left corner. Note the attachment of the levator muscle (arrows) to the pubic bone in axial 1.0, 1.5, and 2.0. Coronal images show the urethra, vagina, and muscles of levator ani and obturator internus (OI). (From DeLancey et al 2003. © DeLancey 2002.)

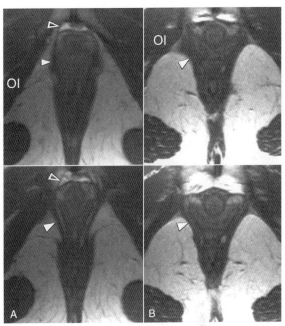

Fig. 5.32 Axial section at level of middle urethra showing difference in levator ani muscle thickness and configuration. In this and subsequent illustrations, scans from two individuals are compared; scans from one individual are displayed on the left, and scans from the other individual are displayed on the right: (A) thin muscle (31-year-old nulliparous woman); (B) thicker muscle (36-year-old nulliparous woman). Note that the muscle is shaped more like a V in A and more like a U in B. Closed arrowhead, right levator ani muscle; open arrowhead, insertion of arcus tendineus fasciae pelvis into pubic bone in B. (From Tunn et al 2003. © DeLancey 2002)

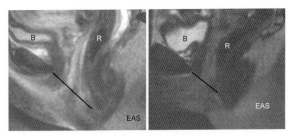

Fig. 5.33 T2-weighted sagittal sections of an 18 year-old woman, para 2, 1 day (left) and 6 months (right) after spontaneous vaginal delivery. The external anal sphincter (EAS) and perineal body that lies ventral to it are much lower in the first day after delivery compared with the anatomy 6 months later and the urogenital hiatus is also larger (line). (From Tunn et al 1999. © DeLancey 2005.)

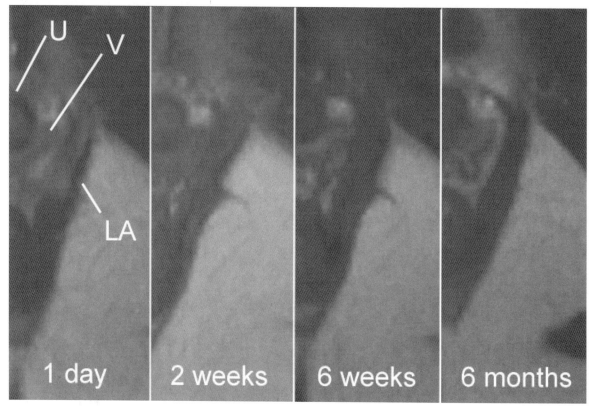

Fig. 5.34 Changes in muscle appearance following birth showing the left side of the pelvis at different time points after delivery. The urethra (U), vagina (V) and levator ani (LA) can be seen. Notice the increasing definition of the structures postpartum, especially the medial portion of the levator ani muscle adjacent to the vagina, which is quite pale 1 day after delivery, but recovers its signal by 6 months. (© DeLancey 2005.)

were recruited. Because the group with stress incontinence were twice as likely to have defects as the continent group, the occurrence of these defects in a group of primiparous women not over-sampled for stress incontinence would be somewhat lower than this figure. However, even if it were half, this still indicates that one in ten women delivering their first infant would have levator damage. In a more recent study, Dietz & Lanzarone (2005) have evaluated women both before and after vaginal birth using 3D ultrasound and have confirmed that these types of injury occur during vaginal delivery.

Among the women with injury to the pubovisceral muscle the amount of muscle injury varies from one individual to another. Some of these injuries involve complete bilateral loss of pubovisceral muscle bulk (see Fig. 5.35) while others have only unilateral loss (Fig.

5.36). There is also variation in the amount of architectural distortion that occurs. Some individuals show major changes in the overall architecture (Fig. 5.37) while others have intact spatial relationships (Fig. 5.38). Whether this represents the difference between a muscle rupture that distorts muscle appearance or denervation that simply results in loss of muscle without deformity, remains to be determined.

What are the mechanisms of levator injury?

There have been several suggestions for why the levator ani muscles might be injured. Information from electrodiagnostic techniques has demonstrated that birth causes changes in mean motor unit duration after vaginal birth (Allen et al 1990) as well as changes in pudendal terminal motor latency. Abnormal tests have

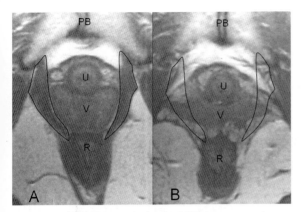

Fig. 5.35 (A) Axial proton density MRI shows normal pubococcygeal muscle with the muscle outlined at the level of the mid-urethra. (B) A similar image from a woman with complete loss of the pubococcygeal muscle (expected location of pubococcygeal muscle shown by outline). PB, pubic bone; R, rectum; U, urethra, V, vagina. (From DeLancey 2005. © DeLancey 2005.)

been seen in women with both prolapse and stress incontinence (Weidner et al 2000). Although the pudendal nerve innervates the voluntary urethral and anal sphincters, it does not innervate the levator ani muscles, which receive their own nerve supply from the sacral plexus (Barber et al 2002). At present it is not clear whether the visible levator defects are from neurological or stretch injury.

Recent computer models have suggested that some muscle damage during the second stage of labour may come from overstretching because those parts of the muscle that are stretched the most are those parts that are seen to be injured (Lien et al 2004). Using a computer model of the levator ani muscle based on anatomy from a normal woman, the degree to which individual muscle bands are stretched could be studied (Fig. 5.39). This analysis revealed that the muscle injured most often, the pubovisceral (pubococcygeal) portion was the portion of the muscle that underwent the greatest degree of stretch, and the second area of observed injury, the iliococcygeal muscle, was the second most stretched muscle. Furthermore, when the portion of the muscle at risk was identified in cross-sections cut in the same orientation as axial MRI scans, the pattern of predicted injury matched the injury seen in MRI (Fig. 5.40). These theoretical findings suggesting stretch-induced injury are supported by studies showing increased insulin-like growth factor-1 splice variants that indicate stretch and overload in women after a first vaginal birth (Cortes et al 2005).

WHAT ARE THE CLINICAL IMPLICATIONS OF LEVATOR ANI MUSCLE INJURY?

There are potentially both direct and indirect ways in which birth-induced levator injury may influence pelvic floor function. Pelvic organ support is provided by the combined action of the levator ani muscles and the endopelvic fascia. The levator ani closes the vagina by creating a high-pressure zone (Guaderrama et al 2005) similar to the high-pressure zones created by the urethral and anal sphincter muscles. The muscles and ligaments must resist the downward force applied on the pelvic floor by the superincumbent abdominal organs and the forces that arise from increases in abdominal pressure during cough, sneeze or from inertial loads placed on them when landing from a jump (for example). This normal-load sharing between the adaptive action of the muscles and the energy efficient action of static connective tissues is part of the elegant load-bearing design of the pelvic floor. When injury to one of these two components occurs, the other must carry the increased demands placed on it. When the muscle is injured, the connective tissue is subjected to increased load. If this load exceeds the strength of the pelvic tissues, they may be stretched or broken, and prolapse may result. This forms a causal chain of events by which pelvic muscle injury may influence pelvic organ prolapse or urinary incontinence. In addition, there is accumulating evidence that women operated on for pelvic organ prolapse or urinary incontinence have higher postoperative failure rates if they have levator ani muscle impairment assessed by biopsy (Hanzal et al 1993) or muscle function testing (Vakili et al 2005) than women who have normal muscles.

Birth-induced levator ani muscle injury may be accompanied by other types of injury that occurred during vaginal birth. A birth that was sufficiently difficult that it resulted in injury to the levator ani muscle may have also created injury to the connective tissue supports. This hypothesis is supported by observations made on the function of the urethral sphincter in women with injured levator ani muscle and also those with intact muscles (Miller et al 2004). In this study of 28 women with normal muscles and 17 women with complete bilateral pubovisceral muscle loss, women with intact muscles generated a greater increase in urethral pressure during a maximal pelvic muscle contraction than those with absent pubovisceral muscles (14 ± 11 vs 6 ± 9 cmH$_2$O) (Table 5.7). This difference in the ability to increase pressure came from the fact that more of the women (86%) were able to elicit a measurable increase (>5 cmH$_2$O) in urethral closure than those with missing

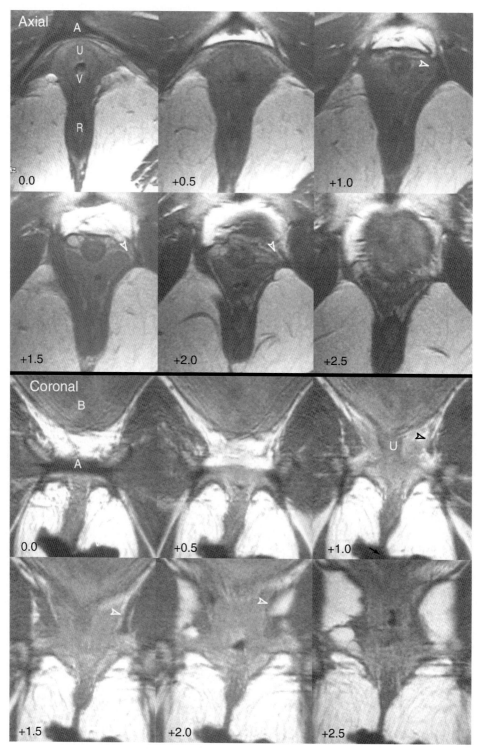

Fig. 5.36 Axial and coronal images from a 34-year-old incontinent primiparous woman showing a unilateral defect in the left puboviseral portion of the levator ani muscle. The arcuate pubic ligament (A), urethra (U), vagina (V), rectum (R), and bladder (B) are shown. The location normally occupied by the puboviseral muscle is indicated by the open arrowhead in axial and coronal images 1.0, 1.5, and 2.0. (From DeLancey et al 2003. © DeLancey 2002.)

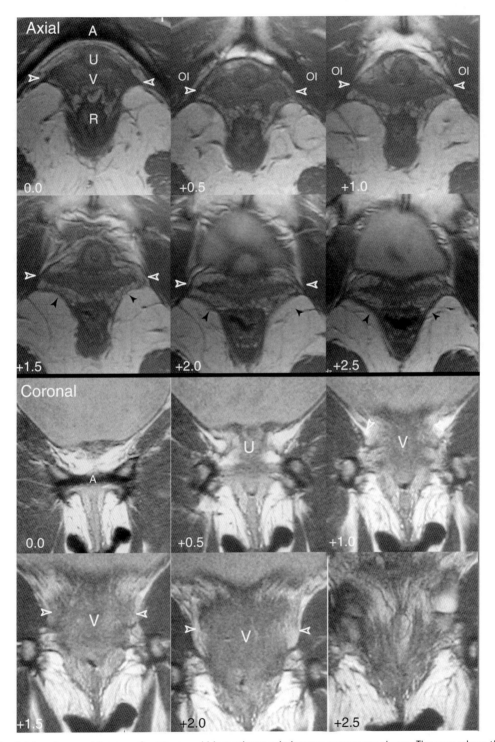

Fig. 5.37   Axial and coronal images of a 38-year-old incontinent primiparous woman are shown. The area where the puboviseral portion of the levator ani muscle is missing (open arrowhead) between the urethra (U), vagina (V), rectum (R), and obturator internus muscle (OI) is shown. The vagina protrudes laterally into the defects to lie close to the obturator internus muscle. A arcuate pubic ligament. (From DeLancey et al 2003. © DeLancey 2002.)

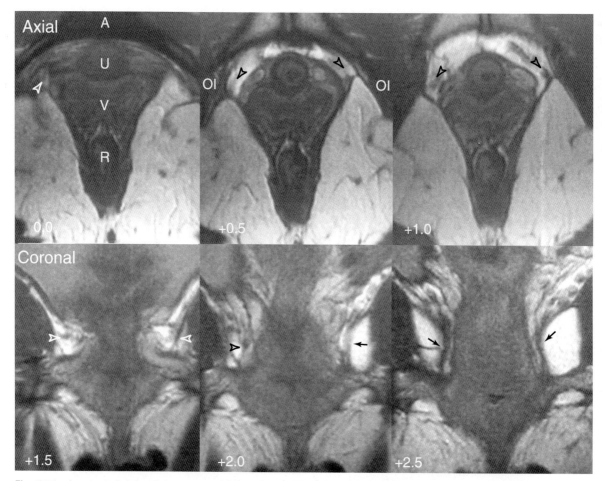

Fig. 5.38   Levator ani defect in a 30-year-old incontinent primiparous woman with loss of muscle bulk but preservation of pelvic architecture. The area where the levator is absent in this woman is shown (open arrowhead) in the axial images and the coronal images 1.5 and 2.0. Note that in contrast to Fig. 5.30, where the vagina lies close to the obturator internus (OI), it has a normal shape. The normal appearance of the levator ani muscle is seen in coronal images 2.0 and 2.5 (arrows). A, arcuate pubic ligament; R, rectum; U, urethra; V, vagina. (From DeLancey et al 2003. © DeLancey 2002.)

muscles (41%); among women that could increase urethral closure pressure, the increase in urethral closure pressure was the same. Women with complete levator muscle loss can volitionally elevate urethral pressure in the absence of the pubovisceral muscle (presumably using their still-intact striated urethral sphincter muscle), but fewer women are able to do this, suggesting the occurrence of sphincter injury as well in a subset of women in this group. This indicates that some women who are unable to contract their levator ani muscles due to muscle (or nerve) injury escape injury to the urethral sphincter (or pudendal nerve), whereas others do not,

and that this phenomenon occurs more often in women with muscle problems.

Issues in rehabilitation

'The injured patient is entitled to know at the outset, in general terms, what [her] injuries are, what the immediate treatment will be, and what may be the expected result' (Committee on Trauma, ACS 1961, p. 16) and 'The fate of the injured person depends to a large extent upon the initial care that [her] injuries receive. Skilled competent care may salvage function in seemingly

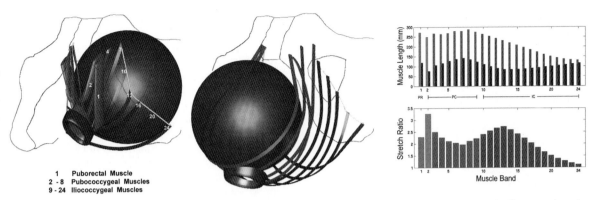

1   **Puborectal Muscle**
2 - 8   **Pubococcygeal Muscles**
9 - 24   **Iliococcygeal Muscles**

Fig. 5.39 On the left is a computer model of selected levator ani muscle bands before birth, with muscle fibres numbered and the muscle groups identified; the middle figure demonstrates muscle band lengthening present at the end of the second stage of labour; on the right is a graphic representation of the original and final muscle (top) and the stretch ratio (bottom), indicating the degree to which each muscle band must lengthen to accommodate a normal-sized fetal head. Note that the pubococcygeal muscle fascicles labelled 'PC2' undergo the greatest degree of stretch and would be the most vulnerable to stretch-induced injury. (From Lien et al 2004, with permission. © Biomechanics Research Laboratory 2005.)

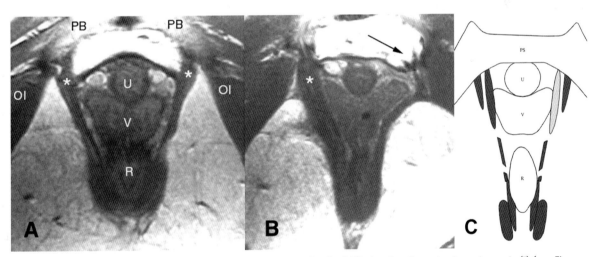

Fig. 5.40 (A) Normal anatomy in an axial mid-urethra proton density MRI showing the pubovisceral muscle (*) (see Fig. 5.28 for orientation). (B) Woman who has lost a part of the left pubovisceral muscle (displayed on the right side of the image, according to standard medical imaging convention) with lateral displacement of the vagina into the area normally occupied by the muscle. The arrow points to the expected location of the missing muscle. The puborectalis is left intact bilaterally. OI, obturator internus; PB pubic bone; R, rectum; U urethra, V vagina. In (C), an axial, mid-urethral section of the model through the arch of the pubic bone (see pubic symphysis [PS], top) and the model levator ani muscles corresponding to those from the patients shown in (A) and (B). Intact muscles are shown in dark grey. Simulated PC2 muscle atrophy is illustrated by the light grey shading of the left-side PC2 muscle. This location is shown to correspond with the location of muscle atrophy demonstrated in Fig. 5.33. R, rectum; U, urethra; V, vagina. (From Lien et al 2004, with permission. © Biomechanics Research Laboratory 2005.)

Table 5.7 Urethral closure pressure data in 28 women with intact pubovisceral muscles and 17 women with absent pubovisceral muscles (Adapted from Miller et al 2004)

	Pubovisceral muscle intact	Pubovisceral muscle absent
Pressure increase >5 cmH$_2$O (%)	86	41
Mean MUCP (SD)	58 (21)	55 (19)
Mean volitional MUCP pressure increase (SD)	14 (11)	6 (9)

MUCP, maximum urethral closure pressure.

hopeless situations; inept care for even a trivial injury may end in disaster.' (Committee on Trauma, ACS 1961, p. 1).

This statement made over 40 years ago articulates an enduring truth about injury management; that is, knowing the type of injury is an important guide to proper treatment. Imaging has now demonstrated specific evidence of localized muscle loss revealing a great variety of injury patterns in different women. At present, we do not know whether birth-induced muscle injury is caused by neurological injury or by muscle rupture. Whether or not there should be similar treatment of these two types of injury or not remains to be determined. Further research is needed to develop effective strategies to answer this question in individual women.

In addition, the nature of a woman's defect later in life may influence the type of therapy selected. Pelvic muscle training can have two effects. First it can improve a woman's skill in using her muscles and second, it can improve the contractile force. Whether or not exercise changes resting urethral function is not known. If the ability to contract a normally-innervated pelvic floor muscle during a cough is lost, for example, a woman can be taught to purposefully contract the muscle. Second, the muscles can be exercised to become stronger through hypertrophy. Therefore, if the normally occurring muscle contraction occurs, but is not strong enough, this muscle can be strengthened and continence improved. Most of a person's time is not spent coughing or jumping. Most of the time, there should be normal 'tone' in the muscle. This tonic activity is similar to the action of postural muscle in the back in that it automatically adjusts to the loads placed upon it. Whether this can be improved is unknown.

At present, the success of muscle training in women with different types of levator ani muscle injury is not clear. If the pubovisceral muscle is missing, then the connections between the pubic bone and the vagina or perineal body are missing. Although the iliococcygeal and puborectal muscles remain, there are presently no data to know whether the success of pelvic muscle training is similar in women with and without muscle injury. This should be a fertile field for research as new imaging modalities make the detection of muscle injury routine.

REFERENCES

Allen R E, Hosker G L, Smith A R B et al 1990 Pelvic floor damage and childbirth: a neurophysiological study. British Journal of Obstetrics and Gynaecology 97:770–779

Barber M D, Bremer R E, Thor K B et al 2002 Innervation of the female levator ani muscles. American Journal of Obstetrics and Gynecology 187:64–71

Committee on Trauma, American College of Surgeons 1961 Early care of acute soft tissue injuries, 2nd edn. W B Saunders, Philadelphia

Cortes E, Fong L F, Hameed M et al 2005 Insulin-like growth factor-1 gene splice variants as markers of muscle damage in levator ani muscle after the first vaginal delivery. American Journal of Obstetrics and Gynecology 193:64–70

DeLancey J O 2005 The hidden epidemic of pelvic floor dysfunction: achievable goals for improved prevention and treatment. American Journal of Obstetrics and Gynecology 192:1488–1495

DeLancey J O, Kearney R, Chou Q et al 2003 The appearance of levator ani muscle abnormalities in magnetic resonance images after vaginal delivery. Obstetrics and Gynecology 101:46–53

Dietz H P, Lanzarone V 2005 Levator trauma after vaginal delivery. Obstetrics and Gynecology 106:707–712

Guaderrama N M, Nager C W, Liu J et al 2005 The vaginal pressure profile. Neurourology and Urodynamics 24:243–247

Halban J, Tandler J 1907 Anatomie und Aetiologie der Genitalprolapse beim Weibe. Wilhelm Braumueller, Wien

Hanzal E, Berger E, Koelbl H 1993 Levator ani muscle morphology and recurrent genuine stress incontinence. Obstetrics and Gynecology 81:426–429

Hoyte L, Schierlitz L, Zou K et al 2001 Two- and 3-dimensional MRI comparison of levator ani structure, volume, and integrity in women with stress incontinence and prolapse. American Journal of Obstetrics and Gynecology 185:11–19

Kearney R, Sawhney R, DeLancey J O 2004 Levator ani muscle anatomy evaluated by origin-insertion pairs. Obstetrics and Gynecology 104:168–173

Kirschner-Hermanns R, Wein B, Niehaus S et al 1993 The contribution of magnetic resonance imaging of the pelvic floor to the understanding of urinary incontinence. British Journal of Urology 72:715–778

Lawson J O 1974 Pelvic anatomy. I. Pelvic floor muscles. Annals of the Royal College of Surgeons of England 54:244–252

Lien K C, Mooney B, DeLancey J O et al 2004 Levator ani muscle stretch induced by simulated vaginal birth. Obstetrics and Gynecology 103:31–40

Mant J, Painter R, Vessey M 1997 Epidemiology of genital prolapse: observations from the Oxford Family Planning Association study. British Journal of Obstetrics and Gynaecology 104: 579–585

Miller J M, Umek W H, DeLancey J O et al 2004 Can women without visible pubococcygeal muscle in MR images still increase urethral closure pressures? American Journal of Obstetrics and Gynecology 191:171–175

Mørkved S, Bø K, Schei B et al 2003 Pelvic floor muscle training during pregnancy to prevent urinary incontinence: a single-blind randomized controlled trial. Obstetrics and Gynecology 101:313–319

Rortveit G, Daltveit A K, Hannestad Y S et al 2003 Norwegian EPINCONT Study.Urinary incontinence after vaginal delivery or cesarean section. New England Journal of Medicine 348:900–907

Sampselle C M, Miller J M, Mims B L et al 1998 Effect of pelvic muscle exercise on transient incontinence during pregnancy and after birth. Obstetrics and Gynecology 91:406–412

Strohbehn K, Ellis J H, Storhbehn J A et al 1996 Magnetic resonance imaging of the levator ani with anatomic correlation. Obstetrics and Gynecology 87:277–285

Tunn R, DeLancey J O, Howard D et al 1999 MR Imaging of levator ani muscle recovery following vaginal delivery. International Urogynecology Journal and Pelvic Floor Dysfunction 10:300–307

Tunn R, DeLancey J O, Howard D et al 2003 Anatomic variations in the levator ani muscle, endopelvic fascia, and urethra in nulliparas evaluated by magnetic resonance imaging. American Journal of Obstetrics and Gynecology 188:116–121

Vakili B, Zheng Y T, Loesch H et al 2005 Levator contraction strength and genital hiatus as risk factors for recurrent pelvic organ prolapse. American Journal of Obstetrics and Gynecology 192:1592–1598

Weidner A C, Barber M D, Visco A G et al 2000 Pelvic muscle electromyography of levator ani and external anal sphincter in nulliparous women and women with pelvic floor dysfunction. American Journal of Obstetrics and Gynecology 183:1390–1399

ACKNOWLEDGEMENT

We gratefully acknowledge support of our research through NIH Grants R01 DK 51405; R01 HD 38665; and P50 HD 44406

Clinical assessment of pelvic organ prolapse

Richard C Bump

BACKGROUND: WHY MEASURE PELVIC ORGAN SUPPORT?

Pelvic organ prolapse (POP) is a common clinical condition, encountered on a daily basis by physiotherapists specializing in the care of women with pelvic floor disorders. By definition female POP is an anatomical condition, the downward displacement of the pelvic organs from their usual anatomical location. This section will consider the standardized, quantitative description of pelvic organ position in women, stressing existing evidence for the reliability and validity of this description. However, it is clear that anatomical changes alone neither fully characterize POP nor define its importance as a health condition for women. The importance of POP is its relationship to functional deficits of the involved organs, which in turn impact overall quality of life.

Women who have POP may describe many clinical symptoms alone or in combination. These include, but are not limited to, urinary incontinence, voiding difficulty, defecatory dysfunction, anal incontinence, vaginal pressure, difficulties with coitus, pelvic pressure, and abdominal and back pain. It is unclear whether the anatomical findings are directly related to these symptoms and either partial or total correction of anatomy is necessary to resolve them. Some women with POP have no symptoms and it is unknown what proportion of these is destined to develop symptoms and/or progression of their anatomic changes. Finally, the long-term anatomical outcomes of most interventions for POP, non-surgical as well as surgical, are often poorly documented, both in the medical literature and in the clinic record.

Each of these unknowns represents a daily clinical challenge for clinicians and a career scientific challenge for researchers dedicated to the field of female pelvic floor disorders. Answers to these challenges depend upon a very basic prerequisite, our ability to reliably measure and record pelvic organ support. Without such a measuring system, we cannot communicate with others across space or with ourselves over time. It is important to emphasize that a measuring system does not define what are critical, clinically important changes in pelvic organ support. However, we are unlikely to ever provide these definitions and correlate anatomy with symptoms if we cannot reliably measure the anatomy.

SUMMARY OF THE PELVIC ORGAN PROLAPSE QUANTIFICATION (POP-Q) SYSTEM

Before 1996, there was no widely accepted system for describing the anatomic position of the pelvic organs. As a result, many reports related to pelvic organ prolapse treatment used undefined and non-validated terms, rendering conclusions questionable and comparisons impossible. One of the most widely referenced systems (Beecham 1980), graded prolapse based on the presumed organ involved (rectum, bladder, urethra, uterus, and small bowel or peritoneal cavity) and mandated a resting, non-straining examination. Both these requirements likely resulted in inaccurate examinations that misidentified the involved segments and underestimated the true extent of the prolapse.

In 1993 an international multidisciplinary committee composed of members of the International Continence Society (ICS), the American Urogynecologic Society (AUGS), and the Society of Gynecological Surgeons (SGS) began work on a standardization document for terminology for female pelvic organ prolapse and pelvic floor disorders. Over the ensuing several years, drafts and revisions of the document were circulated to members of the three societies and validation studies were performed. The final document was formally adopted by the societies in late 1995 and early 1996 and was published in July 1996 (Bump et al 1996).

One part of the standardization document is dedicated to the quantitative description of pelvic organ position. This system quickly became known as the POP-Q, though this designation appears nowhere in the standardization document. The POP-Q borrowed heavily from the several site-specific 'half-way' classifications developed and modified by Baden & Walker (1992). Using the hymen as a precisely identifiable visual landmark for reference, the anatomical locations of six defined vaginal points (two anterior, two posterior, and two superior) (Fig. 5.41) are measured in centimetres above or proximal to (negative number) or below or distal to (positive number) the plane of the hymen, which is defined as zero (0).

Measurements are made only when the full extent of the prolapse has been demonstrated and the document details criteria that can be used confirm this. Additional measurements include the anteroposterior length of both the genital hiatus and perineal body and the total vaginal length (see Fig. 5.41). A vaginal profile can be drawn on a grid once all POP-Q measurements are completed. While the nine-number POP-Q vaginal profile was designated as the preferred way of describing pelvic organ position, the committee recognized the need for a more concise designation of POP. The standardization document therefore also includes an ordinal staging system, with five stages (0 through IV) based on the measurements from the full POP-Q profile (Table 5.8).

Fig. 5.42 represents a clinical data sheet that can be used to record the results of the POP-Q exam, including the nine measurements, stage and substage, and the

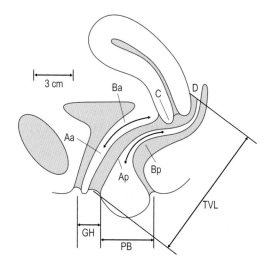

Fig. 5.41 The six vaginal segments (Aa, Ba, C, D, Ap, and Bp), the genital hiatus (GH), perineal body (PB), and total vaginal length (TVL) measured to complete the pelvic organ prolapse quantitation (POP-Q) profile. (From Bump et al 1996, with permission.)

Table 5.8   Ordinal staging system for pelvic organ prolapse, based on the POP-Q system

Stage	Definition
0	No prolapse is demonstrated. Points Aa, Ap, Ba, and Bp are all at −3 and the absolute value of either point C or D is ≤ (TVL−2) cm +6
I	Criteria for stage 0 are not met, but the most distal portion of the prolapse is >1 cm above the hymen (its absolute value is <−1 cm)
II	The most distal portion of the prolapse is ≤1 cm proximal to or distal to the hymen (its absolute value is ≤+1 but ≥−1 cm)
III	The most distal portion of the prolapse is >1 cm below the plane of the hymen but protrudes no further than 2 cm less than TVL (its absolute value is >+1 but < [TVL−2] cm)
IV	Essentially, complete eversion of the total length of the vagina is demonstrated. The distal portion of the prolapse protrudes to at least (TVL−2) cm (its absolute value is ≥ [TVL−2] cm)

type of defect believed to be responsible for any observed prolapse (see below). A grid is also provided to facilitate drawing of the vaginal profile.

LEARNING AND USING THE POP-Q

The full POP standardization document, which includes a detailed description of the measurement technique, is found in Bump et al 1996. However, the POP-Q is much more complicated to describe in words than to demonstrate visually or to perform. An instructional video demonstrating how measurements are taken is available through the AUGS website (www.AUGS.org under the 'Education resources' tab).

The instructional video has been demonstrated to enhance significantly the ability of new users to understand and interpret findings based on the POP-Q examination (Steele et al 1998). Others have demonstrated that the POP-Q system is easily learned and that even inexperienced examiners can obtain reliable measurements after a brief period of instruction and orientation (Hall et al 1996).

The POP-Q system has been recommended for use as a baseline and outcome measure in POP research by the US National Institutes of Health (Weber et al 2001), the AUGS and SGS (Wall et al 1998), and the International Consultation on Incontinence (Brubaker et al 2005). Nonetheless, a recent survey showed that 29.1% of published pelvic floor research used the POP-Q and 23.3% used the similar Baden Walker system from July 2001 to June 2002, while nearly half used either a nonstandard system or did not reference any system (Muir et al 2003).

Because it was developed by societies oriented toward research, the POP-Q is often seen as only a research instrument. But it also has obvious clinical value in that it can significantly enhance the follow-up of patients and the evaluation of treatments. A 2004 report showed that 40.2% of ICS and AUGS members used the POP-Q in their clinical practice (Auwad et al 2004).

REPRODUCIBILITY

Inter and intra-observer reliability

Before its publication, the POP-Q system was evaluated for reproducibility in 240 women in four reports from the USA and Europe (Bump et al 1996). Two of these studies were published as full manuscripts. The first (Hall et al 1996) evaluated inter-observer reliability in 48 subjects using five experienced and two inexperienced physician examiners. Between different examiners, correlations for each of the nine POP-Q measurements were substantial and highly significant. Absolute differences in measurements were not clinically relevant, averaging between 0.04 and 0.40 cm. Staging and substaging agreement was also highly and significantly correlated. The findings with respect to intra-observer reproducibility in 25 patients were similar. Experienced examiners took an average of 2.05 minutes to complete and record the POP-Q exam, while inexperienced examiners averaged 3.73 minutes. Level of experience did not impact the accuracy of the measurements.

The second published report (Kobak et al 1996) determined inter-observer reliability, comparing physician

Pelvic organ prolapse examination record

Point	Definition	Possible range in cm	Value in cm
Aa	Lower anterior vaginal wall	−3 to +3	
Ba	Upper anterior vaginal wall	−3 to +TVL	
C	Cervix or vaginal cuff scar	−TVL to +TVL	
D	Posterior fornix	−TVL to +TVL	
Ap	Lower posterior vaginal wall	−3 to +3	
Bp	Upper posterior vaginal wall	−3 to +TVL	
GH	Genital hiatus	No limit	
PB	Perineal body	No limit	
TVL	Total vaginal length	No limit	

Stage: ☐ 0 ☐ I ☐ II ☐ III ☐ IV

Substage: ☐ a ☐ p ☐ Aa ☐ Ba ☐ Ap ☐ Bp ☐ C ☐ D

Anterior Defect

☐ none ☐ central ☐ left ☐ right ☐ superior ☐ attenuated fascia

Posterior Defect

☐ none ☐ inferior at PB ☐ central ☐ left ☐ right ☐ superior ☐ attenuated fascia

POP-Q Grid

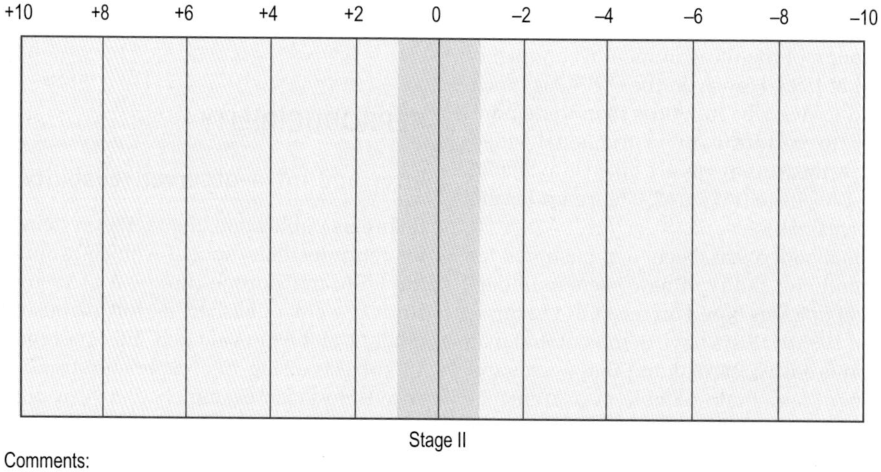

| +10 | +8 | +6 | +4 | +2 | 0 | −2 | −4 | −6 | −8 | −10 |

Stage II

Comments:

Fig. 5.42 Clinical data collection form for the POP-Q examination.

and nurse clinician measurements in 49 women. They found substantial and highly significant correlations between examiners for both the stage of prolapse and for all POP-Q measurements. The high level of agreement between the nurse and physician measurements led the authors to conclude that the most important factors for obtaining accurate and reproducible results were clear definitions and close attention to examination technique.

Variability related to differences in measuring technique

The standardization document stresses that variables of the examination technique should be specified in any report and that efforts should be made to measure the maximum extent of the prolapse. The committee recognized that variations in technique could change measurements and stressed that the patient's confirmation that the maximum prolapse was being observed was an important quality control measure. Obviously, the same technique should be used when serial examinations are performed, especially before and after a therapeutic intervention.

Several techniques of the examination have been demonstrated to have a statistically significant and potentially clinically important effect on POP-Q measurements and staging. Barber et al (2000a) compared supine lithotomy examinations on an examining table to examinations in a semi-upright (45°) position in a birthing chair. Of 133 women, 26% had an increase in one stage and 48% had at least one POP-Q measurement increase by at least 2 cm when examined upright.

Other investigators have confirmed a significant impact of position of measurements. In a seven-site, 16-examiner study involving 133 women, Visco et al (2003) demonstrated significantly greater prolapse across all stages in the standing compared with the lithotomy position. Moreover, the segment of maximum prolapse was different in 18% of patients (95% CI: 16%, 41%). This same group demonstrated that the use of a speculum during the POP-Q exam had minimal impact on the assessment of stage, with 79% of subjects having the same stage with and without a speculum-aided examination. Of those who changed stage, about half increased and half decreased.

Silva et al (2004) examined the impact of position and the state of bladder filling on POP-Q measurements. They confirmed increasing prolapse in the standing compared with the supine position, and further confirmed increasing prolapse with an empty compared with a full bladder. Most women (29 of 50) had their prolapse stage increased going from a supine, full-

bladder examination to a standing, empty-bladder examination: 24 increased by one stage, three by two stages, and two by three stages. Going from supine to standing, 22% (full bladder) to 30% (empty bladder) of women had an increase in stage. Going from full to empty bladder, 34% (supine) to 44% (standing) had an increase in stage.

In contrast to these previous findings, Swift & Herring (1998) did not demonstrate a significant or clinically relevant difference in any POP-Q measurement (correlations between 0.96 and 0.98) or in prolapse stage (identical in 48 of 51 patients) when comparing the results of a lithotomy examination while the patient was performing a maximal Valsalva strain with the results of a standing examination. In both situations, the patients confirmed that the protrusion that bothered them was reproduced during the examination. They concluded that the standing examination was unnecessary as long as the patient was able to strain forcefully and the extent of the protrusion was validated by the patient.

To date, no study has compared the POP-Q results of sitting upright or semi-upright examinations with the results of standing examinations. Importantly, none of these studies reported the clinical impact of their observed changes in POP-Q findings at baseline. It is therefore not clear if these differences actually changed the way the patients were managed. However, it is clear that to be able to measure the anatomical impact of an intervention for POP, the circumstances of the examination should be identical before and after the intervention.

LIMITATIONS OF THE POP-Q

Many of the limitations attributed to the POP-Q system since its introduction are derived from the misconception that the system is meant to identify the precise cause of an individual patient's prolapse, the pelvic organs involved in the prolapse, or the best intervention for the prolapse.

In fact, the system is no more or less than a reproducible, quantitative description of the position of the vaginal segments. It measures where a segment is, not why it is there or how best to change its position. Similarly, the POP-Q measurements do not identify the clinical relevance of a particular stage of prolapse or its relationship to symptoms. However, it does provide a standard measure to facilitate the process of answering many of these unknowns. Analogous to the sphygmomanometer, which measures blood pressure and allows researchers and clinicians to determine the symptoms and impact of high blood pressure as well as the acute and chronic risks and benefits of various treatments, the POP-Q is a measuring tool to be used in our efforts to further our understanding of POP.

The standardization document describes pelvic support in terms of vaginal topography rather than in 'terms such as "cystocele, rectocele, enterocele, or urethrovesical junction" because these terms may imply an unrealistic certainty as to the structures on the other side of the vaginal bulge'. It also stresses that 'functional deficits caused by POP and pelvic floor dysfunction are not well characterized or absolutely established'. A large part of the overall terminology document is dedicated to ancillary techniques for describing or assessing POP, including supplementary physical examination techniques, endoscopy, photography, imaging, surgical observations, pelvic floor muscle testing and symptom surveys. Many of these techniques have unproved clinical use, but the POP-Q can help establish their value. For example, if someone theorizes that a specific defect is responsible for point Aa being at +3 cm, devises a test to identify this defect, and develops an intervention to correct the defect and reposition point Aa to −2 or −3 cm, then validation of the theory, test and intervention would be established if point Aa is actually reliably restored to and maintained in this position.

Scotti et al (2000) have written a detailed critique of the POP-Q system, adding more measures and descriptions of isolated fascial tears and detachments to the system. As one example, the POP-Q is criticized for not including the description of paravaginal (lateral) anterior vaginal wall defects. However, others have demonstrated that the inter- and intra-examiner reliability for the description of these anterior defects is poor (Whiteside et al 2004) and that the findings on physical examination often do not correspond with findings at surgery (Barber et al 1999). The standardization document does mention many supplementary physical examination techniques that may be important for determining optimal treatment, but none of these are essential to actually measuring the position of the vaginal segments. Further, the importance of these additional techniques can be assessed by how they enhance our ability to normalize vaginal position, as measured with the POP-Q.

It has been shown that the six vaginal segments that make up the overall POP-Q vaginal profile do not predict the position of or identify the anatomical structures on the other side of the vaginal wall. Thus, it has been shown that point Aa value is not predictive of urethrovesical junction hypermobility as measured with the Q-tip test (Cogan et al 2002), and that the values for the posterior segment points do not predict the organs involved in the prolapse or the size of a rectocele or enterocele as assessed by cystodefecoperitoneography (Altman et al 2005). Other authors have come to similar conclusions using both contrast fluoroscopy

(Kenton et al 1997) and magnetic resonance imaging (Hodroff et al 2002, Singh et al 2001). Although these are accurate observations, they serve to validate the terminology committee's decision to abandon the '-cele' terminology when describing the anatomical position of the vaginal wall. Moreover, it is unknown if certain identification of the visceral content of a vaginal hernia is important to the successful treatment of the hernia. Proving this value may be difficult, but it would be impossible if the anatomical results could not be measured reliably.

POP-Q USES IN THE MEDICAL RESEARCH

Since their introduction, the POP-Q profile and staging system have been used by many authors in an attempt to clarify the relationships between anatomical findings of prolapse and a variety of pelvic floor symptoms. The system has also contributed to trials that aim to define threshold values for clinically important levels of POP, to define normal levels of support, and to determine the prevalence of, risk factors for, and natural history of POP. Finally, the system has become an important outcome variable in the assessment of various surgical procedures for POP.

Swift et al (2003, 2005) have been at the forefront of efforts to define the anatomical threshold for clinically important POP. First in a single-site study (2003), later confirmed in a multiple-site study (2005), they determined that prolapse at or near the hymen (mid stage 2) 'defined prolapse' or, more correctly, defined the threshold of pelvic support that was clinically important based on patient-recorded symptoms. However, the symptom that was most influential in this determination was 'Can you feel with your hand or see something bulging out of your vagina?', making it inevitable that prolapse at or near the hymen would be the first level at which this criterion would likely be met. Nonetheless, their findings and those of other investigators, legitimately challenge the designation of stage 1 and early stage 2 pelvic organ support as 'prolapse', a term that implies these levels of support represent a disease or abnormality. Swift et al also suggested that a single point, just proximal to or at the hymen should be the dividing line that defines prolapse. However, basing this recommendation primarily on the sensation of a bulge may be too restrictive because functional symptoms possibly related to changes in position of the bladder neck or the rectum may be associated with lesser levels of prolapse.

A thorough review of the literature using the POP-Q to correlate anatomy and function is beyond the scope of this section. However, the availability of the system has facilitated the performance of multiple studies attempting to clarify these relationships (Burrows et al 2004, Ellerkmann et al 2001, Fialkow et al 2002, Heit et al 2002, Mouritsen & Larsen 2003, Tan et al 2005, Tapp et al 2005). Some symptoms, such as vaginal pain and back pain, seem not to be associated with prolapse (Heit et al 2002, Mouritsen & Larsen. 2003). The bimodal relationship between anterior segment prolapse and incontinence (early stage prolapse) and emptying phase symptoms (advanced stage prolapse), while not exact, is fairly widely accepted (Burrows et al 2004, Ellerkmann et al 2001, Tapp et al 2005). Conversely, any relationship between various levels of posterior prolapse with bowel dysfunction and prolapse of any segment with sexual dysfunction is uncertain (Burrows et al 2004, Fialkow et al 2002). Nonetheless, being able to accurately measure pelvic support and correlate those measurements with function is serving to expand our understanding of these complex relationships.

The POP-Q profile and staging system can be used in an observational cross-sectional study design to estimate the point prevalence of various levels of pelvic organ support and to define risk factors for the development of prolapse (Nygaard et al 2004). It can also be used in longitudinal studies to follow the natural progression of POP over time or to assess the impact of various putative inciting factors such as pregnancy (O'Boyle et al 2003) and delivery (O'Boyle et al 2005).

Finally, there are many examples the use of the system as a baseline and outcome measure in surgery for POP. Both the staging system and the numerical values for the individual points can be used to convey the anatomical results of procedures (Barber et al 2000b, Cundiff et al 1997, Cundiff et al 1998). In addition, changes in the genital hiatus and perineal body measurements have been used as an indicator of the correction of perineal descent after successful surgery (Cundiff et al 1997).

SUMMARY

The quantitative measurement of the position of all segments of the vagina and perineum using the ICS/AUGS/SGS POP-Q system has been shown to be reproducible and easy to learn. Clinically, the record of such measures allows health care providers to communicate with each other across space and with themselves across time. The system has also facilitated clinical, basic and translational research in multiple areas related to female pelvic floor disorders. Ultimately this research may help us understand the link between structure and function in the pelvis, improve the outcomes from our treatments, and provide opportunities for prevention of pelvic floor disorders. However, it is important to emphasize that measuring prolapse by any method is only a tool that aids in clinical management and research.

REFERENCES

Altman D, López A, Kierkegaard J et al 2005 Assessment of posterior vaginal wall prolapse: comparison of physical findings to cystodefecoperitoneography. International Urogynecology Journal and Pelvic Floor Dysfunction 16:96–103

Auwad W, Freeman R M, Swift S 2004 Is the pelvic organ prolapse quantitation system (POPQ) being used? A survey of members of the International Continence Society (ICS) and the American Urogynecologic Society (AUGS). International Urogynecology Journal and Pelvic Floor Dysfunction 15:324–327

Baden W, Walker T 1992 Surgical repair of vaginal defects. J B Lippincott, Philadelphia, p 1–7, 51–62

Barber M D, Cundiff G W, Mwidner A C et al 1999 Accuracy of clinical assessment of paravaginal defects in women with anterior vaginal wall prolapse. American Journal of Obstetrics and Gynecology 181:87–90

Barber M D, Lambers A R, Visco A G et al 2000a Effect of patient position on clinical evaluation of pelvic organ prolapse. Obstetrics and Gynecology 96:18–22

Barber M D, Visco A G, Weidner A C et al 2000b Bilateral uterosacral ligament vaginal vault suspension with site-specific endopelvic fascia defect repair for treatment of pelvic organ prolapse. American Journal of Obstetrics and Gynecology 183:1402–1411

Beecham C T 1980 Classification of vaginal relaxation. American Journal of Obstetrics and Gynecology 136:957–958

Brubaker L, Bump R, Fynes M et al 2005 Surgery for pelvic organ prolapse. In: Incontinence. Abrams P, Cardozo L, Khoury S et al (eds) Plymbridge Distributors, Plymouth, UK, p 1371–1401

Bump R C, Mattiasson A, Bø K et al 1996 The standardisation of terminology of female pelvic organ prolapse and pelvic floor dysfunction. American Journal of Obstetrics and Gynecology 175:10–17

Burrows L J, Meyn L A, Walters M D et al 2004 Pelvic symptoms in women with pelvic organ prolapse. Obstetrics and Gynecology 104:982–988

Cogan S L, Weber A M, Hammel J P 2002 Is urethral mobility really being assessed by the pelvic organ prolapse quantification (POP-Q) system? Obstetrics and Gynecology 99:4736

Cundiff G W, Harris R L, Coates K W 1997 Abdominal sacral colpoperineopexy: a new approach for correction of posterior compartment defects and perineal descent associated with vaginal vault prolapse. American Journal of Obstetrics and Gynecology 177:1345–1355

Cundiff G W, Weidner A C, Visco A et al 1998 An anatomic and functional assessment of the discrete defect rectocele repair. American Journal of Obstetrics and Gynecology 179:1451–1457

Ellerkmann R M, Cundiff G W, Melick C F et al 2001 Correlation of symptoms with location and severity of pelvic organ prolapse. American Journal of Obstetrics and Gynecology 185:1332–1338

Fialkow M E, Gardella C, Melville J et al 2002 Posterior vaginal wall defects and their relation to measures of pelvic floor neuromuscular function and posterior compartment symptoms. American Journal of Obstetrics and Gynecology 187:1443–1449

Hall A F, Theofrastous J P, Cundiff G C et al 1996 Inter- and intra-observer reliability of the proposed International Continence Society, Society of Gynecologic Surgeons, and American Urogynecologic Society pelvic organ prolapse classification system. American Journal of Obstetrics and Gynecology 175:1467–1471

Heit M, Culligan P, Rosenquist C et al 2002 Is pelvic organ prolapse a cause of pelvic or low back pain? Obstetrics and Gynecology 99:23–28

Hodroff M A, Stolpen A H, Denson M A et al 2002 Dynamic magnetic resonance imaging of the female pelvis: the relationship with the pelvic organ prolapse quantification staging system. The Journal of Urology 167:1353–1355

Kenton K, Shott S, Brubaker L 1997 Vaginal topography does not correlate well with visceral position in women with pelvic organ prolapse. International Urogynecology Journal and Pelvic Floor Dysfunction 8:336–339

Kobak W H, Rosenberger K, Walters M D 1996 Interobserver variation in the assessment of pelvic organ prolapse. International Urogynecology Journal and Pelvic Floor Dysfunction 7:121–124

Mouritsen L, Larsen J P 2003 Symptoms, bother and POPQ in women referred with pelvic organ prolapse. International Urogynecology Journal and Pelvic Floor Dysfunction 14:122–127

Muir T W, Stepp K J, Barber M D 2003 Adoption of the pelvic organ prolapse quantification system in peer-reviewed literature. American Journal of Obstetrics and Gynecology 189:1632–1636

Nygaard I, Bradley C, Drandt D 2004 For Pelvic organ prolapse in older women: prevalence and risk factors. Obstetrics and Gynecology 104:489–497

O'Boyle A L, O'Boyle J D, Calhoun B et al 2005 Pelvic organ support in pregnancy and postpartum. International Urogynecology Journal and Pelvic Floor Dysfunction 16:69–72

O'Boyle A L, O'Boyle J D, Ricks R E et al 2003 The natural history of pelvic organ support in pregnancy. International Urogynecology Journal and Pelvic Floor Dysfunction 14:46–49

Scotti R J, Flora R, Greston W M et al 2000 Characterizing and reporting pelvic floor defects: the revised New York classification system. International Urogynecology Journal and Pelvic Floor Dysfunction 11:48–60

Silva W A, Kleeman S, Segal J et al 2004 Effects of a full bladder and patient positioning on pelvic organ prolapse assessment. Obstetrics and Gynecology 104:37–41

Singh K, Reid W M N, Berger L A 2001 Assessment and grading of pelvic organ prolapse by use of dynamic magnetic resonance imaging. American Journal of Obstetrics and Gynecology 185:71–77

Steele A, Mallipeddi P, Welgoss J et al 1998 Teaching the pelvic organ prolapse quantitation system. American Journal of Obstetrics and Gynecology 179:1458–1464

Swift S E, Herring M 1998 Comparison of pelvic organ prolapse in the dorsal lithotomy compared with the standing position. Obstetrics and Gynecology 91:961–964

Swift S E, Tate S Z B, Nicholas J 2003 Correlation of symptoms with degree of pelvic organ support in a general population of women: what is pelvic organ prolapse? American Journal of Obstetrics and Gynecology 189:372–379

Swift S, Woodman P, O'Boyle A et al 2005 Pelvic organ support study (POSST): the distribution, clinical definition, and epidemiologic condition of pelvic organ support defects. American Journal of Obstetrics and Gynecology 192:795–806

Tan J S, Lukacz E S, Menefee S A et al 2005 Predictive value of prolapse symptoms: a large database study. International Urogynecology Journal and Pelvic Floor Dysfunction 16:203–209

Tapp K, Connolly A M, Visco A G 2005 Evaluation of Aa point and cotton-tipped swab test as predictors of urodynamic stress incontinence. Obstetrics and Gynecology 105:115–119

Visco A G, Wei J T, McClure L A et al 2003 Effects of examination technique modifications on pelvic organ prolapse quantification (POP-Q) results. International Urogynecology Journal and Pelvic Floor Dysfunction 14:136–140

Wall L L, Norton P, Versi E et al 1998 Evaluating the outcome of surgery for pelvic organ prolapse. American Journal of Obstetrics and Gynecology 178:877–879

Weber A M, Abrams P, Brubaker L et al 2001 The standardization of terminology for researchers in femal pelvic floor disorders. International Urogynecology Journal and Pelvic Floor Dysfunction 12:178–186

Whiteside J L, Barber M D, Paraiso M F et al 2004 Clinical evaluation of anterior vaginal wall support defects: interexaminer and intraexaminer reliability. American Journal of Obstetrics and Gynecology 191:100–104

Chapter 6

Pelvic floor and exercise science

Motor learning

Kari Bø and Siv Mørkved

ABILITY TO CONTRACT THE PELVIC FLOOR MUSCLES

Before starting a training programme of the pelvic floor muscles (PFM) one has to ensure that the patients/clients are able to perform a correct PFM contraction. A correct PFM contraction has two components: squeeze around pelvic openings and inward (cranial) lift (Kegel 1952). Several research groups have shown that over 30% of women are not able to voluntarily contract the PFM at their first consultation even after thorough individual instruction (Benvenuti et al 1987, Bump et al 1991, Bø et al 1988, Kegel 1952). Common mistakes when trying to perform a PFM contraction are listed in

Table 6.1   Common errors in attempts to contract the pelvic floor muscles

Error	Observation
Contraction of outer abdominal muscles instead of the PFM	The person is curving the back, or starts the attempt to contract by 'hollowing'/tucking the stomach inwards (note that a small 'hollowing' can be seen in a correct contraction with the transverse abdominal muscle co-contracting)
Contraction of hip adductor muscles instead of the PFM	A contraction of the muscles of the inner thigh can be seen
Contraction of gluteal muscles instead of the PFM	The person is pressing the buttock together, lifting up from the bench
Stop breathing	The person closes her/ his mouth and holds the breath
Enhanced inhaling	The person takes a deep inspiration often accompanied by contraction of abdominal muscles, and tries erroneously to 'lift up' the pelvic floor by the inspiration
Straining	The person presses downwards. When undressed, the perineum can be seen pressing in a caudal direction. If the person has pelvic organ prolapse, the prolapse may protrude

Table 6.1. Bø et al (1988) and Bø et al (1990a) found that many women contracted other muscles in addition to the PFM, and nine out of 52 were straining instead of lifting. Bump et al (1991) found corresponding results in an American population with as many as 25% of women straining instead of squeezing and lifting. These findings were later supported by Thompson & O'Sullivan (2003) in a population of Australian women.

There may be several explanations why a voluntary PFM contraction is difficult to perform:

- the PFM have a invisible location inside the pelvis;
- neither men nor women have ever learned to contract the PFM and most people would be unaware of the automatic contractions of the muscles;
- the muscles are small and, from a neurophysiologial point of view, therefore more difficult to contract voluntarily;
- the common awareness of these pelvic and perineal area of the body may be associated with voiding and defecation, and straining at toilet is common.

Tries (1990) suggests that there may be a lack of sensory feedback during PFM training in some women, causing:

- problems with feedback from the correct muscles because other muscles are used instead of the PFM;
- insufficient kinaesthetic feedback due to low-intensity contractions in weak PFM;
- lack of or reduced sensation, which may limit the sensory incentive that normally leads to a motor response or reflex preventing leakage.

Motor re-learning depends on sensory feedback (Tries 1990). Following Gentile (1987) learning is in general facilitated by the use of feedback, and the physical therapist (PT) should give external feedback as 'knowledge of results' (KR) as a part of the intervention. KR may compensate for a loss of normal sources for internal feedback in patients with central- or peripheral nerve injuries (Winstein et al 1991). Although many women have reduced innervations in the pelvic floor (e.g. after injury related to pregnancy and delivery), the use of KR may be useful in learning correct PFM contraction.

Our reason for attempting to isolate the PFM contraction from outer pelvic muscles when training the muscles is not because we do not appreciate that all muscles in the body act together and never work in isolation. However, such simultaneous contractions of outer and more commonly used larger muscle groups outside the pelvis may mask the awareness and strength of the PFM contraction. The person erroneously believes he or she is performing a strong contraction, but the PFM are not doing the job. Most importantly, to train and build up a muscle or muscle groups' strength and volume it is mandatory to work specifically with the targeted muscle.

More concerning than the contraction of outer pelvic muscles simultaneously with PFM contraction, is straining. If patients are straining instead of performing a correct contraction, the training may permanently stretch, weaken and harm the contractile ability of the PFM. In addition straining may stretch the connective tissue of fasciae and ligaments, thereby potentially increasing the risk of development of pelvic organ prolapse. Proper assessment of ability to contract the PFM and feedback on performance is therefore mandatory before starting a training programme.

PRACTICAL TEACHING OF CORRECT PFM CONTRACTION

The steps of learning a correct muscle contraction can be separated into five levels.

1. Understand – the patient needs to understand where the PFM are located and how they work (cognitive function).
2. Search – the patient needs time to put this understanding into her or his body. Where is my pelvic floor?
3. Find – the patient must find where the PFM are, but often needs reassurance from the PT of the location.
4. Learn – after having found the PFM, the patient needs to learn how to perform a correct contraction of the PFM. Feedback from the PT is mandatory.
5. Control – after having learned to contract, most subjects still strive for a while to perform controlled and coordinated contractions recruiting as many motor units as possible during each contraction; most people are unable to hold the contraction, perform repetitive contractions or conduct contractions of high velocity or strength.

Basically, four teaching tools can be used to facilitate skill acquisition (Gentile 1972): the therapist can try to verbally indicate key aspects of the task or performance, supplementary visual input can be provided, direct physical contact with the learner might be employed, and the therapist can structure the environmental conditions under which practice is to take place.

To facilitate correct PFM contractions the PT can use different teaching tools

Verbal instructions should be based on knowledge of the function of the PFM, namely to form a structural support and to ensure a fast and strong contraction during abrupt increase in abdominal pressure. One example of a training command is 'squeeze and lift'.

To teach patients the PT might use drawings and anatomical models of the pelvic floor to show the patient where the muscles are located anatomically (Fig. 6.1). We also recommend the PT to demonstrate a correct PFM contraction in standing position, showing that there should be no movement of the pelvis or thighs visible from the outside. The patient can also palpate the

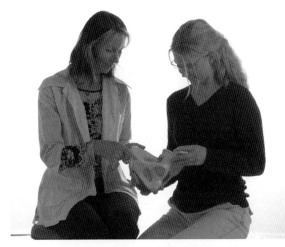

Fig. 6.1 Use of anatomical models or illustrations to teach anatomy and physiology of the pelvic floor. Place the anatomical model in front of the patient's pelvis so she can see the correct location of the organs as they are inside her.

PT's buttocks to feel the difference between gluteal muscle contraction and the relaxed position these muscles should hold during PFM contraction. Allow the patient to ask questions and practice a few contractions for herself.

One way to help patients understand the action of the PFM is to use imagery such as describing the contraction as a lift starting with closure of the doors (squeeze) and from there the elevator is moving upstairs (lift). Another way is to explain the action as eating spaghetti or the action of a vacuum cleaner. Many patients may have general low body awareness and sometimes it is necessary first to focus on the pelvic area and make the patient move the pelvis in different directions by use of outer pelvic muscles (Fig. 6.2). When the patient is familiar with the pelvic area, one can start to focus on the internal pelvic muscles (the PFM).

One way of visualizing where the PFM are located and how they work is to use a skeleton and place the patient's hand as if it was the pelvic floor inside the pelvis. Then the PT presses the hand towards the 'pelvic floor' to make the patient understand the role of the PFM as a structural support for all the pelvic organs and how it should resist increases in abdominal pressure (Fig. 6.3).

Direct physical contact may be used to enhance sensory stimulation and proprioceptive facilitation. An effective position to teach a correct PFM contraction is having the patient sit on an armrest with legs in

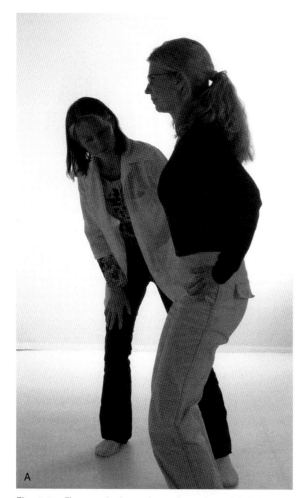

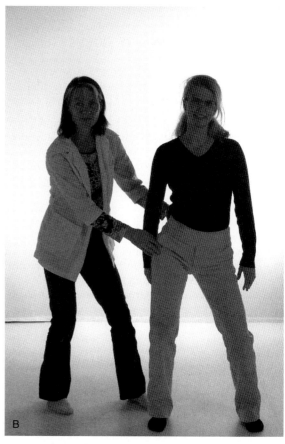

Fig. 6.2 First teach the patient where the pelvis is by practicing movements of the pelvis in anteroposterior direction (A) and sideways (B).

abduction, feet on the floor, straight back and hip flexion. In this position, the patient gets exteroceptive, and for some maybe, proprioceptive stimulus on the perineum/PFM. The patient is then instructed to squeeze and lift away from the chair without rising up, and then relax again (Fig. 6.4). After this instruction the patient is allowed to go to the toilet to empty the bladder. Observation and vaginal palpation then takes place. Fig. 6.5 shows the relationship between the PT and patient with vaginal palpation during attempts to contract the PFM. Both PT and patient give verbal feedback to each other during the contraction. In addition, proprioceptive facilitation may be used during vaginal palpation to enhance contraction of the PFM. The palpation (rectal for men) is also important to give feedback of the strength of the contraction and to make the patient understand that although he or she is con-

tracting correctly it is possible to work much harder. Gentile (1987) claims that in general one of the most important roles of the instructor is to keep the patient's motivation high because practice/training is a premise for learning. A distinction must be made between feedback aiming at giving information about performance or results, and verbal comments to motivate the patient to adherence.

It can be explained to men that if they perform a correct PFM contraction they feel and see a lift of the scrotum. If appropriate, a mirror can be used for both men and women to see the inward lifting movement. However, some people feel uncomfortable observing their genitalia, and the PT must show tact before suggesting this method.

Another way of facilitating learning may be to structure the environmental conditions under which practice

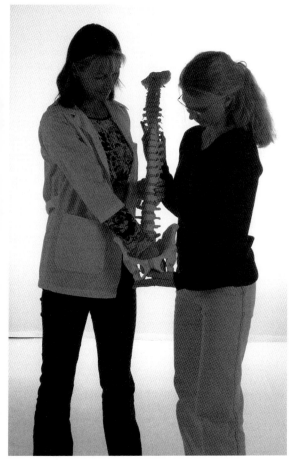

Fig. 6.3 Teaching of the location of the pelvic floor muscles (PFM) as a structural support for the internal organs and how it acts to resist downward movement and increase in abdominal pressure by lifting upwards. The physical therapist presses downwards and the patient holds against the movement mirroring the work of the PFM.

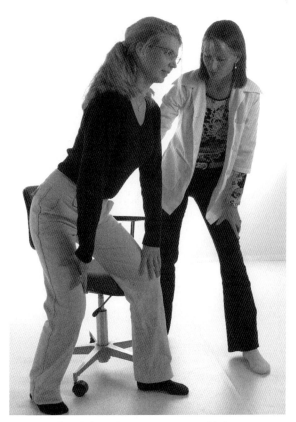

Fig. 6.4 The patient sits on an armrest with legs apart, feet on the floor, flexed hips and straight back with the perineum resting on the armrest. The instruction is to squeeze around the pelvic openings and lift the skin away from the armrest without rising up or putting any pressure on the feet.

is to take place. We emphasize a situation during PFM training, both at home and training groups that allows thorough concentration. One consequence of this is that during group training classes we do not use music when teaching the PFM contractions.

Although as many as 30% may not be able to conduct a correct PFM contraction at the first consultation, we have experienced that most women learn to contract if they are given advice to practice on their own at home for a week. It is important not to strain the patient at the first consultation if she is not able to contract. Ask the patient to exercise on an armrest at home and also ask her or him to try to stop the dribble at the end of the

voiding. However, stopping the urine stream is not recommended in a training protocol, as it may disturb the fine neurological balance between bladder and urethral pressures during voiding. There should be no PFM activity just before (opening of the urethra) and during voiding. Stopping the dribble at the very end of the voiding is therefore only recommended as a test of the ability to contract, and many patients have reported that they have learned to contract the PFM with this method. Another way to improve the awareness of a correct PFM contraction is to contract other circular muscles (e.g. those surrounding the mouth; Liebergall-Wischnitzer et al 2005). The recommendation of all the above mentioned methods to teach PFM contraction is based on clinical experience only. No studies have been found

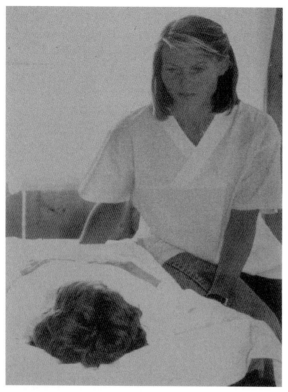

Fig. 6.5 Vaginal palpation is mandatory to give immediate feedback on correctness of the attempt to contract the pelvic floor muscles.

evaluating or comparing the effect of the different teaching methods.

If the patient is still unable to contract the PFM after 1 week of rehearsal on her own, the PT may try general muscle facilitation techniques to stimulate awareness of the PFM. Methods such as fast stretch of the PFM, tapping on the perineum or muscles, pressure/massage techniques or electrical stimulation can be tried out (Brown 2001). However, no studies have yet been found evaluating the effect of such techniques to increase awareness of the PFM or ability to contract. These

recommendations are therefore based on clinical experience only.

Studies using concentric needle electromyography (EMG) in the urethral sphincter and the PFM have demonstrated that there is a co-contraction of the PFM with the use of outer pelvic muscles (gluteal, hip adductor and rectus abdominis) in healthy volunteers (Bø & Stien 1994). In addition, Sapsford & Hodges (2001) used surface EMG and found that there was a co-contraction of the PFM during transversus abdominus (TrA) contraction in healthy volunteers. Therefore, many PTs recommend contractions of outer pelvic muscles and hope for a co-contraction of the PFM if the patient is not able to perform a correct PFM contraction. However, we do not know whether there are such simultaneous co-contractions in persons with pelvic floor dysfunction, and there are no studies showing the effect of interventions for different symptoms of pelvic floor dysfunction using contraction of other muscles than the PFM. If some of the outer pelvic muscles are to be used instead of the PFM, we recommend hip adductor and gluteal muscle contractions and not TrA or other abdominal muscle training because contraction of all the abdominal muscles will increase abdominal pressure (Hodges & Gandevia 2000). In addition, Bø et al (2003) showed that when contracting the TrA, 30% of trained female PTs showed descent of the PFM. Therefore, if there is no co-contraction of the PFM with the abdominal muscle contractions this may strain and weaken the PFM.

High-quality studies in the area of PFM awareness and motor learning should be of high priority and are strongly encouraged in future research. However, it is important that PTs are aware that some subjects may never be able to perform a voluntary PFM contraction. In a study by Bø et al four of 52 patients were still unable to contract after 6 months of PFM training (Bø et al 1990a). Inability to contract the PFM may be due to severe muscle, nerve and connective tissue damage or inability to learn this specific task due to a general low body/muscle/movement awareness. These patients should not spend a lot of time and money with the PT, but should be referred back to their treating general practitioners, urologists or gynaecologists for other treatment options as soon as possible.

REFERENCES

Benvenuti F, Caputo G M, Bandinelli S et al 1987 Reeducative treatment of female genuine stress incontinence. American Journal Physical Medicine 66:155–168

Bø K, Hagen R H, Kvarstein B et al 1990a Pelvic floor muscle exercise for the treatment of female stress urinary incontinence, III: effects of two different degrees of pelvic floor muscle exercise. Neurourology and Urodynamics 9:489–502

Bø K, Larsen S, Oseid S et al 1988 Knowledge about and ability to correct pelvic floor muscle exercises in women with urinary stress incontinence. Neurourology and Urodynamics 7:261–262

Bø K, Kvarstein B, Hagen R et al 1990b Pelvic floor muscle exercise for the treatment of female stress urinary incontinence, II: validity of vaginal pressure measurements of pelvic floor muscle strength and the necessity of supplementary methods for control of correct contraction. Neurourology and Urodynamics 9:479–487

Bø K, Sherburn M, Allen T 2003 Transabdominal ultrasound measurement of pelvic floor muscle activity when activated directly or via a transversus abdominial muscle contraction. Neurourology and Urodynamics 22(6):582–588

Bø K, Stien R 1994 Needle EMG registration of striated urethral wall and pelvic floor muscle activity patterns during cough, Valsalva, abdominal, hip adductor, and gluteal muscle contractions in nulliparous healthy females. Neurourology and Urodynamics 13:35–41

Brown C 2001 Pelvic floor reeducation: a practical approach. In: Corcos J, Shick E, The urinary sphincter. Marcel Dekker, New York, p 459–473

Bump R, Hurt W G, Fantl J A et al 1991 Assessment of Kegel exercise performance after brief verbal instruction. American Journal of Obstetrics and Gynecology 165:322–329

Gentile A M 1972 A working model of skill acquisition with applications to teaching. Quest 17:3–23

Gentile A M 1987 Skill acquisition: Action, movement, and neuromotor processes. In Carr J H, Shepherd P B, Gordon J et al Movement science. Foundations for physiotherapy in rehabilitation. Heinemann Physio Therapy, London, p 93–154

Hodges P W, Gandevia S C 2000 Changes in intra-abdominal pressure during postal and respiratory activation of the human diaphragm. Journal of Applied Physiology 89:967–976

Kegel A H 1952 Stress incontinence and genital relaxation. Clinical Symposia: 4(2):35–51

Liebergall-Wischnitzer M, Hochner–Celnikier D, Lavy Y et al 2005 Paula method of circular muscle exercises for urinary stress incontinence – a clinical trial. International Urogynecological Journal and Pelvic Floor Dysfunction 16:345–351

Sapsford R, Hodges P 2001 Contraction of the pelvic floor muscles during abdominal maneuvers. Archives of Physical Medicine and Rehabilitation 82:1081–1088

Tries J 1990 Kegel exercises enhanced by biofeedback. Journal of Enterostomal Therapy 17:67–76

Thompson J A, O'Sullivan P B 2003 Levator plate movement during voluntary pelvic floor muscle contraction in subjects with incontinence and prolapse: a cross-sectional study and review. International Urogynecology Journal and Pelvic Floor Dysfunction 14(2):84–88

Winstein C J 1991 Knowledge of results and motor learning – implications for physiotherapy. In: Movement science. American Physiotherapy Association, Alexandria, VA, p 181–189

Strength training

Kari Bø and Arve Aschehoug

INTRODUCTION TO THE CONCEPT OF STRENGTH TRAINING FOR PELVIC FLOOR MUSCLES

The pelvic floor muscles (PFM) are regular skeletal muscles and will therefore adapt to strength training in the same way as other muscles (Fig. 6.6). The aim of a strength training regimen is to change muscle morphology by increasing the cross-sectional area, improve neurological factors by increasing the number of activated motor neurons and their frequency of excitation, and improve muscle 'tone' or stiffness (DiNubile 1991) (Fig. 6.7). Specific changes are dependent on the type of exercise and the training programme used, but response to a specific training programme also depends on genetics and hereditary factors (Haskel 1994). However, whenever starting to activate any muscle in the body, physiological changes will occur within the activated muscles. Table 6.2 gives a list of some of the physiological adaptations in the muscle fibre following regular strength training.

Connective tissue is abundant within and around all skeletal muscles including the epimysium, perimysium, and endomysium. These connective tissue sheaths provide the tensile strength and viscoelastic properties ('stiffness') of muscle and provide support for the loading of muscle (Fleck & Kraemer 2004). There is evidence that strength training can increase connective tissue mass, and that intensity of training and load bearing are major factors for effective training. The theoretical rationale for intensive strength training of the PFM is that strength training may build up the structural support of the pelvis by elevating the levator plate to a permanent higher location inside the pelvis and by enhancing hypertrophy and stiffness of the PFM and connective tissue. This would facilitate a more effective co-contraction of the PFM and prevent descent during increases in abdominal pressure. The pelvic floor can be considered as a trampoline with its position inside the pelvis. If the trampoline is stretched and sagging down, it is difficult to jump. However, a firm trampoline gives a quicker response and an effective 'push' upwards (Fig. 6.8).

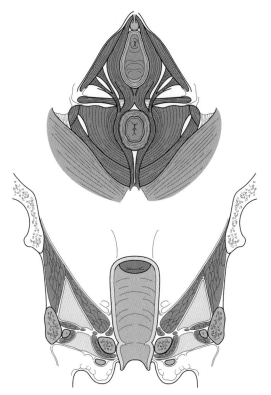

Fig. 6.6 The pelvic floor muscles consist of two muscle layers the pelvic diaphragm (cranial location) and the urogenital diaphragm (caudal location, also named the perineal muscles).

Table 6.2 Muscle fibre adaptation with resistance training (From Kraemer & Fry 1995)

Variable	Muscle's adaptational response
Muscle fibre myofibrillar protein content	↑
Capillary density	↔↓
Mitochondrial volume density	↓
Myoglobin	↓
Succinate dehdrogenase	↔↓
Malate dehydrogenase	↔↓
Citrate synthase	↔↓
3-hydroxyacyl-CoA dehydrogenase	↔↓
Creatine phosphokinase	↑
Myokinase	↑
Phosphofructokinase	↔↓
Lactate dehydrogenase	↔↑
Stored ATP	↑
Stored PC	↑
Stored glycogen	↑
Stored triglycerides	↑ ?
Myosin heavy chain composition	Slow to fast

ATP, adenosine triphosphate, PC, phosphocreatine.

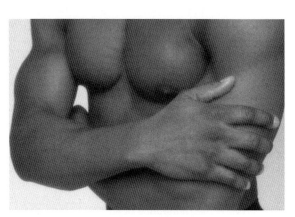

Fig 6.7 Regular strength training develops muscle hypertrophy, and the same has been seen in the pelvic floor muscles.

As most individuals starting a PFM training (PFMT) regimen would be untrained, some improvements would probably occur regardless of the type of training programme applied (Kraemer & Ratamess 2004). Because all PFMT studies have used different training dosage and different outcome measures, it is not possible to compare effects and conclude which training programme is the most effective. It may be considered much easier to improve quality of life (QoL) compared to reducing amount of urinary leakage or increasing muscle hypertrophy. Both general and disease-specific QoL parameters will most likely change because of factors other than the actual training programme (e.g. as a result of information that the condition can be improved or cured, care, support, comfort and motiva-

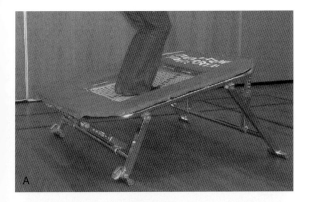

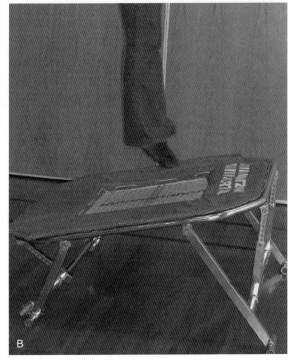

Fig. 6.8 With its location in the bottom of the pelvis the pelvic muscles should act as a trampoline when abdominal pressure is increased. A stiff trampoline gives a quick response to load and pushes upwards.

tion). On the other hand, a change in morphological muscle factors must be due to actual training. In addition, there is a huge difference between a report of 'feeling better' and measurement of cure on a pad test with standardized bladder volume. We will argue that proper training is needed to make a measurable change in muscle morphology and cure symptoms of pelvic floor dysfunction.

TERMINOLOGY AND DEFINITIONS

Muscle strength

Muscle strength is 'the maximal amount of force or torque a muscle or muscle group can generate in a specific movement pattern at a specific velocity of movement' (Knuttgen & Kraemer 1987). To include different muscle actions it has also been defined as the 'maximum force which can be exerted against an immovable object (static/isometric strength), the heaviest weight which can be lifted or lowered (concentric and eccentric dynamic strength), or the maximum torque which can be developed against a pre-set rate limiting device (isokinetic strength)' (Frontera & Meredith 1989).

A **repetition** is one complete movement of an exercise (e.g. one contraction of the PFM). It normally consists of two phases: the concentric muscle action and the eccentric muscle action (Fleck & Kraemer 2004).

A **set** is a group of repetitions performed continuously without stopping or resting. Sets typically range from 1 to 15 repetitions (Fleck & Kramer 2004).

Maximum voluntary contraction – one repetition maximum (1RM)

Knuttgen & Kraemer (1987) described a **maximal voluntary contraction** as 'a condition in which a person attempts to recruit as many fibres in a muscle as possible for the purpose of developing force'. They focus on the importance of the word 'voluntary' because inhibitory mechanisms in the central nervous system (CNS) can limit the recruitment of motor units, and the total number of muscle fibres that will produce the force. An important part of strength training is to diminish the inhibitory mechanisms during maximal effort and allow the person to come as close as possible to total recruitment. The resistance at which the subject can perform only one lift of a free weight and not be able to repeat it is termed the **one repetition maximum (1RM)**. The mass of the free weight that limits the person to ten repetitions would be termed 10RM (Knuttgen & Kraemer 1987). Performing voluntary maximal muscular actions means that the muscles involved must contract against as much resistance as its present fatigue level will allow. This is often referred to as overloading the muscle.

Local muscle endurance

Local muscle endurance is usually defined as either number of repetitions conduced, or duration of sustaining a contraction. Number of repetitions is inversely related to the percentage of 1RM, and varies with training status, sex and amount of muscle mass needed to perform the exercise (Hoeger et al 1990). Fatigue is a necessary component of local muscle endurance training (Kraemer & Ratamess 2004), and increases in maximum strength usually increase local muscle endurance, while muscle endurance training does not improve maximum strength. Training to increase muscle endurance requires the performance of high number of repetitions and minimizing recovery between sets.

Muscle power

Muscle power is the explosive aspect of strength, the product of strength and speed of movement (force × distance)/time (Wilmore & Costill 1999). Power is the functional application of both strength and speed (distance/time), and is the key component of most performances. Knuttgen & Kraemer (1987) explain the interrelationship between power and strength emphasizing that high power development means less than maximal force and maximal force development means low power. Maximum strength is the force developed during contractions of slow-velocity or isometric contractions, and power is developed during high-velocity contractions.

The order in which motor units are recruited is relatively constant and according to the size principle. This means that in light movements using low force, the smaller motor units (low-threshold) motor neurons innervating slow twitch, type I, muscle fibres are always recruited first. With increasing loads the muscle demands more force and progressively higher threshold motor units (type II muscle fibres) are recruited (Fleck & Kraemer 2004). This also applies when the load is constant, but the speed of contraction increases. At higher shortening velocities submaximal forces can be maximum or at least close to maximum (Åstrand et al 2003).

Training to increase muscular power requires two general loading strategies:

1. moderate to high training loads are needed to recruit high-threshold fast twitch motor units for strength, but this implies moderate to slow velocity contractions;
2. incorporation of light to moderate loads performed at an explosive lifting velocity.

These two loading strategies were used in the PFMT programme developed by Bø et al (1990). The patient is asked to contract as close to maximum as possible, try to hold the contraction and then to add 3–4 fast contractions on top of the holding period (Fig. 6.9)

DETERMINANTS OF MUSCLE STRENGTH

There are several determinants of muscle strength.

- **Anatomy**. There is an individual difference in joint angle and lever arm in different muscles. The longer the lever arm the more work the muscle can produce (work = force × lever arm). The most optimal lever arm is difficult to establish in the PFM. A sagging pelvic floor may be more difficult to lift voluntarily, and the expected automatic co-contraction during increased abdominal pressure may be too slow to stop excessive downward movement. Also total number of muscle fibres within a muscle, the cross-sectional area, the distribution of type I and type II muscle fibres (especially in fast dynamic contractions), and the internal muscle architecture are determinants of muscle strength (Åstrand et al 2003). This differs between individuals.

- **Length–tension**. There is an optimal length of which muscle fibres generate maximal force. The total amount of force generated depends on the total number of myosin cross-bridges interacting with active sites on the actin. If a sarcomere or a muscle is stretched or shortened beyond the optimal

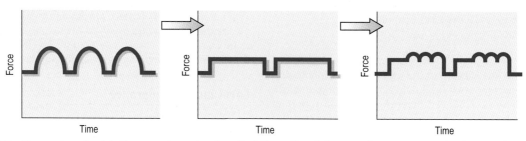

Fig. 6.9 Progression of pelvic floor muscle contraction. First the patient is instructed to contract as hard as possible. Second stage is to hold the contraction, and third stage is to contract as hard as possible, hold the contraction and add 3–4 quick contractions on top of the holding period (third diagram). The latter is meant to recruit fast twitch fibers.

length, less force can be developed (Fleck & Kraemer 2004).

- **Force–velocity.** As the velocity of a movement increases, the maximal force a muscle can produce concentrically decreases. Conversely, as the velocity of movement increases, the force that a muscle can develop eccentrically increases (Fleck and Kraemer 2004).

- **Muscle volume.** There is a highly significant positive correlation between cross-sectional area and maximum strength, especially for experienced athletes (Brechue & Abe 2002). The connection is less pronounced if untrained and in complex exercises because differences in technique can explain a bigger part of the result (Carroll et al 2001).

- **Neural control** (motor unit recruitment and rate of firing) is an important component of muscle strength and a prerequisite for development of muscle hypertrophy (Fleck & Kraemer 2004).

- **Metabolic component** (the rate at which myosin splits ATP) (Fleck & Kraemer 2004).

The two most important factors that can be influenced by strength training are neural adaptations and muscle volume (hypertrophy) (Fleck & Kraemer 2004).

Neural adaptations

Neural factors can be listed as neural drive (recruitment and rate of firing) to the muscle, increased synchronization of the motor units, increased activation of agonists, decreased activation of antagonists, coordination of all motor units and muscles involved in a movement, and inhibition of the protective mechanisms of the muscle (e.g. Golgi tendon organs) (Fleck & Kraemer 2004). When a person attempts to produce a maximal contraction, all available motor units are activated. Force can be increased by recruiting more motor units and an increase in motor unit firing rate. It has been suggested that untrained individuals are not able to voluntarily recruit the highest threshold motor units or maximally activate their muscles (Kraemer et al 1996).

An important part of training adaptation is therefore developing the ability to recruit all motor units in a specific exercise. This is especially important for PFMT because so few People are aware of the PFM or have ever tried to contract PFM voluntarily. Another important neural adaptation to training is a reduction in antagonist activation. For the PFM it is difficult to say which muscles can be considered antagonists. However, abdominal contraction without a PFM contraction may

be an antagonist contraction. An automatic co-contraction of the PFM to counteract any increase in abdominal pressure or the increase from ground reaction force may be considered a goal for training.

The initial quick gains in strength seen after strength training seem to be due to neural adaptation (Sale 1988). A 50% increase in muscle strength within only weeks of training is common. This strength gain is much greater than can be explained by muscle hypertrophy (Fleck & Kraemer 2004). After approximately 8 weeks of regular training, muscle hypertrophy becomes the predominant factor in strength increase, especially in young men. However, muscle hypertrophy also reaches a maximum and plateaus. Then the participants again need to work on neural factors to increase maximum force. Despite minimal changes in muscle fibre size during long-term training in competitive Olympic weightlifters, strength and power increases have been described (Kraemer et al 1996).

Greater loading is needed to increase maximal strength as one progress from intermediate to advanced levels of training and loads greater than 80–85% of 1RM are needed to produce further neural adaptations during advanced resistance training (Kraemer & Ratamess 2004). This is important because maximizing strength, power and hypertrophy may only be accomplished when the maximal numbers of motor units are recruited.

Some of the strength exercises are more difficult to coordinate than others and put the nervous system under greater demands. The potential for neural adaptations to influence the result are therefore higher during such exercises (Chilibeck et al 1998). The more complex bench and leg press movements compared to the not so coordinated difficult arm curl exercise may delay hypertrophy in the trunk and legs (Chilibeck et al 1998).

According to Shield & Zhou (2004) there is in general only a small room for improvement in fully activating the muscles in healthy people. The amount differs with type of contraction (isometric, dynamic), muscle groups, injuries, degenerations and complexity of movements. But there are still disagreements in the amount of activation, and the effect of strength training. Most studies imply a full activation of most muscles is measured with early twitch interpolation techniques, whereas newer more sensitive techniques reveal that even healthy adults routinely fail to fully activate a number of different muscles despite maximal effort (Shield & Zhou 2004). Other factors that can only be explained by neural factors are the cross-education effect seen in unilateral training and the effect where strength is increased after imagined contractions (Åstrand et al 2003).

Hypertrophy

One of the most prominent adaptations to strength training is muscle enlargement. The growth in muscle size is primarily due to an increase in the size of the individual muscle fibre (Fleck & Kraemer 2004). According to Fleck & Kraemer (2004), humans have a potential to hyperplasia, but it does not happen on a large scale and is far from the dominating cause of hypertrophy. An increase in the number of muscle fibres has been shown in birds and mammals, but there are limited data to prove this in humans.

The increase in cross-sectional area is attributed to increased size and number of the contractile proteins (actin and myosin filaments) and the addition of sarcomeres within existing muscle fibres. An increase in non-contractile proteins has also been suggested.

Satellite cells and myonuclei may indicate cellular repair after training and the formation of new muscle cells, and the proportion of satellite cells that appear morphologically active, increases as a result of resistance training (Fleck & Kraemer 2004).

Muscle fibre hypertrophy has been found in both type I and type II fibres after strength training. However, most studies show greater hypertrophy in type II and especially IIa fibres (Green et al 1999). Genetic factors decide whether a person has predominantly type I or type II muscle fibres, and though transitions from type IIb (now named IIx) to type IIa have been found (Green et al. 1999), such changes only seem to happen within fibre type (e.g. not from type II to type I; Fleck & Kraemer 2004). Cessation of training leads to transitions back from IIa to IIb. But even if most studies fail to find changes in the amount of type I fibres, some strength and sprint studies do. Kadi & Thornell (1999) found that there was a significant increase in the amount of MyHC IIa protein and a significant decrease of the amount of MyHC I and IIb in the trapezius muscle of women in the strength group.

Different muscles have different distributions of fibre types and the total number of muscle fibres varies between individuals. Because the number and distribution of muscle fibres do not seem to be the dominant factor for hypertrophy, and it is impossible to evaluate the number and distribution of muscle fibres in an individual without biopsies, types of muscle fibres should be disregarded as a factor when prescribing PFMT. The aim is to target as many motor units as possible in each contraction.

Greater hypertrophy has been associated with high-volume compared to low-volume programmes (Kraemer & Ratamess 2004). Short rest intervals have also been shown to be beneficial for hypertrophy and local muscle endurance (Kraemer & Ratamess 2004). Some studies suggest that a fatigue stimulus with metabolic stress factors has an influence on optimal strength development and muscle growth, even if the mechanisms are unknown. Rooney et al (1994) found that 30 s rest between each lift gave a significant lower strength increase than the same amount of repetitions and loads with no rest between the lifts. Maximal hypertrophy may be best attained by a combination of strength and hypertrophy training. One study showed greater increases in cross-sectional area and strength when training was divided into two sessions a day rather than one (Kraemer & Ratamess 2004).

With the initiation of a strength training regimen, changes in the types of muscle proteins start to take place within a couple of work-outs. This is caused by increased protein synthesis, a decrease in protein degradation, or a combination of both. Protein synthesis is significantly elevated up to 48 hours after exercise (Fleck & Kraemer 2004). However, to demonstrate significant muscle fibre hypertrophy, a longer training time is required (>8 weeks) (Fleck & Kraemer 2004). As studies are demonstrating an elevated muscle protein synthesis after an acute strength training bout (MacDougall et al 1995) the discrepancy seen between increased strength and muscle growth early in a strength training regimen may be more due to methodological problems in measuring small changes in muscle cross-sectional area rather than the traditionally assumed effect of neural adaptation. Another contributing factor that can explain why the role of neural adaptation may be overestimated at the beginning of a strength training programme is an increase of muscle fibre girth at the expense of extracellular spaces (Åstrand et al 2003). In most training studies increase in muscle fibre cross-sectional area range from about 20 to 40% (Fleck & Kraemer 2004). In an uncontrolled PFMT trial Bernstein (1996) found an increase in levator ani thickness of 7.6% at rest and 9.3% during contraction.

Is a voluntary PFM contraction a concentric or isometric muscle action? MRI studies (Bø et al 2001) have shown that there is a movement of the coccyx during PFM contraction. Hence, the contraction is concentric. However, this movement is small and there therefore must be an isometric component of PFMT. It has been suggested that 6 s is necessary to reach maximum contraction. However, holding times between 3 and 10 s are recommended for isometric contractions (Fleck & Kraemer 2004). Daily isometric training is superior to less frequent training, but three training sessions per week will bring significant increases in maximal strength. Isometric training alone with no external weights has been shown to increase protein synthesis 49% and muscular hypertrophy of both type I and type II muscle fibres. Twelve weeks of training increased knee extensor cross-sectional area 8% and muscle iso-metric strength 41% (Fleck & Kraemer 2004). PFM action is eccentric during increases in abdominal pressure.

DOSE–RESPONSE ISSUES

Dose–response issues deal with how much (or how little) exercise is needed to make a measurable training response (Bouchard 2001, Bouchard et al 1994). The dosage can be divided into mode of exercise, frequency, intensity, volume and duration of training. A training response is a progressive change in function or structure that results from performing repeated bouts of exercise, and is usually considered to be independent of a single bout of exercise. However, there is increasing evidence that one bout of exercise can give acute biological responses (Bouchard et al 1994).

Mode of exercise

Mode of exercise refers to type of training (e.g. strength training, flexibility training, cardiovascular training, and all types of specific exercises for different muscle groups). There is only one way to conduct a PFM contraction (squeeze around the pelvic openings and a lift inwards/forwards). However, the exercises can be conducted in different positions and they can be performed as isometric, concentric and eccentric contractions (Fig. 6.10).

Frequency

Frequency of exercise is usually defined as number of training sessions per week in which a certain muscle group is being trained or a particular exercise performed (Fleck & Kraemer 2004). Training with heavy loads increases the recovery time needed before subsequent sessions. Most resistance training studies have used frequencies of 2–3 alternating days per week in previously untrained individuals. Power lifters typically train 4–6 days per week (Kraemer & Ratamess 2004).

Intensity

Intensity of strength training is defined as the percentage of maximum (e.g. any given percentage of maximum or different RM resistances for the exercise; Fleck &

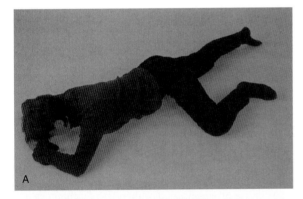

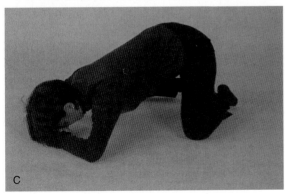

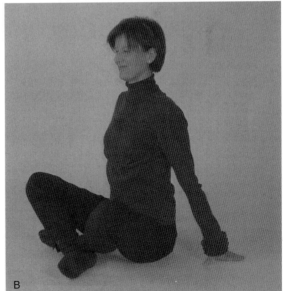

Fig. 6.10 Different positions can be used to vary pelvic floor muscle training.

Kraemer 2004). Intensity is by far the most important factor for effective and quick response to a strength training programme (American College of Sports Medicine 1998). The minimal intensity that has been shown to increase strength in young healthy individuals is 60–65% of 1RM. However, 50–60% of 1RM has been shown to increase strength in special populations (e.g. older women). Performing many repetitions with very light resistance will result in no or minimal strength gain. This is quite contradictory to the recommendations given by Kegel (1956). Although he emphasized to train against resistance, he advised to perform at least 500 contractions per day, and this has been the dominating recommendations for PFMT since then. Today, it is, however, important to use modern evidence-based training principles to gain the best effect. Fewer contractions take less time and may be much more motivating. Hence exercise adherence may increase.

Duration

The duration of the training period (e.g. whether it is 3 weeks or 6 months) influences the results. According to the American College of Sports Medicine (1998) it is reasonable to believe that short-term exercise studies conducted over a few weeks have certain limitations. Several studies have shown that increasing the duration of the exercise period adds substantial improvement in muscle strength.

In a randomized controlled trial (RCT) of PFM strength training to treat female stress urinary incontinence (SUI), Bø et al (1990) demonstrated an increasing PFM strength in the intensive training group throughout the 6-month training period (Fig. 6.11). Short training periods may therefore not elicit the true effect of exercises. The American College of Sports Medicine (1998) recommends that to evaluate the efficacy of various intensities, frequencies and durations of exercise on fitness variables, a 15–20-week duration is an adequate minimum standard.

Training volume is a measure of the total amount of work (joules) performed in a training session, in a week of training, in a month of training or in some other period of time (Fleck & Kraemer 2004). The simplest method to estimate training volume is to summate the number of repetitions performed in a specific time period or the total amount of weight lifted. More precisely it can be determined by calculating the work performed (e.g. total work in a repetition is the resistance multiplied by the vertical distance a weight is lifted).

Periodization is the planned variation in the training volume and intensity (Fleck & Kraemer 2004). Variation is extremely important for continued gains in strength

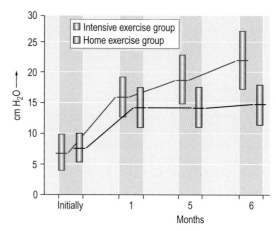

Fig. 6.11 Strength development during 6 months of two different training regimens for the pelvic floor muscles. There is 100% increase in muscle strength during the first month of exercise. After this first initial increase in strength, the group participating in supervised strenuous strength training in a class, further develops muscle strength while the other group exercising at home have no further improvement.

and other training outcomes. For improvements to occur, the programme used should be systematically altered so that the body is forced to adapt to changing stimuli. Variation can be achieved by altering muscle actions (isometric, concentric, eccentric), positions, repetitions, load, resting periods and types of exercises.

Adherence

Adherence (in medical literature often termed compliance) is the extent to which the individual follows the exercise prescription. Adherence is the most important factor influencing outcome and should be reported in all exercise programmes. For theories of adherence and strategies to increase adherence, see Chapter 7.

HOW TO INCREASE MUSCLE STRENGTH AND UNDERLYING COMPONENTS

Four main principles are important in achieving measurable effects of strength training and underlying components: specificity, overload, progression and maintenance.

Specificity

The effect of exercise training is specific to the area of the body being trained (American College of Sports

Medicine 1998, Fleck & Kraemer 2004). Strength training of the arms may therefore have little or no influence on the legs and vice versa. This principle is extremely important when it comes to the PFM. There have been some suggestions that regular physical activity may enhance PFM strength (Bø 2004). However, the prerequisite for this is that the load put on the pelvic floor by the increased abdominal pressure or ground reaction force is counteracted by an adequate response from the PFM. Obviously in women with pelvic floor dysfunction the PFM are not co-contracting in adequate time or with enough strength to counteract the increased load. In such cases the PFM are not trained but overloaded and stretched. There therefore needs to be a balance between the degree of loading and the counteraction of the PFM. A gymnast may have adequate response from the PFM during coughing and light activities. However, landing from a summersault on the bar may be too much load and risk urinary leakage. A small increase in abdominal pressure may therefore be an adequate stimulus for a co-contraction and thereby a 'training effect', while a huge increase may cause PFM descent and stretch and weaken the PFM.

Although studies have shown that there are co-contractions of the PFM with hip adductor, gluteal and different abdominal muscle contractions in healthy subjects (Bø & Stien 1994, Neumann & Gill 2002, Sapsford & Hodges 2001) such contractions may not occur in persons with PFM dysfunction and may be weaker than a specific PFM contraction. One should therefore focus on specific PFMT. In addition, Graves et al (1988) have shown that resistance training should be conducted through a full range of motion for maximum benefit.

Overload

Muscular strength and endurance are developed by the progressive overload principle (e.g. by increasing more than normal the resistance to movement or frequency and duration of activity; American College of Sports Medicine 1998). Muscular strength is best developed by using heavier weights/resistance (that require maximum or near maximum tension development) with few repetitions, and muscular endurance is best developed by using lighter weights with a great number of repetitions (American College of Sports Medicine 1998). There are several ways to overload a muscle or muscle group:

- add weight or resistance;
- sustain the contraction;
- shorten resting periods between contractions;
- increase speed of the contraction;
- increase number of repetitions;

- increase frequency and duration of work-outs;
- decrease recovery time between work-outs;
- alternate form of exercise;
- alternate range to which a muscle is being worked.

The PT can manipulate all the above-listed factors when training the PFM. However, certain important factors are difficult to apply for PFMT (e.g. to add weight and resistance). Plevnik (1985) invented vaginal-weighted cones to make a progression of overload to the PFM (Fig. 12). Vaginal cones come in different shapes and weights and are placed above the levator muscle. The patient is asked to start with a weight that she can hold for 1 minute in standing position. The actual training is to try to stay in an upright position with the cone in place for 20 minutes. When the woman is able to walk around with a weight in place for 20 minutes, a heavier weight should replace the one used to make progression in workload. Although correct from a theoretical exercise science point of view this method can be questioned from a practical point of view. In addition, holding a contraction for a long time may decrease blood supply, cause pain and reduce oxygen consumption (Bø 1995). Many women report that they are unable to hold the cones in place and adherence may be low (Bø et al 1999, Cammu & Van Nylen 1998).

Any magnitude of overload will result in strength development, but heavier resistance loads to maximal or near maximal will elicit a significantly greater training effect (American College of Sports Medicine 1998). Heavy resistance training may cause an acute increase in systolic and diastolic blood pressure, especially when a Valsalva manoeuvre is evoked (American College of Sports Medicine 1998). This is of importance for PFMT

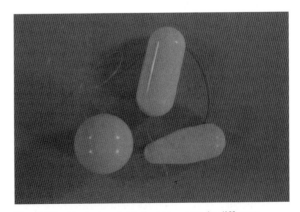

Fig. 6.12 Vaginal weighted cones come in different shapes and with different weights to make progression to pelvic floor muscle training. They were developed by Plevnik in 1985.

because many women tend to erroneously perform a Valsalva manoeuvre when attempting to perform a PFM contraction. As far as we know, there have been no studies so far examining blood pressure during PFMT. However, some women report slight headache, dizziness and discomfort during their first PFMT sessions, and this may be due to an increase in blood pressure or inadequate breathing. Normal breathing during attempts of maximum contractions to contract is almost impossible. Therefore, an emphasis on normal breathing between each contraction is important.

Eccentric (lengthening) exercises are effective in increasing muscle strength (Fleck & Kraemer 2004). However, the potential for skeletal muscle soreness and muscle injury is increased when compared to concentric (shortening) or isometric contractions, particularly in untrained individuals (American College of Sports Medicine 1998, Fleck & Kraemer 2004). Eccentric contractions are also more difficult to perform (require more motor skill and muscle awareness) than concentric or isometric contractions, and are therefore not recommended at the beginning of a PFMT programme.

Progression

The three principles of progression are overload, variation and specificity.

Progressive overload is defined as 'continually increasing the stress placed on the muscle as it becomes capable of producing greater force or has more endurance' (Fleck & Kraemer 2004, p. 7). One of the first reports of progression in strength training is from ancient Greece where Milo, an Olympic 'wrestler' lifted a calf each day until it reached full growth (DiNibule 1991).

The American College of Sport Medicine (2002) recommends that both concentric and eccentric muscle actions are used in strength training programmes. For initial training it is recommended that loads corresponding to 8–12 repetitions maximum are used for novice training. For intermediate to advanced training the recommendation is to use a wider range, from 1–12RM in a periodized fashion, with eventually an emphasis on heavy loading (1–6RM) with rest periods of at least 3 minutes between sets, and with a moderate contraction velocity. Higher volume is recommended for maximizing hypertrophy.

In practice, the principle of progressive overload is the most difficult factor to overcome in PFMT. It is difficult to put weight on the pelvic floor, and therefore other methods needs to be used. In most cases the PT has tried to encourage the woman to contract the PFM as close to maximum as possible. This can be done simultaneously with vaginal palpation (feedback) and with any measurement tool in situ (biofeedback). Using

biofeedback to reach a maximum contraction can be important from an exercise science point of view. Strong verbal encouragement and motivation seem to be very important in reaching maximum effort. However, the PT should always ensure that the patient is performing a correct contraction and not involving other muscles or increasing abdominal pressure too much. Leaving a patient to train alone is likely to result in loss of the overload and progression because only a few individuals can motivate themselves for maximal efforts. Follow-up, either individual training with the PT or in a class, seems to be a prerequisite for effective training.

Bø et al (1990) have developed a method for progression in PFMT (see Fig. 6.9). First the patient learns to contract as hard as possible with no holding period, then the patient is encouraged to hold as long as possible, and the third step is to add 3–4 fast contractions on top of the sustained contraction. After this has been accomplished the PT encourages the patient to contract as hard as possible in each contraction.

One way to produce progression is to ask the patient to contract against progressively increasing gravity going from a lying to a standing position (Fig. 6.13). Clinical experience has shown that most women find that PFM contractions are more difficult to conduct in the squatting position (Fig. 6.14). However, it is important that the patients choose a position in which they are able to perceive the contraction, and also choose a position in which they feel a certain difficulty when training. In this way they stimulate the CNS and hopefully recruit an increasing number of motor units. In a group training setting the different positions are also used for variation in the training programme (Bø et al 1990, 1999). So far, there are no studies comparing the effect of different positions on the development of PFM strength.

Another method to increase progression of the contraction is to use vaginal or rectal devices and ask the patient to hold back when the PT or the patient him or herself withdraws the device. This method implies eccentric muscle contraction and may be a very effective method to increase strength. However, no studies have evaluated a possible effect of such a programme, and one should be aware of the increased risk of injuries and development of muscle soreness in untrained individuals.

There is a need for more research evaluating different ways of adding progressive overload to PFMT.

Initial training status plays an important role in the rate of progression during strength training. Trained individuals have shown much slower rates of improvement than untrained individuals. Kraemer & Ratamess (2004) report that a literature review showed that muscular strength increased approximately 40% in 'untrained', 20% in 'moderately' trained, 16% in

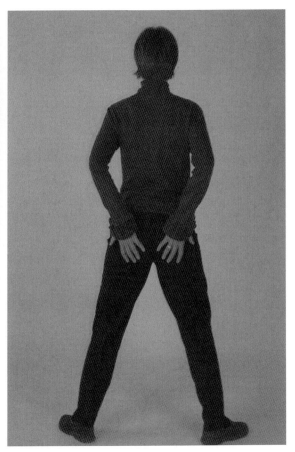

Fig. 6.13 In the standing position the pelvic floor muscles must contract against gravity and is more difficult than in a supine or prone position.

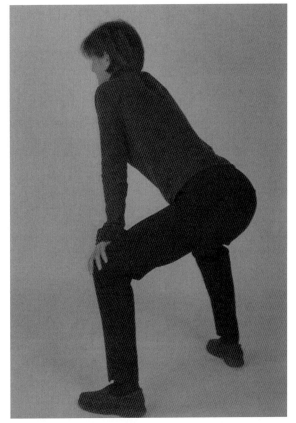

Fig. 6.14 Squatting position is reported to be a difficult position for contracting the pelvic floor muscles and can therefore be used as a progression in loading.

'trained', 10% in advanced and 2% in 'elite' over periods of 4 weeks to 2 years. The only study looking at the development of PFM strength (see Fig. 6.11) showed a 100% increase after 1 month of exercise. This may be explained by the PFM being totally untrained, and shows a huge potential for improvement. In a meta-analysis Rea et al (2003) confirmed statistically greater effect sizes in untrained compared to resistance-trained individuals with respect to training intensity, frequency and volume on progression. As the person approaches his or her genetic ceiling, small changes in strength require large amounts of training time.

Maintenance

Maintenance training is work to maintain the current level of muscular fitness. Cessation of exercise training is often termed 'detraining'. Fleck & Kraemer (2004) described detraining as 'a deconditioning process that affects performance because of diminished physiological capacity'. Detraining from a muscle strengthening programme will reduce muscle girth, muscle fibre size, short-term endurance and strength/power, whereas capillary density, fat percentage, aerobic enzymes and mitochondrial density will increase (Fleck & Kraemer 2004). However, following a shorter period of detraining most individuals would still have higher values for these variables than untrained subjects, and physiological functions return quickly with retraining after the detraining period. Strength may be maintained for up to 2 weeks of detraining in power athletes and in recreationally trained individuals strength loss has been shown to take as long as 6 weeks. However, eccentric force and power seem to be more sensitive to detraining effects over a few weeks (Fleck & Kraemer 2004).

In general, strength gains decline at a slower rate than strength increases due to training. There are few studies, however, investigating the minimal level of exercise necessary to maintain the training effect. A 5–10% loss of muscle strength per week has been shown after training cessation (Fleck & Kraemer 2004). Greater losses has been shown in the elderly (65–75-year-olds) compared to younger people (20–30-year-olds), and for both groups most strength loss was from week 12–31 after cessation of training.

The rate of strength loss may depend on the duration of the training period before detraining, type of strength test used and the specific muscle groups examined. Graves et al (1988) showed that when strength training was reduced from 3 or 2 days a week to at least 1 day a week, strength was maintained for 12 weeks of reduced training. Reducing training frequency therefore does not seem to adversely affect muscular strength as long as intensity is maintained (Fleck & Kraemer 2004). In one study, 24 weeks of heavy resistance training three times a week increased vertical jump ability 13%. Twelve weeks of detraining decreased the ability, but it was still 2% above the pretraining value (Fleck & Kraemer 2004). It is suggested that the ability to perform complex skills involving strength components may be lost if not included in the training programme (Fleck & Kraemer 2004). Electromyography (EMG) studies have shown a change in motor unit firing rate and motor unit synchronization, and that this may cause the initial strength loss in the detraining period. Type II fibres may atrophy to a greater extent than type I fibres during short detraining periods in both men and women (Fleck & Kraemer 2004).

Fleck & Kraemer (2004) concluded that research has not yet indicated the exact resistance, volume, and frequency of strength training or the type of programme needed to maintain the training gains. However, studies indicate that to maintain strength gains or slow strength loss the intensity should be maintained, but the volume and frequency of training can be reduced: 1–2 days a week seems to be an effective maintenance frequency for those individuals already engaged in a resistance training programme (Kraemer & Ratamess 2004)

Only one follow-up study measuring PFM strength after cessation of PFMT has been found. Bø & Talseth (1996) showed that there was no reduction in PFM muscle strength in the intensive training group 5 years after cessation of a RCT: 70% of the women in this group reported strength training of the PFM at least once a week.

RECOMMENDATION FOR EFFECTIVE TRAINING DOSAGE FOR PELVIC FLOOR MUSCLE TRAINING

The American College of Sport Medicine has given the following recommendations for general strength training for adults (American College of Sports Medicine 1998):

- target specific muscles;
- perform 8–12 slow-velocity, close-to-maximum contractions (even fewer repetitions better to optimize strength and power);
- perform three sets per day;

Table 6.3 Recommendations for progression of training for strength, power and hypertrophy in novice participants. (From Kraemer & Ratamess 2004)

	Strength	Power	Hypertrophy
Muscle action	Eccentric and concentric	Eccentric and concentric	Eccentric and concentric
Exercise selection	Single and multiple-joint	Multiple-joint	Single and multiple-joint
Exercise order	High before low intensity	High before low intensity	High before low intensity
Loading	60–70% 1RM	60–70% for strength 30–60% for velocity/technique	60–70% 1RM
Volume	1–3 × 8–12 repetitions	1–3 × 8–12 repetitions	1–3 sets × 8–12 repetitions
Rest intervals	1–2 min	2–3 min for core 1–2 min for others	1–2 min
Velocity	Slow to moderate	Moderate	Slow to moderate
Frequency	2–3 days per week	2–3 days per week	2–3 days per week

- exercises should be conducted 2–3 (4) days a week;
- exercise for more than 5 months of training to show effect.

Table 6.3 shows more specific recommendations for strength training regimens to effectively improve muscle strength, power and hypertrophy (Kraemer & Ratamess 2004). Developing from untrained to intermediate and advanced, the progression is to get closer to maximum contraction and to add more training days per week.

CLINICAL RECOMMENDATIONS

- Make sure the patient is able to perform a correct contraction.

- Ask the patient to contract as hard as possible.
- Progress with sustained contractions, and add contractions with higher velocity as a progression.
- Holding time should be 3–10 s.
- Recommend PFMT every day.
- Encourage and motivate patients to get as close to maximum contraction as possible. Use strong verbal encouragement.
- Advance to eccentric contractions if possible (no data on effect of eccentric training for the PFM).
- Inform the patient that strength training develops in steps and that the largest improvements come during the first training period. After that the patient needs to work harder to achieve further improvement.

REFERENCES

American College of Sports Medicine 1998 The recommended quantity and quality of exercise for developing and maintaining cardiorespiratory and muscular fitness, and flexibility in healthy adults. Medicine and Science in Sports and Exercise 30:975–991

American College of Sports Medicine 2002 Position stand. Progression models in resistance training for healthy adults. Medicine and Science in Sports and Exercise 34:364–380

Åstrand P O, Rodahl K, Dahl H A et al 2003 Textbook of work physiology; physiological basis of exercise. Human Kinetics, Champaign IL

Bernstein I T 1996 The pelvic floor muscles. Doctoral Thesis, Hvidovre Hospital, Department of Urology, University of Copenhagen

Bø K 1995 Vaginal weight cones. Theoretical framework, effect on pelvic floor muscle strength and female stress urinary incontinence. Acta Obstetricia et Gynecologica Scandinavica 74:87–92

Bø K 2004 Urinary incontinence, pelvic floor dysfunction, exercise and sport. Sports Medicine 34(7):451–464

Bø K, Hagen R H, Kvarstein B et al 1990 Pelvic floor muscle exercise for the treatment of female stress urinary incontinence: III. Effects of two different degrees of pelvic floor muscle exercise. Neurourology and Urodynamics 9:489–502

Bø K, Lilleås F, Talseth T, Hedlund H 2001 Dynamic MRI of pelvic floor muscles in an upright sitting position. Neurourology and Urodynamics 20:167–174

Bø K, Stien R 1994 Needle EMG registration of striated urethral wall and pelvic floor muscle activity patterns during cough, valsalva, abdominal, hip adductor, and gluteal muscles contractions in nulliparous healthy females. Neurourology and Urodynamics 13:35–41

Bø K, Talseth T 1996 Long-term effect of pelvic floor muscle exercise 5 years after cessation of organized training. Obstetrics and Gynecology 87:261–265

Bø K, Talseth T, Holme I 1999 Single blind, randomised controlled trial of pelvic floor exercises, electrical stimulation, vaginal cones, and no treatment in management of genuine stress incontinence in women. British Medical Journal 318:487–493

Bouchard C, Shephard RJ, Stephens T 1994 Physical activity, fitness and health. Consensus Statement. Human Kinetics Publishers. Champaign IL

Bouchard C 2001 Physical activity and health: introduction to the dose–response symposium. Medicine and Science in Sports and Exercise 33(6 suppl):S347–S350

Brechue W F, Abe T 2002 The role of FFM accumulation and skeletal muscle architecture in powerlifting performance. European Journal of Applied Physiology 86(4):327–336

Cammu H, Van Nylen M 1998 Pelvic floor exercises versus vaginal weight cones in genuine stress incontinence. European Journal of Obstetrics, Gynecology, and Reproductive Biology 77:89–93

Carroll T J, Riek S, Carson R G 2001 Neural adaptations to resistance training: implications for movement control. Sports Medicine 31(12):829–840

Chilibeck P D, Calder A W, Sale D G et al 1998 A comparison of strength and muscle mass increases during resistance training in young women. European Journal of Applied Physiology and Occupational Physiology 77(1–2):70–175

DiNubile N A 1991 Strength training. Clinics in Sports Medicine 10(1):33–62

Fleck S J, Kraemer W J 2004 Designing resistance training programs. 3rd edn. Human Kinetics. Champaign IL

Frontera W R, Meredith C N 1989 Strength training in the elderly. In: Harris R, Harris S, Physical activity, aging and sports, 1: scientific and medical research. Center for the Study of Aging, Albany, NY, p 319–331

Graves J E, Pollock M L, Leggett S H et al 1988 Effect of reduced frequency on muscular strength. International Journal of Sports Medicine 9:316–319

Green H, Goreham C, Ouyang J et al 1999 Regulation of fiber size, oxidative potential, and capillarization in human muscle by resistance exercise. American Journal of Physiology 276(2 Pt 2):591–596

Haskel W L 1994 Dose–response issues from a biological perspective. In: Bouchard C, Blair S N, Haskell W L Physical activity, fitness and health. Human Kinetics Publishers, Champaign, IL, p 1030–1039

Hoeger W W K, Hopkins D R, Barette S L et al 1990 Relationship between repetitions and selected percentages of one repetition maximum: a comparison between untrained and trained males and females. Journal of Strength and Conditioning Research 4(2):47–54

Kadi F, Thornell L E 1999 Training affects myosin heavy chain phenotype in the trapezius muscle of women. Histochemical Cell Biology 112(1):73–78

Kegel A H 1956 Early genital relaxation. Obstetrics and Gynecology 8(5):545–550

Knuttgen HG, Kraemer W J 1987 Terminology and measurement in exercise performance. Journal of Applied Sport Science Research 1:1–10

Kraemer W J, Fleck S J, Evans W J 1996 Strength and power training: physiological mechanisms of adaptation. Exercise and Sport Science Review 24:363–397

Kraemer W J, Fry A C 1995 Strength testing: development and evaluation of methodology. In: Maud PJ, Foster C, Physiological assessment of human fitness. Human Kinetics, Champaign, IL, p 115–138

Kraemer W J, Ratamess N A 2004 Fundamentals of resistance training: progression and exercise prescription. Medicine and Science in Sports and Exercise 36(4):674–688

MacDougall J D, Gibala M J, Tarnopolsky M A et al 1995 The time course for elevated muscle protein synthesis following heavy resistance exercise. Canadian Journal of Applied Physiology 20(4):480–486

Neumann P, Gill V 2002 Pelvic floor and abdominal muscle interaction: EMG activity and intra–abdominal pressure.

International Urogynecology Journal and Pelvic Floor Dysfunction 13:125–132

Plevnik S 1985 A new method for testing and strengthening pelvic floor muscles. Proceedings of the International Continence Society, 267–268

Rea M R, Alvar B A, Burkett L N et al 2003 A meta-analysis to determine the dose response for strength development. Medicine and Science in Sports and Exercise 35(3):456–464

Rooney K J, Herbert R D, Balnave R J 1994 Fatigue contributes to the strength training stimulus. Medicine and Science in Sports and Exercise 26(9):1160–1164

Sale D 1988 Neural adaptation to resistance training. Medicine and Science in Sports and Exercise 20(5 suppl):135–145

Sapsford R, Hodges P 2001 Contraction of the pelvic floor muscles during abdominal maneuvers. Archives of Physical Medicine Rehabilitation 82:1081–1088

Shield A, Zhou S 2004 Assessing voluntary muscle activation with the twitch interpolation technique. Sports Medicine 34(4):253–267

Wilmore J H, Costill D L 1999 Physiology of sport and exercise. 2nd edn. Human Kinetics, Champaign, IL

Chapter 7

Strategies to enhance adherence and reduce drop out in conservative treatment

Dianne Alewijnse, Ilse Mesters, Job F M Metsemakers and Bart van den Borne

INTRODUCTION

Non-compliance or non-adherence is an important problem of health care interventions and therapy. Many people have difficulties following given health care advice. There is no generally agreed definition of compliance or adherence, and over the past 25 years, several alternative terms have been proposed. Adherence is defined as 'the extent to which patients follow the instructions they are given for prescribed treatments'. The term adherence is intended to be non-judgmental, a statement of fact rather than of blame of the patient, prescriber, or treatment (Haynes et al 2002). We have chosen to use this term here on the understanding that it can include the spirit of patient participation and autonomy. Adherence behaviour is often not a matter of all or nothing, but has to be regarded as a continuum and patients may have many reasons why they adhere completely, partly or not at all. According to the International Classification of Functioning, Disability and Health (ICF), the goal of physical therapy is to improve functions and health and reduce disabilities (www.cdc.gov/nchs). This requires adherence, and consequently behavioural change and active patient participation (Sluijs et al 1993, Steiner & Earnest 2000).

One of the greatest challenges for physical therapists is how to effectively promote adherence behaviour and prevent drop out, with techniques that can easily be implemented in physical therapy and physiotherapeutic pelvic floor muscle training (PFMT) in particular. This chapter provides insight into:

- rationale for a relationship between adherence to and effectiveness of PFMT;

- determinants of adherence to PFMT;
- theories that relate to behavioural change, adherence and drop out;
- a health education programme to promote adherence and prevent drop out;
- evidence-based research on the promotion of adherence to PFMT;
- clinical recommendations on how to promote adherence and prevent drop out in PFMT.

RATIONALE FOR A RELATION BETWEEN ADHERENCE TO AND EFFECTIVENESS OF PELVIC FLOOR MUSCLE TRAINING

Physiotherapeutic PFMT is recommended for women with stress, urge or mixed urinary incontinence. PFMT is targeted to improve the strength, coordination, endurance and number of repetitions of the PFM aiming to improve and cure urinary incontinence. Increased awareness is expected to motivate patients to perform exercise behaviours to reduce disabilities and restore functions and health (Berghmans et al 1998b, Versprille-Fischer 1995).

Three systematic reviews (Berghmans et al 1998a, Berghmans et al 2000, Hay-Smith et al 2001) revealed that there is evidence that PFMT is effective for women with either stress or mixed urinary incontinence, and that favourable results for urge incontinence could be expected. Short-term effect rates (cured or improved by ≥50%) may exceed 70% of participants, while long-term effect rates may reach adequate improvement in 50% when adherence is maintained (Mouritsen 1994, Mouritsen & Schiøtz 2000).

Three studies on long-term effects found that adherence was a significant predictor, both during the period of therapy and thereafter (Bø & Talseth 1996, Chen et al 1999, Lagro-Janssen & Van Weel 1998). In general, the best results and most adequate adherence behaviour were found in women who had intensive training programmes guided by motivated physical therapists as compared to women who were instructed for a short time and then left to train alone (Bø et al 1990, Cammu & Van Nylen 1994, Wall & Davidson 1992, Wyman et al 1998). The effectiveness of PFMT therefore seems dependent on the intensity of the training programme and on adherence to all behavioural aspects of the treatment.

The observations concerning the possible link between adherence and therapy outcome, as well as the need for systematic and planned health education as an adherence-promoting strategy, led to the study of Alewijnse (2002). The study contained a longitudinal randomized controlled trial (RCT) on the effectiveness of PFMT supplemented with a theory-driven health education programme to promote long-term adherence to PFMT. It was hypothesized that better adherence behaviour was related to better therapy outcomes. The study revealed relevant predictors of long-term adherence to PFMT and suggested several clinical recommendations.

In this chapter, this study serves as an illustration on how to analyse determinants of adherence, how to apply theories to promote adherence and prevent drop out in educational interventions, and how to evaluate the effect of such interventions.

DETERMINANTS OF ADHERENCE TO PELVIC FLOOR MUSCLE TRAINING

In a needs assessment to prepare for the development of the PFMT programme with health education intervention, an extensive literature study was conducted and interviews were held with the target population – women with urinary incontinence and physical therapists specialized in PFMT – to provide information about determinants of adherence to PFMT (Alewijnse et al 2002a). Three important findings are illustrated here.

First, the promotion of adherence behaviour is considered to be an integral part of patient education in PFMT. However, patient education in physical therapy, and especially the part of encouraging adherence behaviour, lacks a systematic and theoretically funded behavioural approach (Knibbe & Wams 1994, Sluijs et al 1993). Such an approach is expected to enhance the effectiveness of education (Green & Kreuter 1991, 2004).

Second, there is a difference between short-term supervised adherence, which is the adherence during the period of therapy sessions, and long-term non-supervised adherence, which is the adherence during the period after the therapy sessions have ended and the patient has to train alone. Physical therapists estimate that 64% of patients adhere to exercise regimens and health advice in the short term, but that only 23% do so in the long term (Sluijs & Knibbe 1991). Findings indicate that there is room for improvement (Alewijnse et al 2003a).

Third, it was found that short- and long-term adherence were partly related to different determinants (Box 7.1) (Johnson et al 2000, Knibbe & Wams 1994, Kok & Bouter 1990, Sluijs & Knibbe 1991, Sluijs et al 1993).

Furthermore, targeting health education was also identified as an important determinant of adherence behaviour (Kreuter et al 2000, Sluijs & Knibbe, 1991). This involves tuning the health education messages to the characteristics of the target group involved, so that

> **Box 7.1:** Short- and long-term determinants of adherence to physical therapy
>
> *SHORT-TERM DETERMINANTS*
> - Barriers
>   - forgetting to exercise
>   - difficulty with integrating exercise advice in daily life
>   - lack of time
>   - lack of motivation
> - Feelings of competence
> - Self-efficacy expectations
> - Attitude towards adherence behaviour
> - Feedback
> - Perception of symptoms
>
> *LONG-TERM DETERMINANTS*
> - Social norms
> - Motivation to comply as a result of perceived social norms
> - Self-efficacy expectations
> - Attitude towards outcome expectations
> - Patient's representation of illness and concurrent emotions and self-care strategies (i.e. drinking less, frequent voiding)

information closely links up with adherence determinants such as the perceptions, values and expectations of the target group.

In summary, health education to promote adherence behaviour needs a systematic and theory-driven approach. Educational messages should focus on determinants of both short- and long-term adherence and the information should be targeted at the group of interest.

Theoretical framework for determinants

To categorize and conceptualize variables found important in determining adherence behaviour in a theoretical framework, a social cognition model called the Attitude Social influence self-Efficacy (ASE) model can be used (De Vries et al 1988). According to this model, behavioural change is best predicted by someone's intention to perform that behaviour. The model assumes that behavioural intention is determined by three types of cognitive proximal factors: attitudes, social influences and self-efficacy expectations. Distal variables such as sociodemographic, psychosocial and medical variables are expected to influence behavioural intention through the proximal variables. Barriers and skills play a role when actual behaviour is performed, and this perform-

ance leads to a feedback process that influences the three proximal variables (De Vries & Mudde 1998, Lechner 1998).

According to the ASE model, the key to changing adherence to PFMT is to analyse determinants of the intention to adhere. Knowing what determinants influence this particular intention could help physical therapists to motivate patients to adhere to PFMT. Fig. 7.1 shows how the ASE model is applied (Alewijnse et al 2001) and what determinants have been taken into account in the health education programme (Alewijnse et al 2002a).

The needs assessment revealed several proximal determinants: positive and negative outcome expectations, perceived social norms, modelling, social support, and self-efficacy expectations towards adherence to PFMT. Distal determinants were lay beliefs about incontinence, self-care strategies, illness representation, cultural norms and values, risk perception, prognosis, and perceived severity of symptoms. Barriers were lack of discipline, time and energy, forgetting, stressful situations, (negative) associations with sex, perceiving the pelvic floor as an unconscious body area, difficulties with integrating exercises in daily life, fluctuations in effectiveness, and muscle pain (bladder).

Two types of feedback played a role as well. In terms of internal feedback, progress, symptom distress or impact, self-esteem and body esteem were important for adherence behaviour, while oral feedback, guidance and reinforcement from the therapist and important others seemed external feedback determinants. Two aspects influenced many of the above determinants: knowledge and sex-specific aspects such as perception of the pelvic floor, socialization and gender role (Ashworth & Hagan 1993, Bø et al 1990, Bø 1995b, Burns et al 1993, Cammu et al 1991, Cammu & van Nylen 1994, Castleden et al 1984, Cramer 1995, Dougherty et al 1993, Gallo & Staskin 1997, Hahn et al 1993, Janetzky 1993, Knibbe & Wams 1994, Kok & Bouter 1990, Lagro-Janssen et al 1994, 1995, Lagro-Janssen & Van Weel 1998, Mantle & Versi 1991, Mouritsen et al 1991, Nygaard et al 1990, 1996, O'Dowd 1993, Sluijs & Knibbe 1991, Sluijs et al 1993, Wall & Davidson 1992, Wilson et al 1987, Wyman et al 1998).

THEORIES THAT RELATE TO BEHAVIOURAL CHANGE AND ADHERENCE

The ASE model explains behaviour. Other theories provide insight in how to change behaviour. Promotion of adherence to PFMT for urinary incontinence involves stimulating a behavioural change process in terms of integrating new behaviours in daily life and refraining

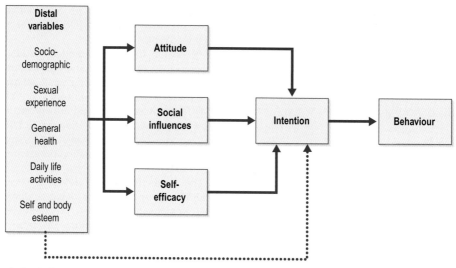

Fig. 7.1 The Attitude Social influence self-Efficacy (ASE) model of behavioural determinants. The dotted line between distal variables and intention indicates a possible direct influence of distal variables on intention.

from behaviours that negatively affect incontinence symptoms. Previous studies have emphasized the importance of positive motivation (Cammu et al 1991, Kok & Bouter 1990, Lagro-Janssen & Van Weel 1998, Mantle & Versie 1991, Sluijs & Knibbe 1991).

The transtheoretical model (TTM) explains behavioural change processes in terms of five motivational stages (pre-contemplation, contemplation, preparation, action and maintenance, Box 7.2) and is appropriate to many health behaviours (Prochaska et al 1992, 1994), including adherence (Willey et al 2000). The TTM emphasizes the dimension of time in behavioural change and provides options to influence behaviour. Each motivational stage is characterized by several behavioural determinants. This means that every stage needs specific methods and strategies to help patients move from one stage to the next.

The following processes are considered key in moving patients from precontemplation to contemplation: consciousness raising, dramatic relief, environmental re-evaluation, self-evaluation and decisional balance.

Consciousness raising indicates that a patient acquires information about the negative aspects of his or her current behaviour (frequent voiding), and the relationship between the advised behaviour and the health problem. Furthermore, patients often become motivated when they realize that their emotions are either aroused (dramatic relief) by internal stimuli (not being able to hold urine) or by external stimuli (smelling

> **Box 7.2:** Stages of behavioural change in the transtheoretical model
>
> - Pre-contemplation – people do not intend to change certain behaviours or adopt new behaviours
> - Contemplation – people are considering a change
> - Preparation – people make active plans to change
> - Action – people have changed, but their behaviour has not yet become a routine
> - Maintenance – people have integrated the altered behaviour in their lives and are trying to sustain it

other people, and relate this to the fear of being smelled). Talking about embarrassing moments or fear of embarrassment might help to proceed to a more action-oriented stage. Urinary incontinence might have an effect on the environment as well. Many patients avoid going out for instance. As a consequence the rest of the family gets isolated as well (environmental re-evaluation). Realization that urinary incontinence negatively affects themselves and others can heighten a patient's motivation to get into action. And finally, weighing up positive and negative outcomes of the advised behaviour (decisional balance) might help patients understand the gains and losses and help them to assign importance to the pros and cons of changing or remaining the way they are. In this context personal values can be discussed (self re-evaluation). For example, how current behaviour and the health problem conflicts with personal values and life goals, such as being independent or the duty to take good care of one's body.

In the attempt to move people from contemplation to preparation the same processes are relevant. Patients start to think seriously about solving their problem. They might want to receive information about treatment options and wonder about their ability to do exercises (self-efficacy expectations). When changing from preparation into action people need a plan to proceed. Confidence in their ability to adhere to the advice remains important in this stage, as well as stimulus control (being cued to perform the advised behaviour) and counterconditioning (altering response to cues that might hinder performance), for example deliberately taking time to do exercises in a stressful situation.

When changing into action, support from others such as a physical therapist, becomes important. Urinary incontinence is often not openly discussed, which might result in patients feeling alone in this respect. Realizing that a support system is available might be important in this stage. In the process from action to maintenance similar key processes can be identified as in the previous transition.

The literature shows that sustaining behaviour is difficult (Haynes et al 2002). The client has to consolidate the change attained and struggles to prevent relapse. Besides previously mentioned processes, reinforcement management might be important. Of course the most rewarding success is a decrease of symptoms. Nevertheless patients should learn that a temporary slip in adherence is not a failure and that they can pick up or intensify the exercise routine again as soon as symptoms reappear or get worse. They have to learn which exercise intensity works best to maintain their success.

As relapse and drop out are inherent to behavioural change, it may occur in any of the motivational stages (Prochaska et al 1992). Motivation is therefore seen as a state of readiness or eagerness to change, which may fluctuate from one time or situation to another (Miller & Rollnick 2002), implying that a person can go back (relapse) and forth between the stages as long as the behavioural change is not internalized. Health education can guide this iterative process.

The TTM is partly related to two other theories, the self-regulation theory (SRT; Leventhal & Cameron 1987, Leventhal et al 1998) and the social cognition theory (SCT; Bandura 1986). The SRT provides insight in adherence as self-management behaviour. It states that active participation of patients is necessary to promote adherence. To give patients more control over their lives and more faith in their own abilities, attention must be paid

to patients' cognitive representations of the illness in relation to coping with the illness and appraisal of the outcomes of behavioural change. The representation of the illness is based on current symptoms, previous experiences with illness, and personal views of health and illness originating from social and cultural influences. This representation also influences the self-care strategies of patients, such as drinking less or frequent voiding (Johnson et al 2000). To appraise the outcomes of adherence behaviour, patients need to evaluate their representations, self-care strategies and outcomes. This, in turn, could enhance patients' self-efficacy and effectiveness in terms of adherence behaviour.

Self-efficacy is a construct derived from the SCT (Bandura 1986). According to the SCT human behaviour can be explained by various expectations of certain behaviour:

- situation-outcome expectations;
- action-outcome expectations; and
- self-efficacy expectations.

In this theory, behaviour is the consequence of continuous interactions between the person, the behaviour and the environment or situation. Another assumption of the SCT is that people not only learn from performing a (new) behaviour and experience the consequences, but also from observing others (vicarious learning or modelling). Bandura (1986) adds the concept of self-control to the theory because people behave on the basis of setting their own goals and strategies for performing a specific behaviour and reward themselves.

HEALTH EDUCATION PROGRAMME

A detailed account of the health education programme to promote adherence to PFMT has been described in Alewijnse et al (2002a). The rationale of this programme was based on the three theories TTM, SRT and SCT. In addition, to stimulate recognition and acknowledgement of behavioural and informational needs, the principle of targeted communication was used as a means to promote adherence behaviour (Kreuter et al 2000, Mullen et al 1985, Sluijs & Knibbe 1991). Consequently, the programme was designed in such a way that women could find appropriate answers to their changing needs for information. Furthermore, attention was payed to women's sex-specific perception of their pelvic floor, to body esteem, and to making explicit the relationship between women's socialization, social position and gender role and their adherence behaviour (Alewijnse et al 2002b, Janetzky 1993, Toner & Akman 2000).

The development of the theory-driven health education programme was based on a problem-solving approach called intervention mapping (Bartholomew et al 2001), in which for each identified determinant specific programme objectives were formulated and appropriate theory-based methods and practical strategies were selected (Alewijnse et al 2002a). For example, for the method of goal setting, the strategy consisted of a filling-in task to write down personal treatment goals, and for the method of modelling, role model stories were the strategy (Bassett & Petrie 1999, Strecher et al 1995). Furthermore, self-evaluation about changes in symptoms was stimulated through the strategies assessment and feedback (Leventhal et al 1998), and reinforcement was provided for positive behaviour changes through self-monitoring of symptoms (Eagly & Chaiken 1993, Skinner 1938).

A minimal, a medium, and a maximum intervention were developed, each following the phases of the physiotherapeutic treatment plan (Knibbe & Wams 1994, Verhulst et al 1994). This enabled investigating what intensity of health education would be necessary to promote adherence effectively. The most important components were reminders in the form of stickers, guidance of adherence as self-management process in the form of a self-help guide, and structured feedback in the form of a counselling scheme for physical therapists, guiding structural oral feedback and reinforcement. The description of the programme of the self-help guide and counselling scheme follows the stages of the TTM as they logically follow the iterative phases of the physiotherapeutic treatment plan (Verhulst et al 1994). The counselling scheme stimulates the systematic addressing of issues, which should have a positive influence on adherence. Table 7.1 presents the content of the self-help guide and the corresponding counselling tasks for physical therapists along the motivational stages of change and phases of the physiotherapeutic treatment plan.

EVIDENCE-BASED RESEARCH ON THE PROMOTION OF ADHERENCE TO PFMT

Pelvic floor muscle training and adherence behaviour

As the Dutch clinical practice guidelines (Berghmans et al 1998b) were not available at the time of the study, a protocol for individual PFMT was prepared in cooperation with the participating physical therapists as a standard for all study conditions (Alewijnse et al 2003a). This written protocol checklist covered all treatment aspects usually applied in PFMT during diagnostic assessment activities, formulation of the treatment plan, commonly given patient education, treatment of exercise therapy and evaluation (Berghmans et al 1998b,

Knibbe & Wams 1994, Verhulst et al 1994, Versprille-Fischer 1995) (Box 7.3).

A schedule for frequency of treatment sessions over time, covering nine sessions of 30 minutes each in 14 weeks, or for additional sessions up to 22 weeks, was added to the protocol. This protocol and treatment frequency reflected usual care in the Netherlands. In addition, physical therapists were asked to complete treatment forms for every patient to evaluate eight treatment goals (Box 7.4).

Twenty-eight physical therapists specialized in the field of PFMT were recruited and trained to use the protocol checklist. For the three experimental conditions, the use of the health education intervention was indicated in this checklist. The specific behaviours trained in PFMT were translated into four performance objectives for adherence to PFMT (Berghmans et al 1998b, Bø et al 1990, Bø 1995a, Lagro-Janssen et al 1995, Miller et al 1998, Mouritsen et al 1991, Nygaard et al 1996, Payne 2000, Versprille-Fischer 1995, Wyman et al 1998). Adherence was thus operationalized as (Alewijnse et al 2003a):

- performing 50 slow (10–30 s) and 50 fast (2–3 s) contractions during daily activities;
- using sudden contractions to prevent leakage (the knack);
- training the bladder when needed;
- integration of the use of the pelvic floor muscles in the daily posture and movement pattern.

Study design

A longitudinal RCT with three interventions and one control condition was conducted (Alewijnse et al 2003a). The control condition consisted of individual PFMT alone, representing usual care. The intervention conditions consisted of PFMT supplemented with one of the three health education interventions.

Primary outcome measures were weekly frequency of wet episodes and number of days per week women had followed the behavioural advice of the physical therapist, both measured with a 7-day diary (Kerssens et al 1996, Nygaard & Holcomb 2000, Wyman et al 1988). Secondary measures included demographics, determinants of adherence behaviour and perceived severity of symptoms. Patients were randomly allocated to one of the four treatment conditions.

One hundred and twenty-nine women with urinary incontinence were included. All women completed self-administered questionnaires and diaries before and directly after therapy, and 3 and 12 months later. Process evaluation forms were completed by both physical therapist and patients.

Table 7.1   Content of the self-help guide and counselling tasks for PFMT therapists along the motivational stages of change and the phases of the physiotherapeutic treatment plan

Physiotherapeutic treatment plan phases	Motivational stages	Chapters of self-help guide	Counselling tasks for PFME therapist
History taking, diagnosis, observation and physical assessment, patient education	Precontemplation & contemplation Contemplation	1. Urinary incontinence: PFMT helps! What's in this guide? Who is who in guide? 2. Urinary incontinence: You can help yourself! What is PFMT, what can you do and when can you expect results?	Create open atmosphere, build confidence Explore lay beliefs, self-care strategies, explain relationship behaviour and symptoms and content of PFMT
Formulation of treatment plan, patient education	Preparation Action	Decide when you want to do your exercises. Personal diary-pages for exercise advice	Weigh pros and cons of exercising, discuss personalized therapy goals and behavioural needs in terms of exercising and toileting and drinking behaviour
Treatment plan	Precontemplation & contemplation Preparation Preparation & action	3. Tackle the problem of incontinence Impact of urinary incontinence Set your own goals, why doing PFMT? 4. Coping with incontinence Discuss incontinence aids; drinking and toileting, toileting diary, toileting behaviour Urgency and PFM Pads and hygiene	Contract start of adherence behaviour, reinforce self-management behaviour Explore adherence behaviour
	Preparation	5. The challenge: make exercising a habit What is regular exercising? What barriers prevent adherence to the advice of your physical therapist?	Discuss personal barriers for adherence and personal solutions

Table 7.1–cont'd   Content of the self-help guide and counselling tasks for PFMT therapists along the motivational stages of change and the phases of the physiotherapeutic treatment plan

Physiotherapeutic treatment plan phases	Motivational stages	Chapters of self-help guide	Counselling tasks for PFME therapist
Evaluation of patient education and feedback knowledge and behaviour	Action and maintenance and relapse prevention	Exercising, does that suit me? Forgetting to exercise; interruptions of daily routine; emotional life events; being too busy; needing social support; am I doing it right?; body esteem; personal circumstances	Reinforce skills and self-efficacy regarding adherence Teach internal feedback Teach facts about incontinence, PFM and the exercises
	(Pre)contemplation	Situations that influence urinary incontinence and the PFM	
Patient education	(Pre)contemplation & preparation	6. Facts and myths about incontinence 7. PFM: muscles to use What are PFM? Sexuality and the pelvic floor. Muscles to exercise Facts and myths about PFMT	Stimulate patient to work from simple to complex behavioural goals Evaluate and reinforce progress
Evaluation of patient education and feedback knowledge and behaviour	Maintenance	8. A dry future Adherence is worth while: how were you when you started and how are you today? Drinking and toileting behaviour. PFME: how did they help you? Self-esteem and body esteem	Promote evaluative filling-in tasks Reinforce skills, self-efficacy and self-esteem Reattribute relapses in positive terms
	Maintenance & relapse prevention	9. Epilogue Addresses and further reading	Discuss risk situations for relapse

PFM, pelvic floor muscles, PFME, pelvic floor muscle exercises, PFMT, pelvic floor muscle training.

Box 7.3: Protocol checklist of physical therapists with all important treatment aspects

DIAGNOSIS, HISTORY TAKING, OBSERVATION, PHYSICAL ASSESSMENT

- Ask about
  - sort of complaint, severity, duration, possible causal factors or underlying pathology, reason for seeking help
  - voiding and defecating frequency, use of sanitary towels
  - other physical or mental health problems, factors that may inhibit recovery and adjustment
  - family situation, social roles, self-care potential
  - sport activities
  - (perception of) sexual life
- Observe
  - posture, standing/sitting balance, muscular movement
  - behaviour and respiration pattern
- Identify
  - impairments, disabilities, participation problems and inhibitory factors for recovery and adaptation
  - what's behind the patient's story?

FORMULATION OF TREATMENT PLAN AND PATIENT EDUCATION

- Formulation of treatment plan
- Discuss and show picture of anatomy and physiology of bladder and pelvic floor muscles and their relation with sexuality
- Explain
  - incontinence, causes and treatment options
  - relationship between drinking, eating and voiding, defecating
  - toilet behaviour and toilet posture
  - influence of thoughts on behaviour
  - influence of psychological and social factors on pelvic floor
  - influence of physical and health factors on wet episodes
  - respiration and movement pattern
  - voiding diary: how and why?

TREATMENT PLAN: EXERCISES FOR AWARENESS OF PFM

- Instruct awareness of
  - PFM
  - relationship between respiration and PFM
  - influence of body posture and movement on PFM
  - influence of abdominal pressure on PFM

TREATMENT PLAN: BASIS OF PFMEs AND BLADDER TRAINING

- Instruct basis: fast twitch (strength) and slow twitch (endurance)
- Check for correct contraction and relaxation of PFM

- Explain working towards a patient-centred amount of slow- and fast-twitch exercises per day
- Instruct basic PFMEs with differentiation in buttock, leg and abdominal muscles
- Check for correct basic PFMEs
- Explain treatment goal of integrating basic PFMEs in daily life activities
- Explain bladder training when necessary and/or timed voiding
- Instruct training to prevent voiding when hearing streaming water

TREATMENT PLAN: MORE PFMEs

- Instruct coordination between respiration and posture
- Instruct all kinds of special PFMEs such as the elevator, the knack and others (Versprille-Fischer 1995)
- Instruct daily life activities with the correct use of the PFM such as vacuum cleaning, bending, lifting etc.
- Provoke: walking stairs, hopping, jumping
- Make exercises heavier: use PFM correctly during fast movements and changing body postures

TREATMENT PLAN: OTHER EXERCISES

- Instruct relaxation exercises
- Instruct respiration exercises
- Instruct and/or improve awareness of posture and movement pattern with exercises

EVALUATION OF PATIENT EDUCATION AND FEEDBACK KNOWLEDGE AND BEHAVIOUR

- Answer questions about given education
- Discuss voiding diary, and repeat it if necessary
- Ask for (problems with) integration of PFMEs in daily life activities
- Discuss (problems with) adherence, provide tips to tackle problems and stimulate patient's problem solving skills
- Refer to other health care providers if necessary

EVALUATION OF PFMT AND FEEDBACK

- Answer questions about exercises
- Answer questions about respiration and posture habits
- Provide feedback on patient's performance of various exercises
- Discuss results of therapy

BASIC PRINCIPLES OF THERAPY

- Steps: thinking, feeling, performing, maintaining
- From no awareness, via awareness to automatism

PFM, pelvic floor muscles; PFMEs, pelvic floor muscle exercises, PFMT, pelvic floor muscle training

> **Box 7.4:** Treatment goals
>
> - Conscious control over the pelvic floor muscles (PFM)
> - Conscious control over the PFM with a differentiation in buttock, leg and abdominal muscles
> - Conscious control over the PFM in functional postures and movements
> - Conscious control over the PFM during daily activities
> - Unconscious control over the PFM during daily activities
> - Normal voiding pattern
> - Wet episodes have decreased or patient is dry
> - Problems with adherence are tackled and resolved

Results

Multiple regression analysis revealed relevant predictors of intention to adhere to PFMT. At the onset of therapy, intention to adhere to PFMT was very positive. Two significant predictors of intention were identified. Amount of urinary loss per wet episode and self-efficacy expectations regarding adherence behaviour, were positively related to intention to adhere to PFMT before the start of therapy (Alewijnse et al 2001).

Sequential multiple regression analyses revealed several significant predictors that predicted up to 50% of variance in long-term adherence behaviour. Positive intention to adhere, high short-term adherence levels and positive self-efficacy expectations, significantly predicted high long-term adherence levels. Furthermore, women with frequent weekly wet episodes before and after therapy, were more likely to have high adherence levels 1 year after therapy than women with fewer losses (Alewijnse et al 2003b)

Process evaluation revealed that interventions were not fully implemented as planned. Consequently, the chosen interventions were less different from each other than expected. The level of completeness for the stickers used as a reminder method for improving adherence behaviour was low and, although unintended, the checklist had stimulated counselling skills from all physical therapists. The self-help guide was used as planned and highly appreciated by physical therapists and patients.

Effect evaluation revealed that the three health education interventions or the self-help guide alone had no additional effect on treatment outcome, adherence behaviour, or on predictors of adherence. In all groups,

the individual PFMT was very successful. Weekly frequency of wet episodes drastically decreased from an average 23 wet episodes to eight losses, and results were maintained from post-test to 1 year follow-up (p < 0.001). One year after therapy, 74.8% of the women (n = 103) were cured or improved by 50% (intention to treat 64.4%, n = 129). Adherence behaviour was very high with most women performing the exercise advice on average 6 days per week at post-test and 4–5 days per week 1 year after therapy (Alewijnse et al 2003a).

Discussion and conclusions

The long-term data (after 1 year), including intention to treat, showed a higher rate of cure and improvement of symptoms than reported in other studies (Hay-Smith et al 2001, Mouritsen & Schiøtz 2000). In addition, adherence results were higher than found in other studies during a 1-year follow-up (Ferguson et al 1990, Janssen et al 2001, Lagro-Janssen et al 1992). Of course, measuring adherence itself could have functioned as a reminder for adherence behaviour (Beurskens et al 1992, Myers & Midence 1998, Windsor et al 1994) as well as participating in a study, but that would have affected all groups equally. Social desirability was high (80%), but equal in all groups. Furthermore, this effect was minimized by using a five-point scale to assess adherence behaviour with three options with reasons for non-adherence.

An important finding was that women with more frequent losses before and after therapy, had a higher adherence level 1 year after therapy than women with less frequent losses. This indicates that women learned to adapt adherence behaviour to their symptoms (Alewijnse et al 2003b). A similar adaptation pattern was found by Burns et al (1993). In contrast to others (Bø & Talseth 1996, Chen et al 1999, Lagro-Janssen & Van Weel 1998), it was not found that women with higher adherence levels had fewer wet episodes at follow-up. It may be that it is much more difficult to reduce symptoms even further when they are already low after therapy (floor effect), which is reflected in the effects remaining stable after post-test regardless of high adherence levels (Alewijnse et al 2003b).

Results suggested that the standardization protocol checklist and evaluation form with treatment goals had resulted in such an optimization of usual care in all conditions, that a written health education could not further improve therapy outcome or adherence behaviour. According to the process evaluation conducted among physical therapists, this protocol had provided a clear structure for therapy content. Furthermore, having to check accomplished treatment goals during each session may have stimulated physical therapists to evaluate progress and subsequently provide reinforcement and feedback (Alewijnse et al 2003a).

CLINICAL RECOMMENDATIONS ON HOW TO PROMOTE ADHERENCE AND PREVENT DROP OUT IN PFMT

Clinical recommendations lie in two categories. Adherence can be promoted by influencing self-efficacy through health education, and by adding several factors to PFMT content and structure.

Promoting self-efficacy behaviour

Self-efficacy appeared a predictor of both short- and long-term adherence to PFMT (Alewijnse et al 2003b). Promoting self-efficacy expectations towards adherence behaviour requires a good and open relationship between the physical therapist and patient (Sluijs & Knibbe 1991). This opens the way to discuss specific adherence problems and risk situations for drop out (Kerssens et al 1999). Possible strategies are to stimulate active learning by shaping new behaviours in simpler units, setting realistic goals, exploring skills and self-efficacy regarding performance and reinforcing integration of adherence behaviour by evaluating and appraising progress (Bandura 1986, Clark & Dodge 1999). Process evaluation results of patients revealed that they expected that written personal exercise advice provided by their physical therapist could enhance their adherence behaviour.

To prevent adherence relapse or drop out because of lack of or disappointing progress, information can be given about situations that temporarily aggravate urinary incontinence symptoms, such as having a cold or being tired or stressed, or about factors that affect control over the pelvic floor muscles such as menstruating or taking sleeping tablets. Patients can also be stimulated to restart adherence behaviour after a relapse or drop out, by advising them to attribute relapses as a normal part of adopting new behaviours rather than as personal failures (Weiner 1985).

It is remarkable that many possible determinants of adherence had been identified in the needs assessment, but only a few were significant predictors of adherence behaviour. Of these, self-efficacy expectations and intention may be influenced through optimized counselling. The written self-help guide had no additional influence on these predictors, though it repeated specific methods to enhance self-efficacy, such as setting realistic and attainable goals and providing feedback, as well as motivational messages. Furthermore, PFMT without

health education intervention had no influence on self-efficacy either (Alewijnse et al 2003b).

For comparison, Kerssens et al (1999) developed and evaluated a training programme for the enhancement of patient education skills in physio therapy aimed at better monitoring of adherence problems during treatment and enhancement of self-efficacy of patients regarding adherence behaviour after treatment, but the programme was not effective either. It therefore seems not necessary to address so many variables in a health education programme added to PFMT for women with urinary incontinence. For other target groups, new analyses of adherence determinants are warranted, but group interviews might be enough to reveal new determinants. Although patients and physical therapists considered a self-help guide a useful addition to therapy, the high adherence levels found by Alewijnse et al (2003b) are more likely explained by the motivating effect of the enthusiasm of the physical therapists as well as the intensively guided therapy sessions. Furthermore, evaluating treatment goals stimulated treatment progress by feedback, and might have made therapy more effective because every following therapy session could start where the former had ended in terms of treatment goals.

Therapy content and structure

The optimal results of Alewijnse et al (2003a) were found with a therapy of normal length. As guidance and counselling by the physical therapist seem to be the most important factors for success, further optimization of treatment outcome and adherence behaviour may be realized by providing reminder therapy for those women who continue to have bothersome symptoms. Practically, this can be established by including extra follow-up treatment sessions or evaluating phone calls (Knibbe et al 1997). Further research should evaluate the effectiveness of reminder therapy, and determine at which moments follow-up sessions or calls could best be provided. In addition, the efficiency of reminder therapy should be evaluated as well, in cooperation with paramedical organizations and insurance companies (Alewijnse et al 2003a).

Although the study of Alewijnse (2003a) lacked evidence about whether the protocol checklist for PFMT had optimized usual care, opinions of participating physical therapists in particular confirmed that they worked more planned and systematically when using the checklist. This checklist was developed in 1997 just before the practice guidelines were published (Berghmans et al 1998b, Messelink et al 2000). So results imply that it is best to follow and further implement current practice guidelines in PFMT, and evaluate the effectiveness of the implementation. To promote implementation (Grol et al 1994, Rogers 1995), the use of such guidelines should be included in the training of physical therapists, in refresher courses on pelvic floor dysfunctions, as well as in workshops during conferences and in PFMT discussion groups. Self-evident, adherence to using guidelines needs promotion with strategies as mentioned in this chapter (Grol et al 1994, Hendriks et al 2000).

CLINICAL RECOMMENDATIONS

- Guide therapy sessions intensively
- Promote self-efficacy
- Include reminder therapy
- Use guidelines
- Evaluate treatment goals explicitly and provide feedback

REFERENCES

Alewijnse D 2002 Urinary incontinence in women. Long-term adherence to and outcome of pelvic floor muscle exercise therapy [thesis]. Unigraphic, Maastricht University

Alewijnse D, Mesters I E P E, Metsemakers J F M et al 2001 Predictors of intention to adhere to physiotherapy among women with urinary incontinence. Health Education Research 16(2):173–186

Alewijnse D, Mesters I E P E, Metsemakers J F M et al 2002a Program development for promoting adherence during and after exercise therapy for urinary incontinence. Patient Education and Counseling 48:147–160

Alewijnse D, van Bavel M A P, Wagemakers M A E 2002b Sekse-specifieke voorlichting: de vertaling naar de praktijk [Sex-specific education: translation into practice]. Tijdschrift voor Gezondheidswetenschappen 4:225–230

Alewijnse D, Metsemakers J F M, Mesters I E P E et al 2003a Effectiveness of pelvic floor muscle exercise therapy supplemented with a health education program to promote adherence among women with urinary incontinence. Neurourology and Urodynamics 22(4):284–295

Alewijnse D, Mesters I E P E, Metsemakers J F M et al 2003b Predictors of long–term adherence to pelvic floor muscle exercise therapy among women with urinary incontinence. Health Education Research 18(5):511–524

Ashworth P D, Hagan M T 1993 Some social consequences of non-compliance with pelvic floor exercises. Physiotherapy 79:465–471

Bandura A 1986 Social foundations of thought and action. Prentice Hall, New York

Bartholomew L K, Parcel G S, Kok G et al 2001 Intervention mapping: designing theory and evidence based promotion programs, 1st edn. Mayfield, Mountain View, CA

Bassett S F, Petrie K J 1999 The effect of treatment goals on patient compliance with physiotherapy exercise programmes. Physiotherapy 85(3):130–137

Berghmans L C M, Hendriks H J M, Bø K et al 1998a Conservative treatment of stress urinary incontinence in women: a systematic review of randomized clinical trials. British Journal of Urology 82:181–191

Berghmans L C M, Bernards A T M, Hendriks H J M et al 1998b Guidelines for the physiotherapeutic management of genuine stress incontinence. Physical Therapy Reviews 3:133–147

Berghmans L C M, Hendriks H J M, de Bie R A et al 2000 Conservative treatment of urge urinary incontinence in women: a systematic review of randomized clinical trials. British Journal of Urology 85:254–263

Beurskens A J H M, Bouter L M, van der Heijden G J M G 1992 Compliance-bepaling bij oefentherapie. Een beoordeling van de beschikbare meetinstrumenten [Assessing compliance with exercise therapy. A review of the available instruments]. Nederlands Tijdschrift voor Fysiotherapie 102(1):2–7

Bø K 1995a Pelvic floor muscle exercise for the treatment of stress urinary incontinence: an exercise physiology perspective. International Urogynecology Journal and Pelvic Floor Dysfunction 6:282–291

Bø K 1995b Adherence to pelvic floor muscle exercise and long-term effect on stress urinary incontinence, a five-year follow-up study. Scandinavian Journal of Medicine, Science and Sports 5:36–39

Bø K, Hagen R H, Kvarstein B et al 1990 Pelvic floor muscle exercise for the treatment of female stress urinary incontinence, III: Effects of two different degrees of pelvic floor muscle exercises. Neurourology and Urodynamics 9:489–502

Bø K, Talseth T 1996 Long-term effect of pelvic floor muscle exercise 5 years after cessation of organized training. Obstetrics and Gynecology 87:261–265

Burns P A, Pranikoff K, Nochajski T H et al 1993 A comparison of effectiveness of biofeedback and pelvic muscle exercise treatment of stress incontinence in older community-dwelling women. Journal of Gerontology 48:M167–M174

Cammu H, Van Nylen M, Derdre M P et al 1991 Pelvic physiotherapy in genuine stress incontinence. Urology 38(4): 332–337

Cammu H, Van Nylen M 1994 Pelvic floor muscle exercises: 5 years later. Urology 45:113–118

Castleden C M, Duffin H M, Mitchell E P 1984 The effect of physiotherapy on stress incontinence. Age and Ageing 13:235–237

Chen H Y, Chang W C, Lin W C et al 1999 Efficacy of pelvic floor rehabilitation for treatment of genuine stress incontinence. Journal of the Formosan Medical Association 98:271–276

Clark N M, Dodge J A 1999 Exploring self-efficacy as a predictor of disease management. Health Education and Behavior 26(1):72–89

Cramer J A 1995 Optimizing long-term patient compliance. Neurology 45(suppl 1):S25–S28

De Vries H, Dijkstra M, Kuhlman P 1988 Self-efficacy: the third factor besides attitude and subjective norm as a predictor of behavioral intentions. Health Education Research 3:273–282

De Vries H, Mudde A N 1998 Predicting stage transitions for smoking cessation applying the attitude–social influence–efficacy model. Psychology and Health 13:369–385

Dougherty M, Bishop K, Mooney R et al 1993 Graded pelvic muscle exercise, effect on stress urinary incontinence. The Journal of Reproductive Medicine 38:684–691

Eagly A H, Chaiken S 1993 The psychology of attitudes. Harcourt Brace Jovanovich, Fort Worth

Ferguson K L, McKey P L, Bishop K R et al 1990 Stress urinary incontinence: effect of pelvic muscle exercise. Obstetrics and Gynecology 75:671–675

Gallo M L, Staskin D R 1997 Cues to action: pelvic floor muscle exercise compliance in women with stress urinary incontinence. Neurourology and Urodynamics 16:167–177

Green L W, Kreuter M W 1991 Health promotion planning, an educational and environmental approach, 2nd edn. Mayfield Publishing Company, Mountain View, CA

Green L W, Kreuter M W 2004 Health Program Planning: An educational and ecological approach with Powerweb bind-in card, 4th edn. McGraw-Hill, Maidenhead, UK

Grol R T P M, Van Everdingen J J E, Casparie A F 1994 Invoering van richtlijnen en veranderingen, een handleiding voor de medische, paramedische en verpleegkundige praktijk [Implementation of guidelines and changes, a handbook for medical, paramedical and nursing practice]. De Tijdstroom, Utrecht

Hahn I, Milsom I, Fall M et al 1993 Long-term results of pelvic floor training in female stress urinary incontinence. British Journal of Urology 72:421–427

Haynes R B, McDonald H, Garg A X et al 2002 Interventions for helping patients to follow prescriptions for medications. The Cochrane Database of Systematic Reviews 2:CD000011

Hay-Smith E J C, Bø K, Berghmans L C M et al 2001 Pelvic floor muscle training for urinary incontinence in women. The Cochrane Database of Systematic Reviews 1:CD001407

Hendriks H J M, Bekkering G E, Ettekoven H et al 2000 Development and implementation of national practice guidelines: a prospect for continuous quality improvement in physiotherapy. Physiotherapy 86:535–547

Hendriks H J M, Bekkering G E, Ettekoven H van et al Introduction to the method of guideline implementation. In: Development and implementation of clinical practice guidelines in physical therapy. In preparation.

Janetzky C R 1993 Fysiotherapie en incontinentie [Physiotherapy and incontinence]. Tijdschrift voor Integrale Geneeskunde 3:270–276

Janssen C C M, Lagro-Janssen A L M, Felling A J A 2001 The effects of physiotherapy for female urinary incontinence: individual compared with group treatment. British Journal of Urology International 87:201–206

Johnson T M, Kincade J E, Bernard S L et al 2000 Self-care practices used by older men and women to manage urinary incontinence: results from the national follow-up survey on self-care and aging. Journal of the American Geriatrics Society 48:894–902

Kerssens J J, Sluijs E M, Knibbe J J et al 1996 Het effect van therapietrouw verhogende strategieën in de fysiotherapie, patiënten van de controlegroep in hoofdlijnen [The effect of adherence-promoting strategies in physiotherapy, patients of the control group in headlines]. Rapport Nivel, Utrecht

Kerssens J J, Sluijs E M, Verhaak P F M et al 1999 Educating patient educators: enhancing instructional effectiveness in physical therapy for low back pain patients. Patient Education and Counseling 37(2):165–176

Knibbe N E, Wams H W A 1994 Met patiëntenvoorlichting methodisch werken aan therapietrouw, weten wat de patiënt beweegt [Working methodologically on adherence with patient education: knowing what moves the patient]. Nederlands Tijdschrift voor Fysiotherapie 2:44–51

Knibbe N E, Knibbe J J, Elvers J W H et al 1997 Rugscholing, wat heeft zin? Onderzoek naar determinanten van advies-en therapietrouw [Back to school, what has sense? Exploring determinants of adherence to advice and therapy]. Nederlands Tijdschrift voor Fysiotherapie 107(3):60–64

Kok J, Bouter L M 1990 Patiëntenvoorlichting door fysiotherapeuten in de eerste lijn [Patient education by the physiotherapist in primary health care]. Nederlands Tijdschrift voor Fysiotherapie 100(2):59–63

Kreuter M, Farrell D, Olevitch L et al 2000 Tailoring health messages, customizing communication with computer technology. Lawrence Erlbaum Associate Publishers, London

Lagro-Janssen A L M, Debruyne F M J, Smits A J A et al 1992 The effects of treatment of urinary incontinence in general practice. Family Practice 9:284–289

Lagro-Janssen A L M, Smits A J A, Van Weel C 1994 Gunstig effect van oefentherapie bij urine-incontinentie in de huisartspraktijk vooral afhankelijk van therapietrouw en motivatie [Favourable effects of exercise therapy for urinary incontinence in the family practice especially dependent on adherence and motivation]. Nederlands Tijdschrift voor Geneeskunde 138:1273–1276

Lagro-Janssen A L M, Breedveldt Boer H P, Van Dongen J J A M et al 1995 NHG-Standaard incontinentie voor urine, Nederlands Huisarts Genootschap M46 [Dutch Clinical Guideline on Urinary Incontinence for family physicians]. Huisarts en Wetenschap 38:71–80

Lagro-Janssen T, Van Weel C 1998 Long-term effect of treatment of female incontinence in general practice. British Journal of General Practice 48:1735–1738

Lechner E H S 1998 Social psychological determinants of health risk behaviors related to cancer and CVD, applications and elaborations of the ASE model [Thesis]. Unigraphic, Maastricht University

Leventhal H, Cameron L 1987 Behavioral theories and the problem of compliance. Patient Education and Counseling 10:117–138

Leventhal H, Leventhal E A, Contrada R J 1998 Self-regulation, health and behavior: a perceptual-cognitive approach. Psychology and Health 13:717–733

Mantle J, Versi E 1991 Physiotherapy for stress urinary incontinence: a national survey. British Medical Journal 302:753–755

Messelink E J, ten Hoope C A, Lieshout G J C M et al 2000 Consensus de overactieve blaas. [Consensus overactive bladder]. Amsterdam

Miller J M, Ashton-Miller J A, DeLancey J O L 1998 A pelvic muscle precontraction can reduce cough-related urine loss in selected women with mild SUI. Journal of the American Geriatric Society 46:870–874

Miller W R, Rollnick S 2002 Motivational interviewing: preparing people for change, 2nd edn. The Guilford Press, New York

Mouritsen L, Frimodt-Møller C, Møller M 1991 Long-term effect of pelvic floor exercises on female urinary incontinence. British Journal of Urology 68:32–37

Mouritsen L 1994 Pelvic floor exercises for female stress urinary incontinence. International Urogynecology Journal and Pelvic Floor Dysfunction 5:44–51

Mouritsen L, Schiøtz H A 2000 Pro et contra pelvic floor exercises for female stress urinary incontinence. Acta Obstetricia et Gynecologica Scandinavica 79:1043–1045

Mullen P D, Green L W, Persinger G S 1985 Clinical trials of patient education for chronic conditions: a comparative meta-analysis of intervention types. Preventive Medicine 14:753–781

Myers L B, Midence K 1998 Methodological and conceptual issues in adherence. In: Myers L B, Midence K (eds) Adherence to treatment in medical conditions. Harwood Academic Publishers, Amsterdam

Nygaard I, DeLancey J O L, Arnsdorf L et al 1990 Exercise and incontinence. Obstetrics and Gynecology 75:848–851

Nygaard I E, Kreder K J, Lepic M M et al 1996 Efficacy of pelvic floor muscle exercises in women with stress, urge, and mixed urinary incontinence. American Journal of Obstetrics and Gynecology 174:120–126

Nygaard I, Holcomb R 2000 Reproducibility of the seven-day voiding diary in women with stress urinary incontinence.

International Urogynecology Journal and Pelvic Floor Dysfunction 11(1):15–17

O'Dowd T C 1993 Management of urinary incontinence in women. British Journal of General Practice 43:426–429

Payne C P 2000 Behavioral therapy for overactive bladder. Urology 55(suppl 5A):3–6

Prochaska J O, DiClemente C C, Norcross J C 1992 In search of how people change, applications to addictive behaviors. American Psychologist 47:1102–1114

Prochaska J O, Velicer W F, Rossi J S et al 1994 Stages of change and decisional balance for 12 problem behaviors. Health Psychology 13(1):39–46

Rogers E M 1995 Diffusion of innovations. The Free Press, New York

Skinner B F 1938 The behavior of organisms. Appleton–Century–Crofts, New York

Sluijs E M, Knibbe J J 1991 Patient compliance with exercise: different theoretical approaches to short-term and long-term compliance. Patient Education and Counseling 17:191–204

Sluijs E M, Van der Zee J, Kok G J 1993 Differences between physical therapists in attention paid to patient education. Physiotherapy Theory and Practice 9:103–117

Steiner J F, Earnest M A 2000 Lingua medica: the language of medication-taking. Annals of Internal Medicine 132(11): 926–930

Strecher V J, Seijts G H, Kok G J et al 1995 Goal setting as a strategy for health behavior change. Health Education Quarterly 22(2):190–200

Toner B B, Akman D 2000 Gender role and irritable bowel syndrome: literature review and hypothesis. The American Journal of Gastroenterology 95(1):11–16

Verhulst F J C M, Van der Burgt M C A, Lindner K 1994 Concretisering van patiëntenvoorlichting in het fysiotherapeutisch handelen. [Making patient education in physiotherapeutic treatment explicit] Nederlands Tijdschrift voor Fyiotherapie 1:10–17

Versprille-Fischer E S 1995 Begeleiding van patiënten met bekkenbodemdysfunctie [Guidance of patients with pelvic floor dysfunctions]. Lemma, Utrecht

Wall L L, Davidson T G 1992 The role of muscular re-education by physical therapy in the treatment of genuine stress urinary incontinence. Obstetrical and Gynecological Survey 47:322–331

Weiner B 1985 An attributional theory of achievement motivation and emotion. Psychological Review 92(4):548–573

Willey C, Redding C, Stafford J et al 2000 Stages of change for adherence with medication regimens for chronic disease: development and validation of a measure. Clinical Therapeutics 22(7):858–871

Wilson P D, Samarrai T A, Deakin M et al 1987 An objective assessment of physiotherapy for female genuine stress incontinence. British Journal of Obstetrics and Gynaecology 94:575–582

Windsor R, Baranowski T, Clark N et al 1994 Evaluation of health promotion, health education and disease prevention programs, 2nd edn. Mayfield, Mountain View, CA

Wyman J F, Choi S C, Harkins S W et al 1988 The urinary diary in evaluation of incontinent women: a test–retest analysis. Obstetrics and Gynecology 71:812–817

Wyman J F, Fantl J A, McClish D K et al 1998 Comparative efficacy of behavioral interventions in the management of female urinary incontinence. American Journal of Obstetrics and Gynecology 179:999–1007

Chapter 8

Lifestyle interventions for pelvic floor dysfunction

Pauline Chiarelli

EVIDENCE OF THE ASSOCIATION BETWEEN LIFESTYLE FACTORS AND PELVIC FLOOR DYSFUNCTION

In examining the relationship between lifestyle factors and pelvic floor dysfunction available evidence is most commonly related to associations between lifestyle factors and urinary incontinence. However, it seems reasonable to assume that lifestyle factors shown to have a strong association with urinary incontinence might also impact on other symptoms of pelvic floor dysfunction.

Epidemiological studies have shown urinary incontinence to be associated with a number of risk factors, some of which might be considered modifiable. Being modifiable, these factors should be of interest when considering the development of interventions aimed at reducing the symptoms of pelvic floor dysfunction. Modifiable risk factors include those factors commonly called lifestyle factors.

This chapter explores the lifestyle factors known to be associated with urinary incontinence as well as the evidence to support the inclusion of lifestyle changes within continence promotion interventions. The chapter also outlines some of the principles of behaviour change/health promotion and how these might best be incorporated within continence promotion interventions to help patients adopt relevant behaviours or make suggested lifestyle changes.

WHAT ARE THE MODIFIABLE FACTORS ASSOCIATED WITH URINARY INCONTINENCE?

Several epidemiological studies have shown a strong association between self reports of urinary incontinence and lifestyle factors such as obesity (Chiarelli et al 1999, Hunskaar et al 2000), smoking (Bump 1992, Tampakoudis et al 1995), dietary factors (Brown et al 1999, Burgio et al 1991) and physical activity (Bø & Borgen 2001 , Nygaard et al 1994).

HOW STRONG IS THE EVIDENCE TO SUPPORT THE IMPACT OF LIFESTYLE CHANGES ON SYMPTOMS OF PELVIC FLOOR DYSFUNCTION?

The International Continence Society (ICS) (Committee10C) examined the evidence relating to the conservative treatment for urinary incontinence in women, including lifestyle interventions (Wilson & Bø 2002). Systematic reviews of the literature pertaining to obesity, physical forces (exercise, work) smoking and dietary factors were examined. Strong evidence in favour of removing or applying suggested behaviours to reduce urinary incontinence was not available.

A summary of the findings of the ICS committee examining several lifestyle interventions and their impact on the management of urinary incontinence are provided here (Wilson & Bø 2002). Using the same search strategy and inclusion and exclusion criteria as implemented by the initial reviewers, an update of the relevant literature examining lifestyle interventions from 2001 to the present has been added (Table 8.1).

In preparing the systematic review, levels of evidence and grades of recommendation were decided for each lifestyle factor reviewed.

Levels of evidence

Abbreviated levels of evidence and grades of recommendations used within the ICS recommendations are as follows:

- Level 1: usually involves one well-designed randomized controlled trial (RCT);
- Level 2: includes at least one good-quality prospective cohort study;
- Level 3: good-quality retrospective case–control study;
- Level 4: includes good-quality case series.

Rating of randomized controlled trials

Methodological quality of RCTs were further rated using the PEDro scale (Maher et al 2003) (Table 8.2).

Grades of recommendation

Grades of recommendation are:

- grade A: consistent level 1 evidence, the recommendation being considered mandatory for placement within a clinical care pathway;
- grade B: based on consistent level 2 or 3 studies or 'majority' evidence from RCTs;
- level C: based on level 4 studies or most evidence from level 2/3 studies;
- level D: evidence is inconsistent/inconclusive or non-existent (Abrams & Committee 2002).

Weight loss

Any increases in BMI must necessarily translate into increases in intravesical and abdominal forces acting upon the pelvic floor. It might be reasonably assumed therefore that increases in BMI contribute to pelvic floor dysfunction and urinary incontinence and that weight loss in obese women might reduce urinary incontinence.

ICS summary and recommendation

The committee determined obesity to be an independent risk factor for incontinence and recommended that massive weight loss significantly decreases urinary incontinence in morbidly obese women, but found scant evidence in relation to the effect of weight loss in women who are moderately obese. Given the evidence of increasing obesity among women, recommendation was also made that weight loss should be included to reduce incontinence (level 1 or 2). The prevention of weight gain was recommended as having a high research priority.

Evidence from recent review

Recent evidence from a large (n = 6424) prospective, longitudinal study supports obesity as contributing to the onset of symptoms of both stress urinary incontinence (SUI) and overactive bladder (OAB) (Dalosso et al 2003) (level 2).

The results of a pilot study by Subak et al (2002) also support weight reduction as contributing to decreased symptoms of incontinence. Although the results of this study are encouraging, the small number of study

Table 8.1   Trials included in the review of lifestyle factors and urinary incontinence

Author and lifestyle factor	Subak et al 2002: weight loss
Study design	Pilot study. Prospective cohort design
n = and inclusion criteria	n = 20 BMI 25–45 kg/m² Self-report UI for at least 3 months, At least four UI episodes per week
Response rate/drop-outs	4 drop-outs 6 women did not complete post-weight reduction follow-up
Measures	BMI = weight loss ≥5% 7-day urinary diary ≥50% reduction in UI episodes per week Symptoms of UI
Results	SUI n = 1 UUI n = 6 MUI n = 3 6 women achieved weight loss of 5% of baseline and all these women achieved reductions in UI ≥50%
Level of evidence provided	Level 3 (numbers too small to be considered a robust study)
Author and lifestyle factor	Dalosso et al 2004: lifestyle factors
Study design	Prospective, longitudinal. study Baseline survey with 12-month follow-up survey
n = and inclusion criteria	n = 12 565 Randomly selected community dwelling, ≥ years of age Not Asian ethnic origin
Response rate/drop-outs	Response rate 65.3%
Measures	UI symptoms questionnaire Food frequency questionnaire Physical activity levels (usual activities compared with those of same age, and vigorous exercise that made them short of breath) Past and current smoking Self-reported height and weight
Results	**Associations with onset of SUI after regression analysis** *Reduced risk associated with:* Consumption of bread daily Similar or more active than others of same age Non-smoking. *Increased risk associated with:* Consumption of carbonated drink at least daily Obesity Current smoking **Association with onset of OAB after regression analysis** *Reduced risk OAB associated with:* Bread daily Overall vegetable intake

Table 8.1 Trials included in the review of lifestyle factors and urinary incontinence—cont'd

Results—cont'd	*Increased risk OAB associated with:* Carbonated drinks > once weekly Low physical activity levels Obesity Current smoking
Level of evidence provided	Level 2
Author and lifestyle factor	Kapoor et al (2004): pelvic floor dysfunction in morbidly obese women
Study design	Prospective case–control study
n = and inclusion criteria	Cases: 20 morbidly obese women awaiting bariatric surgery Controls: 20 age-matched volunteers from a staff medical clinic. No mention of matching by other parameters
Response rate/drop-outs	N/A
Measures	Incontinence impact questionnaire Urogenital distress inventory.
Results	Obese women reported more leaking small amounts of leakage and significantly more leakage with activity than women with normal BMI
Level of evidence provided	Level 3
Author and lifestyle factor	Stach-Lempinen et al (2004)
Study design	Pre-post measures study
n = and inclusion criteria	85 women No diabetes mellitus, no serious concomitant disease, no previous bladder surgery Conservative management: n = 53 Surgical management: n = 27
Response rate/drop-outs	69 completed the study

Measures	UI severity score
	Pre-treatment urodynamics 48-hour home pad test pre and post
	Time/volume chart
	Activity measures in METs:
	(a) At work
	(b) Exercise during leisure
	   (i) little
	   (ii) connected with other hobbies or irregular
	   (iii) regular physical exercise
	Personal activity computer for 7 days pre-treatment and 7 days 1 year post-treatment

Results	Activity levels estimated in METs did not change in the women 1 year after successful treatment (surgical or conservative)
Level of evidence provided	Level 4
Author and lifestyle factor	Bryant et al (2002): caffeine reduction to improve urinary symptoms
Study design	(1) Baseline measures of caffeine consumption in patients with UI (2) RCT comparing bladder training including reduction of caffeine ingestion to 100 mg per day compared with bladder training without reduction of caffeine intake

Table 8.1 Trials included in the review of lifestyle factors and urinary incontinence—cont'd

n = and inclusion criteria	n = 95 Drop-outs control = 9 Experimental group = 12 Total = 21
Measures	Caffeine intake survey 3-day time/volume charts measuring voided volumes, number of voids, leakage episodes All fluids taken including a detailed caffeine list
Results	Significant difference in number of voids/24 h, occasions of urgency/24 h and occasions of leakage/24 h
Level of evidence provided	Assessed as grade 5 on the PEDro scale

BMI, body mass index; MUI, mixed urinary incontinence; OAB, overactive bladder; RCT, randomized controlled trial; SUI, stress urinary incontinence; UUI, urge urinary incontinence; UI, urinary incontinence.

Table 8.2 PEDro quality score of RCT in systematic review

E – Eligibility criteria specified
1 – Subjects randomly allocated to groups
2 – Allocation concealed
3 – Groups similar at baseline
4 – Subjects blinded
5 – Therapist administering treatment blinded
6 – Assessors blinded
7 – Measures of key outcomes obtained from over 85% of subjects
8 – Data analysed by intention to treat
9 – Comparison between groups conducted
10 – Point measures and measures of variability provided

Study	E	1	2	3	4	5	6	7	8	9	10	Total score
Bryant et al (2002)	+	+	–	+	–	–	–	+	–	+	+	5

+, criterion is clearly satisfied; –, criterion is not satisfied; ?, not clear if the criterion was satisfied. Total score is determined by counting the number of criteria that are satisfied, except that scale item 'eligibility criteria specified' is not used to generate the total score. Total scores are out of 10 (Maher et al 2003).

participants detracts from the level of evidence that might be awarded to the results.

Kapoor et al (2004) provide yet more supporting evidence using a case–control study of 20 morbidly obese women and 20 age-matched volunteers from a health centre. Examination of the symptomatology reported by each group showed more episodes of leaking and significantly more leakage on activity among 20 morbidly obese women than among the 20 women in the control group (level 3). However, other than matching for age, there was no mention of matching cases and controls on other important variables, such as parity.

There still seems 'scant, preliminary level 1 evidence that moderately obese women who lose weight have less incontinence than those who don't' (Wilson et al 2002). The grade of recommendation remains unchanged at B.

Physical forces (exercise, work)

As increases in BMI must necessarily translate into increases in abdominal forces acting upon the pelvic floor as well as the bladder itself, it might be reasonably assumed that increases in abdominal pressure that accompanying some sporting or work activities might contribute to pelvic floor dysfunction and urinary incontinence.

ICS summary and recommendation

The examination of the data undertaken by Wilson & Bø (2002) suggested that women who led sedentary lives might be less likely to report urinary incontinence than their physically active counterparts. However, it was clearly stated that this recommendation was not supported by trials that had evaluated the effect of altering or reducing activity levels on urinary incontinence.

Evidence from recent review

A recent review of the literature produced no further evidence to strengthen the earlier recommendation related to work or specific activities. Stach-Lempinen et al (2004) undertook a thorough exploration of activity, sport and fitness levels among 82 incontinent women aged 28–80 years referred to a hospital gynae-cology clinic for treatment of urinary incontinence. Their conclusion was that women seeking treatment for urinary incontinence report similar levels of physical activity as continent women. They further concluded that successful conservative or surgical cure of urinary incontinence did not result in increases in activity levels in the women cured of incontinence in the longer term.

No studies have examined the effect on urinary incontinence of ceasing provocative activities, so the grade of recommendation remains at C.

Smoking

It is commonly held that smokers are more likely than non-smokers to have a chronic cough. Because cough is related to increases in abdominal pressure, coughing might be likely to contribute to the lower urinary tract dysfunction usually associated with genuine SUI (Bump & McLish 1994).

ICS summary and recommendation

In the review of conservative treatment in women, no studies were examined to show that smoking cessation resolves or reduces urinary incontinence (Wilson & Bø 2002). Recommendations evolved from a case–control study and a number of cross-sectional studies and were placed at level C.

Evidence from recent review

More recently a study by Dalosso et al (2003) showed an increased risk for the onset of SUI and OAB over a 1-year study period in women reporting to be current smokers. This was a well-conducted, prospective longitudinal analysis of the relationship between a number of lifestyle factors and the onset of SUI and OAB over a period of 1 year that provides a higher level of evidence supporting the effect of smoking on the development of SUI and OAB (level 2). No studies were found that examined the impact of smoking cessation on symptoms of urinary incontinence. Therefore the grade of recommendation remains at C.

Dietary factors

A number of dietary factors are of interest with regard to the management of incontinence. These include caffeine, overall daily fluid intake, alcohol and diet as a whole. Each of these factors was reviewed individually by Wilson & Bø (2002) in relation to the conservative management of urinary incontinence in women.

Caffeine

Caffeine is the most widely consumed stimulant drug in the world and is well known for its diuretic and stimulant effects (Creighton & Stanton 1990). The updated literature review also provided evidence that carbonated soft drinks should also be considered relevant.

ICS summary and recommendation

Level 1 evidence supporting caffeine reduction as a means to reducing urinary incontinence was scant, and only level 2 and 3 evidence shows caffeine intake to be related to urinary incontinence.

Grade of recommendation for caffeine reduction as part of an intervention to reduce bladder symptoms was placed at B.

Evidence from recent review

Although the study by Bryant et al was available in abstract form for the ICS review (Bryant et al 2000), the study, published in full (Bryant et al 2002) revealed a high drop-out rate that might diminish the power of the statistical analysis within the study. As well as this, there is a blurring of the effects of caffeine reduction on the experience of urgency symptoms because both intervention and control groups underwent a bladder training programme. Despite these shortcomings, a significant difference in number of voids per 24 hours, occasions of urgency per 24 hours and occasions of leakage per 24 hours was reported.

The level of evidence in support of caffeine reduction in the management of urgency, frequency and urge incontinence is strengthening. However, the recommendation remains at level B.

Decreased fluid intake

The average fluid intake of healthy sedentary adults in temperate climates is estimated to be 1220 mL per person per day (Valtin 2001). Incontinent people manipulate their fluid intake, reducing it in an attempt to prevent leakage episodes. Fluid intake is an important factor related not only to urinary incontinence, but also to bowel health, especially as an adjunct to the prevention of constipation.

ICS summary and recommendation

The review team concluded that fluid intake overall plays a minor role in the pathogenesis of urinary incontinence. Allocated levels of evidence were 2–3 and the grade of recommendation was B.

Evidence from recent review

The study by Dalosso et al (2003) supports the ICS recommendation that there is no association between total fluid intake and the onset of either SUI or OAB. The grade of recommendation remains at B.

Alcohol

ICS summary and recommendation and evidence from recent review

There would appear to be no association between alcohol consumption and urinary incontinence. The recommendation is further supported by data from the longitudinal, prospective study of 6424 women by Dalosso et al (2003) who found no association between the consumption of alcohol in various forms, and urinary incontinence.

Carbonated soft drinks

A recent study highlighted association between carbonated soft drinks and bladder symptomatology (Dalosso et al 2003). A significant and independent association between the onset of OAB and SUI and ingestion of carbonated beverages was a surprise finding in this study. Discussions related to associations between overall fluid intake and caffeine ingestion (as with cola beverages) were not supported by the data available.

This study was not available for examination by the ICS review team. Using the same levels of evidence and grades of recommendation, reduction in the consumption of carbonated soft drinks as part of the management of both OAB and SUI is supported by level 2 evidence and should be given a level B recommendation.

Diet

Although diet might be seen to contribute to obesity and constipation, there is only anecdotal evidence to support dietary manipulation in the management of urinary incontinence.

ICS summary and recommendation:

There was no evidence to support any recommendation by the review team related to diet and urinary incontinence.

Evidence from recent review

There has been little evidence to support dietary manipulation in the management of urinary incontinence. The study by Dalosso et al (2003) has provided level 2 evidence that there is a reduced risk of onset of OAB associated with increased consumption of vegetables, chicken and bread as well as a reduced risk of SUI associated with increased consumption of bread. As this is the first study of diet and its association with OAB and SUI, the grade of recommendation is placed at C pending support from other studies.

Constipation

Epidemiological studies have shown associations between constipation and urinary incontinence (Chiarelli et al 2000), and some early studies showed a clear association between straining at stool and pelvic floor dysfunction (Lubowski et al 1988, Snooks et al 1985a). However, there are no studies showing that resolution of constipation reduces episodes of SUI or OAB.

ICS summary and recommendation and evidence from recent review

Although there is evidence to support that chronic straining at stool is a risk factor for urinary incontinence and pelvic organ prolapse, there is no evidence from intervention trials to show that reducing constipation in incontinent patients actually reduces their experience of urinary incontinence (level 2 and 3 evidence, with recommendation: grade C.)

SUMMARY OF LIFESTYLE FACTORS ASSOCIATED WITH URINARY INCONTINENCE

In the light of the evidence provided it seems reasonable that lifestyle interventions aimed at modifying risk factors associated with urinary incontinence might include advice related to reducing body mass index (BMI), constipation, the intake of carbonated beverages and caffeine.

Just as there are models and theories used to predict and improve adherence to health behaviours, there are models and theories that address the processes of behaviour change. A commonly used definition of a theory is: 'Systematically organized knowledge applicable in a relatively wide variety of circumstances, devised to analyse, predict or otherwise explain the nature of behaviour of a specified set of phenomena that could be used as the basis for action' (VanRyn & Heaney 1992).

MOTIVATING LIFESTYLE CHANGES

Knowing about a problem is insufficient to motivate change. Health care professionals commonly believe that simply by telling patients about their condition and its contributing health behaviours is sufficient to motivate individuals toward changing the health behaviours.

Evidence to the contrary would appear to have had little effect on the way health care professionals go about inducing behaviour change in their patients. It is well known that knowledge relating to health risks is not sufficient to encourage people to adopt health behaviours. If knowledge itself were enough, the rates of smoking in developed countries would be minimal.

Individuals are bombarded with enormous amounts of information, which is interpreted through the filters of their past experiences, backgrounds, beliefs, values and attitudes. Human behaviour is complex, and understanding how to encourage behaviour change is even more complex. Many theories have been devised in an attempt to understand and promote changes in health behaviour. All such theories are based on the fact that health is mediated by some behaviour and that health behaviours have the potential to change.

Most behaviour change theories have emerged from the behavioural and social sciences which in turn have borrowed from disciplines such as sociology, psychology, management and marketing. The theories derived from this variety of disciplines can be used to provide a framework or model that might be used to underpin the planning, adoption and evaluation of health behaviours.

Chapter 7 has provided an understanding of behavioural strategies related to patient adherence with prescribed treatment protocols. Although some overlap of strategies might be observed, the models described here are specifically related to health promotion – the adoption of specific health behaviours. In keeping with the evidence presented in relation to continence promotion, modifiable health behaviours that might be discussed with patients include restriction of carbonated (fizzy) drinks and caffeine and maintenance or reduction of BMI. The attention to issues surrounding BMI, must, of necessity, involve dietary manipulation as well as increased activity levels. However, simply telling the patient that weight loss is likely to improve their bladder symptoms is unlikely to have any impact unless behaviour modification strategies are implemented.

Behaviour modification strategies are based on a series of evolving theoretical models. Among the theoretical models that have been developed, some are intended to provide understanding, whereas others are aimed more specifically at developing effective intervention protocols. Those models most used to develop strategies for use at an individual level include the Health Belief Model, Theories of Reasoned Action and Planned Behaviour, the Transtheoretical or Stages of Change Model and the Social Cognitive Theory.

Table 8.3 sets out the health behaviour theories and how they might be implemented to optimise continence promotion/behaviour change/lifestyle interventions.

From the table it is clear to see that the theories presented overlap on a number of issues and in general, have more in common than not.

In summary, the main points emphasized by the collected theories are as follows.

- Knowledge and beliefs about health. While advocating health education, all theories emphasize the role of individualization – personalizing the information so that it is seen by individuals as relevant and pertinent.

- A patient's belief in their own ability to do what is asked. Exploring the patient's feelings of competency in relation to the behaviour and encouraging repeated, well-supervised practice to improve self efficacy and self-esteem.

Table 8.3   Theoretical models of behaviour change and their implications for practice

Theory and authors	Health Belief Model (HBM) (Becker 1974)
Description	One of the earliest attempts to explain health behaviour.
	The HBM extends the use of psychosocial variables to explain preventive health behaviour by delineating people's subjective perceptions or beliefs about their health.
	Numerous studies of the HBM provide substantial empirical support for its usefulness in health education planning.
	Evidence supports the effectiveness of this model in developing continence promotion programmes.
Key concepts	The HBM is based on three essential factors: the readiness of the individual to consider behaviour changes to avoid disease or minimize health risks; the existence of forces in the individual's environment that urge change (cues to action) and make it possible; the behaviours themselves.
	The HBM asserts that to undertake a preventive health action, individuals must believe they are susceptible to the incontinence or that severity of present incontinence is likely to worsen; that incontinence and its sequelae are serious; that the action will be beneficial; and that the benefits will outweigh any costs or disadvantages.
	Barriers to action.
	Cues to action.
	Self efficacy – confidence in performing the intervention.
Implications for practice	*The following concepts should be explored with the patient, and relevant information supplied:*
	Patients' perceptions of susceptibility, seriousness and progress of their condition. Corrected if unrealistic.
	Patients' understanding of the impact the health behaviour is likely to have on their condition.
	Need to agree that the health behaviour will be beneficial and worthwhile.
	Barriers to adoption of the health behaviour need to be explored, allowing the patient to suggest how perceived barriers might be overcome.
	Reminders need to be instigated to encourage the behaviour.
	Patient must demonstrate the required action.
	Must be able to practice repeatedly until proficient.
	Patient encouraged to set initial, attainable goals related to the behaviour.
Theory and authors	Theory of Reasoned Action and Planned Behaviour (Ajzen & Fishbein 1980)
Description	Developed to explain behaviour that is able to be changed.
	Assumes that people make rational, predictable decisions in well-defined circumstances.
	Also assumes that the **intention** to act is the most important determinant of action and all factors relating to the particular action will need to be filtered through the initial intention.
	If personal beliefs and social pressures are strong enough, the intention is likely to translate into action.
	A person's intentions are likely to be greater if they feel they have enough personal control over the behaviour.
Key concepts	Attitude towards the behaviour.
	Outcome expectations.
	Value of outcome expectations.
	Beliefs of others.
	Motive to comply with others.
	Perceived personal control over the behaviour.

Table 8.3   Theoretical models of behaviour change and their implications for practice—cont'd

Implications for practice	*Explore* The patient's attitudes to the required behaviour. What the patient believes the outcome might be. How important the expected outcome is to the patient. What impact others might have on the behaviour (e.g. a family attitude to eating more vegetables). What the patient believes others will think. How much control the patient feels in relation to the behaviour.
Theory and authors	Transtheoretical Model (stages of change) (Prochaska & DiClemente 1984)
Description	Integrates a number of principles and behaviours from other models. Based on the assumption that an intention to act (or behave) immediately precedes that action or behaviour. Looks closely at factors related to the intention to perform rather than the behaviour itself. Assessment of the stage a patient has reached can give an indication of the likelihood that they will comply with intervention requirements. Most patients seeking help have advanced through the initial stages of change and are in contemplation or preparation stage.
Key concepts	*Stages of change* Precontemplation: consciousness raising. Contemplation: recognition of the benefits of change. Preparation: identification of barriers. Action: the programme or intervention. Maintenance: recognition that relapse is a strong possibility.
Implications for practice	Discuss the benefits of behaviour change. Discuss the consequences and progress likely if no changes are instigated. Allow the patient to identify barriers to behaviour change. Can the patient offer solutions to overcome the barriers? Work out tailored intervention. Allow patient to repeat programme components in their own words to ensure understanding Check self-efficacy. Monitor progress closely. Use patient-written records (e.g. diary) rather than self-reports for most variables. Discuss this with the patient and put strategies into place in readiness.
Theory and authors	Social Cognitive Theory (Bandura 1977, 1982)
Description	Addresses underlying determinants of health behaviour as well as change methods. Looks at continuous interplay between individual, environment and behaviour Adds cognitions to the relationships. Organizes cognitive and behavioural elements of behaviour change. Recognizes behavioural reinforcement as external, internal, direct, observational or self-reinforcement. Health care professional seen more as an agent of change than an interventionist by developing patient's personal competencies.

Table 8.3 Theoretical models of behaviour change and their implications for practice—cont'd

Key concepts	*Expectations* Self control: goal-directed behaviour. Observational learning: observing the reward for a particular behaviour. Self efficacy: the belief in the ability to successfully perform the behaviour.
Implications for practice	What does the patient see as a likely outcome from behaviour change? Emphasize short-term, tangible benefits to begin with to booster the sense of self control. Explore the value placed on the outcome especially by peers. Patient must feel confident of self control regardless of the environment. Discuss coping strategies for situations when self control might be less.

- The importance of what is perceived as 'normal' by a patient in relation to the influences and values of their social group. The influence of the patient's social group as a role model, family and peer influences.

- Patients move forward and back along a continuum of change or readiness to change.

- Awareness of the impact of socioeconomic and environmental factors on a patient's ability to adopt specific behaviours.

- The importance of changing a patient's environment or perceptions of the environment when it impacts on their progress (Nutbeam & Harris 2004)

HOW MIGHT LIFESTYLE CHANGES BE ENCOURAGED IN CLINICAL PRACTICE?

Health care professionals tend to make inappropriate assumptions about patients and behaviour change. These are likely to have a negative impact on the outcome of consultation and include such assumptions as: the patient 'should' and therefore 'wants' to change, that 'now' is the best time for the patient to change, that the health care professional is the 'expert' and knows what is best for the patient (Emmons & Rollnick 2001).

To improve the interactions of health care professionals with patients related to behaviour change, an excellent technique for negotiating behaviour change in a clinical setting has been developed by Rollnick & Heather (1992). On close examination, this patient-centred interviewing technique appears to be underpinned by a number of the models described earlier. Originally developed to allow motivational interviewing related to substance abuse, the strategy is easily adaptable to suit any behavioural intervention related to lifestyle changes, and primary care clinicians have

reported that the method is acceptable (Rollnick et al 1997). This method of interviewing has been used successfully by various professions working in the fields of alcohol abuse, diabetes mellitus and tobacco smoking (Rollnick et al 1999, Sellman et al 2001) and a systematic review of the efficacy of method shows it to be superior to other interviewing (Dunn et al 2001).

The technique is based on the concept of readiness to change and the fact that a patient's decision to change behaviour is apt to move forward and back along a continuum (Prochaska & DiClemente 1984, see Table 8.3). This ambivalence is one of the main reasons advice giving has such limited effectiveness. Patients will only accept advice and act upon it when they are ready. They often experience feelings of ambivalence toward behaviour change and using motivational interviewing techniques provides the opportunity to build rapport with the patient and to explore the perceived importance of behaviour change through their eyes, to provide information if necessary, and also explore their feelings of confidence (self-efficacy) related to the change in behaviour.

Motivational interviewing requires interviewing skills that are commonly used by health care professionals such as active listening and empathizing. The use of open and closed questioning is also an important component of motivational interviewing (Emmons & Rollnick 2001).

The theoretical base of the interview strategy places importance on concepts such as readiness (related to the Stages of Change Model) the importance of the behaviour (related to the Health Belief Model), the patient's own concepts of beliefs and outcome expectations (related to the Theory of Planned Behaviour) and the patient's confidence in their ability to change (related to self-efficacy).

The interview strategy outlined by Rollnick can be easily incorporated within a continence promotion intervention. As with any intervention strategy, professional confidence comes with practice and experience.

IS THERE EVIDENCE OF THE USE OF BEHAVIOUR MODELS WITHIN CONTINENCE PROMOTION?

Health care practitioners use behavioural interventions on a daily basis without knowing it. Treatment protocols are regularly issued in 'top down' manner with the health care practitioners assuming that having been given the information, patients will know the importance of changing their behaviour and subsequently proceed to do so. Nothing could be farther from the truth (Rollnick & Heather 1992).

Many continence promotion programmes incorporate behavioural techniques within their programmes in an ad hoc fashion, but it is important to examine the available supporting evidence within continence promotion.

Chiarelli & Cockburn (1999) used the Health Belief Model as a framework to underpin the development of a successfully implemented postnatal continence promotion programme. The study by Chiarelli & Cockburn also employed social marketing strategies in the development of materials used within the programme. There was a significantly positive trend shown in the proportions of women adhering with pelvic floor exercise protocols at adequate levels in the intervention group when compared with those in the control group (p = 0.001 Mantel Haenzel Chi Square).

However, there is little evidence to show other interventions have been based on any of the various models of behaviour change.

When new continence promotion programmes are under development, whether individual treatment protocols for use in a physical therapy practice or continence promotion programmes for use in postnatal women or an aged care setting, it seems rational that they be based on a proven framework such as that provided by the various models. In developing programmes aimed at behaviour change, further formative exploration is necessary to determine various beliefs and perceptions that underlie attitudes, motivation and behaviour. When this has been achieved, more effective health/continence promotion programmes might follow.

CLINICAL RECOMMENDATIONS

The following is the menu of strategies suggested as a framework for the interviewing technique that might

easily be used within a continence promotion consultation (Emmons & Rollnick 2001, Rollnick & Heather 1992).

Establishing rapport/introducing the subject

This provides an understanding of the client's concerns about the suggested change and allows deeper understanding of the behaviour in the context of the person. The use of open-ended questions demonstrates to the patient that you are concerned about 'their story'.

Explore what they know about the behaviour as it relates to them personally.

Raising the subject

It is important here to check that the patient is happy to talk about the subject.

Assessing patient's readiness to change

Ask patients directly how they feel about changing the behaviour. By using such phrases as 'on a scale of one to 10, one being absolutely unwilling and 10 being ready, right now, to give it a go', the patient's readiness to change can easily be assessed.

Provide feedback and raise awareness of the consequences of the behaviour

Objective data can be introduced at this point, the patient's need for more information can be explored and their concerns can be discussed along with their feelings of self-efficacy. Offers of more support should be made at this point, especially if the patient feels little confidence in their ability to achieve the required change.

If there is little readiness to change – this should be acknowledged and questions such as 'what are the things about . . . (the behaviour) . . . that concern you?'

If the patient seems undecided

Describe how other patients have coped in the same situation, but be careful to emphasize that 'the patient knows best' and support them in whatever decision they make. In some instances, the subject is better postponed until the patient indicates more readiness to change.

The brief description is provided here to show how patients might be encouraged to become active collaborators in changing their health behaviours by using a method of empowerment that is underpinned by the most commonly used theories of behaviour change.

It is important that specialized health care providers realise the need for referral to other 'experts in the field'. For example, where weight loss is the desired outcome, brief motivational interviewing within a continence promotion consultation might move the patient toward this behaviour, but referral to a dietician might be in the best interests of the patient.

REFERENCES

Abrams P, Committee A T 2002 Levels of evidence and grades of recommendation. In: Abrams P, Cardozo L, Khouri S et al Incontinence. Health Publication, Plymouth, UK

Ajzen I, Fishbein M 1980 Understanding attitudes and predicting behaviour. Prentice–Hall, Englewood Cliffs, NJ

Bandura A 1977 Social learning theory. Prentice–Hall, Englewood Cliffs, NJ

Bandura A 1982 Self-efficacy mechanism in human agency. American Psychologist 37(2):122–147

Becker M 1974 The health belief model and personal health behaviour. Health Education Monographs 2:324–508

Bø K, Borgen J 2001 Prevalence of stress and urge urinary incontinence in elite athletes and controls. Medicine and Science in Sports and Exercise 33(11):1797–1802

Brown J, Grady D, Ouslander J G et al 1999 Prevalence of urinary incontinence and associated risk factors in postmenopausal women. Obstetrics and Gynecology 94(1):66–70

Bryant C, Dowell C, Fairbrother G et al 2000 A randomized trial of the effects of caffeine on frequency, urgency and urge incontinence. Neurourology and Urodynamics 19:501–502

Bryant C, Dowell C, Fairbrother G 2002 Caffeine reduction education to improve urinary symptoms. British Journal of Nursing 11(8):560–565

Bump R C, McLish D K 1992 Cigarette smoking and urinary incontinence in women. American Journal of Obstetrics and Gynecology 167(5):1213–1218

Bump R, McLish D 1994 Cigarette smoking and pure genuine stress incontinence of urine: a comparison of risk factors and determinants between smokers and non-smokers. American Journal of Obstetrics and Gynaecology 170(2): 579–582

Burgio K L, Matthews K A, Engel B T 1991 Prevalence, incidence and correlates of urinary incontinence in healthy middle aged women. The Journal of Urology 146:1255–1259

Chiarelli P, Brown W, McElduff P 1999 Leaking Urine – prevalence and associated factors in australian women. Neurourology and Urodynamics 18(6):567–577

Chiarelli P, Brown W, McElduff P 2000 Constipation in Australian women: prevalence and associated factors. International Urogynecology Journal and Pelvic Floor Dysfunction 11:71–78

Chiarelli P, Cockburn J 1999 The development of a physiotherapy continence promotion program using a customer focus. Australian Journal of Physiotherapy 45(2):111–120

Creighton S, Stanton S 1990 Caffeine: does it affect your bladder? British Journal of Urology 66(6):613–614

Dalosso H, McGrother C, Matthews R J et al 2003 The association of diet and other lifestyle factors with overactive bladder and stress incontinence: a longitudinal study in women. British Journal of Urology International 92:69–77

Dunn C, Deroo L, Rivara F P 2001 The use of brief interventions adapted from motivational interviewing across behavioural domains: a systematic review. Addiction 96:1725–1742

Emmons K, Rollnick S 2001 Motivational interviewing in health care settings: opportunities and limitations. American Journal of Preventive Medicine 20(1):68–74

Hunskaar S, Arnold E, Burgio K et al 2000 Epidemiology and natural history of urinary incontinence. International Journal of Urogynecology and Pelvic Floor Dysfunction 11:301–319

Kapoor D, Davila G W, Rosenthal R J et al 2004 Pelvic floor dysfunction in morbidly obese women: pilot study. Obesity Research 12(7):1104–1107

Lubowski D, Swash M, Nicholls R J et al 1988 Increases in pudendal nerve terminal motor latency with defaecation straining. British Journal of Surgery 75:1095–1097

Maher C G, Sherrington C, Herbert R D et al 2003 Reliability of the PEDro scale for rating quality of randomized controlled trials. Physical Therapy 83:713–721

Nutbeam D, Harris E 2004 Theory in a nutshell. McGraw-Hill, Sydney

Nygaard I E, Thompson F L, Svengalis S L et al 1994 Urinary incontinence in elite nulliparous athletes. Obstetrics and Gynecology. 84(2):183–187

Prochaska J, DiClemente C 1984 The transtheoretical approach: crossing traditional foundations of change. Don Jones/Irwin, Homewood, IL

Rollnick S, Heather N 1992 Negotiating behaviour change in medical settings. Journal of Mental Health 1(1):25–38

Rollnick S, Butler C, Stott N 1997 Helping smokers make decisions: the enhancement of brief intervention for general medical practice. Patient Education and Counselling 31:191–203

Rollnick S, Mason P, Butler C 1999 Health behaviour change. A guide for practitioners. Churchill Livingstone, Edinburgh

Sellman J D, Sullivan P F, Dore G M et al 2001 A randomized controlled trial of motivational enhancement therapy (MET) for mild to moderate alcohol dependence. Journal of Studies on Alcohol 62(3):389–396

Snooks S J, Barnes P R H, Swash M et al 1985a Damage to the pelvic floor musculature in chronic constipation. Gastroenterology 89:977–981

Stach-Lempinen B, Nygard C, Laippala P et al 2004 Is physical activity influenced by urinary incontinence? British Journal of Obstetrics and Gynaecology 111:475–480

Subak L, Johnson C, Whitcomb E et al 2002 Does weight loss improve incontinence in moderately obese women? International Urogynecology Journal and Pelvic Floor Dysfunction 13:40–43

Tampakoudis P, Tantanassis, T, Grimbizis G et al 1995 Cigarette smoking and urinary incontinence in women – a new calculative method of measuring exposure to smoke. European Journal of Obstetrics, Gynecology and Reproductive Biologyy 63:27–30

Valtin H 2001 Drink at least eight glasses of water a day. Really? Is there scientific evidence for 8x8 per day? American Journal of Physiology. Regulatory, Integrative and Comparative Physiology 283(5):R993–R1004

VanRyn M, Heaney C 1992 What's the use of theory? Health Education Quarterly 19(3):315–330

Wilson P, Bø K 2002 Conservative treatment in women. In: Cardozo L, Abrams P, Khoury S et al Incontinence. Health Publication, Plymouth, UK

Chapter 9

Pelvic floor dysfunction and evidence-based physical therapy

Female stress urinary incontinence

PREVALENCE, CAUSES, PATHOPHYSIOLOGY: TWO VIEWS, ONE DISEASE

Jacques Corcos and Anders Mattiasson

The most fascinating aspect of medicine is its constant evolution over time. This even progression is based on new findings in our laboratories, new data from clinical research, new imaging techniques, and new views and theories. The evolution of concepts has also reached the 'world of incontinence', and a new perspective of stress urinary incontinence (SUI) pathophysiology is proposed here. We have therefore decided to present two different views of pathophysiology in this chapter: one classical, and the other 'revolutionary'. The classical model could be easily criticised because it lacks evidence for most of its basis. However, it has the advantages of clarity and simplicity. The new revolutionary model we are proposing is founded on a new way of thinking about structure and function (cause + consequence) (Mattiasson 2001, 2005).

DEFINITION OF STRESS URINARY INCONTINENCE

Prevalence of SUI in women

Most published surveys on the prevalence of incontinence have evaluated it as a whole. Two recent surveys reporting on urinary incontinence (UI) in Europe and in the USA both defined it as any leakage occurring in the past 30 days (Hunskaar et al 2004, Kinchen et al 2003). Their overall results were congruent, showing an average UI prevalence of 35 and 37%, respectively. In these studies, SUI, at 37 and 42%, respectively, seemed to be the most prevalent type, whereas mixed incontinence was found in 33 and 46%. Similar numbers were obtained in previous surveys (Burgio et al 1991, Hannestad et al 2000, Yarnell et al 1981). However, Hampel et al (1997) undertook a meta-analysis of 48 reports and arrived at a slightly higher SUI incidence of 49%, with only 29% of mixed incontinence.

The difficulties in differentiating between types of incontinence were related to the fact that most studies were based on telephone or direct interviews, making the diagnosis of SUI incomplete since urodynamic tests were not performed.

Some investigators have reported on the severity of incontinence by measuring the frequency of leakage episodes and the quantity of urine lost or both (Diokno et al 1986, Sandvik et al 1993, 2000). These two parameters must be considered as being very subjective because the former derives from the recollection of incidents, which could be difficult for some elderly patients, and the latter is attributed to personal perception, hygiene and coping mechanisms.

What is more significant for caregivers is the 'bothersomeness' of incontinence. Sandvik et al (2000), trying to match 'bothersomeness' and the severity of incontinence, determined that only 20% of incontinent women were 'suffering' from bothersome and severe incontinence.

Age is an important parameter in prevalence, severity, bothersomeness and any other variables studied. SUI occurs mainly in young and perimenopausal women (Hunskaar et al 2004). Mixed incontinence increases beyond menopause and has become the most prevalent type of incontinence in the seventh decade of life.

In conclusion, SUI appears to be the most frequent type of incontinence reported in literature. However, the most relevant prevalence for caregivers should be the number of sufferers who seek treatment, though this number may vary according to the type of treatment offered. Most probably, incontinent patients will more readily accept a non-invasive approach, such as pelvic floor exercises, rather than a surgical procedure, and the number of sufferers seeking therapy may depend on the invasiveness of the intervention proffered. Such studies do not exist according to our readings, and will probably never be conducted, given the complexity of the questionnaires that would be required. These questionnaires should take into consideration several personal parameters as well as a good understanding of the different types of treatment. A large-scale survey therefore seems difficult to perform. However, existing and future epidemiological studies should be analysed, keeping in mind these important considerations that explain why a large number of incontinent patients do not even consult a physician.

CAUSES AND PATHOPHYSIOLOGY OF SUI

The classical view

Urinary incontinence is the end result of one or several important causes. Bladder and sphincter integrity are necessary to assure normal continence in men and women, but globally UI is more frequent in women than in men (Hunskaar et al 2004). Many reasons could account for this gender difference: dissimilarities in the anatomy of the pelvic floor muscles and ligaments supporting the bladder and sphincter, the effect of childbirth and maternal injury on the pelvic structure and sphincter, and the role of hormones which have important receptors in the bladder, sphincter, and vaginal area. Finally, genetic factors not yet well studied could explain racial and familial trends of incontinence.

A classification of the causes of incontinence in women is proposed by Koelbl et al (2002) and is summarized in Box 9.1.

Box 9.1: Classical classification of incontinence

GENERAL CAUSES OF INCONTINENCE
- Congenital anomalies
- Injuries and diseases of the nervous system
- Abnormalities of the bladder itself
  - muscle
  - connective tissue
  - innervation
    - sensory afferents
    - somatosensory control and coordination of the sphincter
- Connective tissue of the lower urinary tract (LUT)
- Ageing

SPECIFIC CAUSES OF INCONTINENCE IN WOMEN
- Genuine stress urinary incontinence (SUI)
  - urethral weakness
  - vaginal relaxation
- Specific contributing factors
  - anatomy of the pelvic floor, levator hiatus, muscle size and strength
  - childbirth and maternal injury
  - vaginal support of the urethra
  - ageing
- Menopause

General and specific causes

Congenital anomalies involve mainly the central nervous system (CNS) (e.g. myelomeningocele, sacral agenesis, severe scoliosis). Most of these lesions produce a neurogenic overactive bladder. However, the lowest lesions, involving the bottom segments of the cord, may lead to cauda equina syndrome with sphincteric deficiency and/or an areflexic bladder. Other congenital anomalies (e.g. bladder extrophy) involve the bladder itself and its sphincter mechanism, which is often only partially developed (Koelbl et al 2002).

Injuries and diseases of the nervous system (e.g. multiple sclerosis, lipomas and other benign or malignant tumours) are additional causes of incontinence. In the same line of thought, incontinence in these situations is mainly due to a neurogenic overactive bladder, but lower lesions, such as disc compression, sacral tumours, sacral injuries, and neuropathies (e.g. diabetes mellitus or toxins) are associated with sphincteric weakness and a hypofunctional bladder. With all these lesions, incontinence is related to overactivity of the detrusor, leading to urgency incontinence, overflow in the case of a hypocontractile detrusor, or SUI if the sphincter is hypofunctional.

Anomalies of the detrusor and its innervation. Connective tissue is not an important component of the normal detrusor because the smooth muscle cells are arranged closely together (Gosling 1997). Connective tissue is increased in the obstructed bladder, suggesting that some smooth muscle fibres convert from a contractile to a collagen synthetic phenotype. Bladder collagen transformation is not seen with ageing. In both these models, denervation is observed, but to a much lesser extent in the ageing bladder. In women with pure SUI, there are no structural alterations of the bladder wall except for the usual changes secondary to ageing.

Effect of pregnancy and delivery on the lower urinary tract (LUT). For the pelvic floor, delivery is probably the most 'stressful' period in a woman's lifetime. However, very little is known about the relationship between delivery, pelvic floor changes and SUI. It is widely recognized that SUI may be a consequence of pregnancy/delivery and that usually pregnancy worsens pre-existing SUI (Hojberg et al 1999).

According to Koebel et al (2002), vaginal delivery might lead to SUI via four major mechanisms.

1. Injury to connective tissue supports by the mechanical process of vaginal delivery.
2. Vascular damage to pelvic structures as a result of compression by the presenting part of the fetus during labour.
3. Damage to the pelvic nerves and/or muscles from trauma during parturition.

4. Direct injury to the urinary tract during labour and delivery. The physiological changes produced by pregnancy may make women more susceptible to these pathophysiological processes.

Pelvic floor muscle strength decreases after delivery. For some authors it returns to the normal range a few weeks later (Peschers et al 1997). For others there is a persistent weakness (Dumoulin et al 2004). Incontinence seems to be linked to several parameters (e.g. forceps use, duration of labour, number of deliveries, pre-existing bladder neck mobility). It also appears that a close relationship exists between epidural analgesia during labour and the severity of pelvic floor injuries (Cutner & Cardozo 1992, Francis 1960). Episiotomies are often reported to worsen post-partum pelvic floor dysfunction. However, evidence is seldom available, and its relationship to SUI is unproven (Hong et al 1988).

Ageing. Incontinence at large is more frequent in the elderly. However, the prevalence of SUI is relatively decreased because of increased mixed incontinence. Ageing in women qualitatively modifies the pelvic floor muscles. Proportional numbers of slow and fast twitch muscle fibres change with age, as reported by Koelbl et al (1989) who biopsied the pelvic floors of elderly women with incontinence. Also, the response to electrical stimulation and electromyography is modified by ageing (Smith et al 1989). These findings are consistent with the two main classical causes of incontinence, intrinsic sphincter deficiency (ISD) and bladder neck/urethral hypermobility. We strongly believe that SUI in women is always associated with sphincteric deficiency. In our opinion, pelvic floor relaxation leading to different degrees of prolapse is only one cause of sphincteric dysfunction. This is supported by the fact that numerous women with pelvic prolapse and/or bladder neck hypermobility are not incontinent and therefore have a competent sphincter. This viewpoint is shared by Chaikin et al (1998) and Kayigil et al (1999).

Bladder neck and urethral hypermobility

To be fully functional, the urethra must be supported by a 'non-elastic' structure, originally the urethra pelvic ligament, which provides a backboard against increasing abdominal forces compressing the urethra. This is the basis for the 'hammock theory' popularized by DeLancey (1994). The loss of such support leads to what is classically called urethral hypermobility or rotational descent of the urethra around the pubic bone. For a long time, this concept was considered to be the main cause of SUI. It was also the basis behind the pressure transmission theory (Athanassopoulos et al 1994, Enhorning 1960), and the later development of 'slings' for the treatment of women with SUI. The relaxation of urethral support can be ascribed to numerous factors, including childbirth, strenuous exercises, pelvic denervation following surgery and trauma, and probably genetic elements that remain to be proven.

The theory of urethral hypermobility is easy to understand, and explains the success of surgery to repair SUI. However, the fact that SUI occurs without a hypermobile urethra and that failure of surgery is not always associated with recurrence of hypermobility leaves plenty of room for a second important pathophysiological concept, intrinsic sphincter deficiency (ISD).

Intrinsic sphincter deficiency

The female urethra is a short but complex organ intimately connected to the bladder and pelvic floor structures. Anatomically, it can be isolated and described very precisely (DeLancey et al 2002), but its functionality cannot be studied separately (Corcos & Schick 2001).

Besides its proximal smooth muscle sphincteric component and its mid-urethra rhabdosphincter, the wall of the urethra comprises an outer muscle coat and an inner epithelial membrane continuous with the bladder urothelium. The outer smooth muscle coat extends throughout the length of the urethra and is essentially made up of longitudinal fibres, whereas circular fibres are rare. The innervation of this coating is mainly parasympathetic, and its function appears to be to shorten and open the urethral lumen during micturation (Ek et al 1977).

The urethral lamina propria covers the entire length of the urethra. It is lined by the urethral urothelium and lies on a rich layer of vascular plexus and mucous glands, which separates it from the smooth muscle layers. The vascular plexus is important for normal continence and has been shown to be highly sensitive to hormone levels in women (Dokita et al 1991, Persson & Andersson 1992). A defect in one of these entities elicits poor closure of the sphincteric urethra and SUI. Loss of sphincteric mass has been clearly demonstrated by different imaging modalities (electromyography, ultrasound and magnetic resonance imaging (Masata et al 2000, Schaer et al 1995, Yang et al 1991).

It is, however, hard to believe that urethral sphincter mechanisms, in continuous use during a lifetime, can spontaneously become anatomically incompetent. Ageing, through mechanisms of nerve and vascular 'injuries', can weaken the sphincter (Koelbl et al 1989). Nerve and vascular injuries, provoked by a lack of hormones (menopause), pelvic surgery, radiation therapy, neuropathies (e.g. diabetes mellitus, toxins), are the most common causes of sphincteric weakness. Furthermore, a relationship probably exists between hypermobility and ISD. Repeated elongation of muscular fibres of the sphincter and surrounding tissues, including the nerves, may be responsible for sphincteric damage.

In conclusion, the classical concept of SUI pathophysiology proposes a model based mainly on two mechanisms: bladder neck mobility and ISD. These two defects can be evoked by several factors, among which pregnancy/delivery and ageing are generally the most important. The two defects have to be considered as being concomitant in all cases of SUI with hypermobility, though ISD can exist alone. Albeit imperfect, this theory has the advantage of clarity and ease of understanding. However, too many elements of the theory remain unclear, opening the door for a more modern, revolutionary pathophysiological hypothesis for SUI.

The revolutionary view

Stress incontinence is a term that has long been quoted to denote a disease described as an insufficiency in the urethra itself or in the surrounding tissues that normally help to close the urethra. As such insufficiency becomes obvious under stress and the concomitant rise in abdominal pressure, we have coined the umbrella term 'stress incontinence' for the involuntary movement of urine from the bladder through the entire urethra. The nature of deviations from the normal state has been described, among other things, as excessive mobility of the urethra (with descent or rotation) accompanying strain and a rise in abdominal pressure known as hypermobility. This has long been thought to be an important etiological factor in stress incontinence. Because such incontinence also occurs in cases without hypermobility, it has been assumed to arise because of insufficiency in the actual urethra wall (i.e. without concomitant hypermobility), and this type of insufficiency has been named ISD. The prevailing view of the underlying pathophysiology is therefore that stress incontinence can arise in both the presence and absence of a hypermobile urethra. In both cases, then, it is taken for granted that the inadequate closing forces on the urethra under strain are the reason why urine can be passed involuntarily. This picture of the changes that lead to stress incontinence is likely incomplete. The reason for the claim is not just that stress incontinence is not a disease in itself, but also the nature of the underlying disorder is not sufficiently well studied or understood.

A reassessment of stress incontinence as a diagnosis

If we free ourselves from the currently-prevailing, consequence-based classification (consequence + cause),

we can instead see a new picture of female incontinence emerging, and this is revolutionary in that it does not merely question the old opinion; it also represents a new model based on pathophysiology in terms of structure and function (cause + consequence). A series of circumstances and observations suggests that this view is correct. The original theoretical model (Mattiasson 2001) is supported by steadily increasing amounts of clinical, experimental and epidemiological data. For female LUT dysfunctional disorders, a portrait is emerging of a disease in the urethra and pelvic floor, a disease that is of a chronic and progressive nature and with two components, insufficient closure and overactivity. The disease might develop during a long period of time, and then continue without symptoms. Childbirth and trauma with consequent denervation of the pelvic floor and sphincter muscles might be important in this context (Swash et al 1985). When symptoms appear, they might or might not be associated with incontinence (i.e. they can be described as wet or dry, respectively). Overactivity in this sense does not only refer to overactive behaviour of the bladder (i.e. the detrusor), but also to overactive opening of the urethra.

Several investigations speak in favour of the presence of urethral overactivity (Farrell & Tynski 1996, Kulseng-Hanssen 2001, Low et al 1989, McGuire 1978, McLennan et al 2001, Vereecken & Proesmans 2000). If we can agree on the presence of such overactivity at the urethral level, urethral insufficiency might well be seen as a mixture of passive insufficiency and overactive opening. In women, this disease can give rise to different symptoms, of which stress incontinence is one. Other symptoms of the same disease could be urgency and urge incontinence, often of course also with involvement of the bladder (see p. 204). The result is therefore completely different from the currently-prevailing approach of proceeding from the occurrence of urine leakage at stress/strain and working backwards to try to construct a pathophysiological basis (Abrams et al 1988, 2002, Koelbl et al 2001).

A disturbed balance between closure and opening at the urethral level actually seems to be the simplest and most logical explanation for a number of different functional disorders of the LUT in women. The underlying pathophysiological state is characterized by insufficient contraction in the musculature of the urethra/pelvic floor, which instead creates the conditions where smooth muscle relaxation can take place (Mattiasson 2001). Our revolutionary view of the disorder that leads to female incontinence in various forms, including stress incontinence, can therefore be described rather simply: a relaxatory mechanism in the urethra, which is manifested in incontinent women by a greater propensity to opening than in continent women and which should be added to the occurrence of insufficient contraction of the urethral/pelvic floor musculature that attempts to close the urethra, is what mediates female incontinence.

A new way of describing the disease in the female LUT that leads, inter alia, to incontinence

We have long been bewildered by the way that stress and urgency incontinence can occur together as mixed incontinence. It is even difficult at times to understand a patient who gives hesitant answers to our questions, which are supposed to help discriminate between stress and urge incontinence. We have also noted that pelvic floor training can be a successful treatment for both stress and urge incontinence as well as mixed incontinence. In addition, we know that two out of three patients with mixed incontinence become free of symptoms after surgery directed solely against the stress component. If we add to this the epidemiological picture that stress incontinence is more common in younger women than mixed and urge incontinence (Hannestad et al 2000) and the fact that the more pronounced stress incontinence they have, the more likely it is that they also have a component of urge incontinence (Bump et al 2003, Teleman et al 2004), then the new picture emerging seems to be much easier to interpret.

A weakness in the pelvic floor musculature has been observed in women with all types and degrees of incontinence. This weakness is progressive and as pronounced in patients with urge and mixed incontinence as in those with stress incontinence (Gunnarsson & Mattiasson 1994, 1999). These observations have provided the foundation for the hypothesis that one and the same disease could lie behind all types of female incontinence, which seems to agree well with the 'integral theory' presented at roughly the same time (Petros & Ulmsten 1993). The close association between different forms of incontinence in women was suggested in this theory to be due to a weakness in the anterior vaginal wall, a lax vagina, which could explain why both an insufficiency in the urethra and mechanical stretching in the tissues of the bladder bottom arise, triggering urges as a consequence.

With an increased degree of insufficiency as a result of trauma, disease, fatigue and/or age, the inability to close with the aid of the musculature of the urethra and/or pelvic floor is greater. At the same time, the influence of an easily-triggered relaxatory mechanism stimulating opening and emptying is stronger. The more powerful the relaxation, the greater is the probability of sensory irritation, which may be due to exposure of the urethral mucous membrane to urine (De

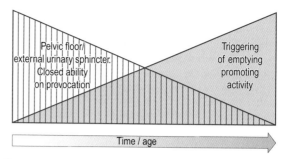

Fig. 9.1 When passive insufficiency in closure of the urethra dominates, then stress incontinence arises. With increasing degrees of insufficiency there is also greater risk of active opening of the urethra, of active relaxation taking effect, and a greater risk of mixed or urge incontinence.

Groat et al 2001), but it could perhaps also be induced solely by motor overactivity, and possibly perceived in both cases at the cerebral level as urgency (Fig. 9.1).

In the description of a new classification system for all LUT disorders, it has been suggested on theoretical grounds that incontinent women could also have a trigger mechanism causing overactivity at the urethral, and not only at the bladder level (Mattiasson 2001). Incontinent women, including those with stress incontinence, also seem to have a quicker opening mechanism of the urethra than their age- and parity-matched continent counterparts (Teleman et al 2003). This means that part of the disorder is due to the urethra opening more easily, or at least more quickly, than in symptom-free women. Another study, conducted in 1996–2001, showed that women with stress incontinence tended to have lower urethral pressure through relaxation when attempting to close by squeezing (Mattiasson & Teleman 2006). Currently available methods for urethral pressure measurements could be criticised, but the pattern of the pressure drop observed in patients agrees well with what is seen experimentally in both animals and humans in vitro and in vivo (Andersson et al 1983, Mattiasson 1984, Radziszewski et al 2003). Strangely, relaxation of the urethral smooth muscle does not seem to have found any place in clinical thinking or action. All we have encountered in the literature is such mechanisms as they concern basic science, never as they relate to the clinical situation, whether in research or for clinical application (Abrams et al 2005, Cardozo & Staskin 2001, Corcos & Schick 2001).

We could therefore describe the interaction between closing and opening forces as a balance, and the disease that causes incontinence, among other things, could be called an imbalance. The relationship between these mechanisms can be visualized in a diagram illustrating

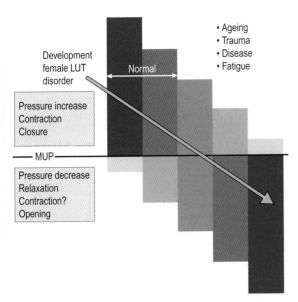

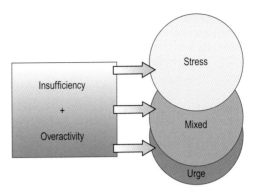

Fig. 9.3 A combination of insufficiency and overactivity (especially urethral overactivity–relaxation) can give rise to several different symptoms. The degree of insufficiency and overactivity determines whether urges will be felt or not. One and the same disease can therefore cause several different symptoms, including some that do not entail urine leakage, for example, urges.

Fig. 9.2 With increasing insufficiency in the musculature that in normal conditions is able to close the urethra, the possibility of opening relaxatory mechanisms becomes significant as two different but interacting mechanisms that can both entail incontinence. The more opening, relaxatory activity there is, the more urges are felt. The loss of contraction and closure can be described in simplified terms as insufficiency, and the rise of opening through relaxation as overactivity initiated at the urethral level. LUT, lower urinary tract; MUP, maximum urethral pressure.

progressive changes with the loss of closing function and the rise of unintentional opening (Fig. 9.2).

It is plausible to envisage that not just trauma and disease, but also, for example, fatigue in the closing musculature could bring about a shift with increasing possibilities of relaxatory activity (Fig. 9.3). Another possibility is that relaxation of the closing musculature at rest, say at night, could lead to a similar shift with a tendency to relaxation/opening and urgency, for example in the form of nocturia.

The new perspective on the disease that causes, inter alia, female incontinence proceeds from a theoretical model that describes the pathophysiological basis for LUT diseases (structure/function + consequences instead of consequences + structure/function) (Mattiasson 2001). It could be summed up as follows.

- It is a chronic progressive disease that may or may not give symptoms.
- Disease, trauma, fatigue and ageing can interact in a negative direction.

- The functional part of the disease consists of a disturbed balance between closing and opening, between storage and emptying functions.
- Insufficiency and overactivity at the level of the urethra and perhaps the bladder are shared features of all female incontinence.
- There are striking similarities in the patterns of functional disorder irrespective of the type of incontinence. Differences in disease and symptomatology seem to be differences of degree rather than kind.
- Impaired pelvic function and an altered structure are found in all types of female incontinence.
- Overactivity can be triggered at different levels and via several mechanisms in the LUT/nervous system, among them urethral smooth muscle relaxation.
- Relaxatory mechanisms in the urethra with a faster than normal opening function are an important part of the functional disorder of the female LUT.
- Unintentional opening of the urethra with pressure drop often occurs in attempts to close by squeezing.
- The more pronounced the stress component, the more likely it is that the patient also has urgency.
- The faster the opening mechanism, the greater the probability that urgency will occur.

It therefore looks as if there are mechanisms in the urethra and pelvic floor that have been interpreted in several studies as probably being of essential significance for urethral function and have not yet been incorporated in the descriptions of normal or abnormal LUT function in the clinical context and therefore reveal a lacuna in the transition between basic science and clinical knowledge. In other words, clinicians need to be trained in applied translational thinking. If the elected generalists in our scientific organizations encourage specialists in different fields to adopt a translational approach, we will almost certainly be successful in establishing a new understanding of disorders of the LUT.

REFERENCES

Abrams P, Blaivas J G, Stanton S L et al 1988 The standardisation of terminology of lower urinary tract function. The International Continence Society Committee on Standardisation of Terminology. Scandinavian Journal of Urology and Nephrology. Supplementum 114:5–19

Abrams P, Cardozo L, Fall M et al 2002 The standardisation of terminology of lower urinary tract function: report from the Standardisation Sub-committee of the International Continence Society. Neurourology and Urodynamics 21(2): 167–178

Abrams P, Cardozo L, Khoury S et al (eds) 2005 Incontinence. Plymbridge Distributors, Plymouth, UK

Andersson K E, Mattiasson A, Sjogren C 1983 Electrically induced relaxation of the noradrenaline contracted isolated urethra from rabbit and man. The Journal of Urology 129(1):210–214

Athanassopoulos A, Melekos M D, Speakman M et al 1994 Endoscopic vesical neck suspension in female urinary stress incontinence: results and changes in various urodynamic parameters. International Urology and Nephrology 26(3): 293–299

Bump R C, Norton P A, Zinner N R et al 2003 Duloxetine urinary incontinence study Group. Mixed urinary incontinence symptoms: urodynamic findings, incontinence severity, and treatment response. Obstetrics and Gynecology 102(1):76–83

Burgio K L, Matthews K A, Engel B T 1991 Prevalence, incidence and correlates of urinary incontinence in healthy, middle-aged women. The Journal of Urology 146(5):1255–1259

Cardozo L, Staskin D (eds) 2001 Book of female urology and urogynaecology. ISIS Medical Media, London. Online. Available: www.dunitz.co.uk

Chaikin D, Rosenthal J, Blaivas J 1998 Pubovaginal fascial sling for all types of stress urinary incontinence: long-term analysis. The Journal of Urology 160(4):1312–1316

Corcos J, Schick E (eds) 2001 The urinary sphincter. Marcel Dekker, New York. Online. Available: www.dekker.com

Cutner A, Cardozo L D 1992 The lower urinary tract in pregnancy and the puerperium. International Urogynecology Journal and Pelvic Floor Dysfunction 3:312–323

De Groat W C, Fraser M O, Yoshiyama M et al 2001 Neural control of the urethra. Scandinavian Journal of Urology and Nephrology. Supplementum (207):35–43, discussion 106–125

DeLancey J O 1994 Structural support of the urethra as it relates to stress urinary incontinence: the hammock hypothesis. American Journal of Obstetrics and Gynecology 170(6): 1713–1720

DeLancey J O, Gosling J, Creed K et al 2002. Gross anatomy and cell biology of the lower urinary tract. In: Incontinence. Abrams P, Cardozo L, Khoury S et al (eds) Plymbridge Distributors, Plymouth, p 17–82. Online. Available: cservs@plymbridge.com

Diokno A C, Brock B M, Brown M B et al 1986 Prevalence of urinary incontinence and other urological symptoms in the noninstitutionalized elderly. The Journal of Urology 136(5):1022–1025

Dokita S, Morgan W R, Wheeler M A et al 1991 NG-nitro-L-arginine inhibits non-adrenergic, non-cholinergic relaxation in rabbit urethral smooth muscle. Life Sciences 48(25):2429–2436

Dumoulin C, Lemieux M C, Bourbonnais D et al 2004 Physiotherapy for persistent postnatal stress urinary incontinence: a randomized controlled trial. Obstetrics and Gynecology 104(3):504–510

Enhorning G 1960 Functional sphincterometry a test for stress incontinence. Urologia Internationalis 10:129–136

Ek A, Alm P, Andersson K E et al 1977 Adrenergic and cholingeric nerves of the human urethra and urinary bladder. A histochemical study. Acta Physiologica Scandinavica 99(3):345–352

Farrell S A, Tynski G 1996 The effect of urethral pressure variation on detrusor activity in women. International Urogynecology Journal and Pelvic Floor Dysfunction 7(2):87–93

Francis W J A 1960 The onset of stress incontinence. The Journal of Obstetrics and Gynaecology of the British Empire 67:899–903

Gosling J A 1997 Modification of bladder structure in response to outflow obstruction and ageing. European Urology 32(suppl 1):9–14

Gunnarsson M, Mattiasson A 1994 Circumvaginal surface electromyography in women with urinary incontinence and in healthy volunteers. Scandinavian Journal of Urology and Nephrology. Supplementum 157:89–95

Gunnarsson M, Mattiasson A 1999 Female stress-, urge- and mixed urinary incontinence are associated with a chronic and progressive pelvic floor/vaginal neuromuscular disorder: an investigation of 317 healthy and incontinent women using vaginal surface electromyography. Neurourology and Urodynamics 18(6):613–621

Hampel C, Wienhold D, Benken N et al 1997 Prevalence and natural history of female incontinence. European Urology 32(suppl 2):3–12

Hannestad Y S, Rortveit G, Sandvik H et al 2000 Norwegian EPINCONT study. Epidemiology of incontinence in the county of Nord-Trondelag. A community-based epidemiological survey of female urinary incontinence: the Norwegian EPINCONT study. Journal of Clinical Epidemiology 53(11): 1150–1157

Hojberg K E, Salvig J D, Winslow N A et al 1999 Urinary incontinence: prevalence and risk factors at 16 weeks of gestation. British Journal of Obstetrics and Gynaecology. 106(8):842–850

Hong P L, Leong M, Selzer V 1988 Uroflowmetric observation in pregnancy. Neurourology and Urodynamics 7:61–70

Hunskaar S, Lose G, Sykes D et al 2004 The prevalence of urinary incontinence in women in four European countries. BJU International 93(3):324–330

Kayigil O, Iftekhar A S, Metin A 1999 The coexistence of intrinsic sphincter deficiency with type II stress incontinence. The Journal of Urology 162(4):1365–1366

Kinchen K S, Burgio K, Diokno A C et al 2003 Factors associated with women's decision to seek treatment for urinary incontinence. Journal of Women's Health 12(7):687–698

Koelbl H, Mostwin J, Boiteux J P et al 2001 Pathophysiology. In: Abrams P, Cardozo L, Khoury S et al (eds) Incontinence. Plymbridge Distributors, Plymouth, p 205–241

Koelbl H, Mostwin J, Boiteux J P et al 2002 Pathophysiology. In: Abrams P, Cardozo L, Khoury S et al (eds) Incontinence. Plymbridge Distributors, Plymouth, p 203–242. Online. Available: cservs@plymbridge.com

Koelbl H, Strassegger H, Riss P A et al 1989 Morphologic and functional aspects of pelvic floor muscles in patients with pelvic relaxation and genuine stress incontinence. Obstetrics and Gynecology 74(5):789–795

Kulseng-Hanssen S 2001 The clinical value of ambulatory urethral pressure recording in women. Scandinavian Journal of Urology and Nephrology. Supplementum (207):67–73

Low J A, Armstrong J B, Mauger G M 1989 The unstable urethra in the female. Obstetrics and Gynecology 75(1):142–143

Masata J, Martan A, Halaska M et al 2000 [Ultrasonography of the funneling of the urethra]. Ceská Gynekologie/Ceská Lékarská Spolecnost J. Ev. Purkyne 65(2):87–90

Mattiasson A 1984 On the peripheral nervous control of the lower urinary tract [thesis]. Lund University, Sweden

Mattiasson A 2001 Characterisation of lower urinary tract disorders: a new view. Neurourology and Urodynamics 20:601–621

Mattiasson A 2005 Classification of lower urinary tract dysfunction. In: Corcos J, Schick E (eds) The neurogenic bladder. Marcel Dekker, London, p 469–480

Mattiasson A, Teleman P 2006 Abnormal urethral motor function is common in female stress, mixed and urge incontinence. Neurourology and Urodynamics 25:703–708

McGuire E J 1978 Reflex urethral instability. British Journal of Urology 50(3):200–204

McLennan M T, Melick C, Bent A E 2001 Urethral instability: clinical and urodynamic characteristics. Neurourology and Urodynamics 20(6):653–660

Persson K, Andersson K E 1992 Nitric oxide and relaxation of pig lower urinary tract. British Journal of Pharmacology 106(2):416–422

Peschers U M, Schaer G N, DeLancey J O et al 1997 Levator ani function before and after childbirth. British Journal of Obstetrics and Gynaecology 104:1004–1008

Petros P E, Ulmsten U I 1993 An integral theory and its method for the diagnosis and management of female urinary incontinence. Scandinavian Journal of Urology and Nephrology. Supplementum 153:1–93

Radziszewski P, Soller W, Mattiasson A 2003 Calcitonin gene-related peptide and substance P induce pronounced motor effects in the female rat urethra in vivo. Scandinavian Journal of Urology and Nephrology 37(4):275–280

Sandvik H, Hunskaar S, Seim A 1993 Validation of a severity index in female urinary incontinence and its implementation in an epidemiological survey. Journal of Epidemiology and Community Health 47(6):497–499

Sandvik H, Seim A, Vanvik A et al 2000 A severity index for epidemiological surveys of female urinary incontinence: comparison with 48-hour pad-weighing tests. Neurourology and Urodynamics 19(2):137–145

Schaer G N, Koechli O R, Schuessler B et al 1995 Improvement of perineal sonographic bladder neck imaging with ultrasound contrast medium. Obstetrics and Gynecology 86(6):950–954

Smith A R, Hosker G L, Warrell D W 1989 The role of partial denervation of the pelvic floor in the aetiology of genitourinary proplapse and stress incontinence of urine. A neurophysiological study. British Journal of Obstetrics and Gynaecology 96(1):24–28

Swash M, Snooks S J, Henry M M 1985 Unifying concept of pelvic floor disorders and incontinence. Journal of the Royal Society of Medicine 78(11):906–911

Teleman P M, Gunnarsson M, Lidfeldt J 2003 Urethral pressure changes in response to squeeze: a population-based study in healthy and incontinent 53- to 63-year-old women. American Journal of Obstetrics and Gynecology 189(4):1100–1105

Teleman P M, Lidfeldt J, Nerbrand C et al 2004 WHILA study group. Overactive bladder: prevalence, risk factors and relation to stress incontinence in middle-aged women. BJOG 111(6):600–604

Vereecken R L, Proesmans W 2000 Urethral instability as an important element of dysfunctional voiding. The Journal of Urology 163(2):585–588

Yang A, Mostwin J L, Rosenshein N B et al 1991 Pelvic floor descent in women: dynamic evaluation with fast MR imaging and cinematic display. Radiology 179(1):25–33

Yarnell J W G, Voyle G J, Richards C J et al 1981 The prevalence and severity of urinary incontinence in women. Journal of Epidemiology and Community Health 35:71–74

PELVIC FLOOR MUSCLE TRAINING FOR STRESS URINARY INCONTINENCE

Kari Bø

INTRODUCTION

In 1948 Kegel (1948) was the first to report pelvic floor muscle training (PFMT) to be effective in the treatment of female urinary incontinence. In spite of his reports of cure rates of over 84%, surgery soon became the first choice of treatment, and not until the 1980s was there renewed interest for conservative treatment. This new interest for conservative treatment may have developed because of higher awareness among women regarding incontinence and health and fitness activities, cost of surgery and morbidity, complications, and relapses reported after surgical procedures (Fantl et al 1996).

Although several consensus statements based on systematic reviews have recommended conservative treatment and especially PFMT as the first choice of treatment for urinary incontinence (Fantl et al 1996, Hay-Smith et al 2001, Wilson et al 2002), many surgeons still seem to regard minimally invasive surgery a better first-line option than PFMT. The scepticism against PFMT may be based on inappropriate knowledge of exercise science and physical therapy, beliefs that there is insufficient evidence for the effect of PFMT, that evidence for long-term effect is lacking or poor, and that women are not motivated to regularly perform PFMT. The aim of this chapter is to report evidence-based knowledge about the above-mentioned points related to PFMT for SUI.

RATIONALE FOR PFMT FOR SUI

To date, there are two main theories of mechanisms on how PFMT may be effective in the prevention and treatment of SUI (Bø 2004):

1. Women learn to consciously contract before and during an increase in abdominal pressure, and continue to perform such contractions as a behaviour modification to prevent descent of the pelvic floor.
2. Women are taught to perform regular strength training over time to build up 'stiffness' and structural support of the pelvic floor.

There is basic research and case–control studies to support both hypotheses.

In addition to these main theories two other theories have been proposed:

3. Sapsford (2001, 2004) claimed that the PFM was effectively trained indirectly by contraction of the internal abdominal muscles, especially the transversus abdominal (TrA) muscle.

Also, many physical therapists claim that there is a fourth theory named 'functional training'

4. 'Functional training of the PFM' means that women are asked to conduct a PFM contraction during different tasks of daily living (Carriere 2002).

Evidence for theory one

By intentional contraction of the PFM before and during an increase in abdominal pressure there is a lift of the pelvic floor in a cranial and forward direction and a squeeze around the urethra, vagina and rectum (DeLancey 1990, 1994a, 1994b, 1997, Kegel 1948). Ultrasonography and MRI studies have verified a lift in a cranial direction and movement of the coccyx in a forward, anterior and cranial direction (Bø et al 2001, Thompson & O'Sullivan 2003). Miller et al (1998) named this voluntary counterbracing-type contraction the 'knack', and in a single-blind randomized controlled trial (RCT), showed that the 'knack' performed during a medium and deep cough reduced urinary leakage by 98.2 and 73.3%, respectively. Cure rate in 'real life' was not reported. Also research on basic and functional anatomy research supports the 'Knack' as an effective manoeuvre to stabilize the pelvic floor (Miller et al 2001, Peschers et al 2001a). However, to date there are no studies on how much strength is necessary to prevent descent during cough and other physical exertions, and we do not know if regular counterbracing during daily activities is enough to increase muscle strength or cause morphological changes of the PFM.

Evidence for theory two

Kegel (1948) originally described PFMT as physiological training or 'tightening up' the pelvic floor. The theoretical rationale for intensive strength training (exercise) of the PFM to treat SUI is that strength training may build up the structural support of the pelvis by elevating the levator plate to a permanent higher location inside the pelvis and by enhancing hypertrophy and stiffness of the PFM and its connective tissue. This would facilitate a more effective automatic motor unit firing (neural adaptation), preventing descent during an increase in abdominal pressure. The pelvic openings may narrow and the pelvic organs are held in place during increases in abdominal pressure. In addition, a pelvic floor located at a higher level inside the pelvis may yield a much quicker and more coordinated response to an increase in abdominal pressure, closing the urethra by increasing the urethral pressure (Constantinou & Govan 1981, Howard et al 2000).

Ultrasound studies have shown that parous women have a more caudal location of the pelvic floor than nulliparous women (Peschers et al 1997). Difference in anatomical placement has also been shown between continent and incontinent women (Miller et al 2001, Peschers et al 2001c).

In an uncontrolled study by Bernstein (1997) a significant increase in muscle volume after training was shown by ultrasound. However, due to the lack of a control group more research is needed to provide conclusive evidence that muscle hypertrophies after PFMT.

None of the strength training RCTs on SUI have evaluated the effect of PFMT on PFM tone or connective tissue stiffness, position of the muscles within the pelvic cavity, their cross-sectional area or neurophysiological function. However, in an uncontrolled trial of PFMT for SUI, Balmforth et al (2004) found that the position of the bladder neck was observed by ultrasound to be significantly elevated at rest, and during Valsalva manoeuvre and squeeze after 14 weeks of supervised PFMT and behavioural modifications. These findings support the hypothesis of mechanisms, but need to be confirmed in a well-designed RCT.

In some studies the patients were tested both subjectively and objectively during physical activity, and had no leakage during strenuous tests after the training period (Bø et al 1990a, 1999, Mørkved et al 2002). Therefore, the effect, most likely was due to improved automatic muscle function and not only ability to voluntary contract before an increase in abdominal pressure.

Evidence for theory three

Sapsford (2001, 2004) suggests that the PFM can be trained indirectly by training the TrA muscle. This is based on an understanding that the PFM are part of the abdominal capsule surrounding the abdominal and pelvic organs. The structures included in this capsule (often referred to as the 'core') are the lumbar vertebrae and deeper layers of the multifidus muscle, the diaphragm, the TrA and the PFM (Sapsford 2001, 2004).

Several studies have shown that different abdominal muscles co-contract during PFM contraction (Bø et al 1990b, Bø & Stien 1994, Neumann & Gill 2002, Peschers et al 2001b, Sapsford et al 2001). In addition, some studies have shown that there is a co-contraction of the PFM during different abdominal muscle contractions in healthy volunteers. Bø & Stien (1994), using concentric needle EMG, found that there was a co-contraction of the PFM during contractions of the rectus abdominis in continent women. Sapsford & Hodges (2001) found that PFM surface electromyography (EMG) increased with TrA contractions in six healthy females, and this was supported by a study of four continent women by Neumann & Gill (2002). In continent women, Sapsford et al (1998) found that a sustained isometric abdominal contraction termed 'hollowing' in which the TrA and internal obliques are contracted increased the urethral pressure as much as a maximal PFM contraction. However, they had also ensured that the women were simultaneously contracting the PFM. Based on these findings, Sapsford (2001, 2004) recommends that incontinence training should begin by training the TrA, rather than the PFM specifically.

To date there are no RCTs comparing the effect of indirect training of the PFM via TrA on SUI with either untreated controls, conscious pre-contraction of the PFM or strength training. However, Dumoulin et al (2004) compared PFMT with PFMT and TrA training, and did not find any further benefit of adding TrA training to the protocol.

Evidence for theory four

In some physical therapist practices the PFMT protocol seems to include only teaching the patients to co-contract the PFM with low load during all daily activities and movements (Carriere 2002). No specific strength training protocol or follow-up training is undertaken. This can be considered using the same theory as use of conscious contraction or 'the knack'. However, unlike the use of a conscious contraction, the idea is that by learning to contract, over time this may become an automatic function and by itself be enough to prevent SUI. Therefore, in 'functional training' the conscious contraction is further developed to be performed in all daily activities where leakage may occur. This means that the woman is asked to contract while lifting, doing housework, playing tennis etc.

Because it is possible to learn to hold a hand over the mouth before and during coughing, it is perhaps possible to learn to pre-contract the PFM before and during simple and single tasks such as coughing, lifting and performing abdominal exercises. However, multiple task activities and repetitive movements such as running, playing tennis, or participating in dance and aerobic activities most likely cannot be conducted with intentional co-contractions of the PFM. To date, there are no basic studies, case–control studies, uncontrolled studies or RCTs to support the use of this kind of functional training of the PFM.

METHODS

Only outcomes from RCTs are included. Computerized search on PubMed, studies, data, and conclusions from Clinical Practice Guideline (AHCPR, USA) (Fantl et al 1996), 2nd and 3rd International Consultations on Incontinence (ICI) (Wilson et al 2002), and Cochrane library of systematic reviews (Hay-Smith et al 2001, Herbison et al 2000) have been used as background sources. Physical therapy techniques to treat SUI include PFMT with or without biofeedback, electrical stimulation and cones (Hay-Smith et al 2001, Herbison et al 2000). Because SUI and urge are different conditions that most likely need different treatment approaches, only studies including female SUI are presented here. Methodological quality of RCTs reporting cure rates assessing the condition with pad tests are judged by use of the PEDro rating scale (Herbert & Gabriel 2002).

EVIDENCE FOR PFMT TO TREAT SUI

Updated and comprehensive systematic reviews on PFMT in the treatment of SUI with detailed tables can be found in the Cochrane library (Hay-Smith et al 2001, Herbison et al 2000) and the three ICI books, so we will not repeat the same detailed tables of each RCT here. We refer to the same studies and newer studies found in our updated search in the text, and urge the reader to stay updated with new studies through the Cochrane library and the PEDro database.

It is difficult to make meaningful comparisons between studies and groups of studies in this area because there is a great heterogeneity between studies. This heterogeneity involves inclusion criteria of the studies (several studies include women with SUI and urge and mixed incontinence), different outcome measures, and different exercise regimens with a huge variety of training dosage. In addition, many researchers have used combined interventions (e.g. electrical stimulation and strength training, bladder training and strength training).

In this textbook, unlike what was done in the Cochrane Collaboration, we have made different decisions with respect to inclusion and exclusion criteria and how to present data.

- First, the Cochrane group made a decision to combine studies with a diagnosis of SUI, urge and mixed incontinence, whereas we have chosen to attempt to report data by separate diagnosis.

- Second, the Cochrane group decided not to analyse data based on measurement of urine loss by pad tests. In our point of view this excludes results from many high-quality studies, and abolishes the opportunity to look at cure rates at the disability level of the International Classifications of Functions (ICF).

- Third, in the Cochrane review, there is no evaluation of the quality of the intervention. There is a dose–response relationship in exercise therapy. Therefore, a thorough discussion of the quality of the intervention is necessary to elaborate a correct cause–effect relationship found or not found in RCTs of PFMT.

One important flaw in PFMT studies is a lack of ability to contract the PFM. Several research groups have shown that over 30% of women are unable to voluntarily contract the PFM at their first consultation even after thorough individual instruction (Benvenuti et al 1987, Bø et al 1988, Bump et al 1991, Kegel 1952). Hay-Smith et al (2001) reported that ability to contract PFM was checked before training in only 15 of 43 RCTs on the effect of PFMT for SUI, urge and mixed incontinence. Common mistakes are to contract other muscles such as abdominals, gluteals and hip adductor muscles instead of the PFM (Bø et al 1988, 1990b). In addition, Bump et al (1991) showed that as many as 25% of women may strain instead of squeeze and lift. If women are straining instead of performing a correct contraction, the training may harm and not improve PFM function. Proper assessment of ability to contract the PFM is therefore mandatory (see Fig. 5.1).

The numerous reports by Kegel with over 80% cure rate comprised uncontrolled studies with the inclusion of a variety of incontinence types and no measurement of urinary leakage before and after treatment. However, since then, several RCTs have demonstrated that PFM exercise is more effective than no treatment to treat SUI (Bø et al 1999, Henalla et al 1989, 1990, Hofbauer et al 1990, Miller et al 1998, Wong et al 1997). In addition, a number of RCTs have compared PFMT alone with either the use of vaginal resistance devices, biofeedback or

vaginal cones (Hay-Smith et al 2001). Of 43 RCTs, only one did not show any significant effect of PFMT on urinary leakage (Ramsey & Thou 1990). Interestingly, in this study there was no check of the women's ability to contract, adherence to the training protocol was poor, and the placebo group contracted gluteal muscles and external rotators of the hips; activities that may give co-contractions of the PFM (Bø et al 1990b, Peschers et al 2001b).

Combined improvement and cure rates

As for surgery (Smith et al 2002) and pharmacology studies (Andersson et al 2002), a combination of cure and improvement measures is often reported. To date there is no consensus on what outcome measure to choose as the gold standard for cure (urodynamic findings of SUI, number of leakage episodes, ≤ 2 g of leakage on pad test [tests with standardized bladder volume, 1-hour, 24-hour, and 48-hour], women's report etc) (Blaivas et al 1997). Subjective cure and improvement rates of PFMT reported in RCTs in studies including groups with SUI and mixed incontinence vary between 56 and 70% (Hay-Smith et al 2001, Wilson et al 2002).

Cure rates for SUI

It is often reported that PFMT is more commonly associated with improvement of symptoms, rather than a total cure. However, short term cure rates of 44–70%, defined as ≤ 2 g of leakage on different pad tests, have been found after PFMT (Bø et al 1999, Dumoulin et al 2004, Henalla et al 1990, Mørkved et al 2002, Wong et al 1997). Table 9.1 describes these studies and Table 9.2. gives the methodological quality of the same studies. The highest cure rates were shown in two single-blind RCTs of high methodological quality. The participants had thorough individual instruction by a trained physical therapist, combined training with biofeedback or electrical stimulation, and close follow-up once or every second week. Adherence was high, and drop-out was low (Dumoulin et al 2004, Mørkved et al 2002). Because biofeedback and electrical stimulation have not shown any additional effect to PFMT in RCTs and systematic reviews (Hay-Smith et al 2001, Wilson et al 2002), one could hypothesize that the key factors for success are most likely close follow-up and more intensive training.

Quality of the intervention – dose–response issues

Because of use of different outcome measures and instruments to measure PFM function and strength, it is

Table 9.1   Cure rates reported as less than 2 g of leakage measured with a variety of pad tests in randomized controlled trials of PFMT to treat SUI

Author	Henalla et al 1989
Design	Randomized to PFMT, interference therapy, oestrogen, or control
n	104 women, mean age with variance not reported
Diagnosis	Urodynamic stress incontinence
Training protocol	PFMT: vaginal palpation, contract PFM 5×/h, hold 5 s; ten sessions once a week with PT Interference: ten sessions with PT, 0–100 Hz, 20 min Oestrogen: Premarin vaginal cream each night for 12 weeks (1.25 mg) Control: no treatment
Drop-outs	4/104, not reported from which groups
Adherence	Not reported
Results	65% cured or >50% reduction
Author	Henalla et al 1990
Design	Randomized to PFMT, oestrogen, control
n	26 postmenopausal women, mean age 54 (49–64)
Diagnosis	SUI on history
Training protocol	6-week intervention PFMT: protocol not explained Oestrogen: Premarin vaginal cream 2 g/night
Drop-outs	Not reported
Adherence	Not reported
Results	*PFMT* 50% cured or >50% reduction *Oestrogen* 0 *Control* 0
Author	Glavind et al 1996
Design	Randomized to PFMT with PT or PFMT with biofeedback
n	40 women, mean age 45 (range 40–48)
Diagnosis	Urodynamic SUI
Training protocol	4-week intervention. Vaginal palpation. Both groups asked to perform PFMT at home at least 3×/day PFMT with PT: individual treatment with PT 3–4×/day PFMT with biofeedback: Individual treatment as above with addition of four times with biofeedback
Drop-outs	PFMT: 25% PFMT with biofeedback: 5%
Adherence	Not reported
Results	*PFMT* 20% cured PFMT with *biofeedback* 58% cured

Table 9.1 Cure rates reported as less than 2 g of leakage measured with a variety of pad tests in randomized controlled trials of PFMT to treat SUI—cont'd

Author	Wong et al 1997
Design	Randomized to clinic-based PFMT or home-based PFMT
n	47 women, mean age 48.8 (SD 9.4)
Diagnosis	Urodynamic SUI
Training protocol	4-week training period Clinic: 8 sessions plus daily PFMT Home: Daily PFMT at home
Drop-outs	Not reported
Adherence	Not reported
Results	No difference between groups. 55% cured
Author	Bø et al 1999
Design	Randomized to PFMT, ES, cones, or control
n	107 women, mean age 49.5 (range 24–70)
Diagnosis	Urodynamic SUI
Training protocol	6-month intervention. Vaginal palpation PFMT: 3×8–12 contractions per day at home. Training diary. Weekly 45-min exercise class. Individual assessment of muscle strength and motivation for further training once a month
Drop-outs	8%
Adherence	93%
Results	*PFMT* 44% cured *Control* 6.7% cured
Author	Mørkved et al 2002
Design	Randomized to PFMT or PFMT with biofeedback
n	103 women, mean age 46.6 (range 30–70)
Diagnosis	Urodynamic SUI
Training protocol	6-month intervention after vaginal palpation Both groups: same amount of exercise and met PT once a week for the first 2 months, then once every second week. Three sets of ten contractions holding 6 s add 3–4 fast contractions on top at each visit Home training: three sets of ten contractions daily Biofeedback: same programme with biofeedback
Drop-outs	8.7%
Adherence	PFMT: 85.3% PFMT + biofeedback: 88.9%
Results	PFMT 69% cured *PFMT + biofeedback* 67% cured

Table 9.1   Cure rates reported as less than 2 g of leakage measured with a variety of pad tests in randomized controlled trials of PFMT to treat SUI—cont'd

Author	Dumoulin et al 2004
Design	Randomized to multimodal PFMT, multimodal PFMT + abdominal training, or control
n	64 women, mean age 36.2 (range 23.3–39)
Diagnosis	Urodynamic SUI
Training protocol	8 weeks PFMT: supervised sessions once a week with PT, 15 min of ES, 25 min of PFMT, home exercise 5 days a week Same PFMT + 30 min of deep abdominal training Control: back and extremities massage
Drop-outs	3.1%
Adherence	Not reported
Results	*PFMT* 70% cured *PFMT + abdominals* 70% cured *Control* 0% cured
Author	Aksac et al 2003
Design	Randomized to PFMT, PFMT with biofeedback, or control group on oestrogen
n	50 women, mean age 52.9 (SD 7.1). 20 in each training group, 10 in control group
Diagnosis	Urodynamic diagnosis of SUI
Training protocol	8 weeks of: PFMT: vaginal palpation, 10 contractions three times daily, hold for 5 s, progressing to 10 after 2 weeks. Weekly office sessions + 'regular' home training Biofeedback: weekly office sessions, use biofeedback at home 3×/week. 20 min with 10-s hold and 20 s rest
Drop-outs	None
Adherence	Not reported
Results	*PFMT* 75% cure, 25% improvement *Biofeedback* 80% cured, 20% improvement *Control* None cured, 20% improvement

ES, electrical stimulation; PFMT, pelvic floor muscle training; PT, physical therapist; SUI, stress urinary incontinence.

impossible to combine results between studies, and it is difficult to conclude which training regimen is the more effective. Also the exercise dosage (type of exercise, frequency, duration and intensity) varies significantly between studies (Hay-Smith et al 2001, Wilson et al 2002). Looking into the studies on SUI patients included in the Cochrane systematic review, duration of the intervention varies between 6 weeks and 6 months, intensity (measured as holding time) varies between 3 and 40 s, and number of repetitions per day between 36 and over 200. Frequency of training is every day in all RCTs (Hay-Smith et al 2001).

Table 9.2   PEDro quality score of RCTs in systematic review

E – Eligibility criteria specified
1 – Subjects randomly allocated to groups
2 – Allocation concealed
3 – Groups similar at baseline
4 – Subjects blinded
5 – Therapist administering treatment blinded
6 – Assessors blinded
7 – Measures of key outcomes obtained from over 85% of subjects
8 – Data analysed by intention to treat
9 – Comparison between groups conducted
10 – Point measures and measures of variability provided

Study	E	1	2	3	4	5	6	7	8	9	10	Total score
Henalla et al 1989	+	+	–	?	–	–	–	+	–	?	+	3
Henalla et al 1990	+	+	?	?	–	–	–	+	?	–	–	2
Glavind et al 1996	+	+	+	+	–	–	–	+	–	+	+	6
Wong et al 1997	–	+	?	+	–	–	–	?	?	–	–	2
Bø et al 1999	+	+	+	+	–	–	+	+	+	+	+	8
Mørkved et al 2002	+	+	+	+	–	–	+	+	+	+	+	8
Aksac et al 2003	+	+	+	+	–	–	–	+	+	+	+	7
Dumoulin et al 2004	+	+	?	+	–	+	+	+	+	+	+	8

+, criterion is clearly satisfied; –, criterion is not satisfied; ?, not clear if the criterion was satisfied. Total score is determined by counting the number of criteria that are satisfied, except that 'eligibility criteria specified' score is not used to generate the total score. Total scores are out of 10.

Bø et al (1990a) have shown that instructor-followed up training is significantly more effective than home exercise. In this study individual assessment and teaching of correct contraction was combined with strength training in groups in a 6-month training programme. The women were randomized to either an intensive training programme consisting of seven individual sessions with a physical therapist, combined with 45 minutes weekly PFMT classes, and three sets of 8–12 contractions per day at home or the same programme except the weekly intensive exercise classes. The results showed a much better improvement in both muscle strength (see Fig. 6.11, p. 126) and urinary leakage in the intensive exercise group: 60% reported to be continent/almost continent in the intensive exercise group compared to 17% in the less intensive group. A significant reduction of urinary leakage, measured by pad test with standardized bladder volume, was only demonstrated in the intensive exercise group (Fig. 9.4).

This study demonstrated that a huge difference in outcome can be expected according to the intensity and follow-up of the training programme and very little effect can be expected after training without close follow-up. It is worth noting that the significantly less effective group in this study had seven visits with a skilled physical therapist and that adherence to the home training programme was high. Nevertheless, the effect was only 17%. More intensive training has also been shown to be more effective in two other RCTs (Glavind et al 1996, Goode et al 2003) and in one non-randomized study (Wilson et al 1987). There is a dose–response issue in all sorts of training regimens (Haskel 1994). Therefore, one reason for disappointing effects shown in some clinical practices or research studies may be due to insufficient training stimulus and low dosage. If low dosage programmes are chosen as one arm in a RCT comparing PFMT with other methods, PFMT is bound to be less effective.

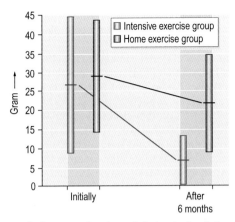

Fig. 9.4 Pad test results showed that only the 'intensive' pelvic floor muscle training group had a statistically significant reduction in urinary leakage. (From Bø et al 1990a, with permission.)

PFMT with biofeedback

Biofeedback has been defined as 'a group of experimental procedures where an external sensor is used to give an indication on bodily processes, usually in the purpose of changing the measured quality' (Schwartz & Beatty 1977). Biofeedback equipment has been developed within the area of psychology, mainly to measure sweating, heart rate and blood pressure during different forms of stress. Kegel (1948) always based his training protocol on thorough instruction of correct contraction using vaginal palpation and clinical observation. He combined PFMT with use of vaginal squeeze pressure measurement as biofeedback during exercise. Today, a variety of biofeedback apparatus are commonly used in clinical practice to assist with PFMT.

In urology or urogynaecology textbooks the term 'biofeedback' is often used to classify a method different from PFMT. However, biofeedback is not a treatment by its own. It is an adjunct to training, measuring the response from a single PFM contraction. In the area of PFMT both vaginal and anal surface EMG, and urethral and vaginal squeeze pressure measurements have been used to make patients more aware of muscle function, and to enhance and motivate patients' effort during training (Hay-Smith et al 2001, Wilson et al 2002). However, one should be aware that erroneous attempts at PFM contractions (e.g. by straining) may be registered by manometers and dynamometers, and contractions of other muscles than the PFM may affect surface EMG activity. Therefore biofeedback cannot be used to register a correct contraction.

Since Kegel first presented his results, several RCTs have shown that PFMT without biofeedback is more effective than no treatment for SUI (Hay-Smith et al 2001, Wilson et al 2002). In women with SUI or mixed incontinence, all but two RCTs have failed to show any additional effect of adding biofeedback to the training protocol for SUI (Aksac et al 2003, Aukee et al 2002, Berghmans et al 1996, Castleden et al 1984, Ferguson et al 1990, Glavind et al 1996, Laycock et al 2001, Mørkved et al 2002, Pages et al 2001, Shepherd et al 1983, Sherman et al 1997, Taylor & Henderson 1986, Wong et al 2001). Berghmans et al (1996) demonstrated quicker progress in the biofeedback group. In the study of Glavind et al (1996) a positive effect was demonstrated. However, this study was confounded by a difference in training frequency, and the effect might be due to a double training dosage, the use of biofeedback, or both. The results support the studies concluding that there is a dose–response issue in PFMT.

Very few of the studies comparing PFMT with and without biofeedback have used the exact same training dosage in the two groups. For example Pages et al (2001) compared 60 minutes of group training five days a week with 15 minutes of individual biofeedback training 5 days a week, and found that the individualized biofeedback training protocol was more effective assessed by the women's report and measurement of PFM strength. When the two groups under comparison receive different dosage of training in addition to biofeedback, it is impossible to conclude what is causing a possible effect. In addition, other factors flaw the results of studies comparing PFMT with and without biofeedback. As PFMT is effective without biofeedback, a large sample size may be needed to show any beneficial effect of adding biofeedback to an effective training protocol. In most published studies comparing PFMT with PFMT combined with biofeedback, the sample sizes are small, and type II error may have been the reason for negative findings (Hay-Smith et al 2001, Wilson et al 2002). However, in the two largest RCTs published, no additional effect was demonstrated from adding biofeedback.

Many women may not like to undress, go to a private room and insert a vaginal or rectal device to exercise (Prashar et al 2000). On the other hand, some women find it motivating to use biofeedback to control and enhance the strength of the contractions when training. Any factor that may stimulate high adherence and intensive training should be recommended to enhance the effect of a training programme. Therefore, when available, biofeedback should be given as an option for home training, and the physical therapist should use any sensitive, reliable and valid tool to measure the contraction force at office follow-up.

PFMT with vaginal weighted cones

Vaginal cones are weights that are put into the vagina above the levator plate (Herbison et al 2000) (see Fig. 6.12, p. 127). The cones were developed by Plevnik (Hay-Smith et al 2001) in 1985. The theory behind their use in strength training is that the PFM are contracted reflexively or voluntarily when the cone is perceived to slip out. The weight of the cone is supposed to give a training stimulus and make women contract harder with progressive weight. In a Cochrane review, combining studies including patients with both SUI and mixed incontinence it was concluded that training with vaginal cones is more effective than no treatment (Herbison et al 2000).

Five RCTs have been found comparing PFMT with and without vaginal cones for SUI (Arvonen et al 2001, Bø et al 1999, Cammu & van Nylen 1998, Laycock et al 2001, Pieber et al 1994). Bø et al (1999) found that PFMT was significantly more effective than training with cones both to improve muscle strength and reduce urinary leakage. In three other studies there were no differences between PFMT with and without cones (Cammu & van Nylen 1998, Laycock et al 2001, Pieber et al 1994). Cammu & van Nylen (1998) reported very low compliance and therefore did not recommend use of cones. Also in the study of Bø et al (1999), women in the cone group had great motivational problems. Laycock et al (2001) had a total drop-out rate in their study of 33%.

The use of cones can be questioned from an exercise science perspective. Holding the cone for as long as 15–20 minutes, as recommended, may result in decreased blood supply, decreased oxygen consumption, muscle fatigue and pain, and recruit contraction of other muscles instead of the PFM. In addition, many women report that they dislike using cones (Bø et al 1999, Cammu & van Nylen 1998). On the other hand, the cones may add benefit to the training protocol if used in a different way: the subjects can be asked to contract around the cone and simultaneously try to pull it out in lying or standing position, repeating this 8–12 times in three series per day, or they can use the cones during progressively graded activities of daily living. In this way, general strength training principles are followed, and progression can be added to the training protocol. Arvonen et al (2001) used 'vaginal balls' and followed general strength training principles. They found that training with the balls was significantly more effective in reducing urinary leakage than regular PFMT.

PFMT or electrical stimulation for SUI?

Rationale and evidence for electrical stimulation for SUI are covered in pp. 171–184. In the present chapter studies comparing PFMT and electrical stimulation and studies combining PFMT and electrical stimulation will be cited.

Hennalla et al (1989), Hofbauer et al (1990) and Bø et al (1999) found that PFMT was significantly better than electrical stimulation to treat SUI. Laycock & Jerwood (1996) and Hahn et al (1991) found no difference, and Smith (1996) found that electrical stimulation was significantly better. Bidmead et al (2002), Goode et al (2003), Hofbauer et al (1990) and Knight et al (1998) found no effect of adding electrical stimulation to PFMT.

Many of the electrical stimulation studies are flawed with small numbers, and future RCTs with better methodological quality should be repeated (Hay-Smith et al 2001, Wilson et al 2002). However, electrical stimulation has shown side-effects (Indrekvam et al 2002) and is less well tolerated by women than PFMT (1999). In addition, Bø & Talseth (1997) found that voluntary PFM contraction increases urethral pressure significantly more than electrical stimulation, and several consensus statements have concluded that strength training is more effective than electrical stimulation in humans (Dudley & Harris 1992, Vuori & Wilmore 1993). Fig. 9.5 shows the difference in effect on urinary leakage measured by pad test with standardized bladder volume after PFMT, electrical stimulation and vaginal-weighted cones and in controls.

Is bladder training equally effective as PFMT for SUI?

The rationale behind bladder training and evidence for bladder training in overactive bladder are discussed in

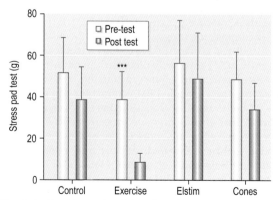

Fig. 9.5 The Norwegian Pelvic Floor Study demonstrated huge and statistically significant improvement pad test results only for the training group. Elstim, electrical stimulation. (From Bø et al 1999, with permission.)

pp. 208–217. One study showed that bladder training had similar effects on SUI and urge incontinence in women (Fantl et al 1991), and another RCT that bladder training had similar effects as PFMT in women with SUI and urge and mixed incontinence (Elser et al 1999). Wilson et al (2002) concluded that these findings required further investigation. To date, there is no clear-cut understanding of how bladder training works, and it is difficult to understand how it can treat SUI if it does not include specific PFM contractions.

Is surgery more effective than PFMT for SUI?

Only one RCT has compared surgery with PFMT as first-line treatment for SUI. In the study of Klarskov et al (1986) the patients had different surgeries according to their problems. The PFMT programme was described as group training with five or more sessions with a physical therapist, and it is not clear whether the participants had vaginal palpation to make sure they were able to contract the PFM correctly. At 4 months the PFMT group was less likely to report cure compared to women who had surgery. However, there was no statistical difference in the proportions reporting cure/improvement. At 12 months 10/24 women in the PFMT group reported satisfaction with the initial therapy versus 19/26 in the surgery group. Adverse effects were reported only in the surgery group, including new urge incontinence, retropubic or pelvic pain or dyspareunia.

Adverse effects of PFMT

Few, if any, adverse effects have been found after PFMT (Hay-Smith et al 2001, Wilson et al 2002). Lagro-Jansson et al (1992) found that one woman reported pain with exercise and three had an uncomfortable feeling during the exercises. Aukee et al (2002) reported no side-effects in the training group, but found that two women interrupted the use of home biofeedback apparatus because they found the vaginal probe uncomfortable. These women were both postmenopausal. In other studies no side-effects have been found (Bø et al 1999).

Long-term effect of PFMT for SUI

Several studies have reported long-term effect of PFMT (Hay-Smith et al 2001, Wilson et al 2002). However, usually women in the non-treatment or less effective intervention groups have gone on to retrieve treatment after cessation of the study period. Therefore, follow-up data are usually reported for either all women or for only the group with the best effect. As for surgery (Black & Downs 1996, Smith et al 2002), there are only few long-term studies including clinical examination (Bø & Talseth 1996, Klarskov et al 1991, Lagro-Janssen

et al 1998). Klarskov et al (1991) assessed only some of the women originally participating in the study. Lagro-Janssen et al (1998) evaluated 88 of 110 women with SUI and urge or mixed incontinence 5 years after cessation of training and found that 67% remained satisfied with the condition. Only seven of 110 had been treated with surgery. Moreover, satisfaction was closely related to compliance to training and type of incontinence, with women with mixed incontinence being more likely to lose the effect. Women with SUI had the best long-term effect, but only 39% of them were exercising daily or 'when needed'.

In a 5-year follow-up, Bø & Talseth (1996) examined only the intensive exercise group and found that urinary leakage was significantly increased after cessation of organized training. Three of 23 had been treated with surgery. Two of these women who had not been cured after the initial training, were satisfied with their surgery, and had no leakage on pad test. The third woman had been cured after initial PFMT. However, after 1 year she stopped training because of personal problems connected to the death of her husband. Her incontinence problems returned and she had surgery 2 years before the 5-year follow-up. She was not satisfied with the outcome after surgery and had visible leakage on cough test and 17 g of leakage on the pad test. Of the women, 56% had a positive closure pressure during cough and 70% had no visible leakage during cough at 5-year follow-up; 70% of the patients were still satisfied with the results and did not want other treatment options.

Cammu et al (2000) used a postal questionnaire and medical files to evaluate the long-term effect on 52 women who had participated in an individual course of PFMT for urodynamic SUI. Eighty-seven percent were suitable for analysis – 33% had had surgery after 10 years. However, only 8% had undergone surgery in the group that had originally had success after training, whereas 62% had undergone surgery in the group initially dissatisfied with training. Successful results were maintained after 10 years in two-thirds of the patients originally classified as successful.

Bø et al (2005) reported current status of lower urinary tract symptoms from questionnaire data 15 years after cessation of organized training. They found that the short term significant effect of intensive training was no longer present: 50% from both groups had interval surgery for SUI, however more women in the less intensive training group had surgery within the first 5 years after ending the training programme. There were no differences in reported frequency or amount of leakage between women who had or had not had surgery, and women who had surgery reported significantly more severe leakage and to be more bothered by urinary incontinence during daily activities than those who had not.

The general recommendations for maintaining muscle strength are one set of 8–12 contractions twice a week (Pollock et al 1998). The intensity of the contraction seems to be more important than frequency of training. So far, no studies have evaluated how many contractions subjects have to perform to maintain PFM strength after cessation of organized training. In a study by Bø & Talseth (1996) PFM strength was maintained 5 years after cessation of organized training with 70% exercising more than once a week. However, number and intensity of exercises varied considerably between successful women (Bø 1995). One series of 8–12 contractions could easily be instructed in aerobic dance classes or recommended as part of women's general strength training programmes. On the other hand, we do not know how a voluntary pre-contraction before an increase in abdominal pressure will maintain or increase muscle strength. In the study of Cammu et al (2000) the long-term effect of PFMT appeared to be attributed to the pre-contraction before sudden increases in intra-abdominal pressure, and not so much to regular strength training. Muscle strength was not measured in their study. Although not taught in the original programme, several women in the study of Bø et al (2005) also had performed pre-contractions of the PFM before and during a rise in abdominal pressure during the long-term follow-up period.

Other programmes

Today there is a lot of interest in PFMT in combination with so-called 'core training' (stabilizing training for the lower spine including mTra and multifidus muscles). Yoga, Pilates, Feldenkrais and Mensendick classes are examples of exercise programmes that may include training of the PFM. All these programmes except yoga (which is much longer established) were developed in the 1920 and 1930s, and as far as this author has been ascertained none originally included PFMT. A search on PubMed in May 2006 did not reveal any RCTs evaluating the effect of such exercise programmes including PFMT in the treatment of pelvic floor dysfunction.

One pilot study has been found training lumbopelvic stability by Pilates for SUI (Savage 2005). In this study ten women with SUI, mean age 48.3 years (range 37–66 years) were randomized to either 12 weeks of PFMT consisting of six individual sessions of 30–45 minutes PFMT plus home training and use of the knack, or to Pilates training combining abdominal, PFMT and breathing exercises. No comparisons of the results between groups were conducted, and it was concluded that a sample size of 42 in each group was needed to see statistical significant differences.

Liebergall-Wischnitzer et al (2005) performed a RCT comparing the 'Paula method' with PFMT. The 'Paula method' is based on a theory that all sphincters in the body work simultaneously, and that by contracting e.g. muscles around the mouth, the PFM will co-contract or be facilitated. However, in the above mentioned trial the PFM were contracted consciously simultaneously with contraction of mouth muscles. No comparisons were done between groups in the report of the results.

Therefore it is not possible to make any conclusions about any of these methods.

In untrained individuals all stimulus for regular training have the potential for improving function, and a focus on and incorporation of PFMT in any fitness programme for women should therefore be welcomed. One should be aware, however, that many women may not be able to perform correct contractions without proper individual instruction. Lack of effect of such general programmes may therefore also be due to incorrect contractions.

Motivation

Several researchers have looked into factors affecting outcome of PFMT on urinary incontinence (Hay-Smith et al 2001, Wilson et al 2002). No single factor has been shown to predict outcome, and it has been concluded that many factors traditionally supposed to affect outcomes such as age and severity of incontinence may be less crucial than previously thought. Factors that appear to be most associated with a positive outcome are thorough teaching of correct contraction, motivation, adherence with the intervention, and intensity of the programme.

Some women may find the exercises hard to conduct on a regular basis (Alewijnse 2002). However, when analysing results of RCTs, adherence to the exercise programme is generally high, and drop-out rate is low (Hay-Smith et al 2001, Wilson et al 2002). In a few studies low adherence and high drop-out rates have been reported (Laycock et al 2001, Ramsey & Thou 1990). Knowledge about behavioural sciences such as pedagogy and health psychology, and ability to explain and motivate patients may be a crucial factor to enhance adherence and minimize drop-outs from training. In some studies such strategies have been followed, and high adherence has been achieved (Alewijnse 2002, Chiarelli & Cockburn 2002). In other studies specific strategies have not been reported, but emphasis has been put on creating a positive, enjoyable and supportive training environment. Group training after thorough individual instruction may be a good concept if lead by a skilled and motivating person (Bø et al 1990a, Bø et al 1999) (Figs 9.6 and 9.7).

PFMT concepts with no drop-outs (Berghmans et al 1996) and adherence over 90% (Bø et al 1999) are possible. In a study of Alewijnse (2002) most women followed advice of training 4–6 times a week 1 year after cessation of the training programme. The following factors predicted adherence with 50%:

- positive intention to adhere;
- high short-term adherence levels;
- positive self-efficacy expectations;
- frequent weekly episodes of leakage before and after initial therapy.

Patients do not comply with treatment for a wide variety of reasons: longlasting and time-consuming treatments, requirement of lifestyle changes, poor client/patient interaction, cultural and health beliefs, poor social support, inconvenience, lack of time, motivational problems and travel time to clinics have been listed (Paddison 2002).

Sugaya et al (2003) used a computerized pocket-size device giving a sound three times a day to remind the person to perform PFMT. To stop the sound the person needed to push a button, and by pushing the button for each contraction, adherence was registered: 46 women were randomly assigned to either instruction to contract the PFM following a pamphlet or with the same pamphlet together with the sound device and instruction on how to use the device. The results showed a significant improvement in daily incontinence episodes and pad

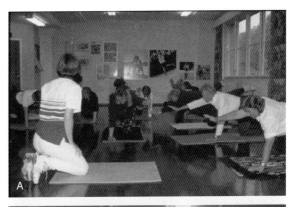

A

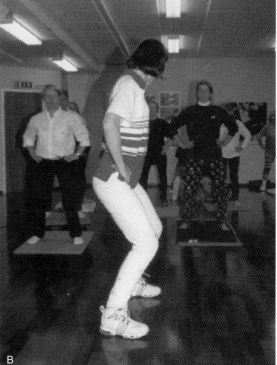

B

Fig. 9.7 In between the pelvic floor muscle strength training other exercises are performed to music. The original class emphasizes strength training of the abdominal (including transversus abdominis), back and thigh muscles in addition to body awareness and relaxation (breathing and stretching) exercises. The class is 60 minutes with 45 minutes of exercising and 15 minutes for information, conversation and motivation for home training.

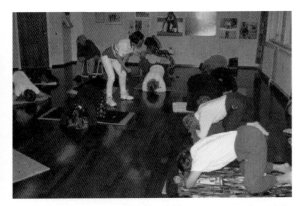

Fig. 9.6 When the patients are able to contract the pelvic floor muscles correctly it can be fun and motivating to conduct the strength training in a class. Group training classes for pelvic floor muscle training was developed by Bø in 1986 and the results of the first randomized controlled trial using group training for stress urinary incontinence was presented in Neurourology and Urodynamics in 1990.

test only in the device group: 48% were satisfied in the device group compared to 15% in the control group. It was reported that patients in the device group felt obliged to perform PFMT when the chime sounded.

CONCLUSIONS

RCTs with high methodological quality, systematic reviews and a Cochrane review have concluded that there is level A evidence that PFMT is more effective than no treatment, sham or placebo treatment for SUI. PFMT is recommended as first-line treatment for SUI. There is no evidence to suggest that adding use of biofeedback, electrical stimulation or vaginal cones brings any additional effect over PFMT alone.

CLINICAL RECOMMENDATIONS

- Teach the patient about the PFM and lower urinary tract function using diagrams, drawings and models.

- Explain a correct PFM contraction. Allow the patient to practice before checking ability to contract.

- Assess PFM contraction.

- If the woman is able to contract, set up an individual training programme to be conducted at home. Aim for close to maximum contraction, building up to 8–12 contractions three times a day. Ask the patient to

suggest where and when exercises should be performed. Supply the patient with an exercise diary or biofeedback with computerized adherence registration. If available, discuss whether use of biofeedback motivates the patient to exercise.

- If the woman is unable to contract try manual techniques such as touch, tapping, massage, and fast stretch or electrical stimulation. Be aware that most patients learn to contract if they are given some time by themselves at home to practice.

- Follow-up with weekly or more often supervised training. Supervised training can be conducted individually or in groups.

- Follow development in PFM function and strength closely with sensitive, reliable, and valid assessment.

- In addition to a strength training regimen ask the patient to pre-contract and hold the contraction before and during coughing, laughing, sneezing, and lifting (conscious pre-contraction, 'the knack').

- Suggested assessment of urinary leakage and quality of life (QoL) before and after treatment:
  - 3-day leakage episodes (Lose et al 1998);
  - leakage index (Bø 1994);
  - pad test (48-hour, 24-hour, 1-hour, short tests with standardized bladder volume) (Lose et al 1998);
  - general and disease-specific QoL questionnaires (SF-37, ICIQ UI SF, Kings College, B-FLUTS) (Corcos et al 2002).

REFERENCES

Aksac B, Semih A, Karan A et al 2003. Biofeedback and pelvic floor exercises for the rehabilitation of urinary stress incontinence. Gynecological and Obstetrical Investigation 56:23–27

Alewijnse D 2002 Urinary incontinence in women. Long term outcome of pelvic floor muscle exercise therapy [thesis]. Maastricht Health Research Institute for Prevention and Care/ Department of Health Education and Health Promotion

Andersson K, Appell R, Awad S et al 2002. Pharmacological treatment of urinary incontinence. In: Abrams P, Cardozo L, Khoury S et al (eds) Incontinence. Plymouth: Plymbridge Distributors, Plymouth p 479–511

Arvonen T, Fianu-Jonasson A, Tyni-Lenne R 2001 Effectiveness of two conservative modes of physiotherapy in women with urinary stress incontinence. Neurourology and Urodynamics 20:591–599

Aukee P, Immonen P, Penttinen J et al 2002 Increase in pelvic floor muscle activity after 12 weeks' training: a randomized prospective pilot study. Urology 60:1020–1024

Balmforth J, Bidmead J, Cardozo L et al 2004 Raising the tone: a prospective observational study evaluating the effect of pelvic

floor muscle training on bladder neck mobility and associated improvement in stress urinary incontinence. Nerourology and Urodynamics 23:553–554

Benvenuti F, Caputo G M, Bandinelli S et al 1987 Reeducative treatment of female genuine stress incontinence. American Journal of Physical Medicine 66(4):155–168

Berghmans L C M, Frederiks C M A, de Bie R A et al 1996 Efficacy of biofeedback, when included with pelvic floor muscle exercise treatment, for genuine stress incontinence. Neurourology and Urodynamics 15:37–52

Bernstein I. 1997 The pelvic floor muscles [thesis]. University of Copenhagen, Hvidovre Hospital, Department of Urology

Bidmead J, Mantle J, Cardozo L et al 2002 Home electrical stimulation in addition to conventional pelvic floor exercises. A useful adjunct or expensive distraction? Neurourology and Urodynamics 21(4):372–373

Black N A, Downs S H 1996 The effectiveness of surgery for stress incontinence in women: a systematic review. British Journal of Urology 78(497):510

Blaivas J G, Appell R A, Fantl J A et al 1997 Standards of efficacy for evaluation of treatment outcomes in urinary incontinence:

recommendations of the urodynamic society. Neurourology and Urodynamics 16(145):147

Bø K 1994 Reproducibility of instruments designed to measure subjective evaluation of female stress urinary incontinence. Scandinavian Journal of Urology and Nephrology 28:97–100

Bø K 1995 Adherence to pelvic floor muscle exercise and long term effect on stress urinary incontinence. A five year follow up. Scandinavian Journal of Medicine and Science in Sports 5:36–39

Bø K 2004 Pelvic floor muscle training is effective in treatment of stress urinary incontinence, but how does it work? International Urogynecology Journal and Pelvic Floor Dysfunction 15:76–84

Bø K, Hagen R H, Kvarstein B et al 1990a Pelvic floor muscle exercise for the treatment of female stress urinary incontinence: III. Effects of two different degrees of pelvic floor muscle exercise. Neurourology and Urodynamics 9:489–502

Bø K, Kvarstein B, Hagen R et al 1990b Pelvic floor muscle exercise for the treatment of female stress urinary incontinence: II. Validity of vaginal pressure measurements of pelvic floor muscle strength and the necessity of supplementary methods for control of correct contraction. Neurourology and Urodynamics 9:479–487

Bø K, Kvarstein B, Nygaard I 2005 Lower urinary tract symptoms and pelvic floor muscle exercise adherence after 15 years. Obstetrics and Gynecology 105(5 Pt 1):999–1005

Bø K, Larsen S, Oseid S et al 1988 Knowledge about and ability to correct pelvic floor muscle exercises in women with urinary stress incontinence. Neurourology and Urodynamics 7(3):261–262

Bø K, Lilleås F, Talseth T et al 2001 Dynamic MRI of pelvic floor muscles in an upright sitting position. Neurourology and Urodynamics 20:167–174

Bø K, Stien R 1994 Needle EMG registration of striated urethral wall and pelvic floor muscle activity patterns during cough, valsalva, abdominal, hip adductor, and gluteal muscles contractions in nulliparous healthy females. Neurourology and Urodynamics 13:35–41

Bø K, Talseth T 1996 Long term effect of pelvic floor muscle exercise five years after cessation of organized training. Obstetrics and Gynecology 87(2):261–265

Bø K, Talseth T 1997 Change in urethral pressure during voluntary pelvic floor muscle contraction and vaginal electrical stimulation. International Urogynecology Journal and Pelvic Floor Dysfunction 8:3–7

Bø K, Talseth T, Holme I 1999 Single blind, randomised controlled trial of pelvic floor exercises, electrical stimulation, vaginal cones, and no treatment in management of genuine stress incontinence in women. British Medical Journal 318:487–493

Bump R, Hurt WG, Fantl JA et al 1991 Assessment of Kegel exercise performance after brief verbal instruction. American Journal of Obstetrics and Gynecology 165:322–329

Cammu H, Van Nylen M 1998 Pelvic floor exercises versus vaginal weight cones in genuine stress incontinence. European Journal of Obstetrical and Gynecological Reproductive Biology 77:89–93

Cammu H, Van Nylen M, Amy J 2000 A ten-year follow-up after Kegel pelvic floor muscle exercises for genuine stress incontinence. British Journal of Urology International 85:655–658

Carriere B 2002 Fitness for the pelvic floor. Georg Thieme Verlag, Stuttgart

Castleden C M, Duffin H M, Mitchell E P 1984 The effect of physiotherapy on stress incontinence. Age and Ageing 13:235–237

Chiarelli P, Cockburn J 2002 Promoting urinary continence in women after delivery: randomised controlled trial. British Medical Journal 324:1241

Constantinou C E, Govan D E 1981 Contribution and timing of transmitted and generated pressure components in the female urethra. Female incontinence. Allan R Liss, New York, p 113–120

Corcos J, Beaulieu S, Donovan J et al 2002 Quality of life assessment in men and women with urinary incontinence. Journal of Urology 168:896–905

DeLancey J 1990 Functional anatomy of the female lower urinary tract and pelvic floor. Neurobiology of incontinence. Ciba Foundation Symposium 151:57–76

DeLancey J 1994a Structural support of the urethra as it relates to stress urinary incontinence: the hammock hypothesis. American Journal of Obstetrics and Gynecology 170:1713–1723

DeLancey J 1994b The anatomy of the pelvic floor. Current Opinion of Obstetrics and Gynecology 6:313–316

DeLancey J 1997 The pathophysiology of stress urinary incontinence in women and its applications for surgical treatment. World Journal of Urology 15:268–274

Dudley G A, Harris R T 1992. Use of electrical stimulation in strength and power training. In: Komi P V (ed) Strength and power in sport. Blackwell Scientific, Oxford, p 329–337

Dumoulin C, Lemieux M, Bourbonnais D et al 2004 Physiotherapy for persistent postnatal stress urinary incontinence: a randomized controlled trial. Obstetrics and Gynecology 104:504–510

Elser D, Wyman J, McLish D et al 1999. The effect of bladder training, pelvic floor muscle training, or combination training on urodynamic parameters in women with urinary incontinence. Neurourology and Urodynamics 18:427–436

Fantl J A, Newman D K, Colling J et al 1996 Urinary incontinence in adults: acute and chronic management. Clinical Practice Guideline, 2, update [96–0682]. Department of Health and Human Services, Public Health Service, Agency for Health Care Policy and Research, Rockville, MD, p 1–154

Fantl J A, Wyman J F, McLish D K et al 1991 Efficacy of bladder training in older women with urinary incontinence. Journal of American Medical Association 265(5):609–613

Ferguson K L, McKey P L, Bishop K R et al 1990. Stress urinary incontinence: effect of pelvic muscle exercise. Obstetrics and Gynecology 75:671–675

Glavind K, Nøhr S, Walter S 1996 Biofeedback and physiotherapy versus physiotherapy alone in the treatment of genuine stress urinary incontinence. International Urogynecological Journal and Pelvic Floor Dysfunction 7:339–343

Goode P, Burgio K L, Locher J L et al 2003 Effect of behavioral training with or without pelvic floor electrical stimulation on stress incontinence in women. A randomized controlled trial. Journal of American Medical Association 290(3):345–352

Hahn I, Sommar S, Fall M 1991 A comparative study of pelvic floor training and electrical stimulation for treatment of genuine female stress urinary incontinence. Neurourology and Urodynamics 10:545–554

Haskel W, Dose 1994 Response issues from a biological perspective In: Bouchard C, Shephard R J, Stephens T (eds) Physical activity, fitness, and health. International proceedings and consensus statement. Human Kinetics, Champaign, IL, p 1030–1039

Hay-Smith E, Bø K, Berghmans L et al 2001 Pelvic floor muscle training fur urinary incontinence in women (Cochrane review). The Cochrane Library, Oxford

Henalla S M, Hutchins C J, Robinson P et al 1989 Non-operative methods in the treatment of female genuine stress incontinence of urine. Journal of Obstetrics and Gynaecology 9:222–225

Henalla S, Millar D, Wallace K 1990 Surgical versus conservative management for post-menopausal genuine stress incontinence of urine. Neurourology and Urodynamics 9(4):436–437

Herbert R, Gabriel M 2002 Effects of stretching before and after exercising on muscle soreness and risk of injury: systematic review. British Medical Journal 325:1–5

Herbison P, Plevnik S, Mantle J 2000. Weighted vaginal cones for urinary incontinence. 1–24 The Cochrane Library, Oxford

Hofbauer J, Preisinger F, Nurnberger N 1990 Der Stellenwert der Physiotherapie bei der weiblichen genuinen Stressinkontinenz. Zeitung Urologie und Nephrologie 83:249–254

Howard D, Miller J, DeLancey J et al 2000 Differential effects of cough, valsalva, and continence status on vesical neck movement. Obstetrics and Gynecology 95:535–540

Indrekvam S, Hunskaar S 2002 Side-effects, feasability, and adherence to treatment during home-managed electrical stimulation for urinary incontinence: a Norwegian national cohort of 3198 women. Neurourology and Urodynamics 21:546–552

Kegel A H 1948 Progressive resistance exercise in the functional restoration of the perineal muscles. American Journal of Obstetrics and Gynecology 56:238–249

Kegel A H 1952 Stress incontinence and genital relaxation. Ciba Clinical Symposium 2:35–51

Klarskov P, Belving D, Bischoff N et al 1986 Pelvic floor exercise versus surgery for female urinary stress incontinence. Urology International 41:129–132

Klarskov P, Nielsen K K, Kromann-Andersen B et al 1991 Long-term results of pelvic floor training for female genuine stress incontinence. International Urogynecology Journal 2:132–135

Knight S, Laycock J, Naylor D 1998 Evaluation of neuromuscular electrical stimulation in the treatment of genuine stress incontinence. Physiotherapy 84(2):61–71

Lagro-Janssen A, Debruyne F, Smiths A et al 1992 The effects of treatment of urinary incontinence in general practice. Family Practice 9(3):284–289

Lagro-Janssen T, van Weel C 1998 Long-term effect of treatment of female incontinence in general practice. British Journal of General Practice 48:1735–1738

Laycock J, Brown J, Cusack C et al 2001 Pelvic floor reeducation for stress incontinence: comparing three methods. British Journal of Community Nursing 6(5):230–237

Laycock J, Jerwood D 1996 Does pre-modulated interferential therapy cure genuine stress incontinence? Physiotherapy 79(8):553–560

Liebergall-Wischnitzer M, Hochner-Celnikier D, Lavy Y et al 2005 Paula method of circular muscle exercises for urinary stress incontinence – a clinical trial. International Urogynecological Journal and Pelvic Floor Dysfunction 16:345–351

Lose G, Fantl J A, Victor A et al 1998 Outcome measures for research in adult women with symptoms of lower urinary tract dysfunction. Neurourology and Urodynamics 17(3):255–262

Miller J M, Ashton-Miller J A, DeLancey J 1998 A pelvic muscle precontraction can reduce cough-related urine loss in selected women with mild SUI. Journal of American Geriatric Society 46:870–874

Miller J, Perucchini D, Carchidi L et al 2001 Pelvic floor muscle contraction during a cough and decreased vesical neck mobility. Obstetrics and Gynecology 97:255–260

Mørkved S, Bø K, Fjørtoft T 2002 Is there any additional effect of adding biofeedback to pelvic floor muscle training? A single-blind randomized controlled trial. Obstetrics and Gynecology 100(4):730–739

Neumann P, Gill V 2002 Pelvic floor and abdominal muscle interaction: EMG activity and intra-abdominal pressure. International Urogynecology Journal and Pelvic Floor Dysfunction 13:125–132

Paddison K 2002 Complying with pelvic floor exercises: a literature review. Nursing Standard 16(39):33–38

Pages I, Schaufele M, Conradi E 2001 Comparative analysis of biofeedback and physiotherapy for treatment of urinary stress incontinence in women. American Journal of Physical Medicine Rehabilitation 80(7):494–502

Peschers U, Schaer G, DeLancey J et al 1997 Levator ani function before and after childbirth. British Journal of Obstetrics and Gynaecology 104:1004–1008

Peschers U, Fanger G, Schaer G et al 2001c Bladder neck mobility in continent nulliparous women. British Journal of Obstetrics and Gynaecology 108:320–324

Peschers U, Gingelmaier A, Jundt K et al 2001b. Evaluation of pelvic floor muscle strength using four different techniques. International Urogynecology Journal and Pelvic Floor Dysfunction 12:27–30

Peschers U, Vodusek D, Fanger G et al 2001a. Pelvic muscle activity in nulliparous volunteers. Neurourology and Urodynamics 20:269–275

Pieber D, Zivkovic F, Tamussino K 1994 Beckenbodengymnastik allein oder mit Vaginalkonen bei pramenopausalen Frauen mit milder und massiger Stressharninkontinenz. Gynecologische Geburtshilfliche Rundsch 34:32–33

Pollock M L, Gaesser G A, Butcher J D et al 1998 The recommeneded quantity and quality of exercise for developing and maintaining cardiorespiratory and muscular fitness, and flexibility in healthy adults. Medicine and Science in Sports and Exercise 30(6):975–991

Prashar S, Simons A, Bryant C et al 2000 Attitudes to vaginal/urethral touching and device placement in women with urinary incontinence. International Urogynecology Journal and Pelvic Floor Dysfunction 11:4–8

Ramsey I N, Thou M 1990 A randomized, double blind, placebo controlled trial of pelvic floor exercise in the treatment of genuine stress incontinence. Neurourology and Urodynamics 9(4):398–399

Sapsford R 2001 The pelvic floor. A clinical model for function and rehabilitation. Physiotherapy 87(12):620–630

Sapsford R 2004 Rehabilitation of pelvic floor muscles utilizing trunk stabilization. Manual Therapy 9:3–12

Sapsford R, Hodges P 2001 Contraction of the pelvic floor muscles during abdominal maneuvers. Archives of Physical Medicine Rehabilitation 82:1081–1088

Sapsford R, Hodges P, Richardson C et al 2001 Co-activation of the abdominal and pelvic floor muscles during voluntary exercises. Neurourology and Urodynamics 20:31–42

Sapsford R, Markwell S, Clarke B 1998 The relationship between urethral pressure and abdominal muscle activity. 7th National CFA conference on incontinence: 102

Savage A M 2005 Is lumbopelvic stability training (using the Pilates model) an effective treatment strategy for women with stress urinary incontinence? A review of the literature and report of a pilot study. Journal of the Association of Chartered Physiotherapists in Women's Health 97:33–48

Schwartz G, Beatty J 1977 Biofeedback: Theory and research. Academic Press, New York

Shepherd A, Montgomery E, Anderson R S 1983 A pilot study of a pelvic exerciser in women with stress incontinence. Journal of Obstetrics and Gynaecology 3:201–202

Sherman R A, Wong M F, Davis G D 1997 Behavioral treatment of exercise induced urinary incontinence among female soldiers. Military Medicine 162(10):690–694

Smith J J 1996 Intravaginal stimulation randomized trial. Journal of Urology 155:127–130

Smith T, Daneshgari F, Dmochowski R et al 2002 Surgical treatment of incontinence in women. In: Abrams P, Cardozo L, Khoury S, et al (eds) Incontinence. Plymbridge Distributors, Plymouth, UK p 823–863

Sugaya K, Owan T, Hatano T et al 2003 Device to promote pelvic floor muscle training for stress incontinence. International Journal of Urology 10:416–422

Taylor K, Henderson J 1986 Effects of biofeedback and urinary stress incontinence in older women. Journal of Gerontological Nursing 12(9):25–30

Thompsen J, O'Sullivan P 2003 Levator plate movement during voluntary pelvic floor muscle contraction in subjects with incontinence and prolapse: a cross-sectional study. International Urogynecological Journal and Pelvic Floor Dysfunction 14:84–88

Vuori I, Wilmore J H 1993 Physical activity, fitness, and health: Status and determinants. In: Bouchard C, Shephard RJ, Stephens T (eds) Physical activity, fitness and health. Consensus statement. Human Kinetics, Champaign, IL, p 33–40

Wilson P D, Bø K, Nygaard I, et al 2002 Conservative treatment in women. In: Abrams P, Cardozo L, Khoury S et al (eds) Incontinence. Plymbridge Distributors, Plymouth, UK, p 571–624

Wilson P D, Samarrai T A L, Deakin M et al 1987 An objective assessment of physiotherapy for female genuine stress incontinence. British Journal of Obstetrics and Gynaecology 94:575–582

Wong K, Fung B, Fung, L C W et al 1997 Pelvic floor exercises in the treatment of stress urinary incontinence in Hong Kong chinese women. ICS 27th Annual Meeting, Yokohama, Japan, p 62–63

Wong K, Fung K, Fung S et al 2001 Biofeedback of pelvic floor muscles in the management of genuine stress incontinence in Chinese women. Physiotherapy 87(12):644–648

ELECTRICAL STIMULATION FOR SUI

Bary Berghmans

INTRODUCTION

When a nerve is stimulated, signals travel both toward the periphery and toward the central nervous system (CNS). Electrical stimulation may elicit responses to these signals, which may come from the CNS or the tissues innervated by the nerve, or the CNS may be modified to reinterpret some signals (Chancellor & Leng 2002, Fall & Lindström 1994).

For lower urinary tract dysfunctions, electrical stimulation is applied particularly to the pelvic floor muscles (PFM), bladder and sacral nerve roots. These kinds of currents have been tested for their potential and ability to support lower urinary tract functions through improvement of strength and/or coordination of the PFM (Hahn et al 1991, Sand et al 1995) and inhibition of detrusor muscle contractions (stimulation of the detrusor inhibition reflex) (Yamanishi & Yasuda, 1998).

Electrical stimulation can be divided into two major forms: neurostimulation and neuromodulation. Neurostimulation of the pelvic floor aims at stimulating motor efferent fibres of the pudendal nerve, which may elicit a direct response from the effector organ, for instance a contraction of the PFM (Eriksen 1989, Fall & Lindström 1991, Scheepens 2003). The object of neuromodulation is to remodel neuronal reflex loops, for instance the detrusor inhibition reflex, by stimulating afferent nerve fibres of the pudendal nerve that influence these reflex loops. Therefore, neuromodulation may elicit an **indi**rect response from the effector organ, for instance detrusor muscle inhibition (Vodusek et al 1986, Weil 2000).

Today it is still difficult to clarify the potential value and benefits of electrical stimulation in the treatment of urinary incontinence, which is the most prevalent form of lower urinary tract dysfunction (Wilson et al 2002) for several reasons.

First, the nomenclature used to describe electrical stimulation has been inconsistent. Stimulation has sometimes been described on the basis of the type of current being used (e.g. faradic stimulation, interferential therapy), but is also described on the basis of the structures being targeted (e.g. neuromuscular electrical stimulation), the current intensity (e.g. low-intensity stimulation, or maximal stimulation), and the proposed mechanism of action (e.g. neuromodulation). In the absence of a clear unequivocal classification of electrical stimulation, the author of this section will make no attempt to classify the interventions that are considered.

Second, in electrical stimulation studies many combinations of current types, amplitudes, types of waveforms, frequencies, intensities, electrode placements etc. are reported (Wilson et al 2002). The lack of a clear biological rationale seems to hamper reasoned choices of electrical stimulation parameters. Additional confusion is created by the relatively rapid developments in the area of electrical stimulation. Even for the same health problem, a wide variety of stimulation devices and protocols have been used (Wilson et al 2002). For example, in the past 20 years or so women with stress urinary incontinence (SUI) have been treated using anything from a single clinic-based episode of maximal stimulation under general anaesthetic for 20 minutes with vaginal and buttock electrodes (Shepherd et al 1984) to ten sessions of interferential therapy at 10–40 Hz with perineal body and symphysis pubis electrodes (Laycock & Jerwood 1993), to 8 weeks of home-based stimulation using a 'new pattern of background low frequency and intermediate frequency with an initial doublet', for 1 hour a day (Jeyaseelan et al 2000, Oldham 1997), to 6 months of low-intensity stimulation at 10 Hz using a vaginal electrode (Knight et al 1998).

Third, although it has been suggested that electrical stimulation as an intervention for urinary incontinence is using the natural neural pathways and micturition reflexes (Fall 1998, Yamanishi et al 1998) and the understanding of both neuroanatomy and neurophysiology of the CNS and peripheral nervous system is increasing, there is still lack of a well-substantiated biological rationale supporting the use of electrical stimulation (Wilson et al 2002).

It has been suggested that electrical stimulation restores continence by:

- strengthening the structural support of the urethra and the bladder neck (Plevnic et al 1991);
- securing the resting and active closure of the proximal urethra (Erlandson & Fall 1977);
- strengthening the PFM (Sand et al 1995);
- inhibiting reflex bladder contractions (Berghmans et al 2002, Fall & Lindström 1994);
- modifying the vascularity of the urethral and bladder neck tissues (Fall & Lindström 1991, 1994, Plevnik et al 1991).

In the context of conservative or non-surgical, non-medical therapy electrical stimulation can be applied using surface electrodes (Appell 1998, Brubaker 2000, Goldberg & Sand 2000, Govier et al 2001, Hasan & Neal 1998, Jabs & Stanton 2001, Siegel 1992, Van Kerrebroeck 1998).

Surface electrodes include:

- transcutaneous electrical stimulation (Berghmans et al 2002, Brubaker 2000, Jabs & Stanton 2001) (i.e. TENS), via suprapubic, sacral or penile/clitoral attachment of electrodes, vaginal/anal plug electrodes, plantar/thigh and similar stimulation, and other surface placement of electrodes such as for interferential or maximum electrical stimulation;

- percutaneous electrical stimulation (Govier et al 2001, Janknegt et al 1997, van Balkan et al 2001) (e.g. posterior tibial nerve stimulation, percutaneous nerve evaluation and acupuncture).

There are two main types of electrical stimulation:

- long-term or chronic electrical stimulation is delivered below the sensory threshold and the device is used 6–12 hours a day for several months (Eriksen 1989);
- maximal electrical stimulation uses a high-intensity stimulus (just below the pain threshold) for a short duration (15–30 minutes) several times a week (or 1–2 times daily) (Jonasson et al 1990).

In addition to office-based electrical stimulation, portable electrical stimulation devices for self-care by patients themselves at home have been developed (Berghmans et al 2002).

Electrical stimulation has been used for patients with SUI, symptoms of urgency, frequency and/or urge urinary incontinence, nocturia, detrusor overactivity and mixed urinary incontinence (Polden & Mantle 1990, Wilson et al 2002).

The mechanism and mode of action may vary depending on the cause of urinary incontinence and the structure being targeted by electrical stimulation. In general, in SUI, electrical stimulation is focused on improvement of the urethral closure pressure (UCP)

and sphincter activation (Fall & Lindström 1994, Sand et al 1995), whereas for patients with urge incontinence the aim seems to be to inhibit reflex bladder contractions (i.e. detrusor overactivity) – bladder inhibition (Berghmans et al 2002).

Also, it is hypothesized by some authors and clinicians that electrical stimulation might be used as a sort of biofeedback procedure in patients who are unaware about how to contract the PFM and are incapable of doing so voluntarily (Smith 1996, Wilson et al 2002). Electrical stimulation might help these patients regain awareness of the PFM. However, we were unable to detect any study that actually tested this hypothesis.

In the rest of this chapter we will address the question about the most appropriate electrical stimulation protocol, whether electrical stimulation is better than no treatment, placebo or control treatment, whether electrical stimulation is better than any other single treatment, and whether or not (additional) electrical stimulation to other (additional) treatments adds any benefit. Finally, we will address the results of electrical stimulation on PFM strength and reported adverse events.

METHODS

The following qualitative summary of the evidence regarding electrical stimulation in patients with SUI is based on RCTs included in three systematic reviews (Berghmans et al 1998, 2000, Hay-Smith et al 2001) with the addition of trials performed after publication of the reviews and/or located through additional electronic searching on PubMed from 1998 till 2005 and the Cochrane Library. We also searched the literature used for the International Consultations on Incontinence (ICI) meetings of 1998, 2001 and 2004; published abstracts were excluded.

EVIDENCE FOR ELECTRICAL STIMULATION TO TREAT SYMPTOMS OF SUI

Table 9.3 provides details of results of all included studies (n = 15, one study consisted of two separate RCTs (Laycock & Jerwood 1993).

The PEDro rating scale was used to classify the methodological quality of the included studies (Table 9.4). The studies had low to high methodological quality.

The most appropriate electrical stimulation protocol

It appeared that there was considerable variation in electrical stimulation protocols with no consistent pattern emerging.

Table 9.3 Randomized controlled trials on electrical stimulation to treat stress urinary incontinence

Author	Blowman et al 1991
Design	2-arm RCT double-blind: PFMT + ES, PFMT + sham ES
Sample size (age range or mean age, SD, years)	14 women (range 33–68)
Diagnosis	Urodynamics, filling cystometry, coughing-induced leakage while standing
Training protocol	PFMT + visual feedback with perineometer 4×/day Home (sham) Surface ES: 60 min/day, perineal & buttocks ES: 10 Hz, 4 s hold/relax, pulsewidth 80 μs, 2 weeks 35 Hz, 15 min/day ES: no contraction, minimal sensation, 4 weeks
Drop outs	1/14 (7%)
Adherence	–
Results	NS decrease median (range) IEF/week in sham ES from 12.5 (1–31) to 6 (0–21); sign. decrease ES from 5 (0–14) to 0 (0–1) Max. perineometer in sham ES median (range) pre/post-treatment from 3.5 (1–5) to 5 (3–13), ES 1 (0–8) to 5 (2–16) No side-effect of (sham) ES reported IEF 0 in 6/7 ES, 1/6 in sham ES Questionnaire after 6 mts: ES no ES 4; sham ES further treatment needed
Author	Bø et al 1999
Design	4-arm RCT: PFMT, ES, VC, no treatment
Sample size (age range or mean age, SD, years)	122 women GSI, mean (range) age 49.5 (24–70)
Diagnosis	Urodynamics, uroflowmetry, cystometry, pad test with standard. bladder volume
Training protocol	PFMT: 8–12 VPFMC 3×/day at home; 1×/week office ES: vaginal intermittent stim, 50 Hz 30 min/day VC: 20 min/day
Drop outs	15/122 (12%) primary analysis & ITT analysis of all
Adherence	Mean (SE) adherence PFMT: 93% (1.5%) ES: 75% (2.8%) VC: 78% (4.4%) PFMT vs ES or VC sign. better, ES vs VC NS

Results	Sign. imp. pre-/post-treament all treatment groups: PFMT vs no treatment sign. diff., p < 0.01)
	   PFMT: 44% cured; no treatment 6.7%
	Change in PFM strength sign. greater in PFMT (p = 0.03), not in ES or VC
	ITT analysis same results PFMT vs no treatment sign. change in pad test after 6 mts, IEF
	   (p < 0.01), Social Activity Index (p < 0.01) and Leakage Index (p < 0.01)
	No urodynamic parameters changed in any group pre-/ post-treatment

Table 9.3 Randomized controlled trials on electrical stimulation to treat stress urinary incontinence—cont'd

Author	Brubaker et al 1997
Design	2-arm RCT: ES, sham ES
Sample size (age range or mean age, SD, years)	148 women, subgroup GSI 60 women mean age 57 (SD 12)
Diagnosis	Urodynamics, micturition diary
Training protocol	ES: transvaginal, 20 Hz, 2/4 s work/rest, pulse width 0.1 μs, bipolar square wave, I 0–100 mA Sham ES same parameters, no I, both groups 8 weeks' treatment
Drop outs	18%
Adherence	ES vs sham ES mean compliance 87% vs 81% at 4 and 8 treatment weeks
Results	ES vs sham ES 6-week 24-h frequency NS 6-week no. of accidents/24 h (average) NS Adequate subj. imp. p = 0.027 QoL NS difference No analysis diaries because of incomplete data
Author	Goode et al 2003
Design	3-arm RCT: ES + PFMT/ BF, PFMT/BF, controls (self-administered PFMT)
Sample size (age range or mean age, SD, years)	200 women, age range 40–78
Diagnosis	Urodynamics, cystometry, micturition diary, QoL questionnaires
Training protocol	PFMT: 1×/2 weeks for 8 weeks, anorectal BF for awareness PFM, hold/relax 20 min, verbal & written instructions for 3×/ day PFMT at home, duration hold/relax max. 10 s each ES: vaginal probe, biphasic, 20 Hz, pulse width 1 ms, hold/relax 1 : 1, I_{max} up to 100 mA 15 min/2 days; Controls: written instructions, booklet
Drop outs	18.2% in PFMT, 11.9% in ES, 37.3% in controls, ITT analysis
Adherence	Not reported
Results	Mean reduction 68.6% PFMT/BF, 71.9% ES + PFMT/BF, 52.5% controls condition In comparison with controls both interventions sign. more effective, but not sign. different from each other (p = 0.60) ES + PFMT/BF sign. better patient self-perception of outcome (p < 0.001) and satisfaction with progress (p = 0.02)
Author	Hahn et al 1991
Design	2-arm RCT: PFMT, ES; if not cured after 6 months other arm offered
Sample size (age range or mean age, SD, years)	20 women mean age 47.2 (range 24–64); 13 women had both arms
Diagnosis	Urodynamics, cystometry, pad test, cystourethroscopy
Training protocol	PFMT Fast P_{max} 5 s hold & relax and slow twitch P_{submax} 2 s hold & relax various positions, 5–10×, 6–8×/day, endurance 30–40 s IFT vaginal probe, alternating pulses 10/20/50 Hz, home device (Contelle) 6–8 h/night

Table 9.3   Randomized controlled trials on electrical stimulation to treat stress urinary incontinence—cont'd

Drop outs	2 IFT after unsuccesful PFMT/13
Adherence	–
Results	Pad test: 5/20 cured 1 treatment course (1 PFMT, 4 IFT) PFMT, IFT sign. imp., in between NS 13 s course sign. improvement, subj. imp. 2 cured/11 imp.; Pad test after 4 years: 4/14 further imp., 8/14 unchanged, 2/14 detoriation
	Subj. imp. 1/14 imp., 8/14 unchanged, 5 det.
Author	Henalla et al 1989
Design	4-arm RCT: PFMT, ES, oestrogens, no treatment
Sample size (age range or mean age, SD, years)	104 women, mean age not stated: age comparable between groups
Diagnosis	GSI urodynamically proven
Training protocol	PFMT with digital feedback by patient + regular PFME 5 s 5×/h; PT 1×/week
	ES: 10 sessions 20 min, 1×/week interferential therapy (IFT) 0–100 Hz, I_{max}
	Oestrogens 2 g + nightly applicator 12 weeks
	No treatment
Drop outs	4%
Adherence	Not stated
Results	No in-between comparisons
	Pad test 50% reduction in 17/26 (65%) PFMT, 8/25 (32%) ES; 3/24 (12%) after 3 mts
	Pad weights reduction in PFMT and ES ($p < 0.02$)
	UI recurrence: 3/17 PFMT and 1/8 ES after 9 mts; 3/3 immediate recurrence after discontinuing oestrogens
Author	Hofbauer et al 1990
Design	4 arm RCT: ES + PFMT, PFMT, ES, sham treatment
Sample size (age range or mean age, SD, years)	43 women mean + SD age 57.5 + 12
Diagnosis	Cystoscopy, cystometry, UPP, micturition diary
Training protocol	ES: constant 3×/wk 10 min for 6 weeks perineal and lumbar electrodes, faradic, $I_{variable}$ until contraction
	PFMT + abd/add 20 min 2×/week + home exercises
	Sham ES
Drop outs	–
Adherence	Not reported
Results	Cured/imp./unchanged: ES + PFMT 3/4/4, PFMT 6/1/4, ES 1/2/8, sham ES 0/0/10 MUCP, FUL, pressure transmission NS changes pre- & post-treatment
Author	Jeyaseelan et al 2000
Design	2-arm RCT: ES, sham ES
Sample size (age range or mean age, SD, years)	27 women GSI, age not reported

Table 9.3 Randomized controlled trials on electrical stimulation to treat stress urinary incontinence—cont'd

Diagnosis	Urodynamics, 7-day micturition diary, 20-min pad test
Training protocol	ES: background low frequency (target slow-twitch fibres) and intermediate frequency with an initial doublet (target fast-twitch fibres), vaginal probe, 1 h/day, 8 weeks Sham ES: 1 250 µs/min for 1 h, I no effect
Drop outs	3/27 (11%)
Adherence	ES: 71–98% Sham ES: 64–100%
Results	Perineometry: PFM strength between & within groups NS changes pre-/post treatment (p = 0.86) Digital assessment: sign. within changes pre/ post treatment Endurance PFM by perineometry: ES 73% + 116% imp, sham ES reduction −6% + 24%, diffence between groups NS Pad test, micturition diary, IIQ: NS changes between groups UDI: ES > reduction than sham ES (p = 0.03)
Author	Knight et al 1998
Design	3-arm RCT: clinic ES + PFMT/BF, home ES + PFMT/BF, PFMT/BF
Sample size (age range or mean age, SD, years)	70 women GSI age range 24–68
Diagnosis	Urodynamics, micturition diary, pad test, perineometry
Training protocol	Baseline treatment: home PFMT after instruction PT, max 10 10/4 s hold/relax, repetitions recorded, max 10 fast twitch contractions, 6×/day; Baseline treatment: nightly low I home ES, vaginal probe, trains of 10 Hz, 35 Hz occasionally, pulse width 200 µs, duty circle 5/5 s Baseline treatment + 16 30-min clinic ES, I_{max}, 35 Hz, pulse width 250 ms, together with voluntary contraction
Drop outs	13/70 (18.6%); 24% in home ES (n.s.), ITT analysis of all
Adherence	Median percentage compliance Home ES (72.5%) PFMT/BF (90%) Difference between groups NS
Results	Pad test after 6 mts: sign. reduction urine loss in all three groups, clinic ES best, after 12 mts > reduction Obj.imp/cured after 6 mts clinic ES (n = 20) vs home ES (n = 19) vs controls (n = 18) 80%/52.8%/72.3% Micturition diaries data incomplete, not analysed PFM strength sign. increase in all groups, biggest in clinic ES (NS)
Author	Luber & Wolde-Tsadik 1997
Design	2-arm RCT double-blind: ES, sham ES
Sample size (age range or mean age, SD, years)	45 women GSI mean age 53.8
Diagnosis	Urodynamics, micturition diary, questionnaire, cotton tip test: hypermobility urethra

Table 9.3 Randomized controlled trials on electrical stimulation to treat stress urinary incontinence—cont'd

Training protocol	ES: 2 × 15 min sessions/day for 12 weeks, home device, pulse width 2 ms, 2/4 s work/rest, freq 50 Hz, I 10–100 mA Sham ES same parameters, I no sensation
Drop outs	1/45 (2.2%)
Adherence	Measured by internal memory home device
Results	NS diff. between groups (ES 20 women, sham ES 24 women in subj. cure/imp, obj. cure (diaries, incontinence questionnaire, urodynamics) No adverse events
Author	Laycock & Jerwood 1993 I
Design	2-arm RCT: ES, PFMT +*TT
Sample size (age range or mean age, SD, years)	46 women, age range 28–59
Diagnosis	Urodynamics proven GSI; digital palpation (grading Oxford scale)
Training protocol	Mean 10 ES–IFT sessions, bipolar, perineal & symphysis pubis, 30 min, I_{max} 1/10–40/40 Hz 10 min each PFMT: 6 weeks 5 MVCs every hour, from 2nd visit VC 10 min, 2×/day
Drop outs	ES: no drop-outs; PFMT 6/23 (26%)
Adherence	After therapy in ES group 1 subject (7%) every day home maintenance PFMT, 6 (40%) nearly every day, 8 (53%) 1×/week
Results	Pad test; sign. decrease (p < 0.003) both groups PFM strength ES sign. imp. (p = 0.0035), PFMT NS Micturition diary IEF sign. decrease in both groups Subj. assessment IEF both groups equally effective Review questionnaire after 2 years > 30% ES maintained imp.
Author	Laycock & Jerwood 1993 II
Design	2-arm RCT: ES, sham ES
Sample size (age range or mean age, SD, years)	30 women age range 16–66
Diagnosis	See Laycock & Jerwood 1993 I
Training protocol	IFT: see Laycock I Sham IFT: no current, rest simular IFT
Drop outs	IFT no drop-outs; sham IFT 4/15 (27%)
Adherence	After therapy in ES group 2 subject (15.4%) every day home maintenance PFMT, 5 (38.5%) nearly every day 4 (30.8%) 1×/week, 2 (15.4%) < 1×/wk
Results	Pad test: IFT mean 56.8% decrease weight pre/post-treatment, sham IFT 21.4%; in between sign. Diff. Perineometer: PFMC sign. increase strength only in IFT Micturition chart: IEF reduction only in IFT, severity. reduction only in IFT Review questionnaire after mean 16 mts 20% IFT maintained imp

Table 9.3 Randomized controlled trials on electrical stimulation to treat stress urinary incontinence—cont'd

Author	Olah et al 1990
Design	2-arm RCT: VC, ES
Sample size (age range or mean age, SD, years)	69 women mean age 43.2 ± 8.9 (VC), 47.9 ± 13.0 (ES)
Diagnosis	Continence–frequency chart 1 week pretreatment, pelvic floor strength with VC, 1 h pad test
Training protocol	VC: 1×/week for 4 weeks, active PFMT with VC 2×/day 15 min, increasing weight after two success occasions ES–IFT 3×/week for 4 weeks; 0–100 Hz, 4 vacuum electrodes, 2 abdominal, 2 thighs, I_{max}, 15 min
Drop outs	15/69 (22%)
Adherence	Not reported
Results	Weekly leakages (g) mean ± SD: VC from 22.0 ± 31.4 to 8.2 ± 14.5 to 3.9 ± 9.4 (after 6 mts), IFT 19.3 ± 22.6 to 7.7 ± 11.7 to 5.3 ± 9.2 (after 6 mts); UI (g) mean ± SD: VC 27.7 ± 38.8 to 14.0 ± 36.7 to 2.8 ± 8.3, IFT from 32.2 ± 49.1 to 10.5 ± 17.3 to 9.7 ± 28.4 (after 6 mts) No difference between groups Cured/improved: VC 4/15 of 24, 10/7 of 24 after 6 mts, IFT 4/23 of 30, 12/15 of 30
Author	Sand et al 1995
Design	2-arm RCT multicentre: ES, sham ES
Sample size (age range or mean age, SD, years)	52 women age mean ± SD 53.2 ± 11.4
Diagnosis	Urodynamic proven GSI, UCP >20 cm H_2O, and LPP > 60 cm H_2O at max. cyst. capacity
Training protocol	Vaginal electrode, ES pulse duration 0.3 ms, I_{max}, first 2 weeks 5/10 s, later 5/5 s hold/relax Sham ES 1 mA max, 15–30 min 2×/day 12 weeks
Drop outs	8/52 (15%)
Adherence	61% used ES >50 out of planned 70 h (80%) vs 89% sham ES
Results	ES vs sham ES after 12 weeks: IEF/24 h, IEF/week, UI during pad test, PFM strength on perineometry sign. better in ES No irreversible adverse events Vaginal irritation/infection/urinary tract infection/pain 14%/11%/3%/9% ES and 12%/12%/12%/6% sham ES
Author	Shepherd et al 1984
Design	2-arm RCT: ES, placebo ES
Sample size (age range or mean age, SD, years)	107 women; 42 SUI (26–72)
Diagnosis	Urodynamic assessment with urethral profilometry and cystometry; cystoscopy under general anaesthesia; measurement of pelvic contraction
Training protocol	1 single session of maximum perineal stimulation while under anaesthesia ES: vaginal and buttock ES; monophasic square wave pulses; I_{max} 40 V, 10–50 Hz; 20 min Placebo ES: same but no current Assessment 6 and 12 weeks post-treatment; questionnaires, pad test, diary, perineometry

Table 9.3 Randomized controlled trials on electrical stimulation to treat stress urinary incontinence—cont'd

Drop outs	12%
Adherence	Not applicable
Results	Only overall results available but authors stated no diff. between diagnostic groups No diff. between groups regarding reduction frequency, severity, pads used, pelvic floor muscle strength, subjective improvement
Author	Smith 1996
Design	2-arm RCT: ES, PFMT
Sample size (age range or mean age, SD, years)	Subgroup GSI (type II) 18 women age range 26–72
Diagnosis	Cystoscopy only when indicated, complex video urodynamic study (i.e. uroflow, UPP, cystometrography, Vasalva, LPP)
Training protocol	ES: 5 s contractions (range 3–15), duty circle 1:2, treatment time 15–60 min 2×/day for 4 mts, I 5–80 mA PFMT: 60 contractions/day, fast & slow twitch
Drop outs	None
Adherence	80%
Results	IEF pads >50% imp, obj.. imp. 44% PFMT, 1/4/5 cured/improved/unchanged 66% ES, 2/4/3 In between no stat. sign. diff.

abd/add, abduction/adduction; BF, biofeedback; diff., difference; ES, electrical stimulation; FUL, functional urethral length; GSI, genuine stress incontinence, IEF, incontinence episode frequency; IFT, interferential therapy; imp, improvement; ITT, intention-to-treat analysis; LPP, leak point pressure; mts, months; MUCP, maximum urethral closure pressure; MVC, maximal vaginal contraction; NS, no significant/not significant; PFMT, pelvic floor muscle training; obj., objective; QoL, quality of life; RCT, randomized controlled trial; sign., significant; stat., statistical; stim., stimulation; subj., subjective; UCP, urethral closure pressure; UI, urinary incontinence; VC, vaginal cone; VPFMC, voluntary pelvic floor maximal contraction.

Interferential therapy was used in three trials (Henalla et al 1989, Laycock & Jerwood 1993, Olah et al 1990). Few trials clearly stated whether direct or alternating currents were being used.

The most commonly used descriptors were frequency and pulse duration. Six trials used a single frequency, ranging from 20 Hz (Brubaker et al 1997, Goode et al 2003) to 50 Hz (Bø et al 1999, Hahn et al 1991, Luber & Wolde-Tsadik 1997, Smith, 1996). Two trials included stimulation at both 10 Hz and 35 Hz (Blowman et al 1991, Knight et al 1998), though the protocols were different, one at combined low and intermediate frequency (Jeyaseelan et al 2000). Other protocols included stimulation at 12.5 Hz and 50 Hz (Sand et al 1995), 10–50 Hz (Shepherd et al 1984), 0–100 Hz (Henalla et al 1989, Olah et al 1990), and finally a 30-minute treatment, including 10 minutes at 1 Hz, 10 minutes 10–40 Hz and 10 minutes at 40 Hz (Laycock & Jerwood 1993). Pulse durations ranged from 0.08 ms (Blowman et al 1991) up to 100 ms (Brubaker et al 1997). Eight trials also detailed the duty cycle used during stimulation. The ratios ranged from 1 : 3 (Bø et al 1999), and 1 : 2 (Brubaker et al 1997, Luber & Wolde-Tsadik 1997) to 1 : 1 (Blowman et al 1991, Knight et al 1998, Goode et al 2003) and two trials alternated between a ratio of 1 : 1 and 1 : 2 (Sand et al 1995, Smith 1996).

Six trials asked women to use the maximum tolerable intensity of stimulation (Bø et al 1999, Brubaker et al 1997, Goode et al 2003, Laycock & Jerwood 1993, Olah et al 1990, Sand et al 1995), and one trial increased output until there was a noticeable muscle contraction (Hofbauer et al 1990). The trial by Knight et al (1998) compared 'low-intensity' and 'maximal-intensity' protocols. The trials by Goode et al (2003), Hofbauer et al (1990) and Knight et al (1998) also asked women to add a voluntary PFM contraction to the stimulated contraction, though in the trial of Knight et al (1998) this was only for the maximal stimulation group.

Current was most commonly delivered via a single vaginal electrode (Bø et al 1999, Brubaker et al 1997,

Table 9.4   PEDro quality score of RCTs in systematic review

E – Eligibility criteria specified
1 – Subjects randomly allocated to groups
2 – Allocation concealed
3 – Groups similar at baseline
4 – Subjects blinded
5 – Therapist administering treatment blinded
6 – Assessors blinded
7 – Measures of key outcomes obtained from over 85% of subjects
8 – Data analysed by intention to treat
9 – Comparison between groups conducted
10 – Point measures and measures of variability provided

Study	E	1	2	3	4	5	6	7	8	9	10	Total score
Blowman et al 1991	+	+	−	+	+	+	+	+	−	−	+	7
Bo et al 1999	+	+	+	+	−	−	+	+	+	+	+	8
Brubaker et al 1997	+	+	+	+	+	−	+	−	−	+	+	7
Goode et al 2003	+	+	+	+	−	−	−	−	+	+	+	6
Hahn et al 1991	+	+	−	+	−	−	−	+	−	+	−	4
Henalla et al 1989	+	+	−	?	−	−	−	+	−	?	+	3
Hofbauer et al 1990	+	+	−	+	−	−	−	+	−	−	−	3
Knight et al 1998	+	+	+	+	−	−	−		+	+	+	6
Jeyaseelan et al 2000	+	+	+	+	−	−	+	+	+	+	+	8
Laycock & Jerwood 1993 I	+	+	−	+	−	−	−	+	−	+	+	5
Laycock & Jerwood 1993 II	+	+	−	+	+	−	−	+	−	+	+	6
Luber & Wolde–Tsadik 1997	+	+	+	+	+	+	+	−	−	+	+	8
Olah et al 1990	+	+	−	+	−	−	−	+	+	+	+	6
Sand et al 1995	+	+	+	+	+	+	+	−	+	+	+	9
Smith 1996	+	+	−	−	−	−	−	+	−	+	+	4
Shepherd et al 1984	+	+	+	+	+	−	+	+	−	−	−	6

+, criterion is clearly satisfied; −, criterion is not satisfied; ?, not clear if the criterion was satisfied. Total score is determined by counting the number of criteria that are satisfied, except that 'eligibility criteria specified' is not used to generate the total score. Total scores are + scores out of 10.

Goode et al 2003, Hahn et al 1991, Knight et al 1998, Luber & Wolde-Tsadik 1997, Sand et al 1995, Smith 1996). One trial used both vaginal and buttock electrodes (Shepherd et al 1984). In three trials external electrodes were used: abdomen and inside thighs (Olah et al 1990), perineal body and symphysis pubis (Laycock & Jerwood 1993), perineal and buttock (Blowman et al 1991); and in two studies the electrode placement was not clearly described (Henalla et al 1989, Hofbauer et al 1990).

The duration and number of treatments was also highly variable. The longest-duration treatment periods included daily treatment at home for 6 months (Bø et al 1999, Hahn et al 1991, Knight et al 1998). Medium-duration treatment periods were based on once-daily treatment at home for 8 weeks every other day (Goode et al

2003) and twice-daily treatment at home for 8 (Brubaker et al 1997) to 12 weeks (Luber & Wolde-Tsadik 1997, Sand et al 1995). The shortest treatment periods were all for clinic-based stimulation, ranging from 10 (Henalla et al 1989, Laycock & Jerwood 1993), to 12 (Olah et al 1990), 16 (Knight et al 1998), and 18 sessions in total (Hofbauer et al 1990).

Comparing two protocols with different intensity of electrical stimulation, Knight et al (1998) found a trend across a range of outcomes including self-report of cure or improvement, pad test, and PFM strength measurement, measured by vaginal squeeze pressure, for women who received clinic-based maximal stimulation to benefit more than women in the low-intensity stimulation group though most differences were not significant.

Is electrical stimulation better than no treatment, control or placebo treatment?

Henalla et al (1989) compared electrical stimulation with no treatment in women with SUI. Eight of the 25 women receiving electrical stimulation were 'objectively' cured or improved (negative pad test or more than 50% reduction in pad test) at 3 months, versus none of the 25 women in the no-treatment group.

One trial compared electrical stimulation with control intervention (women were offered use of the Continence Guard (Coloplast AS, used infrequently by 14 out of 30 controls) in women with SUI (Bø et al 1999): electrical stimulation was better than control intervention for change in leakage episodes over 3 days, using the Social Activity Index and Leakage Index. However, only one of these measures (change in leakage episodes over 3 days) remained significant (p = 0.047) with intention to treat analysis. PFM activity was significantly improved in the electrical stimulation group after treatment, but the change in activity was not significant when compared with controls. There was no difference in the primary outcome measure (i.e. pad test with standardized bladder volume). Two of 30 controls were cured (≦2 g leakage) on the pad test compared to 7/25 in the electrical stimulation group. One of 30 women in the control group reported the condition was 'unproblematic' after treatment versus 3/25 in the electrical stimulation group, but 28/30 and 19/25 wanted further treatment, respectively.

Six trials compared electrical stimulation with placebo electrical stimulation in women with urodynamic SUI (Blowman et al 1991, Hofbauer et al 1990, Jeyaseelan et al 2000, Laycock & Jerwood 1993, Luber & Wolde-Tsadik 1997, Sand et al 1995). Blowman et al (1991) compared electrical stimulation/PFM training (PFMT) versus placebo electrical stimulation/PFMT in

women with urodynamic SUI and for the purposes of analysis this trial was considered to be a comparison of electrical stimulation with placebo electrical stimulation. Hofbauer et al (1990) provided minimal detail of participants, methods and stimulation parameters. Laycock & Jerwood (1993) used clinic based, short-term (ten treatments) maximal stimulation with an interferential current applied with external surface electrodes. In the treatment regimen of Jeyaseelan et al (2000) electrical stimulation consisted of a new stimulation pattern (i.e. background low frequency [to target the slow-twitch fibres] and intermediate frequency with an initial doublet [to target the fast-twitch fibres] applied with a vaginal probe). Three trials were based on daily home stimulation for 6 (Blowman et al 1991), 8 (Jeyaseelan et al 2000) or 12 weeks (Luber & Wolde-Tsadik 1997, Sand et al 1995).

The two most comparable trials in terms of stimulation parameters reported contrasting findings. Sand et al (1995) found that the electrical stimulation group had significantly greater changes in the number of leakage episodes in 24 hours, number of pads used, amount of leakage on pad test, and PFM activity (PFM strength measurement measured by vaginal squeeze pressure) than the placebo stimulation group. In addition the electrical stimulation group had significantly improved subjective measures (e.g. visual analogue measure of severity) than the placebo group. Neither group demonstrated significant change in the quality of life (QoL) measure (SF 36). In contrast, Luber & Wolde-Tsadik (1997) did not find any statistically significant differences between electrical stimulation and placebo electrical stimulation groups for rates of self-reported cure or improvement, objective cure (negative stress test during urodynamics), number of incontinence episodes in 24 hours, or Valsalva leak point pressure.

The other trials generally favoured electrical stimulation over placebo electrical stimulation. Laycock & Jerwood (1993) generally found significantly greater improvements in the electrical stimulation group (pad test, PFM activity, self reported severity), though the decrease in incontinence episodes was not significantly different between the groups after treatment. Blowman et al (1991) found a significant decrease in the number of leakage episodes in the electrical stimulation group only. Hofbauer et al (1990) reported that 3/11 women in the electrical stimulation group were cured/improved (not defined) versus 0/11 in the placebo electrical stimulation group.

Jeyaseelan et al (2000) did not find statistically significant differences between the two study groups when PFM strength was measured by a device measuring vaginal squeeze pressure, but in contrast when strength was assessed using digital assessment a statistical significant difference was found. When endurance was assessed an improvement in favour of the electrical stimulation group was found over time in the electrical stimulation group, but not in the sham electrical stimulation group. The authors suggested that between-group differences may be not significant as a result of the high degree of variance combined with a small sample size. No changes were reported using a pad test or diaries, but a significant change in favour of the electrical stimulation group using the Urogenital Distress Inventory (UDI) score (Jeyaseelan et al 2000).

Is electrical stimulation better than any other single treatment?

Henalla et al (1989) compared electrical stimulation (interferential) with vaginal oestrogens (Premarin). Eight of 25 women in the stimulation group reported they were cured or improved versus 3/24 in the oestrogen therapy group. There was a significant reduction in leakage on pad test in the stimulation group, but not in the oestrogen group. In contrast the maximum urethral closure pressure (MUCP) was significantly increased in the oestrogen group, but not the stimulation group. Long-term follow-up (9 months) found that subjectively 1/8 women in the stimulation group who had reported cure/improvement post-treatment had recurrent symptoms, as did all three women in the oestrogen group once oestrogen therapy ceased.

Comparing electrical stimulation with PFMT, using a pad test as mentioned before, only Bø et al found a statistically significant difference in favour of PFMT. It was not clear if the cure data reported by Hofbauer et al (1990) were derived from a symptom scale or voiding diary; these data were therefore excluded. Only Bø et al measured leakage episodes and QoL (Social Activity Index) in SUI women. There was no statistically significant difference between the groups for either outcome. At 9 months post-treatment, Henalla et al found 3/17 PFMT women and 1/8 in the electrical stimulation group reported recurrent symptoms.

In both trials of Olah et al (1990) and of Bø et al (1999) there was no statistically significant difference between vaginal cones (VC) and electrical stimulation groups for self-reported cure, self-reported cure/improvement or leakage episodes in 24 hours. Bø et al did not find any statistically significant difference between the groups in QoL (Social Activity Index). Olah et al (1990) had to exclude some women from their trial before randomization because they could not use cones in the vagina (e.g. wedging of cones).

Is (additional) electrical stimulation better than other (additional) treatments?

For comparisons of electrical stimulation with biofeedback-assisted PFMT versus biofeedback-assisted PFMT alone versus a control condition reporting was limited to one single trial.

In the study of Goode et al (2003) intention to treat analysis showed that incontinence was reduced by a mean of 68.6% with biofeedback-assisted PFMT, 71.9% with electrical stimulation with biofeedback-assisted PFMT, and 52.5% with the control condition. In comparison with the control group both interventions were significantly more effective, but they were not significantly different from each other (p = 0.60). The electrical stimulation with biofeedback-assisted PFMT had significantly better patient self-perception of outcome (p < 0.001) and satisfaction with progress (p = 0.02).

Two trials compared electrical stimulation in combination with PFMT versus PFMT alone in women with SUI (Hofbauer et al 1990, Luber & Wolde-Tsadik 1997). As both arms in these trials received the same PFMT, the trials are essentially investigating the effect of electrical stimulation. Hofbauer gave minimal detail of participants, methods and stimulation parameters. In a three-arm RCT Knight et al (1998) compared PFMT versus PFMT with home-based low-intensity electrical stimulation versus PFMT with clinic-based maximal-intensity stimulation: 10/21 women in the PFMT group, 9/25 women in the low-intensity stimulation group, and 16/24 in the maximum-intensity stimulation group reported cure or great improvement. All three groups had significant improvements in pad tests after treatment, with no significant differences in the percentage reduction between the groups. Similarly all three groups had improvements in vaginal squeeze pressure, but there were no significant differences in improvement.

Overall Knight et al did not find any clear benefits of electrical stimulation in addition to PFMT. This finding is similar to that of Hofbauer et al (1990) of no significant differences between the groups receiving combined electrical stimulation/PFMT and PFMT alone.

Muscle strength

Several studies reported on PFM strength as an outcome measure (Blowman et al 1991, Bø et al 1999, Laycock & Jerwood 1993, Jeyaseelan et al 2000, Knight et al 1998, Sand et al 1995, Shepherd et al 1984). In all but the first trial in the study of Laycock & Jerwood (1993) a (kind of) device measuring PFM strength by vaginal squeeze pressure was used, with contrasting results between the studies. Laycock & Jerwood did use digital assessment in that trial.

Shepherd et al (1984) did not find any difference of PFM strength between groups, though no statistics were performed to confirm this.

An improvement of PFM strength in both groups (PFMT with electrical stimulation versus PFMT with sham electrical stimulation), with more improvement in the PFMT with electrical stimulation was reported in the study of Blowman et al (1991). However, no statistical tests were performed to test statistical significance.

When digitally tested, Laycock and Jerwood found a pre/post-treatment statistically significant improvement (p = 0.0035) only in the electrical stimulation group (PFMT versus electrical stimulation [interferential therapy]). In this trial they did not report the in-between results. In the second trial they used PFM strength measurement measured by vaginal squeeze pressure to measure PFM strength at PFM maximal contraction and found a significant increase only in the electrical stimulation group.

Sand et al (1995) performed PFM strength measurements using a device measuring vaginal squeeze pressure in 35 patients and 17 controls who used identical sham devices before and after a 15-week treatment period. The active group had a significant improvement in vaginal muscle strength compared to the controls. In the active group mean (± SE) change of vaginal muscle strength (mmHg) before and after treatment was 4.6 ± 1.4, and in the control group 1.1 ± 1.5 (p = 0.02).

Knight et al (1998) found a significant increase of PFM strength in all groups, the biggest being in the electrical stimulation group in a clinical setting. However, there was no significant difference between groups.

In contrast with the electrical stimulation group, Bø et al (1999) reported significant improvement of PFM strength only in the PFMT group (compared with no treatment).

Jeyaseelan et al (2000) did not detect any statistically significant differences between electrical and sham electrical stimulation when PFM strength was measured using a device measuring vaginal squeeze pressure. However, if strength was assessed using digital assessment a statistical significant difference in favour of electrical stimulation was found.

The difference between included studies with respect to outcome of PFM strength, using a device measuring PFM strength by vaginal squeeze pressure can be explained by the huge variation in measurement protocols, devices used, and assessment differences. For instance in the studies of Blowman et al (1991) and Sheperd et al (1984) no statistical tests were performed. Knight et al (1998) and Laycock & Jerwood (1993) did not blind the outcome measurement assessors, while Bø

et al (1999), Jeyaseelan et al (2000) and Sand et al (1995) did.

Adverse events

Four trials (Bø et al 1999, Hahn et al 1991, Sand et al 1995, Smith 1996) reported side-effects related to electrical stimulation, including vaginal irritation, infection, urinary tract infection or pain and/or vaginal bleeding. Sand et al (1995) reported that all adverse events were reversible. Besides the electrical stimulation group, the VC group also reported adverse events in the trial by Bø et al (1999).

CONCLUSION

There is a marked lack of consistency in the electrical stimulation protocols that implies a lack of understanding of the physiological principles of rehabilitating urinary incontinence through electrical stimulation used in clinical practice to treat women with SUI.

In women with SUI:

- there is insufficient evidence to judge whether electrical stimulation is better than no or placebo treatment for women with SUI;
- PFMT seems to be better than electrical stimulation, though conclusive evidence is lacking;
- there is insufficient evidence to determine whether electrical stimulation is better than vaginal oestrogens or VC.

At present it seems that there is no extra benefit in adding electrical stimulation to PFMT.

There is a need for more basic research to find out the working mechanism of electrical stimulation in women with SUI and to determine the best electrical stimulation protocol(s) and outcome measures for such patients.

CLINICAL RECOMMENDATIONS

- Up to now there is no convincing evidence from RCTs that electrical stimulation is a useful treatment in women with SUI, and it is therefore impossible to recommend the most optimal electrical stimulation regimen and protocol.

- A protocol based on the hypothesis that electrical stimulation might help those patients to regain awareness of the PFM who are unaware about how to contract the PFM and are not capable to doing so voluntarily should be considered for testing in a high-quality RCT.

REFERENCES

Appell R A 1998 Electrical stimulation for the treatment of urinary incontinence. Urology 51(suppl 2A):24–26

Berghmans L C M, Hendriks H J, Bø K et al 1998 Conservative treatment of genuine stress incontinence in women: a systematic review of randomized clinical trials. British Journal of Urology 82(2):181–191

Berghmans L C, van Waalwijk van Doorn E, Nieman F et al 2000 Efficacy of extramural physiotherapy modalities in women with proven bladder overactivity: a randomised clinical trial. Neurourology and Urodynamics 19(4):496–497

Berghmans L C, van Waalwijk van Doorn E, Nieman F et al 2002 Efficacy of physical therapeutic modalities in women with proven bladder overactivity. European Urology 41:581–587

Blowman C, Pickles C, Emery S et al 1991 Prospective double blind controlled trial of intensive physiotherapy with and without stimulation of the pelvic floor in the treatment of genuine stress incontinence. Physiotherapy 77:661–664

Bø K, Maanum M 1996 Does vaginal electrical stimulation cause pelvic floor muscle contraction? A pilot study. Scandinavian Journal of Urology and Nephrology. Supplementum 179:39–45

Bø K, Talseth T, Holme I 1999 Single blind, randomised controlled trial of pelvic floor exercises, electrical stimulation, vaginal cones, and no treatment in management of genuine stress incontinence in women. British Medical Journal 318(7182):487–493

Brubaker L 2000 Electrical stimulation in overactive bladder. Urology 55(suppl 5A):17–23

Brubaker L, Benson T, Bent A et al 1997 Transvaginal electrical stimulation for female urinary incontinence. American Journal of Obstetrics & Gynaecology 177:536–540

Chancellor M B, Leng W 2002 The mechanism of action of sacral nerve stimulation in the treatment of detrusor overactivity and urinary retention. In: Jonas U, Grünewald V (eds) New perpectives in sacral nerve stimulation. Martin Dunitz, London

Eriksen B C 1989 Electrostimulation of the pelvic floor in female urinary incontinence [thesis]. University of Trondheim, Norway

Erlandson B E, Fall M 1977 Intravaginal electrical stimulation in urinary incontinence. An experimental and clinical study. Scandinavian Journal of Urology and Nephrology. Supplementum 44:1

Fall M 1998 Advantages and pitfalls of functional electrical stimualtion. Acta Obstetricia et Gynecologica Scandinavica 77(suppl 168):16–21

Fall M, Lindstrom S 1991 Electrical stimulation: a physiologic approach to the treatment of urinary incontinence. The Urologic Clinics of North America 18:393–407

Fall M, Lindstrom S 1994 Functional electrical stimulation: physiological basis and clinical principles. International Urogynecology Journal and Pelvic Floor Dysfunction 5:296–304

Goldberg R P, Sand P K 2000 Electromagnetic pelvic floor stimulation: applications for the gynecologist. Obstetrical & Gynecological Survey 55(11):715–720

Goode P S, Burgio K I, Locher J L et al 2003 Effect of behavioral training with and without pelvic floor electrical stimulation on stress incontinence in women. A randomized controlled trial. The Journal of the American Medical Association 290:345–352

Govier F E, Litwiller S, Nitti V et al 2001 Percutaneous afferent neuromodulation for the refractory overactive bladder: results of a multicenter study. The Journal of Urology 165:1193–1198

Hahn H N, Sommar S, Fall M 1991 A comparative study of pelvic floor training and electrical stimulation for the treatment of genuine female urinary incontinence. Neurourology and Urodynamics 10(6):545–554

Hasan S T, Neal D E 1998 Neuromodulation in bladder dysfunction. Current Opinion in Obstetrics and Gynecology 10:395–399

Hay-Smith E J C, Bø K, Berghmans L C M et al 2001 Pelvic floor muscle training for urinary incontinence in women (Cochrane Review). In: The Cochrane Library, Issue 4. John Wiley, Chichester, UK

Henalla S M, Hutchins C J, Robinson P et al 1989 Non-operative methods in the treatment of female genuine stress incontinence of urine. Journal of Obstetrics & Gynaecology 9(3):222–225

Hofbauer J, Preisinger F, Nurnberger N 1990 Der stelllenwert der physikotherapie bei der weiblichen genuinen stressinkontinenz. Zeitschrift für Urologie und Nephrologie 83:249–254

Jabs C F I, Stanton S L 2001 Urge incontinence and detrusor instability. International Urogynecology Journal and Pelvic Floor Dysfunction 12:58–68

Janknegt R A, Weil E J H, Eerdmans P H A et al 1997 Improving neuromodulation technique for refractory voiding dysfunctions: two-stage implant. Urology 49:358–362

Jeyaseelan S M, Haslam EJ, Winstanley J et al 2000 An evaluation of a new pattern of electrical stimulation as a treatment for urinary stress incontinence: a randomized, double-blind, controlled trial. Clinical Rehabilitation 14:631–640

Jonasson A, Larsson B, Pschera H et al 1990 Short-term maximal electrical stimulation: a conservative treatment of urinary incontinence. Gynecologic and Obstetric Investigation 30(2):120–123

Knight S, Laycock J, Naylor D 1998 Evaluation of neuromuscular electrical stimulation in the treatment of genuine stress incontinence. Physiotherapy 84(2):61–71

Laycock J, Jerwood D 1993 Does pre-modulated interferential therapy cure genuine stress incontinence? Physiotherapy 79:553–560

Luber K M, Wolde–Tsadik G 1997 Efficacy of functional electrical stimulation in treating genuine stress incontinence: A randomized clinical trial. Neurourology and Urodynamics 16:543–551

Olah K S, Bridges N, Denning J et al 1990 The conservative management of patients with symptoms of stress incontinence: a randomized, prospective study comparing weighted vaginal cones and interferential therapy. American Journal of Obstetrics and Gynecology 162(1):87–92

Oldham J 1997 International Patent Patient Publication WO97/47357

Plevnic S, Janez J, Vodusek D B 1991 Electrical stimulation. In: Krane K J, Siroky M B (eds) Clinical neuro-urology. Little–Brown, Boston

Polden M, Mantle J 1990 Physiotherapy in obstetrics and gynaecology. Butterworth Heinemann, Oxford

Sand P K, Richardson D A, Staskin D R et al 1995 Pelvic floor electrical stimulation in the treatment of genuine stress incontinence: a multicenter placebo-controlled trial. American Journal of Obstetrics and Gynecology 173:72–79

Scheepens W A 2003 Progress in sacral neuromodulation of the lower urinary tract. Thesis University of Maastricht, The Netherlands

Shepherd A M, Tribe E, Bainton D 1984 Maximum perineal stimulation: a controlled study. British Journal of Urology 56:644–646

Siegel S W 1992 Management of voiding dysfunction with an implantable neuroprosthesis. Urologic Clinics of North America 19:163–170

Smith J J 1996 Intravaginal stimulation randomized trial. The Journal of Urology 155:127–130

Van Balkan M R, Vandoninck V, Gisolf K W H et al 2001 Posterior tibial nerve stimulation as neuromodulative treatment of lower urinary tract dysfunction. The Journal of Urology 166:914–918

Van Kerrebroeck P E V 1998 The role of electrical stimulation in voiding dysfunction. European Urology 34(suppl 1):27–30

Weil E H J 2000 Clinical and experimental aspects of sacral nerve neuromodulation in lower urinary tract dysfunction. Thesis at University of Maastricht, Maastricht, The Netherlands

Wilson P D, Bø K, Hay-Smith J et al 2002 Conservative treatment in women. In: Abrams P, Cardozo L, Khoury S

et al (eds) Incontinence. Health Publication, Plymouth, p 573–624

Yamanishi T, Yasuda K 1998 Electrical stimulation for stress incontinence. International Urogynecology Journal and Pelvic Floor Dysfunction 9:281–290

Overactive bladder

INTRODUCTION

Anders Mattiasson

Overactive bladder (OAB) is a term used to refer to a type of functional disorder in the lower urinary tract, described with the aid of a group of symptoms, known as a 'syndrome of symptoms'. The term OAB was introduced 1997 and was recognized in 2002 by the International Continence Society (ICS) (Abrams et al 2002). Urgency with or without frequency and/or urge incontinence are the core symptoms that constitute OAB. When the patient is not incontinent the diagnosis is 'OAB dry' (approximately two-thirds), otherwise 'OAB wet' (approximately one-third). Nocturia is often found to be associated.

Overactive bladder is found in a large proportion of the population in the developed countries according to questionnaire and interview studies (Milsom et al 2001, Stewart et al 2003), but it is uncertain how many of the approximately 16% who replied that they have symptoms concordant with OAB really had thought of seeking care.

The prevalence of OAB increases significantly with age. Only 10–15% of all women with stress, urge or mixed incontinence seem to have what can be perceived as urge incontinence. Of the rest, 35–40% have mixed incontinence and 50% have stress incontinence. In total, then, 85–90% could have a stress component, while 50% of incontinent women have an urge component and therefore also belong to the OAB group. To this should then be added the large group who have urgency and frequency, but who are not incontinent, the 'OAB-dry' group.

This chapter focuses on overactivity in women, with special emphasis on the urethra and the pelvic floor. It also discusses general mechanisms such as the balance between the lower urinary tract and the nervous system,

and can therefore be largely extrapolated to the situation in other groups of patients.

Previous classification systems used several designations to describe functional disorders of the bladder, but one of the problems was that the focus was almost exclusively on motor disorders (instability and hyperreflexia) (Abrams et al 1988). If no such urodynamic hyperactivity was found, it was assumed that the disorder was sensory, and was consequently grouped under the heading hypersensitivity. Because of the imperfection of this older system and the difficulties in arriving at a better classification based on pathophysiological criteria in terms of structure and function, it was decided to introduce the symptom-based broad surrogate term OAB (Abrams et al 2002). The definition of OAB, however, also states that organically caused disease should first be ruled out before the diagnosis of OAB is considered. On the other hand it can be said that functional disorders in the lower urinary tract are probably always accompanied by organic changes, even if these are not yet all defined. Functional changes of this kind therefore do not occur in isolation without causing organic changes in affected neurons and target cells/organs. The current classification therefore also means that pathological processes that can result in symptoms of overactivity, but have not yet done so are omitted from the OAB group as can be seen in Fig. 9.8 (Mattiasson 2004).

Interestingly, the scientific community took the opposite course from when it abandoned the organ-specific term 'prostatism' in favour of the more general lower urinary tract symptoms (LUTS) (Abrams 1994). In OAB the panorama of symptoms is instead tied to one organ, the bladder, which might be seen as unfortunate. However, for the patients and their communication with health care staff in the field, such as GPs and district nurses, OAB is a useful term (Fig. 9.9) because patients believe they understand what kind of disorder

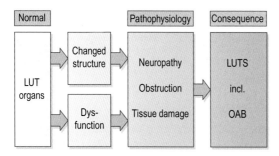

Fig. 9.8 Schematic representation of the development of disease from normality to pathophysiology with or without consequences such as for example lower urinary tract symptoms (LUTS) and/or overactive bladder (OAB) (Based on Mattiasson 2004, with permission.)

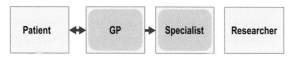

Fig. 9.9 Overactive bladder is a useful term in communication between patients and for example the GP, but is less meaningful for the specialist or researcher who might be more interested in the underlying disease process than in symptoms only.

they have. When differential diagnoses have been considered and diseases that require further investigation and treatment are ruled out, one can start attempts at treatment. For various categories of specialists working for example in gynaecology, urology, paediatrics and geriatrics, OAB is not a particularly useful term.

Whatever the terminology, ever since the initial term 'unstable detrusor' was coined three decades ago, the focus has been on the bladder (Bates et al 1976). Although the bladder plays a central role, it would have been better if a holistic outlook had been adopted instead, considering all the parts of the lower urinary tract at the same time. This means that apart from the bladder and its contents one should look at all other parts of the lower urinary tract, including the outflow, urethra, vagina, pelvic floor and supporting structures, and also consider the nervous system and the lower urinary tract simultaneously. It is only when all the involved parts of the lower urinary tract and the parts of the nervous system that influence the micturition cycle are taken into consideration, as well as all the parts of the micturition cycle, that there is a chance of obtaining a complete picture. With such a covering framework new diagnostic recognition patterns based on pathophysiology in terms of structure and function can be created and identified (Mattiasson 2001, 2004).

OVERACTIVITY AND ORGANIC CHANGES

As long as one regards either nervous structures or muscles as the origin of overactivity, one can speak of neurogenic and myogenic factors. The focus on the bladder that has prevailed for a long time in overactivity is probably also due to the fact that many of the studies have been of an experimental kind and often performed in animals. Myogenic factors have been considered significant by some authors (Brading 1997, Turner & Brading 1997), whereas neurogenic factors at times have been regarded as more important by others (Andersson & Persson 2003, de Groat 1997, Gillespie 2004). In this context myogenic changes mean increased irritability of the detrusor muscle cells, for example, in the form of supersensitivity. Hypoxia as a subsidiary phenomenon in obstruction with bladder wall thickening and decreased blood flow during detrusor contractions has also been assumed to be a potentially important aetiological factor (Brading et al 2004). Both primary and induced changes in the central nervous system (CNS) have been described as important factors in overactivity of the bladder (Steers et al. 1990). A non-neurogenic release from the urothelium has been suggested to be of importance in detrusor overactivity (Yoshida et al 2002). When discussing which factors are more significant, the neurogenic or the myogenic, it is worth considering which two components, wood or oxygen, is most important for the fire.

The relationship between the lower urinary tract and the nervous system is balanced so that it normally permits the two diametrically different functions of filling and voiding urine and allows smooth switches between these functions (Morrison et al 2001). In both modes, filling and voiding, stable conditions are required. The system is at the same time threatened by lability with an increasing degree of filling because an increased readiness to void is built up in the course of filling. There is a clear, but no absolute, correlation between bladder content volume and the appearance of overactivity. With higher degrees of stimulation than normal and/or lowered thresholds for outflow of signals, stimulating the triggering of voiding or promoting voiding activity, conditions exist for speaking about overactivity. This can therefore be afferent or afferent + efferent, and probably only rarely efferent only. As discussed below, it is reasonable to assume that afferent activity is the driving force in the occurrence of overactivity.

When inhibition of the micturition reflex is voluntarily withdrawn micturition should be triggered without delay, and voiding through positive feedback is impelled until voiding is complete. Further lability can easily be added during the filling phase through stimulation   of   excitation-promoting   voiding-stimulating factors and/or loss of functions that have an inhibitory effect on storage-promoting activity. Increasing afferent nervous activity from the bladder to the CNS results in increased motor activation of the striated musculature in the urethral sphincter and the pelvic floor, which can easily be observed, for example, via electromyography (EMG) during cystometry. At the same time, the activity in the voiding-promoting nerves is effectively inhibited. It is also conceivable that the increased activity and increased tension in the external urethral sphincter and in the pelvic floor musculature generate afferent activity, which in turn, at the level of the CNS, has an inhibitory effect on the activation of voiding-promoting mechanisms (Fig. 9.10) (de Groat et al 2001).

In recent years researchers have studied afferent nerves and, as far as it is possible, afferent mechanisms related to the bladder. This has confirmed an abundant innervation superficially in the mucosa and submucosa of the bladder and also demonstrated the existence of interstitial cells, the role of which is unknown, but has been interpreted as an impulse generator, perhaps with a pacemaker-like function (Gillespie et al 2004, Shafik et al 2004). We know in addition that afferent nerves send antidromal axons in an efferent direction (Maggi 1990), probably for regulation of sensory thresholds. Nitrogen oxide (NO), prostaglandins, purines (ATP), and neuropeptides can be of significance for direct communication through the mucosal lining of the bladder (i.e. between the bladder content and superficial nerve endings). Gradually a picture that differs from the traditional view of the function of the bladder is emerging. One difficulty with all these observations, of course, is

that under experimental conditions we know very little about the sensory experience at the level of the CNS that may ensue from stimulation. It is therefore possible that not only the volume of the bladder but also the composition of the urine generates signals that are important for the way the bladder reacts under normal circumstances and in disease (Andersson 2001).

THE ROLE OF THE URETHRA AND THE PELVIC FLOOR

The bladder cannot alone explain all the problems related to overactivity; such activity often seems to be initiated from the urethra/pelvic floor or the nervous system. A broader view is illustrated in Fig. 9.11, which attempts to show a shift of focus in the consideration of lower urinary tract problems of OAB type. From comprising only the bladder, it now includes the outflow part, the urethra, vagina and pelvic floor during both filling and voiding.

When we define overactivity and concomitant urgency as storage-related symptoms, we proceed from the current (old) definition of the different parts of the micturition cycle.

As illustrated in Fig. 9.12 it seems natural to see the switch from storage to voiding at the moment when the storage pattern is stopped in favour of voiding-promoting activity (new). We should consequently include in the voiding phase the pressure drop in the urethra that starts the act of micturition. The overactivity

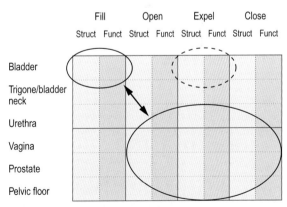

Fig. 9.11   Instead of just looking at the filling and voiding of the bladder, as is now common (e.g. cystometry), the picture can be more all-embracing if one includes outflow with the urethra and surrounding structures. The entire micturition cycle and all parts of the lower urinary tract should be considered when assessing all types of functional disorders.

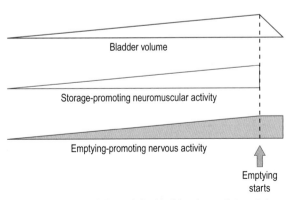

Fig. 9.10   During filling of the bladder the activity of the external sphincter gradually increases. At the same time an increased readiness to empty is built up. A disturbance of the storage-promoting activity can easily change the balance in favour of emptying-promoting activity.

of motor type that occurs during the storage phase and can be interpreted as a premature micturition reflex, normal or not, is by definition voiding activity, and the symptoms that we regard, according to the current definition, as storage-related, could probably better be described as emptying-related. The pressure drop in the urethra for this reason comes into focus as the initial motor event, or one of the initial events, in lower urinary tract activation in connection with micturition, and possibly also in overactivity. Urethral pressure drop has long been neglected or inadequately treated (McGuire 1978). The relaxation of the dominant striated musculature in the urethra is due to inhibited efferent activity during voiding of the bladder.

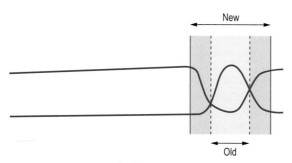

Fig. 9.12 The present (old) and suggested new division of the micturition cycle into storage and emptying phases. The storage pattern is broken when the urethral pressure falls at the initiation of micturition.

What relaxes the smooth musculature is not a question that clinicians have asked, but in experimental studies in vivo and in vitro in both humans and animals, a nerve-mediated relaxation has been found (Andersson et al 1983). If one stimulates the sacral roots of an anaesthetized person with paralysed striated muscles, one can induce a pressure drop in the urethra at the sphincter level (Torrens 1978; Fig. 9.13A). Several substances that can be described as non-adrenergic non-cholinergic (NANC) are interesting as transmitters or neuromodulators, among them nitric oxide (NO), calcitonin gene-related peptide (CGRP), and vasoactive intestinal polypeptide (VIP) (Andersson 2001, Gillespie 2005, Gillespie et al 2004, Radziszewski et al 2003, Fig. 9.13B). This relaxatory activity is probably of great significance for the normal function of the urethra, and it seems likely that these nerves could also be involved in overactivity. It seems that not just smooth musculature but also contracted submucous tissue can be relaxed via the same type of nerves (Mattiasson et al 1985).

Is there anything to suggest that the pelvic floor plays an important part in OAB? The answer is yes. In women with OAB, specifically in those with urge or mixed incontinence an impaired pelvic floor muscle function is found, in the same way as in women with stress incontinence. There is a significant difference in degree of activation compared with continent women of the same age and with an equivalent degree of parity. These findings led to the conclusion that the same disease gives rise to the different symptoms of stress and urge incontinence (Fig. 9.14) (Gunnarsson & Mattiasson 1994, 1999).

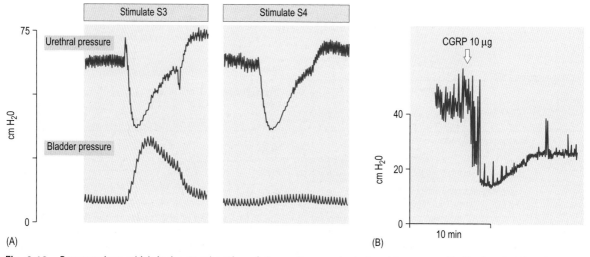

Fig. 9.13 Pressure drop, which is due to relaxation of the urethra, can be induced in an anaesthetized patient in whom the sacral ventral nerve roots are stimulated electrically (A), in rats exposed to intra-arterial injection of the neuropeptide calcitonin gene-related peptide (CGRP) (B). (A from Torrens 1978, with permission, and B from Radziszewski et al 2003, with permission).

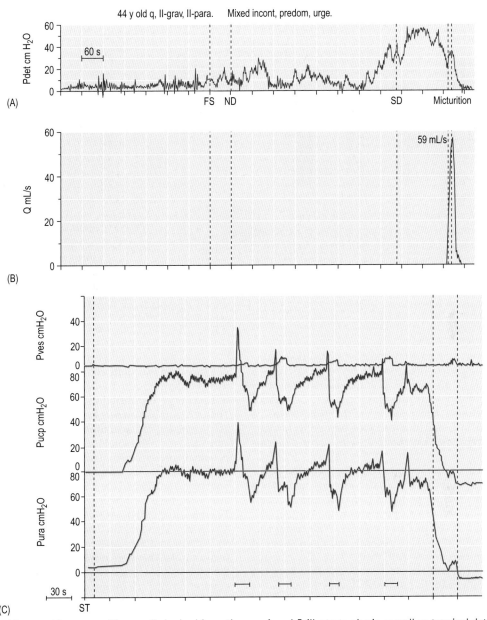

Fig. 9.14 44-year-old woman with so-called mixed incontinence. A and B illustrate phasic as well as terminal detrusor overactivity during cystometry and a forceful emptying reflected by the urinary flow curve with a fast acceleration of flow (steep curve). Pressure measurements in the bladder and the urethra in the high-pressure zone are shown in (C). The patient squeezed repeatedly around a urethral pressure-measuring catheter (bars). The influence of the squeeze procedure on the intra-abdominal pressure was small. An unsuccessful attempt at raised pressure gives way to rapid pressure drop and a slower return to the original pressure level. The pattern is a recurrent finding which is more pronounced the more pronounced the problems the patient has. (Pdet, detrusor pressure; Q, urine flow rate; pucp, urethral closure pressure, pura, intraurethral pressure, pves, intravesical pressure.)

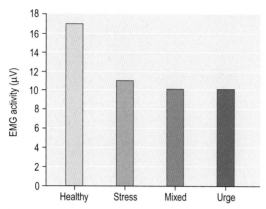

Fig. 9.15 A significant impairment of the maximal electromyographic (EMG) activity of the pelvic musculature when squeezing is seen in women with stress, mixed, and urge incontinence compared with normal matched controls. No differences in the impairment of pelvic musculature function were found in the different incontinent groups. (From Gunnarsson & Mattiasson 1999.)

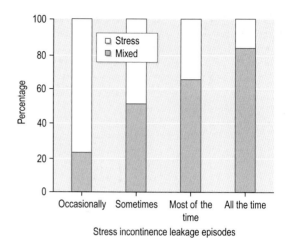

Fig. 9.16 Correlation between the number of stress incontinence leakage episodes and presence of overactive bladder (OAB) symptoms in middle-aged Swedish women. OAB is more prevalent in women with frequent stress leakage episodes. (From Teleman et al 2004, with permission).

Moreover, women with impaired pelvic floor function and impaired squeezing ability seem to have a tendency for a pressure drop in the urethra instead of achieving the desired pressure increase. The balance between closing and opening mechanisms seems to have been lost, and this becomes especially obvious with provocation, for example, with short squeezes (Fig. 9.15).

Even if the pattern of interaction between the pelvic floor musculature and the striated external sphincter is not well charted, we understand that in normal conditions they interact in a purposeful way to maintain continence both at rest and under stress. With rising age, the intraurethral pressure declines and the number of striated muscle fibres and neurons in the external sphincter decreases (Koelbl et al 2001). This does not automatically lead to functional disorders that cause incontinence, but the margins that make it possible to compensate for the consequences of earlier trauma with lesions affecting muscles and nerves, and for diseases, inactivity and fatigue, are reduced, so that incontinence and other symptoms can arise (see Fig. 9.2).

With this decreased ability to close the urethra at rest and under stress, it seems to be easier for opening relaxatory mechanisms to take effect. The more powerful this relaxatory activity is, the more probable that the patient also feels urgency. Insufficiency and overactivity of the urethra and the bladder could therefore be present, in principle, in both female stress, mixed and urge incontinence, albeit in different proportions. Intraurethral

pressure drop was more common than detrusor overactivity in a large group of women with symptoms of OAB wet (i.e. urge and mixed incontinence; Teleman 2003). That stress incontinence to some extent is caused by active opening of the urethra and more powerful relaxatory activity of this kind is combined with an increased potential for sensations such as urgency agrees well with the fact that the more pronounced the stress incontinence is, the more likely it is that it seems to be associated with urge problems (Fig. 9.16; Bump et al 2003, Teleman et al 2004). We also see how the urine flow accelerates significantly faster when micturition has started in incontinent subjects compared with symptom-free controls. The more urgency there is in the picture, the faster the opening mechanism. In women with pronounced symptoms of mixed and urge incontinence, a pronounced detrusor activity is frequently observed, often with 'post-contractions' after voiding is concluded. It is known that urethral instability can occur in symptom-free women, but also and more frequently in combination with urge incontinence (Farrell & Tynski 1996). This detail squares well with the view that urethral relaxation is a central phenomenon in female incontinence.

It has for the reasons given above been suggested that a neuromuscular disorder of the pelvic floor muscles and the urethra presents itself as an overactive opening mechanism. There is a great deal to suggest that the same pathophysiological mechanism is active in both stress and urge incontinence, and the differences could be described as being of degree rather than of kind. Women with urge incontinence perhaps also have an element of stress incontinence, but with a pronounced urge component it can be difficult to detect. It is also conceivable that insufficiency and overactivity are related to the different forms of incontinence as shown in Fig. 9.17.

CONCLUSION

It is possible to combine old opinions with currently established views and new suggestions to arrive at a single, coherent picture of overactivity as long as one retains a holistic outlook and recognizes that overactivity is due to the loss of balance between the lower urinary tract and the nervous system, and that the changes always involve both these parts. The perspective should be cause ± effect instead of the reverse. For the nervous system, overactivity can refer to afferent as well as efferent innervation, and CNS as well as peripheral structures. With a new division of the micturition cycle it is also easy to see why changes on the outflow side (e.g. with weakness in the pelvic floor musculature), can leave scope for mechanisms that initiate

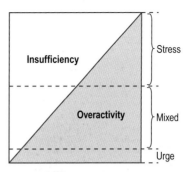

Fig. 9.17 Both urethral insufficiency and lower urinary tract overactivity can be assumed to be present in various proportions in all female stress, urge and mixed incontinence.

opening of the urethra, activation of the micturition reflex, and often also a feeling of urgency. Improved balance is achieved by trying to reverse the course represented by the arrow in Fig. 9.1, p. 168. This can be accomplished with pelvic floor muscle training, drugs, surgery, electric stimulation, or best of all, prophylactic measures so that the journey down the arrow never starts.

REFERENCES

Abrams P 1994 New words for old: lower urinary tract symptoms for 'prostatism'. BMJ 308(6934):929–930

Abrams P, Blaivas J G, Stanton S L et al 1988 The standardisation of terminology of lower urinary tract function. The International Continence Society Committee on Standardisation of Terminology. Scandinavian Journal of Urology and Nephrology. Supplementum 114:5–19

Abrams P, Cardozo L, Fall M et al 2002 The standardisation of terminology of lower urinary tract function: report from the Standardisation Sub-committee of the International Continence Society. Neurourology and Urodynamics 21(2):167–178

Andersson K E 2001 Neurotransmission and drug effects in urethral smooth muscle. Scandinavian Journal of Urology and Nephrology. Supplementum 207:26–34

Andersson K E, Mattiasson A, Sjogren C 1983 Electrically induced relaxation of the noradrenaline contracted isolated urethra from rabbit and man. The Journal of Urology 129(1):210–214

Andersson K E, Pehrson R 2003 CNS involvement in overactive bladder: pathophysiology and opportunities for pharmacological intervention. Drugs 63:2595–2611

Bates P, Bradley W E, Glen E et al 1976 First report on the standardisation of terminology of lower urinary tract function. Urinary incontinence. Procedures related to the evaluation of urine storage: cystometry, urethral closure pressure profile, units of measurements. British Journal of Urology 48:39–42

Brading A F 1997 A myogenic basis for the overactive bladder. Urology 50(6A suppl):57–67

Brading A, Pessina F, Esposito L et al 2004 Effects of metabolic stress and ischaemia on the bladder, and the relationship with bladder overactivity. Scandinavian Journal of Urology and Nephrology. Supplementum (215):84–92

Bump R C, Norton P A, Zinner N R et al 2003 Duloxetine Urinary Incontinence Study Group. Mixed urinary incontinence symptoms: urodynamic findings, incontinence severity, and treatment response. Obstetrics and Gynecology 102(1):76–83

de Groat W C 1997 A neurologic basis for the overactive bladder. Urology 50(suppl 6A):36–52

de Groat W C 2004 The urothelium in overactive bladder: passive bystander or active participant? Urology 64(6 suppl 1):7–11

de Groat W C, Fraser M O, Yoshiyama M et al 2001 Neural control of the urethra. Scandinavian Journal of Urology and Nephrology. Supplementum (207):35–43

Farrell S A, Tynski G 1996 The effect of urethral pressure variation on detrusor activity in women. International Urogynecology Journal and Pelvic Floor Dysfunction 7(2):87–93

Gillespie J I 2004 The autonomous bladder: a view of the origin of bladder overactivity and sensory urge. BJU International 93(4):478–483

Gillespie J I 2005 Inhibitory actions of calcitonin gene-related peptide and capsaicin: evidence for local axonal reflexes in the bladder wall. BJU International 95(1):149–156

Gillespie J I, Markerink-van Ittersum M, de Vente J 2004 cGMP-generating cells in the bladder wall: identification of distinct networks of interstitial cells. BJU International 94(7):1114–1124

Gunnarsson M, Mattiasson A 1994 Circumvaginal surface electromyography in women with urinary incontinence and in healthy volunteers. Scand Journal Urology and Nephrology (Suppl) 157:89–95

Gunnarsson M, Mattiasson A 1999 Female stress, urge, and mixed urinary incontinence are associated with a chronic and progressive pelvic floor/vaginal neuromuscular disorder: an investigation of 317 healthy and incontinent women using vaginal surface electromyography. Neurourology and Urodynamics 18(6):613–621

Koelbl H, Mostwin J, Boiteux J P et al 2001 Pathophysiology. In: Abrams P, Cardozo L, Khoury S et al (eds) Incontinence. Health Publication, Plymouth, UK, p 205–241

Maggi C A 1990 The dual function of capsaicin-sensitive sensory nerves in the bladder and urethra. Ciba Foundation Symposium 151:77–83

Mattiasson A 2001 Characterisation of lower urinary tract disorders: a new view. Neurourology and Urodynamics 20(5):601–621

Mattiasson A 2004 Classification of lower urinary tract dysfunction. In: Corcos J, Schick E (eds) Textbook of the neurogenic bladder – adults and children. Martin Dunitz, London, p 469–480

Mattiasson A, Andersson K E, Sjögren C 1985 Contractant and relaxant properties of the female rabbit urethral submucosa. The Journal of Urology 133(2):304–310

McGuire E J 1978 Reflex urethral instability. British Journal of Urology 50(3):200–204

Milsom I, Abrams P, Cardozo L et al 2001 How widespread are the symptoms of an ovaractive bladder and how are they managed? A population-based prevalence study. BJU International 87(9):760–766

Morrison J, Steers W D, Brading A et al 2001 Neurophysiology and neuropharmacology. In: Abrams P, Cardozo L, Khoury S et al (eds) Incontinence, Health Publication, Plymouth, p 83–163

Radziszewski P, Soller W, Mattiasson A 2003 Calcitonin gene-related peptide and substance P induce pronounced motor effects in the female rat urethra in vivo. Scand J Urol Nephrol 37(4):275–280

Shafik A, El-Sibai O, Shafik A A et al 2004 Identification of interstitial cells of Cajal in human urinary bladder: concept of vesical pacemaker. Urology 64(4):809–813

Steers W D, Ciambotti J, Erdman S et al 1990 Morphological plasticity in efferent pathways to the urinary bladder of the rat following urethral obstruction. The Journal of Neuroscience 10(6):1943–1951

Stewart W F, Van Rooyen J B, Cundiff G W et al 2003 Prevalence and burden of overactive bladder in the United States. World Journal of Urology 20(6):327–336

Teleman P 2003 Urinary incontinence in middle-aged women – a population-based study on prevalence, risk factors and the role of the urethra [thesis, ISBN 91-628-5917-X]. University of Lund, Sweden

Teleman P, Gunnarsson M, Lidfeldt J et al 2002 Urodynamic characterisation of women with naive urinary incontinence: a population-based study in subjectively incontinent and healthy 53–63 years old women. European Urology 42(6):583–589

Teleman P T, Lidfeldt J, Nerbrand C et al 2004 Overactive bladder: prevalence, risk factors and relation to stress incontinence in middle-aged women. BJOG 111(6):600

Torrens M J 1978 Urethral sphincteric responses to stimulation of the sacral nerves in the human female. Urologia Internationalis 33:22–26

Turner W H, Brading A F 1997 Smooth muscle of the bladder in the normal and the diseased state: pathophysiology, diagnosis and treatment. Pharmacology & Therapeutics 75(2):77–110

Yoshida M, Inadome A, Murakami S et al 2002 Effects of age and muscle stretching on acetylcholine release in isolated human bladder smooth muscle [Abstract 160]. The Journal of Urology 167:40

BLADDER TRAINING FOR OVERACTIVE BLADDER

Jean F Wyman

INTRODUCTION

Bladder training has been advocated as a treatment for overactive bladder (OAB) symptoms (e.g. urgency, frequency, urgency incontinence and nocturia) in women since the late 1960s (Jeffcoate & Francis 1966). It has also been recommended as a treatment for mixed urinary incontinence and stress urinary incontinence (Fantl et al 1996, Wilson et al 2005). Bladder training is used in primary and secondary care settings with adult patients who are cognitively and physically intact and highly motivated (Hadley 1986, Wallace et al 2004). The goal of bladder training is to restore normal bladder function through a process of patient education along with a mandatory or self-adjustable voiding regimen that gradually increases the time interval between voidings. How bladder training achieves its effects is unclear (Fantl 1998). Several explanations have been proposed including that bladder training results in:

- improved cortical inhibition over involuntary detrusor contractions (Fantl et al 1981);

- improved cortical facilitation over urethral closure during bladder filling (Fantl et al 1991)

- improved central modulation of afferent sensory impulses (Fantl et al 1991);

- the individual becoming more knowledgeable and aware of the circumstances that cause incontinence and so changing behaviour in ways that increase the 'reserve capacity' of the lower urinary tract system (Fantl et al 1991, Wyman et al 1998).

Bladder training offers the advantages of being simple, relatively inexpensive, and free from unpleasant side-effects (Wyman & Fantl 1991). This makes it particularly attractive for use in older adults, particularly those with high comorbidity who are already on multiple drug regimens and for whom OAB drug therapy, because of its anticholinergic properties, would place them at a higher risk for adverse drug effects (Wyman 2005). Bladder training can be used alone or in combination with drug therapy or with other forms of conservative treatment such as pelvic floor muscle training (PFMT).

This chapter will describe the evidence base for the use of bladder training in the prevention and treatment of OAB in adults. Comment will be made on the systematic literature reviews of bladder training as well as the methodological quality of individual studies. Clinical recommendations on the use of bladder training in OAB with adults will be provided.

BLADDER TRAINING PROTOCOLS

Bladder training consists of three main components: patient education about the bladder, incontinence, and urgency control strategies; a scheduled voiding regimen that gradually extends the inter-voiding intervals (Wallace et al 2004); and positive reinforcement techniques provided by a health care professional (Fantl et al 1996). How these components are delivered varies considerably in practice. In early bladder training protocols, bladder training (also referred to as bladder discipline, bladder drill, bladder re-education, and bladder retraining) was conducted through 5–13 days of hospitalization to ensure mandatory adherence to a strict voiding schedule; voiding off schedule was not permitted even if incontinence resulted (Jeffcoate & Francis 1966). Patients were given anticholinergic drug therapy or sedatives to help cope with severe urgency. In a modification of this approach, Frewen found that patients with less severe symptoms could be treated on an outpatient basis (Frewen 1979, 1980). The duration of the treatment programme, however, increased to 3 months. He added the strategy of self-monitoring by having patients record their micturitions and voided volumes on a voiding chart. Subsequently, Fantl et al (1981) observed that outcomes were similar for patients who received bladder training without the use of anticholinergic drug therapy as for those who did.

A number of variations became incorporated in bladder training protocols as they evolved over the decades. Outpatient programmes became more widespread, varying from 6 to 12 weeks in duration (Wilson et al 2005). Self-adjustable schedules permitted patients to void off schedule with severe urgency if they perceived an incontinent episode was imminent (Wyman & Fantl 1991). Education on urgency suppression strategies such as distraction and relaxation techniques and/or use of pelvic floor muscle contraction provided patients with specific methods to control urgency episodes. Fluid and caffeine modifications might be recommended (Bryant et al 2002); however, in clinical trials this generally has been avoided to test the effect of bladder training as a sole intervention. Alternative delivery strategies have been incorporated into clinical practice or trials such as facsimile machine submission of voiding diaries with weekly telephone feedback (Visco et al 1999), a simplification of the teaching method using a brief written instruction sheet (Mattiassion et al

2003), and use of a programmable electronic voiding timing device (Davila & Primozich 1998).

PREVENTION

There are no studies testing bladder training as a sole intervention in the prevention of OAB in adults. There is therefore no evidence on the effect of bladder training in preventing or delaying OAB on which to base clinical practice decisions (Wilson et al 2005).

TREATMENT

Overview

This section describes the evidence base for bladder training as a treatment for OAB symptoms in adults. Bladder training has been:

- used as a sole treatment;
- compared to another treatment (conservative or pharmacological);
- used as an adjunct treatment in combination with another treatment (conservative or pharmacological); and
- used to enhance the benefit of pharmacological treatment.

Comment will be made on the search strategy and selection criteria used in selecting studies included in the evidence base, the systematic literature reviews on bladder training, as well as the methodological qualities of the included studies as they relate to the type of comparison being made using the PEDro Quality Scale (www.pedro.fhs.edu.au).

The following criteria were used to distinguish levels of evidence based on a modification of criteria proposed by Berghmans et al (2000).

- To conclude there was **strong evidence for or against bladder training** for OAB patients at least three high-quality studies with a PEDro score of 6 or greater were needed.

- The conclusion of **weak evidence for bladder training** required at least three high-quality studies with inconsistent results (e.g. 25–75% considered positive), or at least three low-quality studies with PEDro scores less than 6 with consistent results in favour of bladder training.

- To conclude that there is **weak evidence against bladder training**, there needed to be at least three low-quality studies with consistent results against bladder training on at least one outcome measure (e.g. urgency, urinary frequency, nocturia, or urgency incontinence).

- The conclusion of insufficient evidence was based on low-quality studies with inconsistent results or with fewer than three studies of whatever quality.

The following computerized databases were searched (1980–2005): MEDLINE, CINAHL, and Cochrane Collaboration using keywords urinary incontinence, urgency incontinence, overactive bladder, detrusor overactivity, detrusor hyperactivity, detrusor instability, urgency, frequency, nocturia, conservative management, conservative treatment, nonsurgical treatment, bladder training, behavioural techniques, behavioural therapy, physical therapy, adult, aged, and clinical trial. (In addition, hand searching of journals and International Continence Society's conference proceedings, and reference lists of relevant articles and the recent Cochrane Collaboration review of bladder training were searched for relevant trials.

Studies were included if they met the following criteria:

- bladder training in at least one treatment arm alone;

- comparison of bladder training with another treatment in one arm versus a comparison of the other treatment alone;

- results for participants with urgency incontinence, urodynamic detrusor overactivity (previously diagnosed as detrusor instability), OAB with or without urinary incontinence are reported exclusively or separately from those for participants with mixed urinary incontinence

- published full length report; and

- trial report published in English.

Systematic literature reviews

Several systematic reviews have been published that provide qualitative synthesis with evidence grading on bladder training in the treatment of urinary incontinence or urgency urinary incontinence (Berghmans et al 2000, Wallace et al 2004; Wilson et al 2005). The Cochrane Collaboration published a quantitative analysis of randomized controlled trial (RCT) data (Wallace et al 2004). Each review varies in its objectives, methodology, and the number and type of studies included. These variations contribute to differences in the conclusions regarding the effect of bladder training.

Berghmans et al (2000) focused their review on RCTs that assessed physical therapies including bladder training as well as other forms of conservative therapies used in the treatment of urgency incontinence. Of the nine bladder training trials they located that met inclusion criteria, they concluded that there was only weak evidence to suggest that bladder training is more effective than no treatment, and that bladder training is better than drug therapy.

The Cochrane Collaboration published an updated review that included quantitative analyses of 10 RCTs (n = 1366 participants) on five pre-specified primary outcomes:

- participant's perception of cure of urinary incontinence;
- participant's perception of improvement of urinary incontinence;
- number of incontinent episodes;
- number of micturitions; and
- quality of life (Wallace et al 2004).

Adverse events were also noted.

Their review is limited to RCTs with participants who had urinary incontinence; OAB studies where it could not be determined that participants had urinary incontinence were excluded. However, subanalyses did examine urgency incontinence as a variable. The review focused on testing three hypotheses:

- bladder training is better than no bladder training for the management of urinary incontinence;
- bladder training is better than other treatments (such as conservative or pharmacological); and
- combining bladder training with another treatment is better than the other treatment alone.

The Cochrane Group concluded there was inconclusive evidence to judge the effects of bladder training in both the short and long term. The results of the trials reviewed tended to favour bladder training, especially with urgency incontinence, however the trials were of variable quality, small size, and with wide confidence intervals. They found no evidence of adverse effects. They also concluded that there was not enough evidence to determine whether bladder training was useful as a supplement to another therapy.

The International Consultation on Incontinence (ICI) (Wilson et al 2005) recently updated its systematic review that addressed a broader set of questions than the Cochrane review:

- Can bladder training prevent urinary incontinence?
- What is the most appropriate bladder training protocol?
- Is bladder training better than no treatment, placebo or control treatments for urinary incontinence?
- Is bladder training better than other treatments?

- Does the addition of other treatments add a benefit to bladder training or does the addition of bladder training to other treatments add any benefit?
- What is the effect of bladder training on other LUTS?
- What factors might affect the outcomes of bladder training?

In contrast to the Cochrane review, the ICI included RCTs with participants who had urinary incontinence (urgency, stress, and mixed incontinence) as well as participants who had OAB without urinary incontinence. Fourteen RCTs (n = 1567) were included. The ICI concluded that from the few trials available for women with urgency, stress, and mixed incontinence bladder training is more effective than no treatment, but there was insufficient evidence to draw conclusions on its effect in men. They also found that there was insufficient evidence to draw conclusions on the comparative effectiveness of bladder training and current drug therapy, and the additional benefit of combining drug therapy with bladder training and vice versa. The ICI reported that there was good evidence that bladder training reduces urgency, frequency, and nocturia, and concluded that cognitively intact older persons respond well to bladder training, which appears to have equal benefit in older and younger persons.

Trial comparisons

Fourteen RCTs on bladder training were located; of these, only 10 (n = 1300; majority female) met the criteria for inclusion in this review. A summary of these trials is presented in Table 9.5, with a rating of their quality using the PEDro scale in Table 9.6. Overall, the PEDro rating of these studies ranged from 2 to 9. With the exception of three trials (Fantl et al 1991, Mattiasson et al 2003, Wyman et al 1998), these trials included small sample sizes with groups less than 50 participants.

Bladder training versus no treatment or control

Three RCTs of sufficient methodological quality (PEDro scores ≥5) compared the effect of bladder training to no treatment (Fantl et al 1991, Jarvis & Millar 1980, Yoon et al 2003). The results favoured bladder training in improving incontinent episodes and the symptoms of urgency incontinence as well as urinary frequency, urgency, and nocturia. In one study, bladder training also led to increased voided volumes (Yoon et al 2003). Overall, there is weak evidence that bladder training is more effective than no treatment (control) in controlling OAB symptoms.

Bladder training versus other treatments

Four trials were located in which bladder training was compared to other treatments: PFMT in two studies of sufficient methodological quality (Wyman et al 1998, Yoon et al 2003), and drug therapy in two studies of low quality (Columbo et al 1995, Jarvis 1981). There have been no published trials comparing bladder training to electrical stimulation, incontinence devices, or surgical management.

Bladder training versus bladder training and other treatments The two trials comparing bladder training to PFMT had varying sample sizes. In the one trial with over 50 participants in each treatment arm, slightly less than half of the participants had OAB symptoms (48.5%), whereas the number of women who actually had detrusor overactivity was less than a quarter of the sample (24.5%). Although more women reported they were much or somewhat better with PFMT than bladder training, the difference did not reach statistical significance after treatment or 3 months later. Similarly, although women in the PFMT group had fewer incontinent episodes per day than those in the bladder training group, the difference was not statistically significant at 3 or 6 months post-treatment (Wyman et al 1998). The results in a sufficient-quality RCT that compared an 8-week outpatient bladder training programme to biofeedback-assisted PFMT and a no-treatment control group (Yoon et al 2003) are difficult to interpret because of low power and unclear reporting of incontinent episodes and between-group changes. No significant differences at post-treatment were found between groups on amount of leaked urine on a clinic pad test. The bladder training group was found to result in a significant decrease in micturition and nocturia, and a significant increase in voided volume; the other two groups did not change significantly. With only two trials, small sample sizes and a limited number of OAB participants, there is only weak evidence that bladder training is more effective than PFMT in the treatment for urgency incontinence and OAB.

Two small sample RCTs compared bladder training to drugs that were available before 1995 (Columbo et al 1995, Jarvis 1981) and both are of low methodological quality. One study found that inpatient bladder training as compared to outpatient drug therapy (flavoxate and imipramine) was more effective in reducing OAB symptoms (Jarvis 1981). Columbo et al (1995) found that a 6-week course of 5 mg oxybutynin chloride (immediate release, IR) three times a day had a similar clinical cure rate (e.g. self-reported total disappearance of urgency incontinence, no protective pads, or further treatment) as bladder training. The relapse rate at 6 months was

Table 9.5 Randomized controlled trials on bladder training to treat overactive bladder and/or urgency urinary incontinence

Trial	Bryant et al 2002
Design	2-arm RCT: BT, BT and caffeine reduction
n	95 women and men with urinary symptoms mean age 57 (SD 17)
Diagnosis	Clinical assessment time/volume/ caffeine charts indicating urinary urgency, frequency, with or without urgency incontinence and ingested ≥100 mg caffeine/24 h
Training protocol	4-weekly visits BT programme: increase voiding intervals, maintain or increase fluid intake to 2 L/24 h, urge control techniques, cease 'just in case' voiding
Drop-outs	21/95 (22%)
Adherence	Not assessed
Results	No difference between groups on reduction in incontinent episodes/24 h (p = 0.219) Caffeine reduction with BT led to significantly greater decreases than BT alone in urgency (p < 0.002) and urinary frequency (p = 0.037)
Trial	Columbo et al 1995
Design	2-arm RCT: BT, oxybutynin
n	81 women <65 years with urgency urinary incontinence aged 24–65 years; mean 48.5
Diagnosis	Clinical assessment Cystometry Cystoscopy Post-void urine determination Urine culture Voiding diary
Training protocol	6-week outpatient programme, initial interval based on maximal voiding interval, encouraged to hold urine 30 min beyond initial voiding interval, progressively increase interval every 4–5 days to reach goal of 3–4-h voiding interval; at appointments every 2 weeks, encouragement and BT advice provided
Drop-outs	BT arm: 2/39 (5.1%) Drug arm: 4/42 (9.5%)
Adherence	Not reported
Results	BT arm: 27/37 (73%) clinically cured (e.g. no UUI or pad use) vs drug arm 28/38 (74%) at 6 weeks At 6 months, there were less relapses with BT (1/27) vs drug arm (12/28) BT clinically cured 8/13 (62%) with detrusor overactivity, 6/8 (75%) with low compliance bladder, and 13/16 (81%) with OAB without detrusor overactivity vs drug arm: 13/14 (93%), 6/9 (67%), and 9/15 (60%), respectively Significant increase in first desire BT resolved diurnal frequency 20/29 (69%) and nocturia in 11/18 (61%) BT 17/27 (63%) clinically cured with detrusor overactivity returned to stable bladders vs drug 16/28 (57%)

Table 9.5   Randomized controlled trials on bladder training to treat overactive bladder and/or urgency urinary incontinence—cont'd

Trial	Fantl et al 1991
Design	2-arm RCT: BT, 6-week delayed treatment
n	131 women aged ≥55 years with detrusor overactivity with or without genuine stress incontinence or stress incontinence alone; mean (SD) age 67 (8.5)
Diagnosis	Clinical assessment Urodynamics Voiding diary ≥1 incontinent episode per week
Training protocol	6-week outpatient programme, initial voiding schedule based on urinary diary, typically set at 1-h interval during waking hours only; increased by 30 min depending on schedule tolerance; instructed in urge control strategies; encouraged to avoid voiding off schedule but not prohibited, instructed to empty bladder as completely as possible, instructed to maintain usual fluid intake pattern, keep treatment log; at weekly appointments, positive reinforcement, support, and optimism in successful outcome provided
Drop-outs	8/131 (6%) at 6 weeks 20/131 (15.3%) at 6 months
Adherence	Not reported
Results	At 6-week follow-up: 12% were continent and 75% had reduced their incontinence 50% or better on voiding diary with results maintained at 6 months In OAB group, frequency: improved for those with ≥57 micturitions/week Nocturia: unchanged IIQ scores – improved at 6 weeks and maintained at 6 months
Trial	Jarvis 1981
Design	2-arm RCT: inpatient BT, outpatient drug therapy (flavoxate and imipramine)
n	50 women with detrusor overactivity aged 17–78 years; mean (SD) 46.5 (13.6)
Diagnosis	Clinical assessment Cystometry Cystoscopy
Training protocol	Inpatient BT programme (details not provided)
Drop-outs	5/25 (20%) drug therapy group only
Adherence	Not reported
Results	Greater improvement in BT group: 84% became continent and 76% symptom free vs 56% continent and 48% symptom free in drug therapy group Improvements: frequency 76%, nocturia 81%, urgency, 84%; urgency incontinence, 84%
Trial	Jarvis & Millar, 1980
Design	2-arm RCT: inpatient BT, control (e.g. advised that they should be able to hold urine 4 h, be continent, and allowed home)
n	60 women aged 27–79 years with detrusor overactivity
Diagnosis	Clinical assessment Cystoscopy Urethral dilatation

Table 9.5 Randomized controlled trials on bladder training to treat overactive bladder and/or urgency urinary incontinence—cont'd

Training protocol	Inpatient BT programme: initial voiding schedule typically set at 1.5 h during waking hours only; schedule increases by 30 min daily until 4-h interval reached; instructed to wait to assigned time or be incontinent; encouraged to maintain usual fluid intake and keep a fluid intake record; introduced to patient successfully treated by BT
Drop-outs	None reported
Adherence	Not reported
Results	27/30 (90%) became continent and 25/30 (83.3%) symptom free Improvements noted with frequency 83.3%, nocturia 88.8%, urgency 86.7%, and urgency incontinence 90% which were significantly better than control group (p < 0.01)
Trial	Mattaisson et al 2003
Design	2-arm multicentre RCT: BT and tolterodine, tolterodine alone
n	505 women and men (75% women) ≥18 years with OAB with and without urinary incontinence, median age 63
Diagnosis	Symptoms of OAB including ≥8 micturitions/24 h, urgency with or without urgency incontinence as diagnosed by voiding diary
Training protocol	Brief written instruction sheet on BT, emphasize bladder stretching through delaying urination with goal to reduce urinary frequency to 5–6/24 h, urge control techniques, keep voiding diary every other week to chart progress, no other training or follow-up by study personnel
Drop-outs	391/505 (23%) ITT analysis
Adherence	Subsample of the BT group (n = 95) 68% kept voiding diary for 1 day, 72% at 11 weeks, not reported at 23 weeks; 60% kept diary for 7 days at 1 week, 62% at 11 weeks, and 46/56 (82%) at 23 weeks
Results	BT yielded greater reductions in number of voids/24 h (p < 0.001) and volume voided (p < 0.001) No difference in BT + tolterodine compared to tolterodine alone in number of urgency episodes/24 h, incontinent episodes/24 h, and patient perceptions of symptoms
Trial	Wyman et al 1998
Design	3-arm, 2-site RCT: BT, PFMT, combination therapy
n	204 women aged ≥55 years with detrusor overactivity with or without genuine stress incontinence or stress incontinence alone, mean age 61 (SD 9.7)
Diagnosis	Clinical assessment Urodynamics Voiding diary ≥1 incontinent episode per week
Training protocol	12-week outpatient BT programme: 6-week visits (1st 6 weeks), 6 mailed in logs (2nd 6 weeks) Same training protocol as Fantl et al 1991 above
Drop-outs	11/204 (5.4%) at 12 weeks 16/204 (7.8%) at 3 months
Adherence	57% of office visits 85% adherence to voiding schedule during treatment and 44% to voiding schedule 3 months later

Table 9.5   Randomized controlled trials on bladder training to treat overactive bladder and/or urgency urinary incontinence—cont'd

Results	At 12 weeks, BT + PFMT had less incontinent episodes than BT alone (p = 0.004), but by 24 weeks, no differences noted between groups No differences noted in treatment response by urodynamic diagnosis Women with detrusor overactivity had less symptom distress (p = 0.054) and greater improvement in life impact (p = 0.03) at 12 weeks; no differences at 24 weeks
Trial	Yoon et al 2003
Design	3-arm RCT: BT, PFMT, no treatment
n	50 women aged 35–55 with urinary incontinence
Diagnosis	Clinical assessment 30-min pad test ≥1 g urine loss Voiding diary ≥14 voids/48 h
Training protocol	8-week outpatient programme: gradual increases in voiding intervals
Drop-outs	2/BT (9.5%) 2/14 (14.3%) control
Adherence	Not reported
Results	BT group had greater improvements in urinary frequency and nocturia compared to controls (p < 0.01) BT had significant increase in voided volume whereas this was unchanged in control and PFMT groups (p < 0.01) BT group appeared to have greater reduction in UI scores but not significant No differences between groups for amount of leaked urine

BT, bladder training; IIQ, Incontinence Impact Questionnaire; ITT, intention to treat; PFMT, pelvic floor muscle training; UUI, urge urinary incontinence.

higher for the drug group, while those in the bladder training group showed better maintenance of their results. Overall, the weak evidence available tends to favour bladder training with respect to drug therapy available before 1995.

Four trials compared bladder training alone to bladder training with other treatments including placebo treatments (Bryant et al 2002, Szonyi et al 1995, Wiseman et al 1991, Wyman et al 1998). Three RCTs were of sufficient methodological quality (Szonyi et al 1995, Wiseman et al 1991, Wyman et al 1998), whereas one RCT was low quality (Bryant et al 2002). All trials had small sample sizes with the exception of one (Wyman et al 1998).

One trial compared bladder training alone to bladder training with caffeine reduction in adults (combination therapy) with OAB, and found that the combination intervention was more successful than bladder training in reducing urgency episodes (61 vs 12%, respectively) (Bryant et al 2002). Although the combination therapy group also had a greater reduction in incontinent episodes, this was not statistically significant and could

have been affected by low power. Overall, there is insufficient evidence to determine whether bladder training and caffeine reduction for individuals who consume more than 100 mg caffeine daily is superior to bladder training alone.

In one of the sufficient-quality RCTs with a relatively large sample size, Wyman et al (1998) compared a bladder training programme to combination therapy of bladder training and biofeedback-assisted PFMT. Although 94 participants reported urgency incontinence at baseline, much fewer actually had urodynamically diagnosed detrusor overactivity (n = 38). The combination therapy group had significantly greater improvements in incontinent episodes and quality of life scores at 12 weeks than the bladder training group; however, by 24 weeks there were no group differences. Approximately 3 years later, a similar number in each group sought further treatment. Of the women who had not sought further treatment, fewer were free of leakage episodes in the bladder training group than in the combination therapy group (Wyman et al 1999). There is

Table 9.6 PEDro quality score of RCTs in systematic review

E – Eligibility criteria specified
1 – Subjects randomly allocated to groups
2 – Allocation concealed
3 – Groups similar at baseline
4 – Subjects blinded
5 – Therapist administering treatment blinded
6 – Assessors blinded**
7 – Measures of key outcomes obtained from over 85% of subjects
8 – Data analysed by intention to treat
9 – Comparison between groups conducted
10 – Point measures and measures of variability provided*

Study	E	1	2	3*	4	5	6**	7	8	9	10*	Total score
Bryant et al 2002	+	+	−	+	−	−	−	−	−	+	+	4
Castleden et al 1986	−	+	+	−	−	−	−	+	−	+	−	4
Columbo et al 1995	+	+	−	?	−	−	−	+	−	−	−	2
Fantl et al 1991	+	+	−	+	−	−	−	+	−	+	+	5
Jarvis & Millar, 1980	−	+	+	+	−	−	−	+	?	+	−	5
Jarvis 1981	−	+	−	+	−	−	−	+	?	+	−	4
Mattiasson et al 2003	+	+	?	+	−	−	−	−	+	+	+	5
Szonyi et al 1995	+	+	+	−	+	−	+	−	−	+	+	6
Yoon et al 2003	+	+	?	+	−	−	+	+	−	+	+	6
Wiseman et al 1991	+	+	+	?	+	+	+	+	+	+	+	9
Wyman et al 1998	+	+	+	+	−	−	−	+	−	+	+	5

+ = criterion is clearly satisfied; − = criterion is not satisfied; ? = not clear if the criterion was satisfied. Total score is determined by counting the number of criteria that are satisfied, except that scale item one (eligibility criteria specified) is not used to generate the total score. Total scores are out of 10.
*Based on OAB symptoms (e.g. urinary frequency, nocturia, urinary incontinent episodes).
**Blinded to active vs placebo drug; no studies were able to blind for use of bladder training in protocol.

insufficient evidence to conclude whether combination therapy is superior to bladder training alone. The evidence suggests that combination therapy would be superior immediately after treatment, but the long-term effects are less clear. Because of the relatively small sample size, there are insufficient data to draw definitive conclusions regarding the long-term benefit of bladder training, particularly after 24 weeks; it appears that the combination of bladder training and PFMT may lead to longer term benefit, but additional research is needed.

Bladder training and drug therapy versus drug therapy alone One large sufficient-quality RCT com-

pared bladder training and a more recent OAB drug, tolterodine (2 mg twice daily), to the effect of the drug alone in adults with OAB with and without urgency incontinence (Mattiasson et al 2003). In this trial, bladder training significantly augmented drug therapy resulting in reduced voiding frequency and increased volume per void compared to drug alone. However, there was no difference between groups in their reduction of incontinence episodes and urgency episodes. There is therefore insufficient evidence to conclude whether augmenting newer OAB drug therapy with bladder training is helpful for OAB symptoms. The results tend to favour that bladder training does improve urinary frequency;

it is inconclusive, however, whether it adds any benefit with respect to other OAB symptoms. These results may have been influenced by the method of bladder training, which required less teaching and counselling of patients.

SUMMARY

In summary, the evidence base on bladder training comprises relatively few studies, most with small sample sizes and of moderate methodological quality. There is no evidence to judge the benefit of bladder training in the prevention of OAB, and only weak evidence to judge its effectiveness in treatment. Bladder training may be helpful in the short-term treatment of OAB in women, but evidence regarding its long-term effects is inconclusive. There are limited data to draw conclusions about the effects of bladder training in men; none of the studies that included men incorporated a gender sub-analysis. Also, there is insufficient evidence to judge the benefit of bladder training compared to other conservative treatments and current drug therapy. Few trials have reported on adverse events, and only one has reported on adherence. There is weak evidence to guide choices among bladder training, other conservative treatments, and current drug therapies. The additional benefits of combining bladder training with other treatments were inconsistent, though it appeared to be beneficial to add caffeine reduction to bladder training, and this may also improve outcomes associated with PFMT. The additional benefit of combining bladder training with newer drug therapy was not consistently noted on all OAB symptoms.

CLINICAL RECOMMENDATIONS

Bladder training has no known adverse effects and can be used safely as a first-line treatment for OAB in women. Although it may be helpful for men as well, there is insufficient evidence regarding its use. Its effects might be augmented by adding caffeine reduction for individuals who drink more than 100 mg caffeine daily.

Bladder training programmes can be successfully implemented in both outpatient and inpatient settings depending on the health care delivery system and the services covered. The ICI has recommended that bladder training be initiated by assigning an initial voiding interval based on the baseline voiding frequency (Wilson et al 2005). Typically, this is set at a 1-hour interval during waking hours, though a shorter interval (e.g. 30 minutes or less), may be necessary. The schedule is increased by 15–30 minutes per week depending on tolerance to the schedule (i.e. fewer incontinent episodes than the previous week, minimal interruptions to the schedule, and the individual's control over urgency).

Patient education should be provided about normal bladder control and methods to control urgency such as distraction and relaxation techniques including pelvic floor muscle contraction.

Self-monitoring of voiding behaviour using voiding diaries should also be included to help the clinician determine the patient's adherence to the schedule, evaluate progress, and determine whether the voiding interval should be changed.

Clinicians should monitor progress, determine adjustments to the voiding interval, and provide positive reinforcement at least weekly during the training period.

If there is no improvement after 3 weeks of bladder training, the patient should be re-evaluated with consideration given to other treatment options.

If an inpatient bladder training programme is implemented, a more rigid scheduling regimen with progressive increase of the voiding interval on a daily basis is recommended.

REFERENCES

Berghmans L C M, Hendriks H J M, de Bie R A et al 2000 Conservative treatment of urge urinary incontinence in women: A systematic review of randomized clinical trials. BJU International 85:254–263

Byrant C, Dowell C J, Fairbrother G 2002 Caffeine reduction education to improve urinary symptoms. British Journal of Nursing 11:560–565

Castleden C M, Duffin H M, Gulati R S 1986 Double-blind study of imipramine and placebo for incontinence due to bladder instability. Age and Ageing 15(5):299–303

Columbo M, Zanetta G, Scalambrino S et al 1995 Oxybutynin and bladder training in the management of female urinary urge incontinence: a randomized study. International Urogynecology Journal and Pelvic Floor Dysfunction 6(1):63–67

Davila G W, Primozich J 1998 Prospective randomized trial of bladder retraining using an electronic voiding device versus self administered bladder drills in women with detrusor instability [abstract]. Neurourology and Urodynamics 17(4):324–325

Fantl J A 1998 Behavioral intervention for community-dwelling individuals with urinary incontinence. Urology 51(suppl 2A):30–34

Fantl J A, Hurt W G, Dunn L J 1981 Detrusor instability syndrome: the use of bladder retraining drills with and without anticholinergics. American Journal of Obstetrics and Gynecology 140(8):885–890

Fantl J A, Newman D K, Colling J et al 1996 Urinary incontinence in adults: acute and chronic management. Clinical Practice Guideline, No. 2, 1996 Update. US Department of Health and Human Services, Public Health Service, Agency for Health Care Policy and Research, Rockville, MD

Fantl J A, Wyman J F, McClish D K et al 1991 Efficacy of bladder training in older women with urinary incontinence. JAMA 265(5):609–613

Frewen W K 1980 The management of urgency and frequency of micturition. British Journal of Urology 52:367–369

Frewen W K 1979 Role of bladder training in the treatment of the unstable bladder in the female. Urologic Clinics of North America 6(1):273–277

Hadley EC 1986 Bladder training and related therapies for urinary incontinence in older people. JAMA 18(256):372–379

Jarvis G J 1981 A controlled trial of bladder drill and drug therapy in the management of detrusor instability. British Journal of Urology 53(6):565–566

Jarvis G J, Millar D R 1980 Controlled trial of bladder drill for detrusor instability. British Medical Journal 281(6251): 1322–1323

Jeffcoate T N A, Francis W J 1966 Urgency incontinence in the female. American Journal of Obstetrics and Gynecology 94:604–618

Mattiasson A, Blaakaer J, Hoye K et al 2003 Simplified bladder training augments the effectiveness of tolterodine in patients with an overactive bladder. BJU International 91(1):54–60

PEDro, Physiotherapy Evidence Database. Online. Available: www.pedro.fhs.edu.au

Szonyi G, Collas D M, Ding Y Y, Malone-Lee J G 1995 Oxybutynin with bladder retraining for detrusor instability in elderly people: a randomized controlled trial. Age and Ageing 24(4):287–291

Visco A G, Weidner A C, Cundiff G et al 1999 Observed patient compliance with a structured outpatient bladder retraining program. American Journal of Obstetrics and Gynecology 181(6):1392–1394

Wallace S A, Roe B, Williams K et al 2004 Bladder training for urinary incontinence in adults. Cochrane Database of Systematic Reviews 1:CD001308

Wilson P D, Hay-Smith J, Nygaard I, et al 2005 Adult conservative management. In: Abrams P, Cardozo L, Khoury S et al (eds) Incontinence, volume 2. Health Communications Press, Plymouth, UK, p 855–964

Wiseman P A, Malone-Lee J, Rai G S 1991 Terodiline with bladder retraining for treating detrusor instability in elderly people. British Medical Journal 302:944–946

Wyman J F 2005 Behavioral interventions for the patient with overactive bladder. Journal of Wound, Ostomy, and Continence Nursing, 32(3l):S11–S15

Wyman J F, Fantl J A 1991 Bladder training in ambulatory care management of urinary incontinence. Urologic Nursing 11(3):11–17

Wyman J F, Fantl J A, McClish D K et al 1997 Quality of life following bladder training in older women with urinary incontinence. International Urogynecology Journal 8(4):223–229

Wyman J F, Fantl J A, McClish D K et al 1998 Comparative efficacy of behavioral interventions in the management of female urinary incontinence. American Journal of Obstetrics and Gynecology 179(4):999–1007

Wyman J F, McClish D K, Sale P et al 1999 Long-term follow-up of behavioral interventions in incontinent women [abstract]. International Urogynecological Journal and Pelvic Floor Dysfunction 10(suppl 1):533

Yoon H S, Song H H, Ro Y J 2003 A comparison of effectiveness of bladder training and pelvic muscle exercise on female urinary incontinence. International Journal of Nursing Studies 40:45–50

PELVIC FLOOR MUSCLE TRAINING FOR OAB

Kari Bø

INTRODUCTION

In clinical practice, many patients with overactive bladder (OAB) symptoms are treated with pelvic floor muscle training (PFMT) with and without biofeedback, electrical stimulation, bladder training, or medication, and often many of the interventions are combined. When different methods are combined it is not possible to analyse the cause effect of the different interventions. In most systematic reviews on efficacy of PFMT to prevent and treat urinary incontinence, studies including patients with symptoms or urodynamic diagnosis of stress urinary incontinence (SUI), urgency incontinence and mixed incontinence are combined (Hay-Smith et al 2001, Wilson et al 2002). This makes it impossible to understand the real effect of the different interventions on each condition.

Although there are new theories suggesting PFM dysfunction as a common cause of the two main diagnosis (SUI and urgency incontinence) (Artibani 1997, Mattiasson 1997), the mechanisms behind the PFM dysfunction in each of these diagnoses are not yet thoroughly understood, and pathophysiological factors may be very different (rupture of the pelvic floor and connective tissue during childbirth for SUI, caffeine-induced urgency incontinence in an elderly woman). Optimally, the physical therapy intervention should relate to the underlying pathophysiological condition. PFMT may have different cure and improvement rates for SUI and urgency incontinence, and the combination of heterogeneous patient groups in systematic reviews and meta-analyses may disseminate the real cure rate for each of the diagnoses. In addition, an optimal PFMT protocol may be different for the two conditions due to a different theoretical rationale. In this chapter we will therefore cover studies including only patients with symptoms/diagnosis of OAB. We have excluded the following RCTs:

- Burns et al (1990), Dougherty et al (2002), Lagro-Janssen et al (1992), Sherman et al (1997) – because they included patients with a mixture of diagnoses;
- Burgio et al (1998, 2000, 2002) and Nygaard et al (1996) because they included patients with 'predominantly' urge symptoms, but did not report the results of those with only urge incontinence.

In most of these studies bladder training was also combined with PFMT.

RATIONALE FOR EFFECT OF PELVIC FLOOR MUSCLE TRAINING FOR OVERACTIVE BLADDER

The rationale behind the use of PFMT to treat symptoms of OAB is based on observations from electrical stimulation. Godec et al (1975) studied 40 patients with cysto-metrograms, taken during and after 3 minutes of 20 Hz functional electrical stimulation (FES). The results showed that, during FES, hyperactivity of the bladder was diminished or completely abolished in 31 of 40 patients. One minute after stimulation cessation, the inhibition was still present. Mean bladder capacity also increased significantly, from 151 ± 126 mL to 206 ± 131 mL ($p < 0.05$).

De Groat (1997) noted that during the storage of urine, distension of the bladder produces low-level vesical afferent firing. This stimulates the sympathetic outflow to the bladder outlet (base and urethra), and the pudendal outflow to the external urethral sphincter. He stated that these responses occur by spinal reflex pathways, representing 'guarding reflexes' that promote continence. Sympathetic firing also inhibits the detrusor muscle and bladder ganglia. Morrison (1993) claimed that the excitatory loop through Barringtons's micturition centre is switched on at bladder pressures between 5 and 25 mmHg, whereas the inhibitory loop through the raphe nucleus is active predominantly above 25 mmHg. The inhibition is at the automatic level, with the person not being conscious of the increasing tone in the PFM and urethral wall striated muscles.

Clinical experience tells us that patients can successfully inhibit urgency, detrusor contraction and urinary leakage by walking, crossing their legs, using hip adductor muscles with or without conscious co-contraction of the PFM, or by conscious contraction of the PFM alone. After inhibition of the urgency to void and detrusor contraction, the patients may gain time to reach the toilet and thereby prevent leakage. The reciprocal inhibition reflex runs via cerebral control, recruiting ventral horn motor neurons for voluntary PFM contraction and inhibiting the parasympathetic excitatory pathway for the micturition reflex via Onuf's ganglion. This mechanism has been exploited as part of bladder training regimens (Burgio et al 1998). There may therefore be two main hypotheses for the mechanism of PFMT to treat urgency incontinence:

- intentional contraction of the PFM during urgency, and holding of the contraction till the urge to void disappears;
- strength training of the PFM with longlasting changes in muscle morphology, which may stabilize neurogenic activity.

None of the studies in this field (neither uncontrolled studies or RCTs) have evaluated whether changes in the inhibitory mechanisms really occur after PFMT. In addition, research in this area is relatively new, and there does not seem to be any consensus on the optimal exercise protocol to prevent or treat OAB (Bø & Berghmans 2000). The theoretical basis of how PFMT works in the treatment of OAB therefore remains unclear (Berghmans et al 2000).

METHODS

This systematic review is based on two former systematic reviews (Berghmans et al 2000, Bø & Berghmans 2000) and the literature found in the three International Consensus on Incontinence meetings in 1998, 2001 and 2004. In addition we have conducted an electronic search on PubMed from 1998 till 2004 and the Cochrane library. Only fully published randomized controlled trial (RCTs) including female patients with OAB symptoms (frequency, urgency and urgency incontinence) alone were included. Methodological quality is classified according to the PEDro rating scale, which has been found to have high reliability (Maher et al 2003).

EVIDENCE FOR PELVIC FLOOR MUSCLE TRAINING TO TREAT OVERACTIVE BLADDER SYMPTOMS

Three RCTs using PFMT to treat symptoms of OAB were found (Berghmans et al 2002, Millard 2004, Wang et al 2004). The results of the studies are presented in Table 9.7, and methodological quality in Table 9.8. The studies had moderate to high methodological quality.

Berghmans et al (2002) did not demonstrate any significant effect of their exercise protocol compared to an untreated control group. Wang et al (2004) found that the significant subjective improvement/cure rate of OAB was the same between the electrical stimulation group and in the biofeedback-assisted PFMT group, but lower in the PFMT home training group. Millard (2004) did not show any additional benefit for a simple PFMT protocol (two-page written instruction, no assessment of ability to contract, and no follow-up or supervised training). The effect of PFMT on OAB is therefore questionable.

QUALITY OF THE INTERVENTION: DOSE–RESPONSE ISSUES

Quality of the interventions is difficult to judge because there are no direct recommendations on how PFMT

Table 9.7 Randomized controlled trials on pelvic floor muscle training to treat overactive bladder symptoms

Author	Berghmans et al 2002
Design	4-arm RCT: LUTE, ES, ES + LUTE, no treatment
n	68 women, mean age 55.2 (SD 14.4)
Diagnosis	Ambulatory urodynamics + micturition diary (DAI score ≥0.5 included)
Training protocol	9 treatments once a week + daily home training programme LUTE: bladder retraining, selective contraction of the PFM to inhibit detrusor contraction, 20 s hold, toilet behaviour
Drop-out	10/68 (15%) ITT anlysis of all
Adherence	92% (reported for all groups together)
Results	Significant decrease in DAI score (0.22, p > 0.001), but no difference compared with no treatment
Author	Wang et al 2004
Design	3-arm RCT: PFMT, PFMT with biofeedback, ES
n	120 women, mean age 52.7 (SD 13.7)
Diagnosis	Symptoms of OBA >6 months, frequency ≥8×/day, urge incontinence ≥ once/day
Training protocol	12 weeks Home exercise: based on individual PFM strength 3×/day Same home training in addition office biofeedback twice a week
Drop-out	17/120 (14%)
Adherence	PFMT: 83% PFMT + biofeedback: 75% ES: 79% Home exercise: PFMT: 14.5 days PFMT + biofeedback: 8.5 days
Results	PFMT: urge incontinence resolved 30%, modified 6%, unchanged 64% PFMT/biofeedback: urge incontinence resolved 38%, modified 12%, unchanged 40% Improvement/cured: PFMT 38%, PFMT/biofeedback 50% PFM strength: no significant differences between exercise groups, but between both exercise groups and ES No change in urodynamic parameters Significant change in several QoL measures for different groups
Author	Millard 2004
Design	2-arm RCT: international multicentre, 54 sites: tolterodine, tolterodine + PFMT
n	480 women (75%) and men, mean age 53.4 (SD 17.4)
Diagnosis	Symptoms of OAB ≥6 months: frequency ≥8×/day, urgency and urge incontinence ≥1/24 h
Training protocol	12 weeks Written instruction on PFMT 10 s hold ×15 twice a day; 20 contractions once a day
Drop-out	ITT analysis of all
Adherence	90% on medication in both groups Adherence not reported for PFMT
Results	Both groups had significant reduction in incontinence episodes, numbers of micturitions, urgency episodes, improvement in perception of bladder symptoms No significant difference between groups

DAI score, detrusor activity index formed from results of extramural ambulatory cystometry and micturition diary; ES, electrical stimulation; ITT, intention to treat; LUTE, lower urinary tract exercise; PFMT, pelvic floor muscle training; QoL, quality of life; OAB, overactive bladder.

Table 9.8   PEDro quality score of RCTs in systematic review

E – Eligibility criteria specified
1 – Subjects randomly allocated to groups
2 – Allocation concealed
3 – Groups similar at baseline
4 – Subjects blinded
5 – Therapist administering treatment blinded
6 – Assessors blinded
7 – Measures of key outcomes obtained from over 85% of subjects
8 – Data analysed by intention to treat
9 – Comparison between groups conducted
10 – Point measures and measures of variability provided

Study	E	1	2	3	4	5	6	7	8	9	10	Total score
Berghmans et al 2002	+	+	+	+	–	–	+	+	+	+	+	8
Wang et al 2004	?	+	+	–	–	–	+	+	–	+	–	5
Millard 2004	+	+	+	+	–	–	+	+	+	+	+	8

+, criterion is clearly satisfied; –, criterion is not satisfied; ?, not clear if the criterion was satisfied. Total score is determined by counting the number of criteria that are satisfied, except that scale item one 'eligibility criteria specified' is not used to generate the total score. Total scores are out of 10.

should be conducted to inhibit urgency and detrusor contraction. The published studies have all used different exercise protocols. Berghmans et al (2002) and Millard (2004) included intentional contraction of the PFM to inhibit detrusor contractions in addition to a strength training programme. However, we have no information about how many conducted the exercises in Millard's study, and Berghmans et al (2002) also included bladder training in their protocol. The protocol from Berghmans et al did not show any effect when compared with untreated controls, but if there had been an effect it would not be possible to tell whether this was due to the exercises or the bladder training. In Millard's study (2004) a very weak exercise protocol was conducted. There was no control of ability to contract the PFM, patients were left alone to exercise, and there was no report on adherence to the exercise protocol. The exercise period varied between 9 and 12 weeks in duration in the four RCTs in this area. This may be too short to treat a complex condition such as OAB.

CONCLUSION

The results of published RCTs in this area are difficult to interpret. In general the studies have moderate to high methodological quality, but the exercise protocols may not have been optimal. Because the pathophysiological background for OAB is not clear, it is difficult to plan an optimal training protocol. Based on the theoretical knowledge and symptoms of bladder overactivity it seems reasonable to put more emphasis on the inhibition mechanisms of the PFM contraction, and teaching and follow-up of patients trying to contract the PFM when there is an urge to void. There is a need for more basic research to understand the role of a voluntary PFM contraction in inhibition of the micturition reflex.

CLINICAL RECOMMENDATIONS

- To date there is no convincing evidence from RCTs to support the use of PFMT in the treatment of OAB. There are no training protocols to recommend.

- Clinical experience and basic research show that it may be possible to learn to inhibit detrusor contraction by intentionally contracting the PFM and holding the contraction to stop the urge to void. A protocol based on patients' experiences needs to be tested in a high-quality RCT.

REFERENCES

Artibani W 1997 Diagnosis and significance of idiopathic overactive bladder. Urology 50(suppl 6A):25–32

Berghmans L, Hendriks H, de Bie R A et al 2000 Conservative treatment of urge urinary incontinence in women: a systematic review of randomized clinical trials. BJU International 85(3):254–263

Berghmans L, van Waalwijk van Doorn E, Nieman F et al 2002 Efficacy of physical therapeutic modalities in women with proven bladder overactivity. European Urology 6:581–587

Burgio K, Locher J, Goode P et al 1998 Behavioral vs drug treatement for urge urinary incontinence in older women. A randomized controlled trial. JAMA 280(23):1995–2000

Burgio K, Locher J, Goode P 2000 Combined behavioral and drug therapy for urge incontinence in older women. Journal of American Geriatric Society 48(4):370–374

Burgio KL, Goode PS, Locher JL et al 2002 Behavioral training with and without biofeedback in the treatment of urge incontinence in older women. Journal of American Medical Association 288(18):2293–2299

Burns PA, Pranikoff K, Nochajski T et al 1990 Treatment of stress urinary incontinence with pelvic floor exercises and biofeedback. Journal of American Geriatric Society 38:341–344

Bø K, Berghmans L 2000 Overactive bladder and its treatments. Non-pharmacological treatments for overactive bladder: pelvic floor exercises. Urology 55(suppl 5A):7–11

De Groat W 1997 A neurologic basis for the overactive bladder. Urology 50(suppl 6A):36–52

Dougherty M C, Dwyer J W, Pendergast J F et al 2002 A randomized trial of behavioral management for continence with older rural women. Research and Nursing Health 25:3–13

Godec C, Cass A, Ayala G 1975 Bladder inhibition with functional electrical stimulation. Urology 6 (6):663–666

Hay-Smith J E, Bø K, Berghmans L et al 2001 Pelvic floor muscle training for urinary incontinence in women (Cochrane review). The Cochrane Library, Oxford

Lagro-Janssen A, Debruyne F, Smiths A et al 1992 The effects of treatment of urinary incontinence in general practice. Family Practice 9(3):284–289

Maher C, Sherrington C, Herbert R D et al 2003 Reliability of the PEDRO scale for rating quality of RCTs. Physiotherapy 83(8):713–721

Mattiasson A 1997 Management of overactive bladder – looking to the future. Urology 50(suppl 6A):111–113

Millard R 2004 Clinical efficacy of tolterodine with or without a simplified pelvic floor exercise regimen. Nerourology and Urodynamics 23:48–53

Morrison J 1993 The excitability of the micturition reflex. Scandinavian Journal of Urology and Nephrology 29(suppl 175):21–25

Nygaard I, Kreder K, Lepic M et al 1996 Efficacy of pelvic floor muscle exercises in women with stress, urge, and mixed incontinence. American Journal of Obstetrics and Gynecology 174(120):125

Sherman R, Wong M, Davis G 1997 Behavioral treatment of exercise induced urinary incontinence among female soldiers. Military Medicine 162(10):690–694

Wilson P D, Bø K, Nygaard I et al 2002 Conservative treatment in women. In: Abrams P, Cardozo L, Khoury S et al (eds) Incontinence. Plymbridge Distributors, Plymouth, p 571–624

Wang A, Wang Y, Chen M 2004 Single-blind, randomized trial of pelvic floor muscle training, biofeedback-assisted pelvic floor muscle training, and electrical stimulation in the management of overactive bladder. Urology 63(1):61–66

ELECTRICAL STIMULATION FOR OAB

Bary Berghmans

INTRODUCTION

Clinical experience has shown that an overactive bladder (OAB) function with associated urgency urinary incontinence (UUI) is not amenable to surgical correction (Millard & Oldenburg 1983, Ulmsten 1999). Therefore, it is important to find another satisfactory treatment modality for patients with this problem. Pharmaceutical agents in general lead to disappointing results with success rates of 60–70% for the most effective single agents, but also with more or less side-effects in most patients and poor tolerability in about 15% (Sussman & Garely 2002). The short duration of most clinical trials and the lack of long-term follow-up give little information about the short- and long-term efficacy and acceptability of drugs (Hay-Smith et al 2002). Although combination therapy is claimed to be more successful,

the use of drugs produces many side-effects, inevitably leading to non-compliance and the recurrence of incontinence (Hay-Smith et al 2002, Millard & Oldenburg 1983, Resnick 1998). Besides bladder (re)training and pelvic floor muscle training (PFMT) with or without biofeedback, electrical stimulation (ES) is one of the physiotherapeutic treatment modalities used for the management of women with OAB.

The theoretical basis for how ES actually works in the treatment of OAB remains unclear.

- Is it the change in PFM activity during nervous excitation that automatically should inhibit or better prevent detrusor overactivity (Messelink 1999)?

- Is it a learning process that should make the patient aware of contracting the PFM during urgency to inhibit involuntary detrusor contraction (reciprocal inhibition) (Messelink 1999)?

- Is it that increase in strength of the PFM could provide more inhibition of the overactivity of the bladder (Messelink 1999)?

The different physiotherapeutic treatment modalities are therefore still based on hypotheses for the underlying pathologies causing OAB. However, clinical experience has shown that different physical therapy treatment modalities generally will provide some progress in most individuals with OAB. Improved bladder control can occur even in the cognitively impaired individual (Colling et al 1992, Engel et al 1990, McCormick et al 1990, Schnelle 1990).

RATIONALE FOR ELECTRICAL STIMULATION FOR OVERACTIVE BLADDER

The literature concerning ES in the management of OAB and UUI is difficult to interpret due to the lack of a well-substantiated biological rationale underpinning the use of ES. The mechanisms of action may vary depending on the cause(s) of OAB and the structure(s) being targeted by ES (e.g. PFM or detrusor muscle, peripheral or central nervous system [CNS]). Eriksen (1989), Eriksen & Eik-Nes (1989) and Fall (2000) claimed that ES theoretically stimulates the detrusor inhibition reflex (DIR) and pacifies the micturition reflex, resulting in a decrease of OAB dysfunction. Schmidt (1988) hypothesized that the electrical stimulus activates the pudendal nerve, contracting the PFM and external urinary sphincter. Both Eriksen and Schmidt suggested that ES of the PFM induces a reflex contraction of the striated paraurethral and periurethral muscles, accompanied by a simultaneous reflex inhibition of the detrusor muscle (Weil 2000). This reciprocal response depends on a preserved reflex arc through the sacral micturition reflex centre. To obtain a therapeutic effect of pelvic floor stimulation in women with OAB, peripheral innervation of the PFM must at least be partially intact (Eriksen 1989). This means that, when increasing stimulation is applied on the nerve, there is improved contraction of the muscles, resulting in more efficient detrusor inhibition (Schmidt 1988).

However, according to Weil (2000), detrusor inhibition is not the result of activating somatosensory efferents of the pudendal nerve (Schulz-Lampel 1997). Schultz-Lampel (1997) holds the β-fibres of the sacral nerve afferents responsible for the electrically-induced inhibition of detrusor contraction. Electrical inhibition of detrusor contractions is induced by pudendal afferent β-fibres from the urinary sphincter and/or pelvic floor (Schulz-Lampel 1997). As these fibres are large in diameter, these nerve cells can be depolarized with minimal amounts of energy. Therefore, ES should not be applied through muscle contraction, nor should excess energy be applied to produce depolarization of the smaller nerve fibres, such as B and unmyelinated C-fibres, which result in a painful sensation (Weil 2000).

It is suggested that ES therapy alone, both external or internal, inhibits the parasympathetic motor neurons to the bladder and enables an effective reduction or inhibition of detrusor activity by stimulation of (large diameter) afferents of the pudendal nerve (Eriksen 1989, Eriksen & Erik-Nes 1989, Fall 2000, Fall & Lindström 1994, Weil 2000).

EVIDENCE FOR ELECTRICAL STIMULATION TO TREAT OVERACTIVE BLADDER (SYMPTOMS)

Not many studies have been performed regarding the efficacy of ES for OAB (Wilson et al 2002). Our review revealed only weak evidence on the efficacy of ES alone or in combination with PFMT for women with UUI (Berghmans et al 2000). However, these findings did not prove the ineffectivity of ES as a treatment modality for bladder overactivity as a whole. It was our assumption that the lack of efficacy is most likely caused by methodological flaws such as heterogeneity of study groups and suboptimal research designs.

Electrical stimulation for OAB is provided by clinic-based mains-powered machines or portable battery-powered stimulators (Fig. 9.18). Also in this area, ES offers a seemingly infinite combination of current types, waveforms, frequencies, intensities, electrode placements, ES probes, etc. (Fig. 9.19). Without that clear biological rationale mentioned above, it is difficult to make reasoned choices of ES parameters. Hence, as in ES studies for stress urinary incontinence (SUI), we see a wide variety of stimulation devices and protocols being used for OAB.

This chapter reviews the evidence in women comparing non-surgical ES with no treatment, placebo ES and comparisons of different ES protocols. It also includes

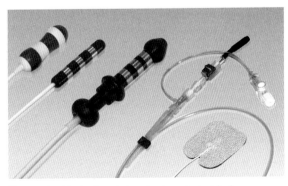

Fig. 9.18 Vaginal, rectal and external electrical stimulation probes.

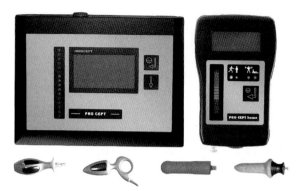

Fig. 9.19   Office-bound and home devices for electrical stimulation.

trials comparing non-surgical ES with any other single intervention (e.g. magnetic stimulation, PFMT, weighted vaginal cones, surgery, medication) and trials comparing ES with any other combined intervention versus that other combined intervention alone.

METHODS

Three systematic reviews (Berghmans et al 1998, 2000; Hay-Smith et al 2001) have been published that include trials relevant to this chapter. The following qualitative summary of the evidence regarding ES is based on the trials included in all previous systematic reviews with the addition of trials performed after publication of the reviews and/or located through additional searching. This search was conducted in the same fashion as for ES in women with SUI (see p. 188).

To be included in this chapter a trial needed to (a) be a RCT, (b) include women with OAB or UUI symptoms, and (c) compare different ES protocols or investigate the effect of ES versus no treatment, placebo treatment, or any other single treatment, with any other combined intervention versus that other combined intervention. Published abstracts and reporting trials in progress were excluded.

Quality of data

The two trials by Yamanishi et al (2000a, 2000b), the trial by Soomro et al (2001) and Walsh et al (2001) included both men and women with OAB and urinary incontinence. It is possible that the effects of ES might be different between sexes (due to difference in electrode placement for example). So, although some of these studies included a large number of women with OAB

and/or UUI symptoms and reported significant objective and/or subjective results in favour of ES in comparison to no or placebo treatment, for reason of heterogeneity of inclusion criteria (i.e. differences in gender), we decided not to use these studies for the analysis of results where they did not perform subgroup analysis or did not differentiate the effects of treatment in women versus men. Only the study of Yamanishi et al (2000a) could partly be used where the authors did report results from subgroups according to sex.

Table 9.9 provides details of results of all included studies (n = 9). The PEDro rating scale was used to classify the methodological quality of the included studies (Table 9.10). The studies had low (n = 2), moderate (n = 1) to high (n = 6) methodological quality.

Quality of the intervention dose–response issues

Some ES protocols were poorly reported, lacking detail of stimulation parameters, devices and methods of delivery. However, on the basis of the details that have been reported it appeared that there was considerable variation in ES protocols. Also the ES dosage (type of current, frequency, duration and intensity) varies significantly between studies (Hay-Smith et al 2001, Wilson et al 2002). Looking into the studies on OAB patients included in the Cochrane systematic review, duration of the intervention varies between 4 months of daily stimulation (Smith 1996) and a single episode of stimulation (Bower et al 1998), intensity varies between 5 mA and maximal tolerable intensity, and duration of each session varies between 20 minutes to several hours. Frequency of stimulation is once or twice every day in all RCTs except in Smith's trial (1996) (Wilson et al 2002).

Despite the many clinical series that have been reported, the common issues of patient selection, dose–response and electrical parameters remain unsolved.

Patient selection criteria should most likely have to include neurophysiological sacral arc testing and assessment of detrusor muscle status, because some forms of muscle dysfunction respond less to neural inhibitory effects (Brubaker 2000).

Also, there is still no consensus on how much stimulation is required for an optimal effect (Brubaker 2000). Currently, most RCTs use an intensity of current to achieve a maximally tolerable motor response of the pelvic floor (Brubaker 2000). But it is still unknown whether or not a contraction of the pelvic floor is really necessary to achieve detrusor inhibition or just excitation of pudendal afferents is sufficiently effective for this kind of inhibition.

Table 9.9   Randomized controlled trials on electrical stimulation to treat overactive bladder and/or urgency urinary incontinence symptoms

Author	Berghmans et al 2002
Design	4-arm RCT: LUTE, ES, ES + LUTE, no treatment
n	68 women mean (SD) age 55.2 (14.4)
Diagnosis	Ambulatory urodynamics + micturition diary (DAI score ≥0.5 included)
Training protocol	9 treatments once a week daily home programme LUTE: bladder retraining, selective contraction of the PFM to inhibit detrusor contraction, 20 s hold, toilet behaviour
Drop out	10/68 (15%) ITT analysis of all
Adherence	92% (reported for all groups together)
Results	Dunnett's t-test: ES compared to no treatment significant difference in decrease in DAI score (0.23, $p = 0.039$), other treatment groups no difference compared with no treatment
Author	Bower et al 1998
Design	3-arm RCT: LF ES, HF ES, sham ES
n	80 women; 49 OAB, 31 sensory urge; mean (SD) age 56.5 (16.9)
Diagnosis	Urodynamics (cystometry)
Training protocol	LF ES: transcuteneous 10 Hz, pulse width 200 µs, sacral placement, I_{max} HF ES: 150 Hz, 200 µs, suprapubic placement, I_{max} Sham ES (placement at random); 1 session during filling cystometry
Drop out	None
Adherence	Not applicable
Results	OAB: sham ES no sign. change first desire to void ($p = 0.69$), MCC & detrusor pressure idem; both active ES groups reduction max. detrusor pressure, sign. increase first desire to void, no change MCC; no change in detrusor pressure at first desire to void; 44% in both active ES groups stable Sensory urgency: sign. increase first desire to void only in 150 Hz active ES; MCC increase only in sham ES
Author	Brubaker et al 1997
Design	2-arm RCT: ES, sham ES
n	148 women, subgroup OAB 28 women, mean (SD) age 57 (12)
Diagnosis	Urodynamics, micturition diary
Training protocol	ES: transvaginal, 20 Hz, 2/4 s work/rest, pulse width 0.1 ms, bipolar square wave, I 0–100 mA Sham ES: same parameters, no I Both groups 8 weeks' treatment
Drop out	18%
Adherence	ES vs sham ES mean compliance 87% vs 81% at 4- and 8-weeks' treatment

Table 9.9   Randomized controlled trials on electrical stimulation to treat overactive bladder and/or urgency urinary incontinence symptoms—cont'd

Results	ES vs sham ES 54% (n = 33) OAB pretreatment reduced to 27% (n = 16) post-treatment (p = 0.0004) vs sham ES 47% (n = 28) to 42% (p = 0.22) 24-h frequency NS 6-week no. of accidents/24 h (average) NS Adequate subj. imp p = 0.027 QoL difference NS No analysis diaries because of incomplete data
Author	Smith 1996
Design	2-arm RCT: ES, propantheline bromide
n	Subgroup detrusor instability 38 women age range 44–73
Diagnosis	Cystoscopy only when indicated, complex video urodynamic study (i.e. uroflow, UPP, cystometrography, Vasalva LPP)
Training protocol	Study group (SG) ES: 5 s contractions (range 3–15), duty circle 1 : 2, treatment time 15–60 min twice daily for 4 mts, I 5-max 25 mA Control group (CG) propantheline bromide 7.5–45 mg 2–3×/day; written/verbal instructions timed voiding & bladder retraining
Drop out	None
Adherence	>80%
Results	CG: IEF 50% imp. SG ES: IEF 72% imp. including 4 patients cured, > bladder capacity trend both groups No imp. urodynamic variables In between no stat. sign. diff.
Author	Soomro et al 2001*
Design	2-arm RCT: ES, oxybutynin
n	43 patients: 30 women, 13 men mean (SD) age 50 (15)
Diagnosis	OAB symptoms SF-36 QoL, Bristol urinary symptom questionnaire Clinical assessment: urodynamics, urinalysis, urine cytology
Training protocol	ES: transcutaneous, 2 self-adhesive pads bilateral perianal region (S2/3 dermatome), I variable tickling sensation, 20 Hz, 200 µs, continuous, 6 h daily Oxybutynin: 2.5 mg orally 2×/day, titrated to 5 mg orally 3×/day by day 7
Drop out	Not reported
Adherence	Not reported
Results	Overall no differences between groups in symptoms, urodynamic data or SF-36 QoL, side-effects
Author	Walsh et al 2001*
Design	2-arm RCT: ES, sham ES
n	146 patients: 111 women, 35 men with urgency incontinence; mean (range) age 47 (17–79)

Table 9.9 Randomized controlled trials on electrical stimulation to treat overactive bladder and/or urgency urinary incontinence symptoms—cont'd

Diagnosis	Clinical assessment: history and examination, urinalysis, pelvic ultrasonography, cystourethroscopy, urodynamics; ES: n = 74: DI/DH/SU 28/18/ 28; sham ES n = 72: 27/17/28
Training protocol	Both groups: transcutaneous neurostimulator, bilateral S3 dermatomes ES: antidromic S3 neurostim, 10 Hz, 200 μs, continuous mode, I_{max} Sham ES: no current Comparison 1st and 2nd cystometry fill, and between groups
Drop out	None
Adherence	Not applicable
Results	ES: pre/post-stimulation sign. greater mean volume bladder capacity at first desire to void (+57.3), strong desire to void (+68.4), urge (+55.2) and max. capacity (+59.5) (p = 0.0002) Sham ES: no changes
Author	Wang et al 2004
Design	3-arm RCT: PFMT, PFMT with biofeedback, ES
n	120 women mean (SD) age 52.7 (13.7)
Diagnosis	Symptoms of OAB >6 months, frequency ≥8x/day, urge incontinence ≥1x/day
Training protocol	12 weeks, home exercise based on individual PFM strength 3x/day Same home training in addition office biofeedback twice a week
Drop out	17/120 (14%)
Adherence	PFMT: 83% PFMT + biofeedback: 75% ES: 79% Home exercise: PFMT: 14.5 days PFMT + biofeedback: 8.5 days
Results	PFMT: urge incontinence resolved 30%, modified 6%, unchanged 64% PFMT/biofeedback: resolved 38%, modified 12%, unchanged 50% ES: resolved 40%, modified 11.5%, unchanged 48.5% Imp./cured: PFMT 38%, PFMT/biofeedback 50%, ES 51.5% PFM strength: diffs NS between exercise groups, but between both exercise groups and ES in favour exercise groups No change in urodynamic parameters Significant change in several QoL measures for different groups between ES and PFMT/biofeedback no sign diffs in imp./reduction rate, between ES and PFMT yes
Author	Yamanishi et al 2000a**
Design	2-arm RCT: ES, sham ES
n	68 patients; 39 women, 29 men; mean (SD) age 70 (11.2)
Diagnosis	Urinalysis, urine cytological examination, clinical assessment, neurological, anatomical, urodynamics (cystometrogram, cystometry)

Table 9.9 Randomized controlled trials on electrical stimulation to treat overactive bladder and/or urgency urinary incontinence symptoms—cont'd

Training protocol	ES: alternating 10 Hz pulses, 1 ms pulse duration, I_{max} tolerable, in women vaginal plug, 15 min 2×/day for 4 weeks
Drop out	12%
Adherence	Not reported
Results	IEF sign. less in ES, not in sham, sign. diff. intergroup favour of ES, favouring ES sign. intergroup change in nocturia (p = 0.03), same for QoL (p = 0.045), sign greater MCC and first desire to void in ES vs sham ES; trend favouring ES daily frequency of pad changes (p = 0.06); Subgroup analysis of self-report of cure/ imp. according to sex: in women sign. diff. in favour ES (p = 0.0091) in no. of cured/imp.
Author	Yamanishi et al 2000b*
Design	2-arm RCT: ES, MS
n	32 patients: 17 women, 15 men; mean (SD) age 62.3 (16.6)
Diagnosis	Urodynamics (cystometrogram, cystometry)
Training protocol	ES: home and office bound device; alternating 10 Hz pulses, 1 ms pulse duration, I_{max} tolerable, in women vaginal plug, 15 min 2×/day for 4 weeks MS: continuous, low-impedance coil, armchair type seat, perineum centre of coil, I_{max}, 10 Hz, maximum output 100% setting of at least 270 J
Drop out	None
Adherence	Not reported
Results	No sign. intergroup diffs between groups for MCC and bladder capacity at first desire to void OAB cured in 3/15 (20%) in MS, 0/17 in ES >50 mL increase MCC in 13/15 in MS, 6/17 in ES No adverse events in either group

*Not included in analysis of results because of inclusion of both women and men.
**Partly included in results for subgroup analysis according to gender.
diff. difference; DAI score, detrusor activity index formed from results of extramural ambulatory cystometry and micturition diary; DI/DH/SU, detrusor instability, detrusor hyperactivity, stress urinary incontinence; ES, electrical stimulation; HF, high frequency; IEF, incontinence episode frequency; imp, improvement; ITT, intention-to-treat analysis; LF, low frequency; LPP, leah point pressure, mts, months; MCC, maximum cystometric capacity; MS, magnetic stimulation; NS no significant/not significant; PFM, pelvic floor muscle; QoL, quality of life RCT, randomized controlled trial; sign. significant; stat, statistical; stim., stimulation; UPP, urethral pressure profile.

Electrical parameters

Current

Although it appeared that all ES trials in this chapter used alternating current only four trials specifically stated this as biphasic (Berghmans et al 2002), bipolar (Brubaker et al 1997), and biphasic pulsed current (Smith 1996, Wang et al 2004).

Pulse shape

The first three trials and the trials of Yamanishi (2000a, 2000b) were the only ones to detail the pulse shape: rectangular (Berghmans et al 2002); square (Brubaker et al 1997, Yamanishi et al 2000a, 2000b); symmetrical (Wang et al 2004); asymmetrical (Smith 1996); balanced with two second ramp up and one second ramp down.

Table 9.10   PEDro quality score of RCTs in systematic review

E – Eligibility criteria specified
1 – Subjects randomly allocated to groups
2 – Allocation concealed
3 – Groups similar at baseline
4 – Subjects blinded
5 – Therapist administering treatment blinded
6 – Assessors blinded
7 – Measures of key outcomes obtained from over 85% of subjects
8 – Data analysed by intention to treat
9 – Statistical comparison between groups conducted
10 – Point measures and measures of variability provided

Study	E	1	2	3	4	5	6	7	8	9	10	Total score
Berghmans et al 2002	+	+	+	+	–	–	+	+	+	+	+	8
Bower et al 1998	+	+	–	+	+	+	?	+	+	+	+	8
Brubaker et al 1997	+	+	+	+	+	–	+	–	–	+	+	7
Smith 1996	+	+	–	–	–	–	–	+	–	+	+	4
Soomro et al 2001	+	+	–	–	–	–	–	+	?	–	+	3
Walsh et al 2001	+	+	–	+	+	–	–	+	+	+	+	7
Wang et al 2004	?	+	+	–	–	–	+	+	–	+	–	5
Yamanishi et al 2000a	+	+	–	+	+	+	+	+	–	+	+	8
Yamanishi et al 2000b	+	+	+	?	–	–	–	+	+	+	+	6

+, criterion is clearly satisfied; –, criterion is not satisfied; ?, not clear if the criterion was satisfied. Total score is determined by counting the number of criteria that are satisfied, except that scale item one 'eligibility criteria specified' is not used to generate the total score. Total scores are out of 10.

Frequency

Nine trials gave details of the frequencies used and these ranged from 10 Hz (Bower et al 1998, Walsh et al 2001, Wang et al 2004, Yamanishi et al 2000a, 2000b) to 20 Hz (Brubaker et al 1997, Soomro et al 2001), a combination of 12.5 and 50 Hz (Smith 1996), 150 Hz (Bower et al 1998), and a random frequency of 4–10 Hz (Berghmans et al 2002).

Pulse duration

Pulse durations were also reported in nine trials, and these were 0.1 ms (Brubaker et al 1997), 0.2 ms (Berghmans et al 2002, Bower et al 1998, Soomro et al 2001, Walsh et al 2001), 0.3 ms (Smith 1996), 0.4 ms (Wang et al 2004) and 1 ms (Yamanishi et al 2000a, 2000b).

Duty circle

Two trials used a duty cycle ratio of 1:2 (Brubaker et al 1997, Smith 1996); in one trial this was 2:1 (Wang et al 2004).

Intensity of stimulation

Intensity of stimulation progressed from 5 to 25 mA in the trial by Smith (1996). Seven trials used the maximum tolerable intensity (Berghmans et al 2002, Bower et al 1998, Brubaker et al 1997, Walsh et al 2001, Wang et al 2004, Yamanishi et al 2000a, 2000b). In the trial of Soomro et al (2001) patients were asked to control the amplitude of intensity to produce a tickling sensation.

Mode of delivery of current

Current was most commonly delivered by a vaginal electrode (Berghmans et al 2002, Brubaker et al 1997, Smith 1996, Wang et al 2004, Yamanishi et al 2000a, 2000b) and over S3 sacral dermatomes (Walsh et al 2001), though one trial used external surface electrode placements with two electrodes over S2–3 sacral foramina or two electrodes just above the symphysis pubis (Bower et al 1998). Transcutaneous ES was applied bilaterally over the perianal region using two self-adhesive electrodes (Soomro et al 2001).

Duration and number of treatments

The duration and number of treatments was also highly variable. The longest treatment period was 4 months of daily stimulation (Smith 1996). Medium-duration treatment periods were based on twice daily stimulation for 4 (Yamanishi et al 2000a), 8 (Brubaker et al 1997), 9 (Berghmans et al 2002), or 12 weeks (Wang et al 2004). In the crossover trial of Soomro et al (2001) after randomization patients received 6 weeks of ES for 6 hours daily or oxybutynin. After a washout period of 2 weeks they started in the second arm of treatment for another 6 weeks. The shortest treatment period consisted of a single episode of stimulation after the voiding phase of cystometry before filling was repeated (Bower et al 1998).

Is ES better than no treatment, control or placebo treatment?

In a four-arm RCT in 83 women with detrusor overactivity, Berghmans et al (2002) investigated the effect of no treatment, ES alone, a combination of PFMT and bladder training alone (which in this study was defined as lower urinary tract exercises), and ES in combination with lower urinary tract exercises. An important fact in this study was that women in the ES group received not only weekly office-bound ES, but also a twice daily ES programme with a home device that also measured patient's compliance of use of ES. The main outcome measures were change in the Detrusor Overactivity Index (DAI) (Berghmans et al 2002), the Incontinence Impact Questionnaire (Berghmans et al 2001) and the adapted Dutch Incontinence Quality of Life questionnaire (DI-QOL). The no-treatment group showed no significant change at all pre- to post-treatment. In comparison with no treatment, there was a significant

improvement in the ES alone group for the DAI (Berghmans et al 2002). The ES-alone group turned out to have statistically significant lower self-professed impact of incontinence on daily life activities (Berghmans et al 2001). Using the DI-QOL ES alone improved self-professed incontinence control in daily life activities.

Yamanishi et al (2000a) investigated maximum-intensity stimulation delivered daily for 4 weeks in 29 men and 39 women with detrusor overactivity. There was significantly more improvement in a number of outcomes in the ES group compared with the placebo ES group post-treatment (i.e. nocturia, number of leakage episodes, number of pad changes, quality of life score [using a questionnaire chart recording 0 = delighted, 1 = mostly satisfied, 2 = dissatisfied and 3 = mostly dissatisfied or unhappy], urodynamic evidence of improvement in detrusor overactivity, self-report of cure or improvement). For a single outcome, self-report of cure/improvement, subgroup analysis on the basis of gender was reported. Women in the active ES group were much more likely to report cure/improvement than women in the placebo ES group.

Bower et al (1998) used a single stimulation episode given after the voiding phase of cystometry and before bladder filling was repeated. The results were reported separately for women with detrusor overactivity and those with urgency. For women with detrusor overactivity both stimulation groups (10 Hz, sacral electrodes and 150 Hz, symphysis pubis electrodes) showed significant improvements in urodynamic measures when compared with the placebo stimulation group (i.e. reduction in maximum detrusor pressure, increase in first desire to void, proportion of women with a stable bladder). However, there were no significant differences between stimulation and placebo groups for change in maximum cystometric capacity or detrusor pressure at first desire to void. Fewer measures were reported for women with urgency. The only significant findings were a significant increase in first desire to void in the 150 Hz group, and a significant increase in the maximum cystometric capacity in the placebo ES group.

One further trial (Brubaker et al 1997) that compared ES with placebo ES in a group of women with urodynamic stress incontinence, detrusor overactivity or both, conducted a subgroup analysis on the basis of diagnosis and found that women with pretreatment detrusor overactivity who received active stimulation were significantly less likely to have urodynamic evidence of detrusor overactivity after treatment.

Due to availability of only a single study in women comparing ES with no treatment and the variation in stimulation protocols comparing ES with placebo stimulation it is difficult to interpret the findings of trials. However, for women with detrusor overactivity there is an absolute trend in favour of active stimulation over no treatment or placebo stimulation.

Is ES better than any other single treatment?

In a three-arm RCT in 103 women with OAB Wang et al (2004) compared the effects of ES with PFMT and with biofeedback-assisted PFMT (BAPFMT). Assessment was performed pre- and post-treatment using the King's Health Questionnaire for subjective cure/improvement, and urinary symptoms such as urgency, diurnal frequency, urgency incontinence, dysuria, nocturia for more objective outcomes. As secondary outcomes PFM strengthening and urodynamic data were used. More study details can be found in Table 9.5.

Wang et al (2004) did not find any statistically significant difference between the groups for self-reported cure or cure/improvement. PFMT women had statistically significantly fewer leakage episodes per day. Although there were no statistically significant differences in the general health perception, incontinence impact, role limitation, physical limitation, social limitation, sleep/energy and personal relationship, domains of the quality of life measure (King's Health Questionnaire), the ES group had statistically significantly better scores after treatment for emotions and severity measures, compared to the exercise regimens and in total score compared to PFMT only. Some women using ES reported discomfort during treatment.

The trial of Smith (1996) compared ES and medication (propantheline bromide) in women with detrusor overactivity with or without urodynamic stress incontinence. He did not find any statistically significant differences in outcome (self-reported improvement and urodynamic parameters) between the two groups.

With only a few single trials comparing ES with PFMT, BAPFMT, or medication there is insufficient evidence to determine whether ES is better than PFMT, BAPFMT, propantheline bromide, anticholinergic or antimuscarinic therapy in women with detrusor overactivity.

Is (additional) ES better than other (additional) treatments?

No studies were found to answer this question, so no conclusion can be drawn about whether or not there is any benefit of adding ES to another treatment modality in women with OAB.

CONCLUSIONS

ES protocols and designs in studies for women with OAB and/or UUI symptoms are largely inconsistent. One reason for this is insufficient understanding of the physiological rationale of the working mechanism and basic principles of ES used in clinical practice to treat these women.

There is some evidence to judge that an intensive programme of office bound and home ES is better than no or placebo treatment for women with OAB and/or UUI symptoms. However, some of the relevant studies in this area included both women and men, making interpretation of results for women only difficult.

There is insufficient evidence to determine whether ES is better than PFMT, BAPFMT or medication in women with OAB and/or UUI symptoms.

At present no studies have investigated the extra benefit of adding ES to other treatment (modalities).

There is a need for more basic research to find out the working mechanism of ES in women with OAB and/or UUI symptoms and to determine the best ES protocol(s) for these patients.

CLINICAL RECOMMENDATIONS

- If available, ES should be applied both in clinical practice and at the patient's home – may be as the treatment of first choice in this diagnostic group. So far, it is impossible to recommend the most optimal ES regimen and protocol. But if ES is applied, do use an intensive (parameters, number of sessions, duration of therapy) ES regimen with both clinical office and home devices. A protocol, that has proven to be effective (Berghmans et al 2002, Fall & Madersbacher 1994), consisted of the following parameters:
  - stochastic frequency 4–10 Hz; frequency modulation 0.1 s;
  - intensity I_{max};
  - pulse duration 200–500 µs;
  - biphasic, duty circle 13 s 5/8;
  - shape of current rectangular;
  - number and time schedule of sessions daily at home 2 × 20 min/day; office 1 × 30 min/week;
  - duration of treatment period 3–6 months.

- Use intravaginal probes for ES therapy only after inspection and digital intravaginal examination to assess integrity of vaginal tissue and to avoid adverse events of ES use.

- Follow-up with weekly or more often supervised training. Supervised training must be conducted individually.

- At follow-up, get as much feedback as possible from the patient about compliance, performance, potential side-effects and adverse events. Micturition diaries are useful and should be filled out regularly to provide feedback to the patient and to monitor progress.

- Try to use ES devices that measure compliance of use electronically. During the office-bound sessions use these data to provide feedback to the patient and to support motivation to continue ES at home.

REFERENCES

Berghmans L C M, Hendriks H J, Bø K et al 1998 Conservative treatment of genuine stress incontinence in women: a systematic review of randomized clinical trials. British Journal of Urology 82(2):181–191

Berghmans L C M, Nieman F, van Waalwijk van Doorn E S C et al 2001 Effects of physiotherapy, using the adapted Dutch I-QOL in Women with urge urinary incontinence (UUI) [Abstract 62 IUGA 2001]. International Urogynecology Journal and Pelvic Floor Dysfunction 12(suppl 3):S40

Berghmans L C M, van Waalwijk van Doorn E S C, Nieman F et al 2000 Efficacy of extramural physiotherapy modalities in women with proven bladder overactivity: a randomised clinical trial. Neurourology and Urodynamics 19(4):496–497

Berghmans L C M, van Waalwijk van Doorn E S C, Nieman F et al 2002 Efficacy of physical therapeutic modalities in women with proven bladder overactivity. European Urology 41:581–587

Bower W F, Moore K H, Adams R D et al 1998 A urodynamic study of surface neuromodulation versus sham in detrusor instability and sensory urgency. Journal of Urology 160(6 pt 1):2133–2136

Brubaker L 2000 Electrical stimulation in overactive bladder. Urology 55(5A suppl):17–23

Brubaker, L, Benson T, Bent A et al 1997 Transvaginal electrical stimulation for female urinary incontinence. American Journal of Obstetrics and Gynecology 177:536–540

Colling J C, Ouslander J, Hadley B J et al 1992. Patterned urge–response toileting for incontinence. Oregon Health Sciences University, Portland, OR

Engel B T, Burgio L D, McCormick K A et al 1990 Behavioral treatment of incontinence in the long-term care setting. Journal of the American Geriatrics Society 38(3):361–363

Eriksen B C 1989 Electrostimulation of the pelvic floor in female urinary incontinence [thesis]. University of Trondheim, Norway

Eriksen B C, Eik-Nes S H 1989 Long-term electrical stimulation of the pelvic floor: primary therapy in female stress incontinence? Urologia Internationalis 44:90

Fall M 2000 Reactivation of bladder inhibitory reflexes – an underestimated asset in the treatment of overactive bladder. Urology 55(5a):29–30

Fall M, Lindstrom S 1994 Functional electrical stimulation: physiological basis and clinical principles. International Urogynecology Journal and Pelvic Floor Dysfunction 5:296–304

Fall M, Madersbacher H 1994 Peripheral electrical stimulation. In: Mundy A R, Stephenson T P, Wein A J (eds) Urodynamics – principles, practice and application, 2nd edn. Churchill Livingstone, Edinburgh, pp 495–520

Hay-Smith E J, Herbison P, Morkved S 2001 Physical therapies for prevention of incontinence in adults (Cochrane Protocol). Update Software, Oxford

Hay-Smith J, Herbison P, Ellis G et al 2002 Anticholinergic drugs versus placebo for overactive bladder syndrome in adults. The Cochrane Database of Systematic Reviews (3):CD003781

McCormick K A, Celia M, Scheve A et al 1990 Cost-effectiveness of treating incontinence in severely mobility-impaired long-term care residents. QRB Quality Review Bulletin 16(12):439–443

Messelink E J 1999 The overactive bladder and the role of the pelvic floor muscles. British Journal of Urology 83:31–35

Millard R J, Oldenburg B F 1983 The symptomatic, urodynamic and psychodynamic results of bladder re-education programs. The Journal of Urology 130:715–719

Resnick N M 1998 Improving treatment of urinary incontinence. JAMA 280:2034–2035

Schmidt R 1988 Applications of neurostimulation in urology. Neurourology and Urodynamics 7:585–592

Schnelle J F 1990 Treatment of urinary incontinence in nursing home patients by prompted voiding. Journal of the American Geriatrics Society 38(3):356–360

Schultz-Lampel D 1997 Neurophysiologische Grundlagen und klinische Anwendungen der sacralen Neuromodulation zur Therapie von Blasenfunktionsstörungen (Habilitationsschrift). Fakultätsklinik Witten/Herdecke, Wuppertal

Smith J J 1996 Intravaginal stimulation randomized trial. The Journal of Urology 155:127

Soomro N A, Khadra M H, Robson W et al 2001 A crossover randomized trial of transcutaneous electrical nerve stimulation and oxybutynin in patients with detrusor instability. The Journal of Urology 166:146–149

Sussman D, Garely A 2002 Treatment of overactive bladder with once-daily extended release tolterodine or oxybutynin: the antimuscarinic clinical effectiveness trial (ACET). Current Medical Research and Opinion 18(4):177

Ulmsten U I 1999 The role of surgery in women. Abstract presented at the symposium 'Freedom' at the 14th Annual Meeting of EAU, Stockholm, Sweden, April 7–11

Walsh I K, Thompson T, Loughridge W G et al 2001 Non-invasive antidromic neurostimulation: a simple effective method for improving bladder storage. Neurourology and Urodynamics 20(1):73–84

Wang A C, Wang Y Y, Chen M C 2004 Single-blind, randomized trial of pelvic floor muscle training, biofeedback-assisted pelvic floor muscle training, and electrical stimulation in the management of overactive bladder. Urology 63(1):61–66

Weil E H J 2000 Clinical and experimental aspects of sacral nerve neuromodulation in lower urinary tract dysfunction [thesis]. University of Maastricht, Maastricht, The Netherlands

Wilson P D, Bø K, Hay-Smith J et al 2002 Conservative treatment in women. In: Abrams P, Cardozo L, Khoury S et al (eds) Incontinence. Health Publication, Plymouth, p 573–624

Yamanishi T, Yasuda K, Sakakibara R et al 2000a Randomized, double-blind study of electrical stimulation for urinary incontinence due to detrusor overactivity. Urology 55:353–357

Yamanishi T, Sakakibara R, Uchiyama T et al 2000b Comparative study of the effects of magnetic versus electrical stimulation on inhibition of detrusor overactivity. Urology 56:777–778

Pelvic organ prolapse

James Balmforth and Dudley Robinson

INTRODUCTION

Urogenital prolapse occurs when there is a weakness in the supporting structures of the pelvic floor allowing the pelvic viscera to descend and ultimately fall through the anatomical defect. Although usually not life-threatening, prolapse is often symptomatic and is associated with a deterioration in quality of life and may be the cause of bladder and bowel dysfunction. Extended life expectancy and an expanding elderly population mean that prolapse is an increasingly prevalent condition, especially because the average woman now spends over one-third of her life in the postmenopausal state.

The lifetime risk of having surgery for prolapse is 11%; one-third of these procedures are operations for recurrent prolapse (Olsen et al 1997). Surgery for urogenital prolapse accounts for approximately 20% of elective major gynaecological surgery and this increases to 59% in elderly women. The economic cost of urogenital prolapse is considerable with figures from the USA revealing a total expenditure of $1012 million in 1997. Vaginal hysterectomy accounted for 49%, pelvic floor repairs for 28% and abdominal hysterectomy for 13% of costs (Subak et al 2001).

The incidence of urogenital prolapse increases with age. Approximately 50% of all women over the age of 50 years complain of symptomatic prolapse (Swift 2000). One-third of all hysterectomies in postmenopausal women and 81% of vaginal hysterectomies (representing about 16% of all hysterectomies) are performed for prolapse. The yearly incidence of hysterectomy for prolapse peaks in the 65–69-year age group at around 30 per 10 000 (Al-Allard & Rochette 1991).

Urogenital prolapse is more common following childbirth, but is frequently asymptomatic. Studies have estimated that 50% of parous women have some degree of urogenital prolapse, and of these 10–20% are symptomatic (Progetto Menopausa Italia Study Group 2000, Samuelsson et al 1999). Only 2% of nulliparous women are reported to have prolapse, and this is usually uterine rather than vaginal (Samuelsson et al 1999).

CLASSIFICATION

Urogenital prolapse has traditionally been classified anatomically depending on the site of the defect and the presumed pelvic viscera involved, and by degree. A large number of different grading systems have been used. Intra- and inter-observer variability is significant with these traditional prolapse grading systems and this makes them unsuitable for research purposes.

Traditional anatomical site prolapse classification is as follows.

- **Urethrocele:** prolapse of the lower anterior vaginal wall involving the urethra only.

- **Cystocele:** prolapse of the upper anterior vaginal wall involving the bladder. Generally there is also associated prolapse of the urethra and the term cystourethrocele is used.

- **Uterovaginal prolapse:** prolapse of the uterus, cervix and upper vagina.

- Enterocele: prolapse of the upper posterior wall of the vagina usually containing loops of small bowel. An anterior enterocele may be used to describe prolapse of the upper anterior vaginal wall following hysterectomy.

- Rectocele: prolapse of the lower posterior wall of the vagina involving the anterior wall of the rectum.

The other problem with these terms is that they imply an unrealistic certainty as to the structures on the other side of the reproductive tract bulge. This is a false assumption, particularly in women who have had previous prolapse surgery.

POP-Q prolapse scoring system

As a result of these acknowledged problems with this traditional approach, the International Continence Society (ICS) has produced a standardized prolapse scoring system, termed the POP-Q, to assess urogenital prolapse more objectively (see Fig. 5.39) (Abrams et al

1988). The POP-Q system has been adopted by major organizations including the ICS, the British and American Urogynecologic Societies, and the NIH as an accepted method of describing pelvic support and comparing examinations over time and after interventions. The POP-Q has been shown to have reproducibility in several centres when the examination is conducted in a standardized fashion.

The system describes the measurement of fixed points on the anterior and posterior vaginal walls, cervix and perineal body, against a fixed reference point, which can be consistently and precisely identified. The hymen is the fixed point of reference used throughout the POP-Q system because it provides a precisely identifiable landmark for reference. Although it is recognized that the plane of the hymen is somewhat variable depending upon the degree of levator ani dysfunction, it remains the best landmark available. Measurements are performed in the left lateral position at rest and at maximal Valsalva manoeuvre, therefore providing an accurate and reproducible method of quantifying urogenital prolapse. Because of the uncertainty as to the structures on the other side of the reproductive tract bulge, the terms 'anterior vaginal wall prolapse', 'posterior vaginal wall prolapse' and 'apical prolapse' are preferred.

FASCIAL SUPPORTS OF THE PELVIC VISCERA

The muscles of the pelvic floor are described in more detail in Chapter 3. Let us consider the fascial supports of the pelvic viscera, which consist of the urogenital diaphragm, perineal body and endopelvic fascia and pelvic ligaments. The role played by connective tissue in providing support, and the natural 'variation' that exists in the mechanical strength of such tissue has been emphasized by recent studies (Dietz et al 2005).

Urogenital diaphragm

The urogenital diaphragm (perineal membrane) is a triangular sheet of dense fibrous tissue spanning the anterior half of the pelvic outlet, which is pierced by the vagina and urethra. It arises from the inferior ischiopubic rami and attaches medially to the urethra, vagina and perineal body, therefore supporting the pelvic floor.

Perineal body

The perineal body lies between the vagina and the rectum and provides a point of insertion for the muscles of the pelvic floor. It is attached to the inferior pubic rami and ischial tuberosities through the urogenital diaphragm and superficial transverse perineal muscles. Laterally it is attached to the fibres of the pelvic diaphragm and posteriorly it inserts into the external anal sphincter and coccyx.

Pelvic fascia

The endopelvic fascia is a meshwork of collagen and elastin that represents the fused adventitial layers of the visceral structures and pelvic wall musculature. Condensations of the pelvic fascia are termed ligaments and these play an important part in the supportive role of the pelvic floor.

Pelvic ligaments

The parametrium, composed of the uterosacral and cardinal ligaments, attach the cervix and upper vagina to the pelvic sidewall. The uterosacral ligament forms the medial margin bordering the pouch of Douglas, while the cardinal ligaments attach the lateral aspects of the cervix and vagina to the pelvic sidewall over the sacrum. The former is composed mostly of smooth muscle whereas the cardinal ligaments contain mostly connective tissue and the pelvic blood vessels (Campbell 1950, DeLancey 1992, Range & Woodburne 1964). The round ligaments are not thought to have a role in supporting the uterus, though they may help to maintain anteversion and anteflexion; the broad ligaments are simply folds of peritoneum and provide no support.

The upper one-third of the vagina is supported by the downward extension of the cardinal ligaments whereas the middle third is supported by lateral attachments to the arcus tendineus fasciae pelvis, which is a condensation of the obturator and levator fasciae (Bartscht & DeLancey 1988). These supports suspend the anterior vaginal wall across the pelvis, the layer of fascia anterior to the vagina being called the pubocervical fascia. Posterolaterally the vagina is attached to the endopelvic fascia over the pelvic diaphragm and sacrum by the rectovaginal septum (fascia of Denonvilliers), which extends caudally into the perineal body and cranially into the peritoneum of the pouch of Douglas. The lower one-third is attached anteriorly to the pubic arch by the perineal membrane, posteriorly to the perineal body and laterally to the medial aspect of levator ani.

AETIOLOGY OF PELVIC ORGAN PROLAPSE

Pregnancy and childbirth

The increased incidence of prolapse in multiparous women would suggest that pregnancy and childbirth have an important impact on the supporting function of the pelvic floor. Damage to the muscular and fascial supports of the pelvic floor and changes in innervation contribute to the development of prolapse.

Studies that examine the association of prolapse with pregnancy implicate vaginal delivery as an important risk factor. In the Oxford Family Planning Association Prolapse Epidemiology Study (Mant et al 1997) parity was the strongest risk factor for the development of prolapse with an adjusted relative risk of 10.85 (4.65–33.81). Although the risk increased with increasing parity, the rate of increase slowed after two deliveries. Samuelsson et al (1999) also found statistically significant associations of increasing parity and maximum birth weight with the development of prolapse.

The opening within the levator ani muscle through which the urethra and vagina pass (and through which prolapse occurs) is called the urogenital hiatus of the levator ani. It is bounded ventrally (anteriorly) by the pubic bones, laterally by the levator ani muscles and dorsally (posteriorly) by the perineal body and external anal sphincter. The normal baseline activity of the levator ani muscle keeps the urogenital hiatus closed: it squeezes the vagina, urethra and rectum closed by compressing them against the pubic bone and it lifts the floor and organs in a cephalic direction. The pelvic floor may be damaged during childbirth causing the axis of the levator muscles to become more oblique and creating a funnel that allows the uterus, vagina and rectum to fall through the urogenital hiatus.

The biochemical properties of connective tissue may also play an important role in the development of prolapse. In addition the proportion of connective tissue to muscle within the pelvic floor tends to increase with increasing age and therefore muscle, once damaged by childbirth, may never regain its full strength. There are data that link clinical, laboratory, and genetic syndromes of abnormalities of collagen to pelvic organ prolapse (POP) (Al-Rawizs & Al-Rawizs 1982, Jackson 1996, Marshman et al 1987, Norton et al 1992). In addition, Rinne & Kirkinen (1999) linked POP in young women with a history of abdominal hernias, suggesting a possible connection with abnormal collagen.

Mechanical changes within the pelvic fascia have also been implicated in the causation of urogenital prolapse. During pregnancy the fascia becomes more elastic and therefore more likely to fail. This may explain the increased incidence of stress incontinence observed in pregnancy and the increased incidence of prolapse with multiparity.

Denervation of the pelvic floor musculature has been shown to occur following childbirth (Snooks et al 1986), though gradual denervation has also been demonstrated in nulliparous women with increasing age. The effects were greatest, however, in those women who had documented stress incontinence or prolapse (Smith et al 1989). Furthermore, histological studies have revealed changes in muscle fibre type and distribution suggesting denervation injury associated with ageing and also following childbirth. It would therefore appear that partial denervation of the pelvic floor is part of the normal ageing process, which may be accelerated by pregnancy and childbirth.

Hormonal factors

The effects of ageing and those of oestrogen withdrawal at the time of the menopause are often difficult to separate. Rectus muscle fascia has been shown to become less elastic with increasing age and less energy is required to produce irreversible damage. There is also a known reduction in skin collagen content following the menopause. Work looking at the expression of oestrogen, progesterone and androgen receptors in the levator ani muscles in 55 women undergoing pelvic surgery showed no expression of oestrogen receptors in levator ani muscle fibres, though androgen and progesterone receptors were identified in both the muscle and stromal cells. Interestingly all types of receptor were identified in the levator ani fascia (Copas et al 2001). The distribution of oestrogen receptors throughout the urogenital tract has also been studied with both α and β receptors being found in the vaginal walls and uterosacral ligaments of premenopausal women, but the latter was absent in the vaginal walls of postmenopausal women (Chen et al 1999). This study is supported by further work demonstrating oestrogen receptors in both the cardinal and uterosacral ligaments and there would appear to be a positive correlation with the number of postmenopausal years (Lang et al 2003).

Constipation

Chronically increased intra-abdominal pressure caused by repetitive straining will exacerbate any potential weaknesses in the pelvic floor and is also associated with an increased risk of prolapse (Lubowski et al 1988). In one case–control study, constipation and straining at stool as a young adult before the onset of recognized POP was significantly more common in women who subsequently developed POP (61%) than in women who did not develop pelvic floor dysfunction (PFD) (4%) (Spence-Jones et al 1994).

Smoking

Chronic chest disease resulting in a chronic cough leads to an increase in abdominal pressure and therefore exposes the pelvic floor to greater strain. Over a period of time this will theoretically exacerbate any defects in the pelvic floor musculature and fascia leading to prolapse. There is a lack of good-quality evidence to support this however.

Obesity

Obesity is another condition associated with chronically increased abdominal pressure (Bump et al 1992). Some studies have demonstrated significant relationships between increasing weight and body mass index and the risk of POP or surgery for POP (Mant et al 1997, Progetto Menopausa Italia Study Group 2000); others have not demonstrated this correlation.

Exercise

Increased stress placed on the musculature of the pelvic floor will exacerbate pelvic floor defects and weakness, therefore increasing the incidence of prolapse. Consequently heavy lifting and exercise as well as sports such as weight lifting, high-impact aerobics and long-distance running increase the risk of urogenital prolapse. A study using the Danish National Registry of Hospitalized Patients included over 28 000 assistant nurses aged 20–69 who are traditionally exposed to repetitive heavy lifting. Their risk of surgery for prolapse and herniated lumbar disc was compared to the risk in over 1.6 million same-aged controls (Jorgensen et al 1994). The odds ratio for the nurses compared to controls was 1.6 (1.3–1.9) for prolapse surgery and 1.6 (1.2–2.2) for disc surgery, suggesting that heavy lifting is a significant risk factor.

Previous Pelvic Surgery

Pelvic surgery may also have an effect on the incidence of urogenital prolapse. Continence procedures elevating the bladder neck, but may lead to defects in other pelvic compartments. Burch colposuspension, by fixing the lateral vaginal fornices to the ipsilateral ileopectineal ligaments, leaves a potential defect in the posterior vaginal wall, which predisposes to rectocele and enterocele formation (Wiskind et al 1992). In a 5-year follow-up study of women 36% had cystoceles, 66% rectocele, 32% enterocele and 38% uterine prolapse. A further series of 109 women with vaginal vault prolapse reported that 43% had previously undergone Burch colposuspension. Overall 25% of women required further surgery for prolapse following Burch colposuspension.

Needle suspension procedures and sacrospinous ligament fixation are also associated with an increased incidence of recurrent prolapse (Bump et al 1996).

The association between prolapse and previous hysterectomy is not as clear. Swift (2000) demonstrated a significant association of prolapse with a previous history of hysterectomy or prolapse surgery. One large series reported vaginal vault prolapse 9–13 years after hysterectomy in 11.6% of women who had the hysterectomy for prolapse and in 1.8% of women who had the hysterectomy for benign disease (Marchionni et al 1999). However, other factors such as the ageing process and oestrogen withdrawal following the menopause may also have an important role.

CLINICAL PRESENTATION

Symptoms

Most women complain of a feeling of discomfort or heaviness within the pelvis in addition to a 'lump coming down'. Symptoms tend to become worse with prolonged standing and towards the end of the day. They may also complain of dyspareunia, difficulty in inserting tampons and chronic lower backache. In cases of third-degree prolapse there may be epithelial ulceration and lichenification that results in a symptomatic vaginal discharge or bleeding.

Pelvic organ prolapse may be associated with lower urinary tract symptoms of urgency and frequency of micturition in addition to a sensation of incomplete emptying, which may be relieved by digitally reducing the prolapse. One study noted that most women with symptomatic prolapse still void effectively (Coates et al 1997). FitzGerald found that preoperative voiding studies with the prolapse reduced by a pessary was the best predictor of normalization of residuals postoperatively (FitzGerald et al 2000).

A chronic urinary residual and associated recurrent urinary tract infections may be associated with severe anterior vaginal wall prolapse. Posterior vaginal wall prolapse may be associated with difficulty in opening the bowels with some women complaining of tenesmus and having to digitate to defecate.

EXAMINATION

For gynaecological purposes, women are usually examined in the left lateral position using a Simms' speculum or in a supine position. Digital examination when standing allows an accurate assessment of the degree of urogenital prolapse and in particular vaginal vault support. An abdominal examination should also be performed to exclude the presence of an abdominal or pelvic tumour, which may be responsible for the vaginal findings.

Differential diagnosis includes vaginal cysts, pendunculated fibroid polyp, urethral diverticulum or a chronic uterine inversion.

INVESTIGATION

Urodynamic studies or a post-micturition bladder ultrasound should be performed in women who also complain of concomitant lower urinary tract symptoms to exclude a chronic residual due to associated voiding difficulties. In such cases a mid-stream specimen of urine should be sent for culture and sensitivity.

Subtracted cystometry, with or without videocystourethrography, will allow identification of underlying detrusor overactivity, and it is important to exclude this before surgical repair. In cases of significant anterior vaginal wall prolapse stress testing should be carried out by asking the patient to cough while standing. Because occult urodynamic stress incontinence may be unmasked by straightening the urethra following anterior colporrhaphy this should be simulated by the insertion of a ring pessary or tampon to reduce the cystocele. Studies have described an occult stress incontinence rate after various methods of reducing the prolapse during preoperative testing of 23–50% (Chaikin et at 2000, Gallentine & Cespedes 2001). If stress incontinence is demonstrated then a continence procedure such as colposuspension or insertion of tension-free vaginal tape (TVT) may be the more appropriate procedure.

In cases of severe prolapse in which there may be a degree of ureteric obstruction it is important to evaluate the upper urinary tract either with a renal tract ultrasound or intravenous urogram. An anterior vaginal wall prolapse may be responsible for mild to moderate irritative urinary symptoms, but if these symptoms are severe or recurrent cystoscopy should be performed to exclude a chronic follicular or interstitial cystitis.

TREATMENT

Prevention

In general any factor that leads to chronic increases in abdominal pressure should be avoided. Consequently care should be taken to avoid constipation, which has been implicated as a major contributing factor to urogenital prolapse in developed countries (Spence-Jones et al 1994). In addition the risk of prolapse in patients with chronic chest pathology such as obstructive airways disease and asthma should be reduced by effective management of these conditions. Hormone replacement therapy may theoretically also decrease the incidence of prolapse, though to date no studies have tested this effect.

Smaller family size and improvements in antenatal and intra-partum care have been implicated in the primary prevention of urogenital prolapse. The role of caesarean section may also be important, though studies examining outcome in terms of incontinence and symptomatic prolapse have had mixed results. One large study of over 21 000 Italian women demonstrated a significant association between vaginal delivery and subsequent uterine prolapse, but not with delivery of a baby weighing over 4500 g (Progetto Menopausa Italia Study Group 2000). To date, specific risk-reduction strategies relating to the management of women in labour, have not been studied sufficiently to identify them as beneficial. Similarly, antenatal and postnatal pelvic floor muscle training has not yet been shown to conclusively reduce the incidence of prolapse, though there are logical reasons to think that it may be protective.

Physical therapy

Pelvic floor exercises may have a role in treating women with symptomatic prolapse, but there are no objective evidence-based studies to support this.

Intravaginal devices

Intravaginal devices are available in a wide variety of sizes and designs (Fig. 9.20). Their availability and ease of fitting offer a further conservative line of therapy for those women who are not candidates for surgery. Consequently they may be used in younger women who have not yet completed their family, during pregnancy and the puerperium, and also for those women who may be unfit for surgery. Clearly this may include the elderly, though age alone should not be seen as a contraindication to surgery. In addition a pessary may offer symptomatic relief while awaiting surgery.

Ring pessaries made of silicone or polythene are currently the most frequently used. They are available in a number of different sizes (52–120 mm) and are designed to lie horizontally in the pelvis with one side in the posterior fornix and the other just behind the pubis, therefore supporting the uterus and upper vagina. Fitting is usually done by trial and error. A properly fitted pessary should allow a finger to fit between the pessary and the vaginal wall, therefore aiding and ensuring easy removal. Wood (1992) advises starting with the largest pessary that can be comfortably admitted into the introitus, but does not protrude out of the orifice. A vaginal lubricant is usually applied to the

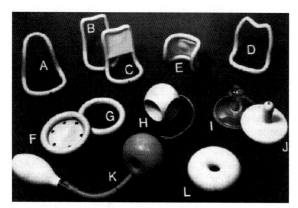

Fig. 9.20   Selection of different vaginal pessaries.

Box 9.2: Operations for pelvic organ prolapse

ANTERIOR COMPARTMENT DEFECTS
- Anterior colporrhaphy: correction of cystourethrocele.
- Paravaginal repair: correction of cystourethrocele

POSTERIOR COMPARTMENT DEFECTS
- Posterior colporrhaphy: correction of rectocele and deficient perineum
- Enterocele repair: correction of enterocele

APICAL PROLAPSE
- Vaginal hysterectomy: uterovaginal prolapse – may be combined with anterior and posterior colporrhaphy
- Vaginal vault suspensions
  - Sacrospinous ligament fixation for vaginal vault prolapse
  - Abdominal sacrocolpopexy for vaginal vault prolapse

pessary surface to minimize the discomfort of fitting. Pretreatment with vaginal oestrogen for 2–3 weeks before insertion is the best way to enhance vaginal lubrication and decrease atrophy and thereby minimize discomfort at the time of fitting.

Pessaries should be changed every 6 months and long-term use may be complicated by vaginal ulceration, therefore a low-dose topical oestrogen may be helpful for postmenopausal women.

Ring pessaries may be useful in the management of minor degrees of urogenital prolapse, but in severe cases, and vaginal vault prolapse a shelf pessary may be more appropriate. These can be difficult to insert and remove and their usage is becoming less common, especially as they preclude coitus.

Surgery

Surgery offers definitive treatment of urogenital prolapse (Box 9.2). It offers the best chance of a long-term cure, but as with all forms of surgical treatment it is not entirely risk free. In particular the risk of postoperative dyspareunia, both short term and occasionally as a long-term complication, need to be discussed. As in other forms of pelvic surgery patients should receive prophylactic antibiotics to reduce the risk of postoperative infection, as well as thromboembolic prophylaxis in the form of low-dose heparin and anti-thromboembolic (TED) stockings. All women should also have a urethral catheter inserted at the time of the procedure unless there is a particular history of voiding dysfunction when a suprapubic catheter may be more appropriate. This allows the residual urine volume to be checked following a void without the need for re-catheterization.

Women having pelvic floor surgery are positioned in the lithotomy position with hips abducted and flexed. To minimize blood loss local infiltration of the vaginal epithelium is performed using 0.5% lidocaine and 1/200 000 adrenaline, though care should be taken in patients with coexistent cardiac disease. At the end of the procedure a vaginal pack may be inserted and removed on the first postoperative day.

Recurrent urogenital prolapse

Approximately one-third of operations for urogenital prolapse are for recurrent defects (Olsen 1997). Recurrent prolapse may occur following both abdominal and vaginal hysterectomy, previous vaginal repair and continence surgery. Women with intrinsically weak connective tissue are at increased risk (Al-Rawizs & Al-Rawizs 1982, Marshman et al 1987). In such cases the vaginal epithelium may be scarred and atrophic making surgical correction technically more difficult and increasing the risk of damage to the bladder and bowel. The risk of postoperative complications such as dyspareunia secondary to vaginal shortening and stenosis is also increased.

In recent years there has been an increasing interest in the use of biological and synthetic surgical meshes to reinforce traditional reconstructive techniques. These materials theoretically offer additional support in cases where the endopelvic fascia and vaginal epithelium are intrinsically weak.

The use of prosthetic mesh was pioneered by general surgeons for the repair of abdominal wall hernias and adapted for use in vaginal surgery. However, unlike the anterior abdominal wall, the vagina is a tubular structure and it is important not to compromise vaginal capacity, elasticity or sensation if sexual function is to be adequately retained. In reconstructive pelvic surgery, biological and synthetic prostheses have been commonly employed for suspending the vaginal vault as part of an abdominal sacrocolpopexy operation since this was first described by Lane in 1962. Reinforcement of the anterior and posterior vaginal walls with mesh as part of a vaginal pelvic floor repair is a more recent phenomenon (Julian 1996). There is emerging evidence to suggest a role for the use of surgical meshes in vaginal repair surgery, but the ideal material and patient group have yet to be firmly established. In one of the very few randomized controlled trials to be conducted in this area of interest, Sand demonstrated significantly lower recurrence rates at 12-month follow-up in 161 women with cystoceles (140 primary and 21 recurrent) undergoing fascial plication with mesh reinforcement of the anterior vaginal wall (25%) compared to those undergoing fascial plication alone (43%). No mesh-related complications were reported during this trial (Sand et al 2001). Elsewhere, the published incidence of mesh-related complications varies greatly. Dyspareunia is a common complication associated with the use of synthetic mesh and may be associated with erosion into the vagina, lower urinary tract and rectum. Erosion rates as high as 25% and cases of severe dyspareunia precluding the resumption of sexual intercourse have been reported (De Tayrac et al 2002). Attempting to reverse adverse effects associated with the use of non-absorbable synthetic prostheses can prove very difficult.

Synthetic prosthetic meshes may be classified into types I to IV according to the type of material, pore size and whether they are monofilament or multifilament (Amid 1997). Current evidence favours the use of type I polypropylene meshes on the basis of lower infection and erosion rates, but there is a desperate need for further randomized controlled trials to determine long-term efficacy and potential morbidity associated with the use of these materials. Although the use of mesh is becoming more common it should be reserved for those patients with recurrent defects in specialist pelvic floor reconstructive surgery units.

CONCLUSION

Although not life-threatening, urogenital prolapse is responsible for much morbidity and impairment of quality of life. With approximately 50% of elective gynaecological operations being performed for correction of urogenital prolapse the economic considerations are also considerable. Although conservative measures may be useful in the management of mild symptomatic prolapse, surgery offers the definitive treatment. Women should be carefully assessed with regard to their symptoms and how these impact on their quality of life before any surgical treatment. As with surgery for female stress incontinence, the primary procedure offers the greatest probability of success, and it is important that women are given realistic figures on the likely outcome of surgical intervention. The large number of surgical procedures described is indicative of the fact that there is no perfect solution and this is reflected in the number of patients who present with recurrent prolapse. Such women should be managed in tertiary units by surgeons with a specialist interest in pelvic floor reconstructive surgery. The use of synthetic meshes to augment traditional prolapse repair operations is an exciting development, but as yet there is little robust evidence to support its widespread use.

REFERENCES

Abrams P, Blaivas JG, Stanton SL et al 1988 The International Continence Society Committee on Standardization of Terminology. The standardization of terminology of lower urinary tract function. Scandinavian Journal of Urology and Nephrology 114S:5–19

Al-Allard P, Rochette L 1991 The descriptive epidemiology of hysterectomy, province of Quebec. Annals of Epidemiology 1:541–549

Al-Rawizs S, Al-Rawizs T 1982 Joint hypermobility in women with genital prolapse. Lancet 26:1439–1441

Amid P 1997 Classification of biomaterials and their related complications in abdominal wall surgery. Hernia 1:15–21

Bartscht K D, DeLancey J O L 1988 A technique to study cervical descent. Obstetrics and Gynecology 72:940–943

Bump R C, Hurt W G, Theofrastous J P et al 1996 Randomized prospective comparison of needle colposuspension versus endopelvic fascia plication for potential stress incontinence prophylaxis in women undergoing vaginal reconstruction for stage III or IV pelvic organ prolapse. American Journal of Obstetrics and Gynecology 175:326–335

Bump R C, Sugerman H J, Fantl F A et al 1992 Obesity and lower urinary tract function in women: effect of surgically induced weight loss. American Journal of Obstetrics and Gynecology 167:392–399

Campbell R M 1950 The anatomy and histology of the sacrouterine ligaments. American Journal of Obstetrics and Gynecology 59:1–12

Chaikin D C, Groutz A, Blaivas J G 2000 Predicting the need for antiincontinence surgery in continent women undergoing repair of severe urogenital prolapse. The Journal of Urology 163:531–534

Chen G D, Oliver R H, Leung B S et al 1999 Oestrogen receptor α and β expression in the vaginal walls and uterosacral ligaments of premenopausal and postmenopausal women. Fertility and Sterility 71(6):1099–1102

Coates K W, Harris R L, Cundiff G W et al 1997 Uroflowmetry in women with urinary incontinence and pelvic organ prolapse. British Journal of Urology 80:217–221

Copas P, Bukovsky A, Asbury B et al 2001 Oestrogen, progesterone and androgen receptor expression in levator ani muscle and fascia. Journal of Women's Health & Gender–based Medicine 10:785–795

DeLancey J O L 1992 Anatomic aspects of vaginal eversion after hysterectomy. American Journal of Obstetrics and Gynecology 166:1717–1728

De Tayrac R, Gervaise A, Fernandez H 2002 Tension-free polypropylene mesh for vaginal repair of severe anterior vaginal wall prolapse. International Urogynecology Journal and Pelvic Floor Dysfunction 13(1):S41

Dietz H P, Hansell N K, Grace ME et al 2005 Bladder neck mobility is a heritable trait. BJOG 112(3):334–339

FitzGerald M P, Kulkarni N, Fenner D 2000 Postoperative resolution of urinary retention in patients with advanced pelvic organ prolapse. American Journal of Obstetrics and Gynecology 183:1361–1364

Gallentine M L, Cespedes R D 2001 Occult stress urinary incontinence and the effect of vaginal vault prolapse on abdominal leak point pressures. Urology 57:40–44

Hagen S, Stark D, Maher C et al 2004 Conservative management of pelvic organ prolapse in women. Cochrane Database of Systematic Reviews (2):CD003882

Jackson S R, Avery N C, Tarlton J F et al 1996 Changes in metabolism of collagen in genitourinary prolapse Lancet 347:1658–1661

Jorgensen S, Hein H O, Gyntelberg F 1994 Heavy lifting at work and risk of genital prolapse and herniated lumbar disc in assistant nurses. Occupational Medicine 44:47–49

Julian T M 1996 The efficacy of Marlex mesh in the repair of severe recurrent vaginal prolapse of the anterior mid vaginal wall. American Journal of Obstetrics and Gynecology 175:1472–1475

Lane F E 1962 Repair of posthysterectomy vaginal vault prolapse. Obstetrics and Gynecology 89:501–506

Lang J H, Zhu L, Sun Z J et al 2003 Oestrogen levels and oestrogen receptors in patients with stress urinary incontinence and pelvic organ prolapse. International Journal of Gynaecology and Obstetrics 80:35–39

Lubowski D Z, Swash M, Nichols J et al 1988 Increases in pudendal nerve terminal motor latency with defecation straining. The British Journal of Surgery 75:1095–1097

Mant J, Painter R, Vessey M 1997 Epidemiology of genital prolapse: observations from the Oxford Family Planning Association study. British Journal of Obstetrics and Gynaecology 104:579–585

Marchionni M, Bracco G L, Checcucci V et al 1999 True incidence of vaginal vault prolapse: thirteen years experience. The Journal of Reproductive Medicine 44:679–684

Marshman D, Percy J, Fielding I et al 1987 Rectal prolapse: relationship with joint mobility. The Australian and New Zealand Journal of Surgery 545:827–829

Norton P, Boyd C, Deak S 1992 Collagen synthesis in women with genital prolapse or stress urinary incontinence. Neurourology and Urodynamics 11:300–301

Olsen A L, Smith V G, Bergstrom J O et al 1997 Epidemiology of surgically managed pelvic organ prolapse and urinary incontinence. Obstetrics and Gynaecology 89:501–506

Progetto Menopausa Italia Study Group 2000 Risk factors for genital prolapse in non-hysterectomised women around menopause: results from a large cross-sectional study in menopausal clinics in Italy. European Journal of Obstetrics, Gynecology, and Reproductive Biology 93:125–140

Range R L, Woodburne R T 1964 The gross and microscopic anatomy of the transverse cervical ligaments. American Journal of Obstetrics and Gynecology 90:460–467

Rinne K M, Kirkinen P P 1999 What predisposes young women to genital prolapse? European Journal of Obstetrics, Gynecology, and Reproductive Biology 84:23–25

Samuelsson E C, Victor F T A, Tibblin G 1999 Signs of genital prolapse in a Swedish population of women 20 to 59 years of age and possible related factors. American Journal of Obstetrics and Gynecology 180:299–305

Sand P K, Koduri S, Lobel R W et al 2001 Prospective randomised trial of Polyglactin 910 mesh to prevent recurrences of cystoceles and rectoceles. American Journal of Obstetrics and Gynecology 185:1229–1307

Smith A R B, Hosker G L, Warrell D W 1989 The role of partial denervation of the pelvic floor in the aetiology of genitourinary prolapse and stress incontinence. A neurophysiological study. British Journal of Obstetrics and Gynaecology 96:24–28

Snooks S J, Swash M, Henry M M et al 1986 Risk factors in childbirth causing damage to the pelvic floor innervation. International Journal of Colorectal Disease 1:20–24

Spence–Jones C, Kamm M A, Henry M M et al 1994 Bowel dysfunction: a pathogenic factor in uterovaginal prolapse and urinary stress incontinence. British Journal of Obstetrics and Gynaecology 101:147–152

Swift S E 2000 The distribution of pelvic organ support in a population of female subjects seen for routine gynecologic health care. American Journal of Obstetrics and Gynecology 183:277–285

Subak L L, Waetjen E, van den Eeden S et al 2001 Cost of pelvic organ prolapse surgery in the United States. Obstetrics and Gynecology 98:646–651

Wiskind A K, Creighton S M, Stanton S L 1992 The incidence of genital prolapse after the Burch colposuspension. American Journal of Obstetrics and Gynecology 167:399–404

Wood N 1992 The use of vaginal pessaries for uterine prolapse. The Nurse Practitioner 17:31–38

PELVIC FLOOR MUSCLE TRAINING IN PREVENTION AND TREATMENT OF POP

Kari Bø and Helena Frawley

INTRODUCTION

Because of its location inside the pelvis, the pelvic floor muscles (PFM) are the only muscle group in the body capable of giving structural support to the pelvic organs and the pelvic openings (urethra, vagina and anus) (Fig. 9.21). It is estimated that approximately 50% of women lose some of the supportive mechanisms of the pelvic floor due to childbirth, leading to different degrees of pelvic organ prolapse (POP) (Brubaker et al 2002). Samuelsson et al (1999) studied 487 women 20–59 years of age attending routine gynaecology assessment and found that 30.8% presented with some degree of POP. They showed that prevalence of POP was associated with age, parity, and PFM weakness as measured by vaginal palpation (Samuelsson et al 1999). DeLancey

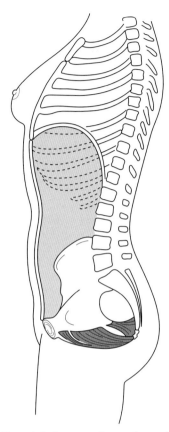

Fig. 9.21 The pelvic floor muscles are located inside the pelvis and form a structural support for internal organs.

et al (2003) demonstrated that women with POP generated 43% less force and had more atrophy of the PFM than women without POP.

Prolapse may be asymptomatic until the descending organ is through the introitus, and therefore POP may not be recognized until it is advanced (Brubaker et al 2002). In some women the prolapse advances rapidly, whereas in others it remains stable for many years. There are no published studies on the natural history of POP. Although historically most clinicians have considered that POP does not seem to regress (Brubaker et al 2002), recently Handa et al (2004) found that prolapse is not always chronic and progressive, and spontaneous regression is common, especially for minor prolapse. The risk of development of prolapse increases with age. Therefore as women live longer, there may be an increase in prevalence of POP in the elderly population (Thakar & Stanton 2002).

Pathophysiological and etiological factors causing prolapse are not yet totally understood (Brubaker et al

2002, Thakar & Stanton 2002), therefore rationales for appropriate methods to prevent and treat the condition are difficult to recommend. However, as many authors consider that stress urinary incontinence (SUI) and POP share similar pathophysiologies (Bump & Norton 1998), proven guidelines for intervention with PFM training (PFMT) for SUI may conceptually apply to POP.

Treatment options for POP are surgery, use of mechanical support (pesssary), lifestyle interventions, and PFMT (Brubaker et al 2002, Thakar & Stanton 2002). According to Brubaker et al (2002) the indication for treatment of POP is uncertain. Although systematic reviews and randomized controlled trials (RCTs) have shown convincing effect of PFMT for stress and mixed urinary incontinence (Hay-Smith et al 2001, Wilson et al 2002), there seems to be a paucity of research for other conditions caused by pelvic floor dysfunction.

Thakar & Stanton (2002) suggested that PFMT may limit the progression of and alleviate mild symptoms of prolapse such as low back pain and pelvic pressure. However, they stated that PFMT would not be useful if the prolapse extends to or beyond the vaginal introitus. Also Davila (1996) suggested that 'Kegel exercises' may alleviate mild prolapse symptoms only. None of the above-mentioned authors, however, referred to any studies to support their recommendations of PFMT for POP. In a Cochrane review (Hagen et al 2004b), no completed RCTs of PFMT for POP were found, but two RCTs and one pilot trial in progress were cited.

A survey of UK women's health physical therapists showed that several women attending physical therapy practice presented with a mixture of pelvic floor dysfunctions such as SUI and prolapse, and that 92% of the physical therapists assessed and treated women with POP (Hagen et al 2004a). The most commonly used treatment was PFMT with and without biofeedback. However, there were no available guidelines for treatment of POP in clinical practice.

RATIONALE FOR PELVIC FLOOR MUSCLE TRAINING IN PREVENTION AND TREATMENT OF POP

There are two main hypotheses of mechanisms of how PFMT may be effective in the prevention and treatment of SUI (Bø 2004), and the same theories may apply for a possible effect of PFMT to prevent and treat POP. The two hypotheses are:

1. women learn to consciously contract before and during increases in abdominal pressure (also termed 'bracing' or 'performing the knack'), and continue to

perform such contractions as a behaviour modification to prevent descent of the pelvic floor;

2. women are taught to perform regular strength training to build up 'stiffness' and structural support of the pelvic floor over time (Bø 2004). There is basic research, case–control studies, and RCTs to support both hypotheses in the prevention and treatment for SUI.

Conscious contraction (bracing or 'performing the knack') to prevent and treat POP

Research on basic and functional anatomy supports conscious contraction of the PFM as an effective manoeuvre to stabilize the pelvic floor (Miller et al 2001, Peschers et al 2001). However, to date there are no studies on how much strength or what neuromotor control strategies are necessary to prevent descent during cough and other physical exertions, or how to prevent gradual descent due to activities of daily living or over time. Furthermore it is not known if regular counterbracing during daily activities is enough to increase muscle strength or cause morphological changes of the PFM. There are no studies investigating the use of counterbracing/the knack in the prevention or treatment of POP. An interesting, but difficult hypothesis to test is whether women at risk of POP can prevent development of prolapse by performing the knack during every rise in abdominal pressure. Because it is possible to learn to hold one's hand over the mouth before and during coughing, it is perhaps possible to learn to pre-contract the PFM before and during simple and single tasks such as coughing, lifting and isolated exercises such as performing abdominal exercises. However, multiple task activities and repetitive movements such as running, playing tennis, aerobics and dance activities can not be conducted with intentional co-contractions of the PFM.

Strength training

The theoretical rationale for intensive strength training (exercise) of the PFM to treat POP is that strength training may build up the structural support of the pelvis by elevating the levator plate to a permanently higher location inside the pelvis and by enhancing hypertrophy and stiffness of the PFM and connective tissue. This would facilitate a more effective automatic motor unit firing, thus preventing descent during increases in abdominal pressure. The training may also lift the pelvic floor and thereby the protruding organs in a cranial direction. The pelvic openings may narrow and the pelvic organs may be held in place during abdominal pressure rises (Bø 2004).

Bernstein et al (1997) found a significant increase in muscle volume after training shown by ultrasound. Balmforth et al (2004) showed that the position of the bladder neck as observed by ultrasound, was significantly elevated at rest, with Valsalva manoeuvre and with squeeze after 14 weeks of supervised PFMT and use of the knack. The findings of Bernstein et al (1997) and Balmforth et al (2004) support that morphological changes occur after PFMT and support this hypothesized mechanism, but need to be confirmed in high-quality RCTs. The only two intervention studies of PFMT to treat POP found in this literature review measured neither PFM strength nor morphological changes.

As described by DeLancey (1993) in his 'boat in dry dock' concept (see Fig. 1.2, p. 2), the connective tissue support of the pelvic organs fails if the PFM relax or are damaged, and organ descent occurs. This underpins the concept of elevation of the PFM and closure of the urogenital hiatus as important elements in conservative management of POP. Using transabdominal ultrasound to assess PFM movement, Thompson & Sullivan (2003) found an inability to elevate the levator plate was a feature of women with POP, significantly more so than in women with SUI. Women with POP were more likely to exhibit a downward movement when attempting to contract the PFM. The ability to re-train this faulty motor control strategy was considered to be important.

Gosling (1996) has drawn the analogy of the role of muscle tone in supporting joints (the loss of which leads to joint instability) to muscle tone supporting pelvic organ viscera. He suggested the principles were the same, therefore the influence of muscle contractility to support pelvic organs is likely to far outweigh the contributions from passive structures such as pelvic fascia and ligaments.

The relationship between enlarged urogenital hiatus and POP was highlighted over 50 years ago by Berglas & Rubin (1953) (Fig. 9.22). In their landmark schematic diagram, the extent of the levator hiatus is shown to increase with a more vertical inclination of the levator plate. In this sketch, the hiatus area reflects the area between the medial borders of the levator ani from the symphysis pubis to the anococcygeal raphe. The relationship between enlarged levator hiatus and prolapse has been observed by several authors in more recent years (DeLancey & Hurd 1998, Ghetti et al 2005, Hoyte et al 2001, Singh et al 2003), and while it is not known whether this is cause or effect, reducing the size of the hiatus would seem to offer greater organ support. A PFM contraction has been shown to reduce the transverse and anteroposterior hiatus dimensions in women with SUI (Hextall et al 1999), and to reduce the levator ani muscle hiatus in women with prolapse (Ghetti et al

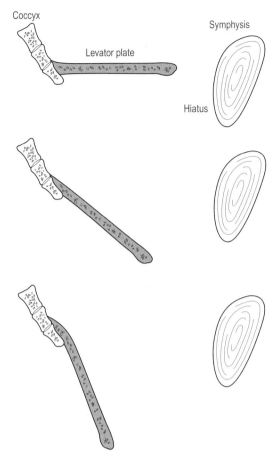

Coccyx

Levator plate

Symphysis

Hiatus

Fig. 9.22 The relationship between lengthening of the levator hiatus and the vertical inclination of the levator plate. (From Berglas & Rubin 1953, with permission.)

2005) but it is not known if the size of the hiatus changes following PFMT intervention in women with SUI or POP.

The relationship of some aspects of PFM function to prevalence has been studied by Slieker-ten Hove et al (2004). In the evaluation of PFM contractility, this study found no relationship between prolapse severity and PFM strength as measured by digital palpation; however, a significant trend towards increased POP with PFM relaxation, use of extra-pelvic muscles, and perineal descent was noted. In addition, this study found a significant relationship between the severity of prolapse and PFM coordination during coughing, as measured by perineal descent, presence of prolapse and urine loss. The clinical importance of these elements, as well as other aspects of PFM function and neuromotor control in assessment and treatment of POP is not yet known.

Surgery for POP is common, with a lifetime risk of undergoing a single operation for either prolapse or incontinence (POPUI) by age 80 of 11.1% (Olsen et al 1997). Surgery for prolapse is not successful for all women. Rates of recurrence of POP after surgery are not known precisely because many women do not re-present for repeat surgery, despite the recurrence of POP. Rates of re-operation for POP vary between 29.2% (Olsen et al 1997) and 58% (Whiteside et al 2004). Clark et al (2003) found the only significant risk factor for re-operation for POPUI was previous surgery for POPUI. Whiteside et al (2004) found women aged younger than 60 years and with more advanced prolapse were predictive of prolapse recurrence. However, Swift et al (2001) found that increasing age, as well as a history of hysterectomy and previous POP surgery were predictive of severe POP. The differences in risk factors may be explained by different study populations.

Some authors consider PFMT to be a useful adjunct to surgery (Bidmead & Cardozo 2001, Kegel 1956); however, these recommendations have been based on clinical impression only. As POP repair surgery can be considered as only a compensatory mechanism (Whiteside et al 2004), additional support may come from rehabilitation of a key element that cannot be improved with surgery (i.e the levator ani muscles). Carey & Dwyer (2001) considered PFM weakness as the most significant factor in the pathogenesis of POP, suggesting that more than surgical repair of fascia or ligaments is required if effective long-term support of POP is to be achieved.

Studies investigating the role of PFMT in partnership with (uro)gynaecological surgery are only beginning to emerge, and many questions remain unanswered. Knowledge of specific patient attributes such as activity levels, general well-being and specific PFM function in women undergoing first or repeat POP is lacking. Furthermore, the effect of POP surgery on PFM function is not known. Does repair of deficient connective tissue allow the PFM which support the pelvic organs, to work more efficiently by providing a firmer base, or improved alignment? Or does the process of surgery inhibit or compromise PFM action, at least in the short term?

DeLancey & Hurd (1998) noted that the size of the urogenital hiatus was larger after several failed POP operations than after successful surgery or a single failure. A recent retrospective study (Vakili et al 2005) investigated the contributions of PFM strength and genital hiatus as factors in POP surgical failure. In this study, PFM contraction strength was assessed by digital palpation and genital hiatus width was measured according to the POP-Q system (distance from the middle of the external urethral meatus to the inferior hymenal ring). At a mean of 5 months postoperatively, recurrence of POP following surgery was correlated with a reduced PFM contraction strength and an increased genital hiatus. Whether reduction of the hiatus width in response to PFMT can reduce recurrence of POP after surgery has not been shown. Differences between vaginal, abdominal and laparoscopic surgery, and their effect on the PFM are also not known.

EVIDENCE FOR PFMT IN THE PREVENTION AND TREATMENT OF POP

This section is divided into three parts:

1. lifestyle interventions;
2. PFMT in primary and secondary prevention and as treatment of POP;
3. PFMT to prevent recurrence after prolapse surgery.

Methods

Computerized searches in PubMed, the Cochrane library, and PEDro were undertaken using the words pelvic organ prolapse or genital prolapse in combination with pelvic floor muscle training, pelvic muscle training, or physical activity. In addition, hand searches from reference lists of general literature on POP were conducted. Methodological quality of randomized controlled trials (RCTs) was rated with the PEDro scale (Maher et al 2003) The scale is based on the Delphi list, and its reliability is supported empirically (Maher et al 2003).

Lifestyle interventions

To date, we have been unable to find any RCTs or uncontrolled intervention studies addressing the effect of lifestyle interventions in the prevention and treatment of POP. Some studies have identified lifestyle risk factors associated with POP, including heavy lifting (Jørgensen et al 1994), constipation and straining at stool (Spence-Jones et al 1994), chronic pulmonary disease (Rinne & Kirkinen 1999) and obesity (Hendrix et al 2002).

A study by Ottesen et al (2003) considered a mixture of lifestyle interventions and exercise on women who had POP surgery. These authors compared POP recurrence rates following vaginal surgery in a retrospective group of patients (who underwent a 'normal' convalescence period, median 6 weeks) with a prospective group of patients who were advised to return to normal activities much sooner. The 6-month postoperative subjective recurrence was 22% in the former group compared to 17% at 1 year postoperatively in the latter. Only 40% of patients in the retrospective study received instructions in PFMT from a specialized physical therapist. The percentage in the prospective group who received instruction was not stated, other than that all patients were advised to perform PFMT. The authors concluded that as POP recurrence rates were not altered significantly by early return to normal activities, perhaps the risk of recurrence might be better reduced through improved instructions on how to do PFMT and how to use PFM contractions before and during increases in abdominal pressure, as well as prophylactic initiatives to protect the pelvic floor. However, due to the limitations in the design, it cannot be concluded from this study what the role of PFMT in the prevention of recurrence is, nor when is the ideal time or dosage to recommence exercises postoperatively.

Quality of the intervention: dose–response issues

As no RCTs have been found based on the outcomes of lifestyle interventions alone on the outcomes of POP, no comment on the quality of the intervention can be made. There is currently no evidence for addressing lifestyle interventions for women with POP, but as recommendations on these exist for women with SUI (Wilson et al 2002), future studies may establish a causal link to POP, and intervention studies may establish a benefit in addressing these risk factors in POP.

PFMT in primary and secondary prevention and as treatment of POP

No studies were found for primary prevention of POP. One uncontrolled study and one RCT were found for treatment of prolapse. In the uncontrolled study, Mimura et al (2000) followed 32 women with rectocele greater than 2 cm below 'the expected line' at proctography. The patients received biofeedback-assisted PFMT with a nurse every 2–3 weeks, usually for four to five sessions. Twenty-five women met for follow-up assessment (drop-out 22%). The results showed that complete resolution of symptoms was achieved in 12%. At follow-up 14 patients (56%) felt that their constipation had improved a little and 11 (34%) felt that it had improved a lot.

Piya-Anant et al (2003) conducted both a cross-sectional study in 682 women and an intervention study of 654 of the same women (mean age 67 years, SD ± 5.6): 70% in the cross-sectional study were diagnosed with POP – 30% were classified as severe and 40% as having mild prolapse. The women were randomly allocated to either an experimental or a control group. Women in the experimental group were taught to contract the PFM 30 times after a meal every day. Women not able to contract were asked to return to the clinic once a month until they could perform correct contractions. In addition, they were advised to increase their intake of vegetables and fruit and to drink at least 2 L of water daily to prevent constipation. There were follow-up visits every 6 months throughout the 2-year intervention period. The results showed that the intervention was only effective in the group with severe prolapse. The rate of worsening of POP was significantly greater in the control group than the PFMT group: 72.2% versus 27.8%, respectively. Methodological quality of the study is shown in Table 9.11. The methodological score was 4/10, therefore the results should be viewed with some caution.

Quality of the intervention: dose–response issues

The intervention in the Piya-Anant et al (2003) study is not described in detail, but women were taught a correct contraction of the PFM. However, the method used to assess correctness of the PFM contraction was not described. Duration and intensity of the contraction were not described and there was neither assessment of adherence to the exercise protocol nor measurement of PFM strength. In addition there was co-intervention with change of nutrition and water intake. This may have improved constipation and excessive straining at stool in some women. However, no data were presented on constipation or straining. The evaluation method and classification categories of POP applied by Piya-Anant et al (2003) were poorly described and there were no references to studies showing that the evaluation systems used had been tested for responsiveness, intra- or inter-test reliability, or validity.

Evidence for PFMT to prevent recurrence after prolapse surgery

The Cochrane review investigating conservative management of POP (Hagen et al 2004b) identified two studies in progress that included PFMT following prolapse surgery. Both of these studies have included lifestyle interventions in addition to PFMT as part of the treatment group protocol. Therefore there are currently no completed RCTs that have shown the effect of PFMT as the sole intervention to prevent POP recurrence postoperatively.

Jarvis et al (2005) studied the effect of PFMT and bladder/bowel training on women undergoing surgery for POPUI with a RCT of 60 women: 30 women were randomized to each of the treatment and control groups. The intervention consisted of PFMT, functional bracing of PFM before rises in abdominal pressure, bladder/bowel training and advice to reduce straining during voiding and defecation. Subjects in the treatment group received the intervention 'package' from a physical therapist on three occasions: 2–4 weeks preoperatively, day 2 postoperatively and at 6 weeks postoperatively. A blinded investigator measured outcomes at 12 weeks postoperatively. All subjects demonstrated improved scores postoperatively in the outcomes of urinary leakage (paper towel test), urinary symptoms and quality of life scores (both assessed by King's Health Questionnaire), and 48-hour voiding diary. The treatment group demonstrated significantly larger pre- to postoperative differences than the control group in the urinary symptom and quality of life scores, and the voiding diary outcomes. Postoperatively, subjects in the treatment group demonstrated an increase in maximum vaginal squeeze pressure compared with subjects in the control group, who showed a decrease in squeeze pressure. The authors recommended preoperative instruction and postoperative reinforcement by a physical therapist for women undergoing surgery for POPUI.

Although the surgical population in this study comprised a mixture of prolapse-only, incontinence-only, and combined-POPUI surgery, most subjects in both groups had prolapse-only surgery, so these results from the physical therapy intervention may be generalizable to a prolapse surgery population. However, no prolapse-specific assessment or outcome measures were reported, therefore the effect of the intervention on the presence of any prolapse signs or symptoms postoperatively is not known. Methodological quality of the study is shown in Table 9.11. The methodological score was 6/10, therefore the effectiveness of the treatment can be accepted with reasonable confidence.

The second study referred to in the Cochrane review is currently investigating the effect of pre- and postoperative physical therapy for women undergoing vaginal POP surgery or hysterectomy (Frawley et al as cited in Hagen et al 2004b). This single-blinded RCT will enrol 50 women, randomizing 25 women to receive a combination of PFMT and lifestyle modifications. Outcomes will be assessed at 12 months postoperatively. The study follow-up period ceased in 2006, and results of the trial will be available in late 2007.

Quality of intervention: dose–response issues

The study by Jarvis et al (2005) provided a low but pragmatic level of intervention to the treatment group. The frequency of intervention was three visits. The home programme of PFM exercises was stated as 'individualized' with four sets of home exercises per day plus performance of functional bracing at appropriate times. No other details of the intensity of exercise or compliance with home training were provided. PFM

Table 9.11   PEDro quality score of RCTs in systematic review

E – Eligibility criteria specified
1 – Subjects randomly allocated to groups
2 – Allocation concealed
3 – Groups similar at baseline
4 – Subjects blinded
5 – Therapist administering treatment blinded
6 – Assessors blinded
7 – Measures of key outcomes obtained from over 85% of subjects
8 – Data analysed by intention to treat
9 – Statistical comparison between groups conducted
10 – Point measures and measures of variability provided

Study	E	1	2	3	4	5	6	7	8	9	10	Total score
Piya-Anant et al 2003	+	+	?	+	–	–	+	–	–	+	–	4
Jarvis et al 2005	+	+	+	+	–	–	+	–	?	+	+	6

+, criterion is clearly satisfied; –, criterion is not satisfied; ?, not clear if the criterion was satisfied. Total score is determined by counting the number of criteria that are satisfied, except that scale item one 'eligibility criteria specified' is not used to generate the total score. Total scores are out of 10.

contraction was assessed and trained by continence physical therapists, so the correctness of the intervention can be assumed. Assessment of PFM strength was recorded via digital palpation and manometry, but no results for digital palpation were provided. Limited results of the manometry scores were provided, which restricts interpretation of the clinical significance of the pre- to post-operative changes in PFM strength. Despite these limitations, the PFMT intervention resulted in a positive outcome at 12 weeks postoperatively, which represents an encouraging direction for future surgical plus PFMT studies.

Several surveys of rehabilitation guidelines including PFMT for patients undergoing POP or POPUI surgery have highlighted the variations in consensus among clinicians (Frawley et al 2005, Hibner et al 2004, Ottesen et al 2001). In the absence of evidence to guide these clinical protocols for POP surgery patients, questions remain regarding optimal rehabilitation, activity restriction, exercise resumption, and PFMT regimens.

CONCLUSION

To date there are few published RCTs to support PFMT in the prevention and treatment of POP. However, there is a strong rationale that PFMT may be effective both in prevention and treatment. Because PFMT has no known side-effects, has been shown to be effective in RCTs and systematic reviews to treat SUI and mixed incontinence (Hay-Smith et al 2001, Wilson et al 2002), and many women present with both POP and UI, it is our opinion that physical therapists should continue to treat POP patients with PFMT. Although POP may occur in the anterior/middle/posterior compartments, the pelvic floor should be considered as a single unit in the treatment of POP (Thakar & Stanton 2002). As occult SUI may be a common side-effect of pessary use and surgery (Brubaker et al 2002, Clemons et al 2004, Maher et al 2004), PFMT should also be advocated in combination with these other treatments. Until information from RCTs showing a positive effect of PFMT to prevent recurrence of prolapse is available, it is recommended that women undergoing POP surgery receive instruction from a specialized physical therapist in PFMT to support the prolapse repair and protect against recurrence or development of de-novo pelvic floor symptoms. There is an urgent need for high-quality RCTs with appropriate training protocols to evaluate the effect of PFMT to prevent and treat POP.

CLINICAL RECOMMENDATIONS FOR TREATMENT

• Include questions about POP symptoms in history taking.

- Assess for POP by use of the POP-Q or simply register the prolapse during straining in cm above or below the hymen. Record the position used because it may affect reproducibility of the measurement. An upright position may be necessary to reproduce the extent of the prolapse that bothers the patient (Visco et al 2003).

- Explain rationale for PFMT in the prevention and treatment of prolapse.

- After thorough instruction of how to perform a correct PFM contraction, check ability to contract.

- Assess PFM strength and ability to elevate the pelvic floor.

- Implement outcome measures to measure effect of intervention for POP symptoms. Suggested outcome measures for POP quality of life and symptom distress/bother could include:
  - the Prolapse Quality of Life (P-QoL) (Digesu et al 2005);
  - the Pelvic Floor Distress Inventory (PFDI) (Barber et al 2001);
  - the Pelvic Floor Impact Questionnaire (PFIQ) (Barber et al 2001);
  - the Urogenital Distress Inventory (Shumaker et al 1994);
  - symptoms and bother in POP (Mouritsen & Larsen 2003).

- Follow clinical recommendations for PFMT for SUI and lifestyle modifications as may be relevant for each woman.

- If no reduction of prolapse severity nor symptom bother after 3 months of supervised training, refer back to the gynaecologist for further management.

REFERENCES

Balmforth J, Bidmead J, Cardozo L et al 2004 Raising the tone: a prospective observational study evaluating the effect of pelvic floor muscle training on bladder neck mobility and associated improvement in stress urinary incontinence [abstract 111]. Neurourology and Urodynamics 23(5):553–554

Barber M D, Kuchibhatla M N, Pieper C F et al 2001 Psychometric evaluation of 2 comprehensive condition-specific quality of life instruments for women with pelvic floor disorders. American Journal of Obstetrics and Gynecology 185(6):1388–1395

Berglas B, Rubin I C 1953 Study of the supportive structures of the uterus by levator myography. Surgery, Gynecology & Obstetrics 97:677–692

Bernstein I 1997 The pelvic floor muscles [thesis]. University of Copenhagen

Bidmead J, Cardozo L 2001 Preparation for surgery. In: Cardozo L, Staskin D (eds) Textbook of female urology and urogynaecology. Isis Medical Media, London, p 469–478

Bø K 2004 Pelvic floor muscle training is effective in treatment of female stress urinary incontinence, but how does it work? International Urogynecology Journal and Pelvic Floor Dysfunction 15(2):76–84

Brubaker L, Bump R C, Jacquetin B et al 2002 Pelvic organ prolapse. In: Abrams P, Cardozo L, Khoury S et al (eds) Incontinence, 2nd edn. Health Publication, Plymouth, p 243–266

Bump R C, Norton P A 1998 Epidemiology and natural history of pelvic floor dysfunction. Obstetrics and Gynecology Clinics of North America 25(4):723–746

Carey M P, Dwyer P L 2001 Genital prolapse: vaginal versus abdominal route of repair. Current Opinion in Obstetrics and Gynecology 13(5):499–505

Clark A L, Gregory T, Smith V J et al 2003 Epidemiologic evaluation of reoperation for surgically treated pelvic organ prolapse and urinary incontinence. American Journal of Obstetrics and Gynecology 189(5):1261–1267

Clemons J, Aguilar V, Tillinghast T et al 2004 Patient satisfaction and changes in prolapse and urinary symptoms in women who were fitted successfully with a pessary for pelvic organ prolapse. American Journal of Obstetrics and Gynecology 190:1025–1029

Davila G W 1996 Vaginal prolapse: management with nonsurgical techniques. Postgraduate Medicine 99(4):171–185

DeLancey J O 1993 Anatomy and biomechanics of genital prolapse. Clinical Obstetrics and Gynecology 36(4):897–909

DeLancey J O, Hurd W W 1998 Size of the urogenital hiatus in the levator ani muscles in normal women and women with pelvic organ prolapse. Obstetrics and Gynecology 91(3):364–368

DeLancey J O L, Kearney R, Umek W et al 2003 Levator ani muscle structure and function in women with prolapse compared to women with normal support. Neurourology and Urodynamics 22(5):542–543

Digesu G A, Khullar V, Cardozo L et al 2005 P-QOL: a validated questionnaire to assess the symptoms and quality of life of women with urogenital prolapse. International Urogynecology Journal and Pelvic Floor Dysfunction 16(3):176–181

Frawley H C, Galea M P, Phillips B A 2005 Survey of clinical practice: pre- and postoperative physiotherapy for pelvic surgery. Acta Obstetricia et Gynecologica Scandinavica 84:412–418

Ghetti C, Gregory W T, Edwards S R et al 2005 Severity of pelvic organ prolapse associated with measurements of pelvic floor function. International Urogynecology Journal and Pelvic Floor Dysfunction 16(6):432–436

Gosling J A 1996 The structure of the bladder neck, urethra and pelvic floor in relation to female urinary continence. International Urogynecology Journal 7(4):177–178

Hagen S, Stark D, Cattermole D 2004a A United Kingdom-wide survey of physiotherapy practice in the treatment of pelvic organ prolapse. Physiotherapy 90:19–26

Hagen S, Stark D, Maher C et al 2004b Conservative management of pelvic organ prolapse in women. Cochrane Database of Systematic Reviews (2):CD003882

Hahn I, Myrhage R 1999 Bekkenbotten. Bygnad, funktion och traning. AnaKomp AB, Goteborg, Sweden, p 39

Handa V L, Garrett E, Hendrix S et al 2004 Progression and remission of pelvic organ prolapse: a longitudinal study of menopausal women. American Journal of Obstetrics and Gynecology 190(1):27–32

Hay-Smith E J, Bø K, Berghmans L C et al 2001 Pelvic floor muscle training for urinary incontinence in women. Cochrane Database of Systematic Reviews 1:CD001407

Hendrix S L, Clark A, Nygaard I et al 2002 Pelvic organ prolapse in the Women's Health Initiative: gravity and gravidity. American Journal of Obstetrics and Gynecology 186(6):1160–1166

Hextall A, Bidmead J, Cardozo L et al 1999 Assessment of pelvic floor function in women with genuine stress incontinence: a comparison between ultrasound, digital examination and perineometry. Neurourology and Urodynamics 18(4):325–326

Hibner M, Cornella J, Magrina J 2004 Weight lifting and physical activity limits in patients after anti-incontinence and anti-prolapse surgery [abstract 648]. International Continence Society/International Urogynecology Association, Paris

Hoyte L, Schierlitz L, Zou K et al 2001 Two- and 3-dimensional MRI comparison of levator ani structure, volume, and integrity in women with stress incontinence and prolapse. American Journal of Obstetrics and Gynecology 185(1):11–19

Jarvis S K, Hallam T K, Lujic S et al 2005 Peri-operative physiotherapy improves outcomes for women undergoing incontinence and or prolapse surgery: Results of a randomised controlled trial. Australian and New Zealand Journal of Obstetrics and Gynaecology 45(4):300–303

Jørgensen S, Hein H O, Gyntelberg F 1994 Heavy lifting at work and risk of genital prolapse and herniated lumbar disc in assistant nurses. Occupational Medicine (Oxford) 44(1):47–49

Kegel A H 1956 Early genital relaxation – new technic of diagnosis and nonsurgical treatment. Obstetrics and Gynecology 8(5):545–550

Maher C, Carey M, Adams E et al 2004 Surgical management of pelvic organ prolapse in women (review). The Cochrane Library, Issue 4

Maher C G, Sherrington C, Herbert R D et al 2003 Reliability of the PEDro scale for rating quality of randomized controlled trials. Physiotherapy 83:713–721

Miller J M, Perucchini D, Carchidi L T et al 2001 Pelvic floor muscle contraction during a cough and decreased vesical neck mobility. Obstetrics and Gynecology 97(2):255–260

Mimura T, Roy A J, Storrie J B et al 2000 Treatment of impaired defecation associated with rectocele by behavioral retraining (biofeedback). Diseases of the Colon and Rectum 43:1267–1272

Mouritsen L, Larsen J P 2003 Symptoms, bother and POPQ in women referred with pelvic organ prolapse. International Urogynecology Journal and Pelvic Floor Dysfunction 14:122–127

Olsen A L, Smith V J, Bergstrom J O et al 1997 Epidemiology of surgically managed pelvic organ prolapse and urinary incontinence. Obstetrics and Gynecology 89(4):501–506

Ottesen M, Moller C, Kehlet H et al 2001 Substantial variability in postoperative treatment, and convalescence recommendations following vaginal repair. A nationwide questionnaire study. Acta Obstetricia et Gynecologica Scandinavica 80(11):1062–1068

Ottesen M, Sorensen M, Kehlet H et al 2003 Short convalescence after vaginal prolapse surgery. Acta Obstetricia et Gynecologica Scandinavica 82(4):359–366

Peschers U M, Fanger G, Schaer G N et al 2001 Bladder neck mobility in continent nulliparous women. BJOG 108(3):320–324

Piya-Anant M, Therasakvichya S, Leelaphatanadit C et al 2003 Integrated health research program for the Thai elderly: prevalence of genital prolapse and effectiveness of pelvic floor exercise to prevent worsening of genital prolapse in elderly women. Journal of the Medical Association of Thailand 86(6):509–515

Rinne K M, Kirkinen P P 1999 What predisposes young women to genital prolapse? European Journal of Obstetrics, Gynecology, and Reproductive Biology 84(1):23–25

Samuelsson E C, Arne Victor F T, Tibblin G et al 1999 Signs of genital prolapse in a Swedish population of women 20 to 59 years of age and possible related factors. American Journal of Obstetrics and Gynecology 180:299–305

Singh K, Jakab M, Reid W M et al 2003 Three-dimensional magnetic resonance imaging assessment of levator ani morphologic features in different grades of prolapse. American Journal of Obstetrics and Gynecology 188(4):910–915

Shumaker S A, Wyman J F, Uebersax J S et al 1994 Health-related quality of life measures for women with urinary incontinence: the Incontinence Impact Questionnaire and the Urogenital Distress Inventory. Continence Program in Women (CPW) Research Group. Quality of Life Research 3(5):291–306

Slieker-ten Hove M C P, Vierhout M E, Bloembergen H et al 2004 Distribution of pelvic organ prolapse (POP) in the general population; prevalence, severity, etiology and relation with the function of the pelvic floor muscles [abstract 4]. Neurourology and Urodynamics 23(5/6):401–402

Spence-Jones C, Kamm M A, Henry M M et al 1994 Bowel dysfunction: a pathogenic factor in uterovaginal prolapse and urinary stress incontinence. BJOG 101(2):147–152

Swift S E, Pound T, Dias J K 2001 Case–control study of etiologic factors in the development of severe pelvic organ prolapse. International Urogynecology Journal and Pelvic Floor Dysfunction 12(3):187–192

Thakar R, Stanton S 2002 Management of genital prolapse. BMJ 324(7348):1258–1262

Thompson J A, O'Sullivan P B 2003 Levator plate movement during voluntary pelvic floor muscle contraction in subjects with incontinence and prolapse: a cross-sectional study and review. International Urogynecology Journal and Pelvic Floor Dysfunction 14(2):84–88

Vakili B, Zheng Y T, Loesch H et al 2005 Levator contraction strength and genital hiatus as risk factors for recurrent pelvic organ prolapse. American Journal of Obstetrics and Gynecology 192:1592–1598

Visco A G, Wei J T, McClure L A et al 2003 Effects of examination technique modifications on pelvic organ prolapse quantification (POP-Q) results. International Urogynecology Journal and Pelvic Floor Dysfunction 14(2):136–140

Whiteside J L, Weber A M, Meyn L A et al 2004 Risk factors for prolapse recurrence after vaginal repair. American Journal of Obstetrics and Gynecology 191:1533–1538

Wilson P D, Bø K, Hay-Smith J et al 2002 Conservative treatment in women. In: Abrams P, Cardozo L, Khoury S et al (eds): Incontinence, 2nd edn. Health Publication, Plymouth, p 571–624

Pelvic pain

Helena Frawley and Dr Wendy Bower

DEFINITIONS AND CLASSIFICATION OF DIFFERENT FORMS

Chronic pelvic pain has been defined as 'non-malignant pain perceived in structures related to the pelvis of either men or women. In the case of documented nociceptive pain that becomes chronic, the pain must have been continuous or recurrent for at least 6 months. If non-acute pain mechanisms are documented, then the pain may be regarded as chronic irrespective of the time period. In all cases, there may be associated negative cognitive, behavioral and social consequences' (Fall et al 2004).

This definition forms the basis of the classification system illustrated in Table 9.12. Pelvic pain syndrome has a separate definition, proposed by Abrams et al (2002) and adopted by Fall et al (2004) as 'the occurrence of persistent or recurrent episodic pelvic pain associated with symptoms suggestive of lower urinary tract, sexual, bowel or gynecological dysfunction. There is no proven infection or other obvious pathology'.

Part of the complexity of pelvic pain is that it can be diffuse and felt in more than one area, therefore the description of pelvic pain should always specify location, duration, identifiable pathology, and other relevant pelvic comorbidities (Williams et al 2004). Pelvic pain may be reported in the anterior abdominal wall below the level of the umbilicus, the spine from T10 (ovarian and testes nerve supply) or T12 (nerve supply to pelvic musculoskeletal structures) to S5, the perineum, and all of the external and internal tissues within these reference zones.

Pelvic pain can be further subclassified into pelvic pain syndromes of muscular origin, which includes perineal pain syndrome (Abrams et al 2002, Fall et al 2004) and pelvic floor muscle (PFM) pain syndrome, the latter defined as 'the occurrence of persistent or recurrent episodic pelvic floor pain with associated trigger points that is either related to the micturition cycle or associated with symptoms suggestive of lower urinary tract, or sexual dysfunction. There is no proven infection or other obvious pathology' (Fall et al 2004).

It has been postulated that pelvic floor pain arises from spasm or tension in one or more of the pelvic muscles (levator ani, coccygeus, piriformis), and/or referred pain in their attachments to the sacrum, coccyx, ischial tuberosities or pubic rami (Howard 2000a).

Sexual dysfunction and pain are two symptoms of PFM dysfunction (Messelink et al 2005). Pelvic pain of PFM origin has been variously labelled as coccygodynia (De Andres & Chaves 2003, Thiele 1937), levator (spasm) syndrome (McGivney & Cleveland 1965, Smith 1959), tension myalgia of the pelvic floor (Sinaki et al 1977), pelvic floor spasticity (Kuijpers & Bleijenberg 1985) urethral/anal sphincter dyssynergia (Whitehead 1996), vaginismus (Masters & Johnson 1970) and shortened pelvic floor (FitzGerald & Kotarinos 2003).

This chapter considers pelvic pain and/or related dysfunction originating (or considered to be originating) in the PFM (and their bony attachments, fascia and ligaments), including both deep (levator ani) and superficial (perineal muscle) layers. Dysfunction may be primarily from the PFM, occur secondary to visceral changes (lower urinary tract, reproductive tract or anorectum), or be referred from other pelvic somatic (cutaneous and muscular) structures. It is often difficult to differentially diagnose pain originating from deep muscular structures from that emanating from visceral structures because the symptoms are often similar due to anatomical proximity and shared innervation, hence pain can be perceived in either location (Perry 2003).

NEUROANATOMY

The PFM structures receive somatic innervation from the pudendal nerve (S2–S4) and sacral nerve roots (S3–S5) (Barber et al 2002). The pelvic viscera are innervated by parasympathetic efferent neurons arising from the intermediolateral cell column at spinal levels S2–S4 (Rogers 1998). Pain from viscera is transmitted through the inferior hypogastric plexus and onwards via either the hypogastric, pelvic splanchnic or sacral splanchnic nerves. Nociceptive information may also travel with

Table 9.12   Classification of chronic pelvic pain syndromes. Reprinted from Fall et al 2004, with permission

Chronic pelvic pain (new definition)	Pelvic pain syndrome	Urological	Painful bladder syndrome	Interstitial cystitis
			Urethral pain syndrome	
			Penile pain syndrome (new definition)	
			Prostate pain syndrome (Adapted from NIH)	
			Scrotal pain syndrome	Testicular pain syndrome (new definition)
				Post-vasectomy pain syndrome (new definition)
				Epididymal pain syndrome (new definition)
		Gynaecological	Endometriosis-associated pain syndrome (new definition)	
			Vaginal pain syndrome	
			Vulvar pain syndrome	Generalized vulvar pain syndrome (ISSVD 1999)
				Localized vulvar pain syndrome (ISSVD 1999)
				Vestibular pain syndrome (ISSVD 1999)
				Clitoral pain syndrome (ISSVD 1999)
		Anorectal	Proctalgia fugax	
			Anorectal pain syndrome (new definition)	
			Anism	
		Neurological	Pudendal pain syndrome (new definition)	
		Muscular	Perineal pain syndrome	
			Pelvic floor muscle pain syndrome (new definition)	
	Well-defined conditions that produce pain, examples include:	Urological	Infective cystitis	
			Infective prostatitis	
			Infective urethritis	
			Infective epididymo-orchitis	
		Gynaecological	Endometriosis	
		Anorectal	Proctitis	
			Haemorrhoids	
			Anal fissure	
		Neurological	Pudendal neuropathy	
			Sacral spinal cord pathology	
		Other	Vascular	
			Cutaneous	
			Psychiatric	

the ovarian vessels or the superior rectal artery. For a more detailed explanation of the neuroanatomy and neurobiology of the pelvis, see Ch. 4.

PREVALENCE AND INCIDENCE

The true prevalence and incidence of PFM pain syndrome alone or coexisting with other chronic pelvic pain conditions is unknown. Prevalence of chronic pelvic pain of multisystem aetiology (visceral, somatic, pyscho-neurological) has been estimated at 3.8% of all women (Howard 2003) or 14.7% of women aged 18–50 years (Mathias et al 1996). Prevalence estimates of pelvic pain syndromes that overlap with PFM pain syndrome may be indicative of PFM pain prevalence. Vaginismus, for example, has been reported to affect up to 21% of women younger than 30 years (Laumann et al 1999). Jamieson & Steege (1996) found higher prevalence figures in their study of women aged 18–45 years, with 90% reporting dysmenorrhea, 46% reporting dyspareunia, 39% reporting pelvic pain and 12% reporting irritable bowel syndrome.

AETIOLOGY AND PATHOPHYSIOLOGY

Acute PFM pain may result from overzealous or unaccustomed exercise (DeLancey et al 1993), but the reason(s) why pain would be chronically maintained in the PFM are not clear. It seems necessary to look beyond the PFM in isolation, and consider the interrelationships with nearby viscera, and the unique and complex peripheral and central neural control that influences this region, as depicted in Fig. 9.23.

Abnormal muscle tone

A physiological and mechanical explanation of muscle tone is presented in Fig. 9.24. Here, muscle tone has two components: the viscoelastic component, which is independent of nervous activity, and the contractile component, which is caused by activation of motor units. It is possible that abnormalities of both the viscoelastic and the contractile component may contribute to abnormality in PFM tension. Other terms denoting muscle tension linked to muscle pain, include spasm and cramp. There is no generally accepted definition of the term 'spasm' and no consensus concerning how to differentiate severe muscle contractions from cramps, chronic muscle tension, or spasm.

Mense et al (2001, p. 111) offer the following definition of muscle spasm: 'electromyographic (EMG) activity that is not under voluntary control and is not dependent on posture. It may or may not be painful'. However if the contraction is painful, it is often called a 'cramp'. Reissing et al (2004, p. 9) used a working definition of spasm in their study of vaginismus as 'an invol-

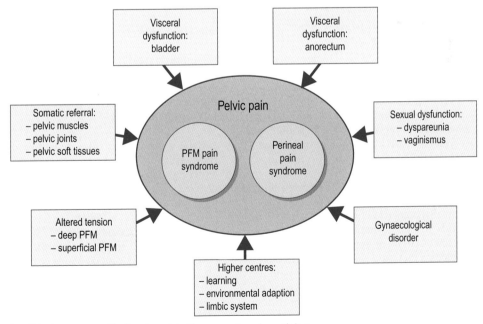

Fig. 9.23   Possible factors contributing to pelvic floor muscle pain aetiology.

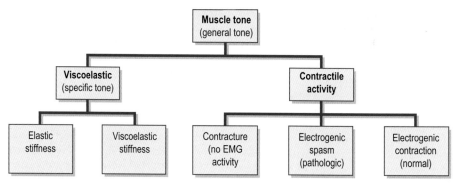

Fig. 9.24 Relationship among terms commonly used to characterize muscle tension: tone, stiffness, contracture and spasm (Reprinted from Mense et al 2001, with permission).

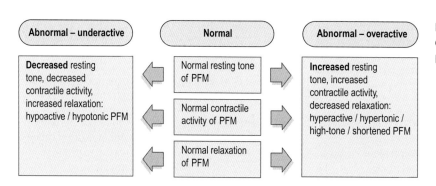

Fig. 9.25 Terminology used to describe normal and abnormal pelvic floor muscle activity.

untary contraction of some or all of the PFM which prevents examination'.

Several terms have been used to denote abnormal PFM tone or activity linked to PFM pain syndromes. These appear in Fig. 9.25. This chapter will adopt the International Continence Society (ICS) recommended term 'overactive PFM' (Messelink et al 2005) to denote a condition where the resting tone of the PFM may be elevated, the contractile activity (voluntary or involuntary) of the PFM may be increased, or the relaxation control may be reduced.

Not all authors agree with the presumed causal link between PFM pain and overactivity. Mense et al (2001) cited clinical and physiological studies indicating that muscle pain tends to inhibit, not facilitate, voluntary and reflex contractile activity of the same muscle. These authors acknowledge that sufficient spasm can cause pain, but something other than the muscle pain is causing the spasm. It could be that the presence of trigger points within a muscle may contribute to the palpable findings, the pain, and the variable degree of spasm measured in the muscle.

Pelvic floor muscle pain and overactivity

It has not been clearly established whether pain in the PFM causes the overactivity, or whether the overactivity causes the pain. Despite this, several factors have been postulated to potentiate PFM overactivity and pain, including the following:

- skeletal muscle overload – repetitive or sustained (Everaert et al 2001);
- tethering of fascia overlying skeletal muscle;
- trigger points (see below);
- local inflammation (Segura et al 1979);
- infection (Chung et al 2001);
- trauma (Butrick 2000);
- pelvic surgery (Zermann et al 1998);
- psychosomatic conditions (Pauls & Berman 2002);
- alterations in neural control (Butrick 2003, Perry 2003, Zermann et al 1999, 2001a, 2001b):
  - spinal cord wind-up, hyperalgesia;
  - convergence in the dorsal horn, upregulation, central sensitization;

- dichotomizing neurons;
- increase in excitotoxic neurotransmitters;
- cross-communication between visceral and somatic structures.

Relationship of PFM pain and myofascial trigger points

Several authors have linked PFM pain with myofascial pain syndrome (Butrick 2000, Howard 2003). A myofascial pain syndrome is a regional pain syndrome characterized by the presence of myofascial trigger points (Mense et al 2001). The clinical characteristics of trigger points include:

- spot tenderness in a nodule that is part of a palpably tense band of muscle fibres;
- patient recognition of the pain that is evoked by pressure on the tender spot;
- pain referral in a pattern that is characteristic of that muscle;
- a local twitch response;
- painful limitation of active and passive range of motion;
- some weakness in that muscle.

The regions of referred pain caused by trigger points in the levator ani and perineal muscles include the coccyx, anal area, lower part of the sacrum and genital structures (Travell & Simons 1992). There is no generally accepted aetiology for myofascial pain syndrome. It is proposed that macrotrauma or microtrauma events may disturb the normal or weakened muscle through muscle injury or sustained muscle contraction, leading to trigger points and myofascial pain syndrome. Signs and symptoms of myofascial pain syndromes resemble other musculoskeletal entities, so differential diagnosis can be difficult. In up to 88% of female patients with pelvic pain, such trigger points can be identified within the PFM group and also in the abdominal wall and hip girdle (FitzGerald & Kotarinos 2003). Despite support in the literature for the link between PFM pain and trigger points, causation has not been proven.

Impact of an overactive PFM on bladder and bowel function and sexual activity

The effect of PFM overactivity on the urinary tract is dynamic. Symptoms include hesitancy or difficulty initiating a void, slow or intermittent urine flow, pain with micturition, significant postvoid residual urine, urgency, frequency and urethral sphincter hyperalgesia (Meadows 1999, Weiss 2001, Zermann et al 1999). A significant number of patients also have a diagnosis of interstitial cystitis (FitzGerald & Kotarinos 2003).

Functional obstruction to complete emptying of the bladder associated with non-relaxation of the PFM generates increased detrusor pressures (Yeung 2001). Further PFM activity is triggered in an effort to prevent additional detrusor pressure rise. Eventually the micturition reflex becomes destabilized during bladder filling, evidenced on urodynamic investigation as an overactive bladder and on a frequency–volume chart as frequent low-volume voids. Pelvic floor muscle contraction is a common method to inhibit urgency, but in patients with PFM overactivity it is likely that little additional pressure will be generated because the muscle is in its shortened range. Prescription of PFM exercises to increase urethral closure pressure and maximize detrusor inhibition is likely to be inappropriate because it can exacerbate both pain and muscle imbalance.

Patients with PFM overactivity perceive appropriate perineal fullness and fecal urge but have trouble passing stools. There is delayed initiation of evacuation, prolonged duration of passage of stool and incomplete emptying of the rectum when compared to control subjects (Halligan et al 1995). Smaller more acute straining angles are seen in symptomatic patients than in normal defecation attempts, a direct consequence of a slowly or non-relaxing PFM (Kuijpers & Bleijenberg 1985, Lee et al 1994). As a consequence defecation may be painful and mechanically difficult, often requiring external assistance (Bleijenberg & Kuijpers 1987). Constipation is common in patients with PFM overactivity and can precipitate further anorectal pathology, such as anal fissures and hemorrhoids. Anal manometry indicates essentially normal readings for both resting and squeeze pressure (Halligan et al 1995). However, on straining there is no obvious perineal descent and marked EMG activity in place of relaxation in puborectalis and the external anal sphincter (Bleijenberg & Kuijpers 1987).

Pelvic floor muscle overactivity has been associated with vaginal and sexual pain and therefore impaired sexual activity or dysfunction.

Prevention

No studies addressing the prevention of PFM pain or overactivity have been found to date.

Summary

Pelvic floor muscle pain and/or PFM overactivity are prevalent and complex conditions that present a challenge to the clinician and the researcher. The exact condition or symptom being addressed should be described precisely, recognizing that overlap with other pelvic pain syndromes commonly occurs. Little is known regarding the aetiology and pathophysiology of PFM pain syndrome. Further studies are required to address the basic mechanisms of PFM pain and/or overactivity, and to inform effective therapy.

ASSESSMENT OF PFM PAIN AND OVERACTIVITY

There are no widely accepted clinical guidelines on the assessment of pelvic pain syndromes originating specifically from the PFM, though several clinical practice overviews are available (FitzGerald & Kotarinos 2003, Howard 2000b, 2003, Howard & El-Minawi 2000, Shelly et al 2002). There are neither assessment scales nor psychometric outcome measures known to have been tested specifically for PFM pain/PFM overactivity. It is desirable that any aspect of PFM dysfunction is evaluated using valid, reliable and responsive outcome measures.

Assessment techniques and outcome measures used in studies evaluating pelvic pain (and the effect of intervention) frequently borrow from other chronic pain fields or continence domains, and adapt these to make the measures relevant to the presenting symptoms. Commonly used pain scales in PFM assessment include the visual analogue scale (Wallerstein 1984) and the McGill Pain Questionnaire (Melzack 1975). A scale proposed by Marinoff & Tuner (1991) for dyspareunia combines both a subjective pain and functional limitation rating, but has not been tested psychometrically.

The subjective history and objective physical assessment of PFM pain should be comprehensive and relevant to the presenting symptoms while keeping in mind the coexistence of possibly one or several other pelvic pain syndromes. A thorough biopsychosocial history should be taken. The psychosocial component may require multidisciplinary input, especially with respect to depression, which is one of several predictors of pain severity in women with chronic pelvic pain and is a significant indicator of response to treatment (Howard 2003). As pain is often the predominant symptom, a thorough pain history should include the site of pain confirmed by a pain diagram, the duration of pain, nature of onset or precipitating event, the pain characteristics, and response of pain to activity and associated symptoms (Hopwood 2000). It has been reported that pain from a shortened PFM may be perceived as aching or cramping in the coccygeal region or as a heavy feeling in either the vagina or rectum (FitzGerald & Kotarinos 2003, Meadows 1999, Shelly et al 2002) and is often exacerbated after activities that stretch the PFM (Segura et al 1979) and by sitting (Markwell 1998). Some patients report non-specific tenderness or referred pain in the perineum or labia (Schmidt & Vapnek 1991).

Both PFM pain and PFM activity should be specifically assessed. If no abnormality can be identified in the PFM that is responsible for the pain, and the symptoms cannot be clinically reproduced, assessment should expand to structures that may refer pain to the PFM. These include nearby muscles, joints, viscera and the central nervous system. It has been stated that 'the muscle in which the pain and tenderness is located often serves only as a starting point for finding the source of the pain' (Mense et al 2001, p. 84).

Much information may be gathered by objective assessment, but the validity, reliability, responsiveness and generalizability of this information is limited by a lack of normative data especially in subjects with PFM pain/overactivity. Despite this, the information that is gathered by careful assessment is of prime clinical usefulness, and may lead the way to the development of robust assessment tools and normative values of PFM activity. Basic PFM observation and objective assessment should be performed as described on pp. 50–55.

In the assessment of a patient with pelvic pain, particular emphasis is placed on muscle resting tone, contractile activity, ability to relax, and the presence of pain. Sensitive and careful examination is vital. A suggested process to elicit useful information in the physical assessment is as follows:

1. Visually inspect the perineum at rest. The genital hiatus may appear small and the perineal body displaced anteriorly if the PFM are in a shortened position.

2. Observe PFM contraction, relaxation and bearing down. Movement associated with PFM contraction may be absent due to an elevated resting level of tone, or display obvious change in recruitment patterning, timing and proprioception. Incomplete, abnormal (discordant) or absent relaxation may be observed following attempted contraction, or the woman may need to attempt relaxation several times before the PFM activity subsides. Bearing down may be absent or result in an indrawing. Early fatigue may be noted. On attempted location and isolation of a PFM contraction, accessory muscle activity is frequently seen in the thigh muscles, hips, buttocks and thorax. It may be helpful to note the presence or absence of PFM indrawing with a volitional cough, though this is difficult to measure objectively.

3. Check sensation/neurological integrity: the anal wink reflex may be absent due to an already contracted PFM.

4. Palpate the external tissues, sites of possible pain referral and the perineum. Palpation of the external

genitalia and perineum is systematic and considers tissue quality, sensation, temperature and tenderness. Thickening of subcutaneous connective tissues around perineal or suprapubic trigger points, or their regions of pain referral, may be identified on palpation as altered tissue bulk, contour, elasticity and temperature, along with variation in colour (FitzGerald & Kotarinos 2003). Possible referral sites such as the abdomen may become hyperalgesic and display trophic changes such as oedema, altered blood flow, subcutaneous thickening or muscle atrophy. A device has been reported that assesses sensitivity to light touch in women with urogenital pain (Pukall et al 2004) and is reliable in the evaluation of vestibular pain.

5. Palpate the internal vagina/rectum. This examination should always be performed very gently, with a single, well-lubricated digit. There is known to be a higher prevalence of previous sexual abuse among patients with functional disorders in comparison to patients with organic disease (Jacob & DeNardis 1998), with genitourinary symptoms being one of the most common somatic complaints (Drossman 1994). Clinicians should be aware of this association when assessing women with pelvic pain. The clinician should evaluate:

   – Presence of pain. Identify and record site, nature and whether it is localized or diffuse. The aim is to reproduce the patient's pain, at a mild intensity only. Severity of pain can be rated on a visual analogue scale. A five-point scale has been reported (Whitmore et al 1998), but there are no reports on the validity of this scale as a scoring system for PFM tenderness, but it has been used in a clinical trial (Oyama et al 2004).

   – Pelvic floor muscle tone. Mense et al (2001) suggest a qualitative definition of muscle tone, determined by the compliance (compressibility) of a muscle. This is assessed by pressing a finger into a muscle belly to determine how easily it indents and how 'springy' it is. Stiffness and elasticity are assessed according to the ease of muscle indentation and return to original shape. This assessment method has not been tested for validity with respect to the PFM. Other scales reported to be relevant to the PFM are yet to undergo validity and/or reliability testing (Devreese et al 2004, Hetrick et al 2003, Lamont 1978, Reissing et al 2004).

   – Muscle contractile activity. Interpretation of measurements obtained is limited by lack of normative data, however various tools may contribute information regarding PFM contraction:

   ○ Digital palpation. See Chapter 5, p. 51, with particular emphasis on the qualitative aspects of PFM contractility, symmetry and coordination. Per vaginum or per rectum palpation can be used in assessment.

   ○ Surface electromyography (sEMG). From the earlier definition of muscle tone, it follows that muscle spasm can be measured by EMG activity, provided other non-contractile sources of muscle stiffness have been identified. Although some studies have reported good reliability and predictability of different PFM conditions using sEMG evaluation (Glazer et al 1999), other studies have found that sEMG is neither diagnostic of condition nor agrees with palpation findings of per vaginum spasm or increased PFM tone (Engman et al 2004, Reissing et al 2004, van der Velde & Everaerd 1999). Surface EMG can also be used per rectum or via electrodes attached to the perianal skin.

   ○ Manometry. Reports on the use of vaginal manometry in the evaluation of PFM pain or overactivity are scarce. One study used vaginal manometry to screen for PFM 'hypertonicity' (Jarvis et al 2004). These authors defined hypertonicity as vaginal resting pressure of greater than 40 cmH$_2$O. This group of authors also reported a case study of a patient with pelvic pain due to painful and overactive PFM, again using vaginal manometry as an assessment tool and an outcome measure (Thomson et al 2005). Anal manometry has been used more frequently than vaginal manometry, predictably for studies assessing anal sphincter activity in subjects with pelvic floor dyssynergia (PFD) and anorectal pain (levator ani syndrome and proctalgia fugax) (Palsson et al 2004).

   ○ Transperineal and transabdominal ultrasound. No studies have been found that used realtime ultrasound as an assessment tool in patients with PFM pain or overactivity.

   – Spasm. Pelvic floor muscle spasm may be present during the examination, and may be associated with pain. Reissing et al (2004, p. 9) describe spasm occurring during digital palpation as: 'a prolonged muscle contraction not relieved by reassurance'. However this description is not standardized terminology. Spasm may be invoked by vigorous examination; therefore it is paramount to assess the PFM carefully. Spasm may occur involuntarily or be provoked by a voluntary PFM contraction attempt and therefore override the voluntary attempt.

– Relaxation of the PFM. PFM relaxation has been defined as the diminution or termination of PFM contraction (Messelink et al 2005) and is always tested after a contraction. The ICS-proposed qualitative rating scale has three levels: absent, partial, complete. To date this scale has not been tested for validity nor reliability. Another scale for PFM relaxation is described as 3 for active (good) relaxation after active contraction, 2 denotes hypertonic muscle with temporary relaxation after elongation, and 1 indicates a spastic muscle, unable to relax even after passive elongation (De Ridder et al 1998). This scale has been reported to be reliable in a population of patients with multiple sclerosis. It is assumed that elongation is achieved by stretching the PFM, but the technique to perform this assessment has not been described.

If a comprehensive pelvic floor assessment reveals neither PFM overactivity nor elicits reproduction of the patient's symptom(s), further assessment must address structures that have the potential to refer pain to the PFM. A detailed explanation of the mechanisms of how pain is referred from other muscles, nearby joints, viscera and the central nervous system is beyond the scope of this chapter but addressed comprehensively by Mense et al (2001). It is common to find obturator internus, psoas, gluteal, abdominal and piriformis muscle abnormality and pain in patients with PFM pain (Doggweiler-Wiygul & Wiygul 2002, FitzGerald & Kotarinos 2003, Hetrick et al 2003, Segura et al 1979, Shelly et al 2002). It is prudent to consider pudendal nerve entrapment in all patients with PFM pain, and to review pelvic girdle instability in peri- and postnatal women because these problems may present as or contribute to, the presentation of PFM pain.

The importance of assessing beyond the immediate pelvic floor structures for dysfunction located in other musculoskeletal structures that may impact on the local system has been highlighted (Baker 1993, Brown 2000, Doggweiler-Wiygul & Wiygul 2002, FitzGerald & Kotarinos 2003, Howard 2000a, Prendergast & Weiss 2003, Shelly et al 2002, Weiss 2001). Once neurophysiological adaptation to the chronic local pain has occurred, the sensitized sacral spinal cord is vulnerable to, and influenced by other organs and muscles that converge onto the same nerves (somatovisceral convergence) or by general factors that increase nerve sensitivity. Dysfunction in other pelvic muscles (abdominal, gluteal, thigh) may therefore perpetuate PFM pain and dysfunction.

If no somatic or visceral structure can be identified as contributing to the patient's symptom(s), further assessment of non-organic pelvic pain as the primary disease or pain per se as the primary disease is appropriate (Siddall & Cousins 2004). This may incorporate psychological and/or psychosexual evaluation and should be performed by an appropriately skilled person.

OUTCOME MEASURES

There are no current guidelines for the selection of outcome measures appropriate for the assessment and treatment of patients with PFM pain or overactivity. Due to the heterogenous nature of presentations of PFM pain syndromes, outcome measure selection may be guided by visceral or somatic perspectives. Hence guidelines from the ICS (Lose et al 2001) or chronic (non-pelvic) pain outcome guidelines may be followed, such as the IMMPACT recommendations (Turk et al 2003). The core domains recommended for clinical trials of chronic pain treatment efficacy and effectiveness include measurement of pain, physical functioning, emotional functioning, participant ratings of global improvement, symptoms and adverse events, and participant disposition (Turk et al 2003).

A comprehensive selection of useful outcome measures relevant to disease-specific (bladder) and general pain has been published (Hanno et al 2005). Other tools exist that include measurements or questions on possible PFM-related pain complaints (Litwin et al 1999, Rosen et al 2000, Pukall et al 2004). The clinician and researcher should carefully consider the appropriateness of the selected outcome measure to the patient or population under review, considering reliability, validity and responsiveness to change of the particular tool being used. Outcomes should be selected that reflect both subjective and objective measures. To date, no outcome measures have been specifically tested for applicability to a PFM pain/overactivity population.

SUMMARY

Further research is needed to determine the extent to which muscle dysfunction can lead to or exacerbate pain, and the extent to which pain and/or guarding may lead to muscle dysfunction. Consensus regarding assessment of the dysfunction, whether it is pain alone, overactivity alone, or a combination of both, is urgently required. Reference data of normal PFM activity against which abnormalities in activity may be compared are lacking. Development and testing of robust assessment tools and outcome measures will facilitate well-designed, high-quality intervention studies to measure PFM pain and overactivity.

REFERENCES

Abrams P, Cardozo L, Fall M et al 2002 The standardisation of terminology of lower urinary tract function: report from the Standardisation Sub-committee of the International Continence Society. American Journal of Obstetrics and Gynecology 187(1):116–126

Baker P K 1993 Musculoskeletal origins of chronic pelvic pain. Diagnosis and treatment. Obstetrics and Gynecology Clinics of North America 20(4):719–742

Barber M D, Bremer R E, Thor K B et al 2002 Innervation of the female levator ani muscles. American Journal of Obstetrics and Gynecology 187(1):64–71

Bleijenberg G, Kuijpers H C 1987 Treatment of the spastic pelvic floor syndrome with biofeedback. Diseases of the Colon and Rectum 30(2):108–111

Brown J S 2000 Faulty posture and chronic pelvic pain. In: Howard F M, Perry C P, Carter J E et al (eds) Pelvic pain: diagnosis and management. Lippincott Williams & Wilkins, Philadelphia, p 363–380

Butrick C W 2000 Discordant urination and defecaton as symptoms of pelvic floor dysfunction. In: Howard F M, Perry C P, Carter J E et al (eds) Pelvic pain: diagnosis and management. Lippincott Williams & Wilkins, Philadelphia, p 279–299

Butrick C W 2003 Interstitial cystitis and chronic pelvic pain: new insights in neuropathology, diagnosis, and treatment. Clinical Obstetrics and Gynecology 46(4):811–823

Chung A K, Peters K M, Diokno A C 2001 Epidemiology of the dysfunctional urinary sphincter. In: Corcos J, Schick E (eds) The urinary sphincter. Marcel Dekker, New York, p 183–191

De Andres J, Chaves S 2003 Coccygodynia: a proposal for an algorithm for treatment. Journal of Pain 4(5):257–266

De Ridder D, Vermeulen C, De Smet E et al 1998 Clinical assessment of pelvic floor dysfunction in multiple sclerosis: urodynamic and neurological correlates. Neurourology and Urodynamics 17(5):537–542

DeLancey J O, Sampselle C M, Punch M R 1993 Kegel dyspareunia: levator ani myalgia caused by overexertion. Obstetrics and Gynecology 82(4 Pt 2 Suppl):658–659

Devreese A, Staes F, de Weerdt W et al 2004 Clinical evaluation of pelvic floor muscle function in continent and incontinent women. Neurourology and Urodynamics 23(3):190–197

Doggweiler-Wiygul R, Wiygul J P 2002 Interstitial cystitis, pelvic pain, and the relationship to myofascial pain and dysfunction: a report on four patients. World Journal of Urology 20(5):310–314

Drossman D A 1994 Physical and sexual abuse and gastrointestinal illness: what is the link? [comment]. American Journal of Medicine 97(2):105–107

Engman M, Lindehammar H, Wijma B 2004 Surface electromyography diagnostics in women with partial vaginismus with or without vulvar vestibulitis and in asymptomatic women. Journal of Psychosomatic Obstetrics and Gynecology 25:281–294

Everaert K, Devulder J, De Muynck M et al 2001 The pain cycle: implications for the diagnosis and treatment of pelvic pain syndromes. International Urogynecology Journal and Pelvic Floor Dysfunction 12(1):9–14

Fall M, Baranowski A P, Fowler C J et al 2004 EAU guidelines on chronic pelvic pain. European Urology 46(6):681–689

FitzGerald M P, Kotarinos R 2003 Rehabilitation of the short pelvic floor. I: Background and patient evaluation. International Urogynecology Journal and Pelvic Floor Dysfunction 14(4):261–268

Glazer H I, Romanzi L, Polaneczky M 1999 Pelvic floor muscle surface electromyography. Reliability and clinical predictive validity. Journal of Reproductive Medicine 44(9):779–782

Halligan S, Bartram C I, Park H J et al 1995 Proctographic features of anismus. Radiology 197(3):679–682

Hanno P, Baranowski A, Fall M et al 2005 Painful bladder syndrome (including interstitial cystitis). In: Abrams P, Cardozo L, Khoury S et al (eds) Incontinence: 3rd edn. Health Publication, Plymouth, UK, p 1455–1520

Hetrick D C, Ciol M A, Rothman I et al 2003 Musculoskeletal dysfunction in men with chronic pelvic pain syndrome type III: a case–control study. Journal of Urology 170(3):828–831

Hopwood M B 2000 Collection of historical data. In: Abram S E, Haddox J D (eds) The pain clinic manual, 2nd edn. Lippincott Williams & Wilkins, Philadelphia, p 33–36

Howard F M 2000a Pelvic floor pain syndrome. In: Howard F M, Perry C P, Carter J E et al (eds) Pelvic pain: diagnosis and management. Lippincott Williams & Wilkins, Philadelphia, p 429–432

Howard F M 2000b Physical examination. In: Howard F M, Perry C P, Carter J E et al (eds) Pelvic pain: diagnosis and management. Lippincott Williams & Wilkins, Philadelphia, p 26–42

Howard F M 2003 Chronic pelvic pain. Obstetrics and Gynecology 101(3):594–611

Howard F M, El-Minawi A M 2000 Taking a history. In: Howard F M, Perry C P, Carter J E et al (eds) Pelvic pain: diagnosis and management. Lippincott Williams & Wilkins, Philadelphia, p 7–25

Jacob M C, DeNardis M C 1998 Sexual and physical abuse and chronic pelvic pain. In: Steege J F, Metzger D A, Levy B S (eds) Chronic pelvic pain: an integrated approach. WB Saunders Company, Philadelphia, p 13–24

Jamieson D J, Steege J F 1996 The prevalence of dysmenorrhea, dyspareunia, pelvic pain, and irritable bowel syndrome in primary care practices. Obstetrics and Gynecology 87(1):55–58

Jarvis S K, Abbott J A, Lenart M B et al 2004 Pilot study of botulinum toxin type A in the treatment of chronic pelvic pain associated with spasm of the levator ani muscles. Australian and New Zealand Journal of Obstetrics and Gynaecology 44(1):46–50

Kuijpers H C, Bleijenberg G 1985 The spastic pelvic floor syndrome. A cause of constipation. Diseases of the Colon and Rectum 28(9):669–672

Lamont J A 1978 Vaginismus. American Journal of Obstetrics and Gynecology 131(6):633–636

Laumann E O, Paik A, Rosen R C 1999 Sexual dysfunction in the United States: prevalence and predictors [see comment] [erratum appears in JAMA 1999 281(13):1174]. JAMA 281(6):537–544

Lee H H, Chen S H, Chen D F et al 1994 Defecographic evaluation of patients with defecation difficulties. Journal of the Formosan Medical Association 93(11–12):944–949

Litwin M S, McNaughton-Collins M, Fowler F J Jr et al 1999 The National Institutes of Health chronic prostatitis symptom index: development and validation of a new outcome measure. Chronic Prostatitis Collaborative Research Network. Journal of Urology 162(2):369–375

Lose G, Fantl J A, Victor A et al 2001 Outcome measures for research in adult women with symptoms of lower urinary tract dysfunction. Standardization Committee of the International Continence Society. Acta Obstetrica et Gynecologica Scandinavica 80(11):979–980

Marinoff S C, Turner M L 1991 Vulvar vestibulitis syndrome: an overview. American Journal of Obstetrics and Gynecology 165(4 Pt 2):1228–1233

Markwell S 1998 Functional disorders of the anorectum and pain syndromes. In: Sapsford R, Bullock-Saxton J, Markwell S (eds) Women's health: a textbook for physiotherapists. W B Saunders, London, p 357–382

Masters W H, Johnson V E 1970 Human sexual inadequacy. Little, Brown and Company, Boston

Mathias S D, Kuppermann M, Liberman R F et al 1996 Chronic pelvic pain: prevalence, health-related quality of life, and economic correlates. Obstetrics and Gynecology 87(3):321–327

McGivney J Q, Cleveland B R 1965 The levator syndrome and its treatment. Southern Medical Journal 58:505–510

Meadows E 1999 Treatments for patients with pelvic pain. Urologic Nursing 19(1):33–35

Melzack R 1975 The McGill pain questionnaire: major properties and scoring methods. Pain 1(3):277–299

Mense S, Simons D G, Russell I J (ed) 2001 Muscle pain: understanding its nature, diagnosis and treatment. Lippincott Williams & Wilkins, Philadelphia

Messelink E J, Benson J T, Berghmans L C M et al 2005 Standardization terminology of pelvic floor muscle function and dysfunction: report from the pelvic floor clinical assessment group of the International Continence Society. Neurourology and Urodynamics 24:374–380

Oyama I A, Rejba A, Lukban J C et al 2004 Modified thiele massage as therapeutic intervention for female patients with interstitial cystitis and high-tone pelvic floor dysfunction. Urology 64(5):862–865

Palsson O S, Heymen S, Whitehead W E 2004 Biofeedback treatment for functional anorectal disorders: a comprehensive efficacy review. Applied Psychophysiology and Biofeedback 29(3):153–174

Pauls R N, Berman J R 2002 Impact of pelvic floor disorders and prolapse on female sexual function and response. Urologic Clinics of North America 29(3):677–683

Perry C P 2003 Peripheral neuropathies and pelvic pain: diagnosis and management. Clinical Obstetrics and Gynecology 46(4):789–796

Prendergast S A, Weiss J M 2003 Screening for musculoskeletal causes of pelvic pain. Clinical Obstetrics and Gynecology 46(4):773–782

Pukall C F, Binik Y M, Khalife S 2004 A new instrument for pain assessment in vulvar vestibulitis syndrome. Journal of Sex and Marital Therapy 30(2):69–78

Reissing E D, Binik Y M, Khalife S et al 2004 Vaginal spasm, pain, and behavior: an empirical investigation of the diagnosis of vaginismus. Archives of Sexual Behavior 33(1):5–17

Rogers R M 1998 Basic pelvic neuroanatomy. In: Steege J F, Metzger D A, Levy B S (eds) Chronic pelvic pain: an integrated approach. W B Saunders Company, Philadelphia, p 31–58

Rosen R, Brown C, Heiman J et al 2000 The Female Sexual Function Index (FSFI): a multidimensional self-report instrument for the assessment of female sexual function. Journal of Sex and Marital Therapy 26(2):191–208

Schmidt R A, Vapnek J M 1991 Pelvic floor behavior and interstitial cystitis. Seminars in Urology 9(2):154–159

Segura J W, Opitz J L, Greene L F 1979 Prostatosis, prostatitis or pelvic floor tension myalgia? Journal of Urology 122(2):168–169

Shelly B, Knight S, King P B et al 2002 Pelvic pain. In: Laycock J, Haslam J (eds) Therapeutic management of incontinence and pelvic pain. Springer–Verlag, London, p 156–189

Siddall P J, Cousins M J 2004 Persistent pain as a disease entity: implications for clinical management. Anesthesia and Analgesia 99(2):510–520

Sinaki M, Merritt J L, Stillwell G K 1977 Tension myalgia of the pelvic floor. Mayo Clinic Proceedings 52(11):717–722

Smith W T 1959 Levator spasm syndrome. Minnesota Medicine 42(8):1076–1079

Thiele G H 1937 Coccygodynia and pain in the superior gluteal region and down the back of the thigh: causation by tonic spasm of the levator ani, coccygeus and piriformis muscles and relief by massage of these muscles. JAMA 109(16):1271–1275

Thomson A J, Jarvis S K, Lenart M et al 2005 The use of botulinum toxin type A (BOTOX) as treatment for intractable chronic pelvic pain associated with spasm of the levator ani muscles. BJOG 112(2):247–249

Travell J G, Simons D G 1992 Pelvic floor muscles. In: Travell J G, Simons D G (eds) Myofascial pain and dysfunction: the trigger point manual, vol 2, the lower extremities. Williams & Wilkins, Baltimore, p 111–131

Turk D C, Dworkin R H, Allen R R et al 2003 Core outcome domains for chronic pain clinical trials: IMMPACT recommendations. Pain 106(3):337–345

van der Velde J, Everaerd W 1999 Voluntary control over pelvic floor muscles in women with and without vaginistic reactions. International Urogynecology Journal and Pelvic Floor Dysfunction 10(4):230–236

Wallerstein S L 1984 Scaling clinical pain and pain relief. In: Bromm B (eds) Pain measurement in man: neurophysiological correlates of pain. Elsevier, New York

Weiss J M 2001 Pelvic floor myofascial trigger points: manual therapy for interstitial cystitis and the urgency-frequency syndrome. Journal of Urology 166(6):2226–2231

Whitehead W E 1996 Functional anorectal disorders. Seminars in Gastrointestinal Disease 7(4):230–236

Whitmore K, Kellog-Spadt S, Fletcher E 1998 Comprehensive assessment of pelvic floor dysfunction. Issues in Incontinence Fall:1–10

Williams R E, Hartmann K E, Steege J F 2004 Documenting the current definitions of chronic pelvic pain: implications for research. Obstetrics and Gynecology 103(4):686–691

Yeung C K 2001 Pathophysiology of bladder function. In: Gearhart J, Rink R, Mouriquand P (eds) Pediatric urology. W B Saunders, Philadelphia, p 453–469

Zermann D H, Ishigooka M, Doggweiler R et al 1999 Neurourological insights into the etiology of genitourinary pain in men. Journal of Urology 161(3):903–908

Zermann D H, Ishigooka M, Doggweiler R, Schmidt R A 1998 Postoperative chronic pain and bladder dysfunction: windup and neuronal plasticity – Do we need a more neurological approach in pelvic surgery? Journal of Urology 160(1):102–105

Zermann D H, Ishigooka M, Schmidt R A 2001a Pathophysiology of the hypertonic sphincter or hyperpathic urethra. In: Corcos J, Schick E (eds) The urinary sphincter. Marcel Dekker, New York, p 201–222

Zermann D H, Manabu I, Schmidt R A 2001b Management of the hypertonic sphincter or hyperpathic urethra. In: Corcos J, Schick E (eds) The urinary sphincter. Marcel Dekker, New York, p 679–686

TREATMENT OF PFM PAIN AND/OR OVERACTIVITY

Helena Frawley and Dr Wendy Bower

A search of Cochrane databases for evidence of effectiveness of interventions for PFM pain or overactivity failed to find any reviews regarding PFM exercise interventions, use of adjunctive therapies, or lifestyle modifications for PFM pain/overactivity. The PEDro database reported two papers: a systematic review of chronic pelvic pain (CPP) in women (Kirste et al 2002) and one randomized controlled trial (RCT) (Peters et al 1991). Tables 9.13 and 9.14 summarize findings from the very few RCTs in this area.

Kirste et al (2002) concluded that no treatment of choice emerged, though a flexible biopsychosocial approach seemed the most promising for patients with

Table 9.13 Randomized and controlled trials on treatments for pelvic floor muscle pain and/or pelvic floor muscle overactivity

Author	Bergeron et al 2001
Design	3-arm RCT (block randomized): CBT, sEMG BFB, surgery (vestibulectomy)
n	87 enrolled, 9 refused allocation group (7 from surgery, 1 from each of CBT and BFB), leaving 78 women
Diagnosis	Dyspareunia due to VVS
Treatment protocol	CBT: 8 × 2 h group sessions over 12 weeks, including education, muscle relaxation, breathing, PFM exercises, vaginal dilators, distraction & imagery, skills training BFB: 8 × 45 min BFB sessions over 12 weeks, plus 2× day home use of sEMG unit
Drop-out	13: 3 from surgery group; 10 from BFB group ITT analysis supported general trends of analysis by treatment-received outcomes
Adherence	Treatment adherence defined as complying with ≥70% of homework sessions: CBT: 65%, BFB: 57%
Results	Study completers: all groups had significant pain reduction at post-treatment and 6-month follow-up, surgery most significant reduction (surgery: 68.2%; BFB 34.6%; CBT 39.3%) All groups: equally positive and significant improvement in psychological adjustment and sexual function
Author	Peters et al 1991
Design	2-arm RCT: laparoscopy + psychological, integrated approach
n	106 women: 1st arm: n = 49, mean age 35.7 years, duration of pain 3 years; 2nd arm: n = 57, mean age 35.5 years, duration of pain 4 years
Diagnosis	CPP excluding obvious organic causes Status of PFM pain or tone not detailed for all subjects Positive pain trigger points in 24% of each arm, unclear if abdominal or PFM trigger points
Treatment protocol	49% of patients in integrated approach received assessment of abdominal and PFM Content of treatment specified as 'advice' or 'treatment'. Some patients received PT + other treatment in integrated approach
Drop-out	None specified
Adherence	Not specified
Results	Significantly greater reductions in pain (general pain experience, disturbance of daily activities, associated symptoms), p < 0.01, in integrated approach group Not clear what effect of PT treatment alone was

BFB, biofeedback; CBT, cognitive behavioural therapy; CPP, chronic pelvic pain; integrated approach, multidisciplinary or multimodal intervention, not always including physiotherapy assessment/treatment; PFM, pelvic floor muscle; sEMG, surface electromyography; VVS, vulvar vestibulitis syndrome.

CPP. Physical therapy treatments may add sensory awareness and change body attitude, movement synergy and dysfunctional respiration patterns. Cognitive–behavioural stress management intervention may be indicated in a subsample of patients.

Peters et al (1991) compared two different approaches in women with non-specific CPP of at least 3 months' duration. Randomization was to either laparoscopy (standard procedure) group (n = 49) or to an integrated approach (n = 57), which included physical therapy and

Table 9.14   PEDro quality score of RCT in systematic review

E – Eligibility criteria specified
1 – Subjects randomly allocated to groups
2 – Allocation concealed
3 – Groups similar at baseline
4 – Subjects blinded
5 – Therapist administering treatment blinded
6 – Assessors blinded
7 – Measures of key outcomes obtained from over 85% of subjects
8 – Data analysed by intention to treat
9 – Statistical comparison between groups conducted
10 – Point measures and measures of variability provided

Study	E	1	2	3	4	5	6	7	8	9	10	Total score
Bergeron et al 2001	+	+	+	+	–	–	+	+	+	+	+	8
Peters et al 1991	+	+	+	+	–	–	–	+	+	+	+	7

+, criterion is clearly satisfied; –, criterion is not satisfied; ?, not clear if the criterion was satisfied. Total score is determined by counting the number of criteria that are satisfied, except that scale item one 'eligibility criteria specified' is not used to generate the total score. Total scores are out of 10.

dietary, environmental and psychological input: 49% of subjects in the integrated group received unspecified physical therapy. Based on outcomes measuring pain, presence of associated symptoms and functional limitations, subjects in the integrated therapy approach performed better than the laparoscopy group, but a breakdown of the results from those receiving physical therapy alone was not provided.

LIFESTYLE INTERVENTIONS

Several published studies have included lifestyle modifications and/or behavioural interventions, predominantly patient education, stress reduction techniques (improved sleep patterns, breathing relaxation exercises), hygiene and dietary factors as part of a multimodal intervention for PFM pain/overactivity (Bergeron et al 2001, King et al 1991, Peters et al 1991, Weijmar Schultz et al 1996). The nature of studies that combine interventions, and the lack of outcomes measuring the effect of each specific lifestyle intervention, precludes evaluation of benefit.

COGNITIVE BEHAVIOURAL INTERVENTIONS

Cognitive–behavioural treatments are effective in reducing the suffering of patients with chronic pain,

but it is not known which cognitive–behavioural treatment works for which patient (Vlaeyen & Morley 2005). A theoretical model of cognitive and behavioural pain therapy applicable to patients with CPP has been proposed (Reiter 1998) that combines pain control techniques and activities to reduce disability and promote wellness (including physical exercise).

A randomized study comparing effectiveness of three different treatment regimens (surface electromyography [sEMG] biofeedback, group cognitive–behavioural therapy [GCBT] and surgery) for patients with dyspareunia due to vulvar vestibulitis syndrome (VVS) has been reported (Bergeron et al 2001). Kegel exercises, education and counselling were included in the GCBT arm. From the outcomes of this study, all therapies appeared to be effective treatments for patients with dyspareunia due to VVS, with the surgical group attaining the greatest improvement in pain reduction. As the GCBT included multiple therapies, the value of any one therapy alone is not clear. In addition, lack of comparison with a control group limits interpretation of the effectiveness of any one of the compared therapies on its own.

Partially- or non-randomized studies have investigated the use of cognitive behavioural therapy for PFM pain related to sexual dysfunction (Seo et al 2005, Weijmar Schultz et al 1996). Although positive results were reported for the interventions, application of findings is limited due to the study designs.

EXERCISE

Incorporation of general exercise into a specific PFM therapeutic approach may be useful because patients suffering chronic pain are often deconditioned. Patients with pain perceive an equivalent level of exertion at a significantly lower level of performance because of both central (cardiorespiratory) and peripheral (strength and recruitment) factors (Harding et al 1998). Aerobic conditioning, strengthening exercises directed to the trunk and limbs, postural correction and emphasis on function rather than impairment may be important in the recovery from CPP (Baker 1993, FitzGerald & Kotarinos 2003, Shelly et al 2002). To date no studies of such treatments specific to PFM pain/overactivity have been found.

Pelvic floor muscle exercises

As presence of painful PFM spasm and/or overactivity are frequently identified in patients presenting with CPP, most reported PFM exercise regimens have used a de-training focus (Shelly et al 2002), based on the principle that an overactivated muscle should not be further loaded with active exercise until normal, pain-free range and contractile activity have been restored. Relaxation exercises are often combined with a cognitive–behavioural approach involving imagery and de-sensitization.

Methods used to regain normal movement or contractile activity to the shortened and/or painful PFM include contract/relax, reciprocal inhibition and proprioceptive neuromuscular facilitation (FitzGerald & Kotarinos 2003). The application and evidence of effectiveness of these techniques is limited by a lack of knowledge regarding PFM agonist/antagonist relationships, neuromotor control of the PFM and its synergists, and investigation of these interventions in isolation from other techniques. Normal muscle function in chronic pain conditions may also be restored via graduated loading, with less emphasis on avoidance of pain and more emphasis on restoring normal muscle (contractile) activity. Once normalization is restored, PFM stabilizing or strengthening exercises facilitate maintenance of normal function and prevention of recurrence of pain/overactivity. There is currently no evidence to support this assumption in the case of PFM pain.

MANUAL THERAPY

Several studies investigating a range of manual therapy or exercise interventions for PFM pain/overactivity have been reported, with varying degrees of methodological quality (Bergeron et al 2001, FitzGerald & Kotarinos 2003, King et al 1991, Oyama et al 2004, Thiele 1937, Weiss 2001). Some studies had more than two arms, and others combined several conservative therapies into the treatment arm, rendering it difficult to evaluate the effectiveness of exercise or manual therapy directed to the PFM alone.

VOIDING AND DEFECATION TRAINING

Women with PFM overactivity are likely to have co-existing bladder and bowel dysfunction, and therapy should seek to normalize use of both systems. Patients are initially instructed in routine hydration to overcome voluntary dehydration, create sufficient urine to normalize bladder capacity and minimize constipation. Voiding at regular intervals with a supported posture conducive to PFM relaxation is instituted. Bowel management may be indicated if stool is passed less than second-daily or with pain or difficulty, or the patient has either poor rectal awareness or fecal soiling. Treatment then aims to optimize emptying mechanics of both the bladder and bowel. The specific goals are to achieve consistent relaxation of the pelvic floor throughout voiding/defecation, normalize urine flow pattern, ameliorate postvoid residual urine and facilitate resolution of voiding symptoms and or fecal soiling. Strategies to achieve these goals require combination therapy, generally with a sizeable investment of time over a long period. No studies have been found that identified voiding or defecation training techniques in isolation from other interventions to improve PFM pain or overactivity.

ADJUNCTIVE THERAPIES

Biofeedback modalities

Surface electromyography

Surface EMG has been popular in several studies in recent years (Bergeron et al 2001, Glazer 2000, Glazer et al 1995, McKay et al 2001), particularly in its application to PFM pain and overactivity impacting on sexual function, but few studies have employed an RCT design, so interpretation of findings is limited. The study by Bergeron et al (2001) adopted randomization to sEMG biofeedback group, but no control group was used. Post-treatment results showed that subjects receiving the sEMG intervention had improved pain and sexual function outcomes compared with pre-treatment levels, but pain reduction percentage was less than that achieved in the surgical and GCBT groups.

Use of sEMG as a biofeedback treatment for anal sphincter contractile abnormalities has been reviewed by Bassotti et al (2004). Their recommendations were limited due to the small number of high-quality trials in the area, and were not differentiated between sEMG and other types of biofeedback, but the modality seemed promising in the treatment of pelvic floor dyssynergia (PFD).

Surface EMG may be a useful modality in the treatment of some PFM pain/overactivity disorders because the therapy may assist re-education of the contractile element of muscle tone; however, this modality does not address the viscoelastic contribution to muscle tone. Attention to both aspects that contribute to muscle tone may be required to alleviate the pain/overactivity and provide long-term relief. The sequence of applying the therapies might logically be that muscle extensibility and eradication of trigger points should precede a programme that encourages active muscle contraction and relaxation (Kotarinos 2003). Generally, muscles that are in a contracted state are stretched before active exercise is commenced. Lack of controlled studies in this area limit the strength of recommendation of sEMG as an independent modality in the treatment of PFM pain or overactivity disorders.

Manometry

Manometry records intravaginal or intra-anal squeeze pressure. No studies have been found that used vaginal manometry as a treatment in patients with PFM pain or overactivity.

The use of anal manometry to treat PFD and anorectal pain has been evaluated in a systematic review by Palsson et al (2004). Only one non-randomized controlled clinical trial (Ger et al 1993), and two uncontrolled trials were found. Using published guidelines to rate the clinical efficacy of psychophysiological interventions (La Vaque et al 2002), the authors of the systematic review (Palsson et al 2004) assigned a level of evidence rating of level 2 (possibly efficacious) to the use of pressure biofeedback as a treatment of anorectal pain. For patients with PFD-type constipation treated with biofeedback (combined outcome of sEMG and pressure), the overall average probability of a successful treatment outcome was 62.4%; however, there were insufficient data to warrant such calculation for a treatment outcome for anorectal pain.

Ultrasound imaging

Transabdominal and transperineal realtime ultrasound are relatively new biofeedback modalities for the PFM. The onscreen image of bladder neck (transperineal) or bladder base (transabdominal) resting position and movement (surrogate markers for PFM activity) displays the elevation and depression components of the PFM to the patient. An overactive PFM may display minimal excursion of movement on attempted contraction and relaxation and hence may theoretically be retrained to relax to a lower resting position following contraction. However, no studies have yet investigated the role of ultrasound as a biofeedback tool in patients with PFM pain or overactivity.

Electrical stimulation

Electricity has been a pain treatment modality for many centuries. Today, the most common mechanism for applying therapeutic electricity is via transcutaneous electrical nerve stimulation (TENS).

Transcutaneous electrical (nerve) stimulation

The rationale of the effectiveness of TENS for analgesia is based on the gate control theory of pain modulation. The application of TENS has been studied extensively. Its use as an analgesic therapy for chronic, non-pelvic pain conditions has been evaluated in a Cochrane review (Carroll et al 2001). The results of this review were inconclusive because the published trials did not provide sufficient information on the stimulation parameters that are most likely to provide optimum pain relief or long-term effectiveness. The use of TENS for PFM pain conditions or PFM overactivity has not been investigated.

Muscle re-education and pain relief

Electrogalvanic stimulation (EGS) and electrical muscle stimulation (ES) induce a sustained contraction, followed by muscle fatigue and eventual release of the spasm.

Use of EGS applied per rectum for patients with levator syndrome was first reported in the literature in 1982, and several studies appeared in the following decade (Billingham et al 1987, Ger et al 1993, Hull et al 1993, Morris & Newton 1987, Nicosia & Abcarian 1985, Oliver et al 1985, Sohn et al 1982). Reported success rates ranged from 40 to 90%, but the retrospective nature of the studies and the lack of both objective measures and control groups limits generalizability of the findings.

A small number of studies have reported the use of EGS or ES for anorectal pain, vaginal/sexual PFM pain and levator spasm (Fitzwater et al 2003, Nappi et al 2003, Park et al 2005, Seo et al 2005). The results are encouraging, but the uncontrolled study designs, wide range of populations studied and treatment protocols, and concurrent use of other modalities, limit interpretations of findings. Further high-quality trials are required to evaluate the benefits of electrical stimulation – both analgesic and muscle activation – for PFM pain and overactivity.

Magnetic field therapy

The use of pulsed electromagnetic fields (PEMF) for pelvic pain of various origin has been described in a small uncontrolled study (Jorgensen et al 1994). Study design limitations restrict assessment of this therapy for patients with PFM pain/overactivity. Static magnetic field therapy for CPP in patients has been investigated in a small double-blind pilot study (Brown et al 2002). The primary pain site was the abdomen with PFM status unknown, so the findings from this study can not be taken to apply to PFM pain/overactivity. The effect of magnetic field therapy on a well-defined PFM pain/overactivity population has not been investigated.

Vaginal dilators

Dilators range in size, shape and materials, and graduate in diameter to allow progressive application throughout a course of therapy. The indications for the use of vaginal dilators are to stretch or mobilize contracted or inflexible soft tissues and to act as a desensitizing tool to progressively reduce fear and apprehension of the ability of the vaginal tissues to accommodate coital function. There are no published guidelines on the optimal method of application, but clinicians often introduce the tool to a patient and encourage continuation as part of home therapy.

Vaginal dilators have been used as part of a multimodal approach directed to PFM pain or overactivity (Bergeron et al 2002, Seo et al 2005) with positive outcomes of combined therapy. A Cochrane review (Denton & Maher 2003) evaluated the use of vaginal dilators in women following pelvic radiotherapy. They found that the use of vaginal dilators to prevent stenosis had level II C evidence. Another Cochrane review (McGuire & Hawton 2003) evaluated interventions for vaginismus, but no studies measuring pain outcomes or PFM contractile activity were reported. Two trials were reviewed that included systematic desensitization with positive benefit to coital function reported. On the basis of the limited evidence reviewed, no recommendations of treatment could be made.

Application of heat

Superficial heat may be applied via hot packs (hot water bottle, moist compress), heating pads (electric, chemical or gel pack), or hydrotherapy. One small controlled study considered the effect of immersion in a warm bath on resting pressures in the anal canal in a group of patients with anorectal pain (mixed diagnoses) compared to a group of volunteers without pain (Dodi et al 1986). Results were positive for the therapy in the pain group, but more rigorously designed studies are required to further test this intervention.

Deep heat may be applied via diathermy (shortwave, microwave) or ultrasound. Ultrasound is the preferred treatment for most painful disorders, especially those arising from soft tissues and ligaments because it has greater penetration and also non-thermal effects, such as increasing extensibility of tissues, so is helpful in treating trigger points. It also has the advantage of being safe around metal and useful over small areas (Vasudevan 1997).

The benefit of therapeutic ultrasound has been evaluated with reference to acute perineal pain postpartum. Based on first principles, the application of ultrasound to treat chronic PFM pain or overactivity suggests a possible benefit, but studies investigating this aspect are limited. The penetration depth of the ultrasound current to the target tissue in PFM pain syndromes needs evaluation before further intervention studies using this modality are proposed. One retrospective study has investigated the effect of ultrasound on interstitial cystitis-associated pain (Lilius et al 1973). While favourable results were reported, application of findings is limited due to the study design.

Application of cold

Application of cold is a common and practical treatment for pain, but is used less often in chronic pain conditions than in acute pain conditions. Despite this, it may potentially be useful due to its analgesic effect, particularly when acute-on-chronic flare-ups of pain are experienced, such as postcoital pain. No studies have been found in which cryotherapy has been applied to chronic PFM pain or overactivity.

PAIN MANAGEMENT

Perception of visceral (organ) and somatic (muscular) pain may be governed by differing neurological mechanisms. Pelvic pain can receive contributions from both sources. This may explain why some pain management strategies known to be or not be effective for chronic non-pelvic muscular pain syndromes may differ in their effect on chronic PFM pain syndromes. There is insufficient knowledge regarding these issues at present.

No studies were found that specifically addressed PFM pain in isolation from PFM overactivity. Often no organic dysfunction can be identified at which to direct local treatment. The clinician must be able to refer the patient for psychosocial treatment if required. If treatment of the pain per se is considered the primary focus, principles of chronic pain management should be followed (Siddall & Cousins 2004). The efficacy of the multidisciplinary approach to chronic pain treatment has been reported (Flor et al 1992).

SUMMARY OF TREATMENT STUDIES

The most promising modalities for treating PFM pain/ overactivity seem to lie in the application of manual therapy techniques for reducing muscle tension, PFM exercises to reinforce normal muscle contraction and relaxation, the supplementary use of sEMG or manometry to achieve this goal, and possibly electrical stimulation for pain relief and assisted muscle activation and release. Patient advice, education regarding recognition of aggravating factors and encouragement to adhere to home programmes of exercise would seem important elements in the success of therapy. Cognitive–behaviour therapy and pain management are likely to be required to supplement these other methods.

SUMMARY

There is a significant lack of studies addressing the basic elements of PFM therapy for pelvic pain or muscle overactivity. In most cases study quality limits confident conclusion about treatment efficacy. There is an obvious need for standardized terminology, for studies that consider homogeneous patient groups, single and combination therapies, studies that apply valid and reliable outcome measures, and RCTs to confidently assign evidence to the effectiveness of the intervention.

CLINICAL RECOMMENDATIONS TO DATE

- A comprehensive assessment incorporating a biopsychosocial approach.

- Evaluate the PFM for the presence of overactivity, trigger points, and reduced elasticity. Aim to reproduce and quantify the patient's symptoms.

- Explain the rationale for proposed treatment modalities. Interventions that may be applied include cognitive–behavioural therapy, PFM relaxation and re-education exercises, manual therapy, adjunctive therapies and pain management.

- Direct treatment to the presenting symptoms and address objective findings.

- If there is no response to treatment within a reasonable time frame (allow 3–4 months), refer the patient for either psychosocial evaluation or pain management.

REFERENCES

Baker P K 1993 Musculoskeletal origins of chronic pelvic pain. Diagnosis and treatment. Obstetrics and Gynecology Clinics of North America 20(4):719–742

Bassotti G, Chistolini F, Sietchiping-Nzepa F et al 2004 Biofeedback for pelvic floor dysfunction in constipation. BMJ 328(7436):393–396

Bergeron S, Binik Y M, Khalife S et al 2001 A randomized comparison of group cognitive–behavioral therapy, surface electromyographic biofeedback, and vestibulectomy in the treatment of dyspareunia resulting from vulvar vestibulitis. Pain 91(3):297–306

Bergeron S, Binik Y M, Khalife S 2002 In favor of an integrated pain-relief treatment approach for vulvar vestibulitis syndrome. Journal of Psychosomatic Obstetrics and Gynaecology 23(1):5–6

Billingham R P, Isler J T, Friend W G et al 1987 Treatment of levator syndrome using high-voltage electrogalvanic stimulation. Diseases of the Colon and Rectum 30(8):584–587

Brown C S, Ling F W, Wan J Y et al 2002 Efficacy of static magnetic field therapy in chronic pelvic pain: a double-blind pilot study. American Journal of Obstetrics and Gynecology 187(6):1581–1587

Carroll D, Moore R A, McQuay H J et al 2001 Transcutaneous electrical nerve stimulation (TENS) for chronic pain. Cochrane Database of Systematic Reviews 3:CD003222

Denton A S, Maher E J 2003 Interventions for the physical aspects of sexual dysfunction in women following pelvic radiotherapy. Cochrane Database of Systematic Reviews 1: CD003750

Dodi G, Bogoni F, Infantino A et al 1986 Hot or cold in anal pain? A study of the changes in internal anal sphincter pressure profiles. Diseases of the Colon and Rectum 29(4):248–251

FitzGerald M P, Kotarinos R 2003 Rehabilitation of the short pelvic floor. II: treatment of the patient with the short pelvic floor. International Urogynecology Journal and Pelvic Floor Dysfunction 14(4):269–275, discussion 275

Fitzwater J B, Kuehl T J, Schrier J J 2003 Electrical stimulation in the treatment of pelvic pain due to levator ani spasm. Journal of Reproductive Medicine 48(8):573–577

Flor H, Fydrich T, Turk D C 1992 Efficacy of multidisciplinary pain treatment centers: a meta-analytic review. Pain 49(2):221–230

Ger G C, Wexner S D, Jorge J M et al 1993 Evaluation and treatment of chronic intractable rectal pain – a frustrating endeavor [see comment]. Diseases of the Colon and Rectum 36(2):139–145

Glazer H I 2000 Dysesthetic vulvodynia. Long-term follow-up after treatment with surface electromyography-assisted pelvic floor muscle rehabilitation. Journal of Reproductive Medicine 45(10):798–802

Glazer H I, Rodke G, Swencionis C et al 1995 Treatment of vulvar vestibulitis syndrome with electromyographic biofeedback of pelvic floor musculature. Journal of Reproductive Medicine 40(4):283–290

Harding V R, Simmonds M J, Watson P J 1998 Physiotherapy for chronic pain. Online. Available: www.iasp-pain.org

Hull T L, Milsom J W, Church J et al 1993 Electrogalvanic stimulation for levator-syndrome – how effective is it in the long-term. Diseases of the Colon and Rectum 36(8):731–733

Jorgensen W A, Frome B M, Wallach C 1994 Electrochemical therapy of pelvic pain: effects of pulsed electromagnetic fields (PEMF) on tissue trauma. European Journal of Surgery (suppl 574):83–86

King P M, Myers C A, Ling F W et al 1991 Musculoskeletal factors in chronic pelvic pain. Journal of Psychosomatic Obstetrics and Gynaecology 12(suppl):87–98

Kirste U, Haugstad G K, Leganger S et al 2002 Chronic pelvic pain in women [Norwegian]. Tidsskrift for Den Norske Laegeforening 122(12):1223–1227

Kotarinos R K 2003 Pelvic floor physiotherapy in urogynecologic disorders. Current Women's Health Reports 3(4):334–339

La Vaque T J, Hammond D C, Trudeau D et al 2002 Template for developing guidelines for the evaluation of the clinical efficacy of psychophysiological interventions. Applied Psychophysiology and Biofeedback 27(4):273–281

Lilius H G, Oravisto K J, Valtonen E J 1973 Origin of pain in interstitial cystitis. Effect of ultrasound treatment on the concomitant levator ani spasm syndrome. Scandinavian Journal of Urology and Nephrology 7(2):150–152

McGuire H, Hawton K 2003 Interventions for vaginismus.[update of Cochrane Database Syst Rev. 2001;(2):CD001760; PMID: 11406006]. Cochrane Database of Systematic Reviews 1: CD001760

McKay E, Kaufman R H, Doctor U et al 2001 Treating vulvar vestibulitis with electromyographic biofeedback of pelvic floor musculature. Journal of Reproductive Medicine 46(4):337–342

Morris L, Newton R A 1987 Use of high voltage pulsed galvanic stimulation for patients with levator ani syndrome. Physiotherapy 67(10):1522–1525

Nappi R E, Ferdeghini F, Abbiati I et al 2003 Electrical stimulation (ES) in the management of sexual pain disorders. Journal of Sex and Marital Therapy 29(suppl 1):103–110

Nicosia J F, Abcarian H 1985 Levator syndrome. A treatment that works. Diseases of the Colon and Rectum 28(6):406–408

Oliver G C, Rubin R J, Salvati E P et al 1985 Electrogalvanic stimulation in the treatment of levator syndrome. Diseases of the Colon and Rectum 28(9):662–663

Oyama I A, Rejba A, Lukban J C et al 2004 Modified thiele massage as therapeutic intervention for female patients with interstitial cystitis and high-tone pelvic floor dysfunction. Urology 64(5):862–865

Palsson O S, Heymen S, Whitehead W E 2004 Biofeedback treatment for functional anorectal disorders: a comprehensive efficacy review. Applied Psychophysiology and Biofeedback 29(3):153–174

Park D H, Yoon S G, Kim K U et al 2005 Comparison study between electrogalvanic stimulation and local injection therapy in levator ani syndrome. International Journal of Colorectal Disease 20(3):272–276

Peters A A, van Dorst E, Jellis B et al 1991 A randomized clinical trial to compare two different approaches in women with chronic pelvic pain. Obstetrics and Gynecology 77(5):740–744

Reiter R C 1998 Evidence-based management of chronic pelvic pain. Clinical Obstetrics and Gynecology 41(2):422–435

Seo J T, Choe J H, Lee W S et al 2005 Efficacy of functional electrical stimulation-biofeedback with sexual cognitive–behavioral therapy as treatment for vaginismus. Urology 66:77–81

Shelly B, Knight S, King P B et al 2002 Pelvic pain. In: Laycock J, Haslam J (eds) Therapeutic management of incontinence and pelvic pain. Springer–Verlag, London, p 156–189

Siddall P J, Cousins M J 2004 Persistent pain as a disease entity: Implications for clinical management. Anesthesia and Analgesia 99(2):510–520

Sohn N, Weinstein M A, Robbins R D 1982 The levator syndrome and its treatment with high–voltage electrogalvanic stimulation. American Journal of Surgery 144(5):580–582

Thiele G H 1937 Coccygodynia and pain in the superior gluteal region and down the back of the thigh: causation by tonic spasm of the levator ani, coccygeus and piriformis muscles and relief by massage of these muscles. JAMA 109(16):1271–1275

Vasudevan S V 1997 Physical rehabilitation in managing pain. Online. Available: www.iasp-pain.org

Vlaeyen J W, Morley S 2005 Cognitive-behavioral treatments for chronic pain: what works for whom? Clinical Journal of Pain 21(1):1–8

Weijmar Schultz W C, Gianotten W L, van der Meijden W I et al 1996 Behavioral approach with or without surgical intervention to the vulvar vestibulitis syndrome: a prospective randomized and non-randomized study. Journal of Psychosomatic Obstetrics and Gynecology 17(3):143–148

Weiss J M 2001 Pelvic floor myofascial trigger points: manual therapy for interstitial cystitis and the urgency-frequency syndrome. Journal of Urology 166(6):2226–2231

Female sexual dysfunction

Alessandra Graziottin

ASSESSMENT

Women's sexuality has only recently emerged as a central concern after years of neglect in the medical world. The current challenge is to blend together the biological, psychosexual and context-related components of women's sexual response in a comprehensive and meaningful scenario (Basson et al 2000, 2004). In this perspective, the role of pelvic floor function and dysfunction is of the highest importance (Alvarez & Rockwell 2002, Bourcier et al 2004, Graziottin 2001a, 2005a).

Levator ani's tone, strength and performance is a major contributor to vaginal receptivity, vaginal responsiveness, coital competence and pleasure (for both partners), and for the orgasmic muscular response. Indirectly, pelvic floor disorders (PFD) may impair genital arousal and, through a negative feedback, may affect the potential for physical and emotional satisfaction, and for sexual desire and mental arousal, thus potentially affecting the whole of a woman's sexual response, particularly when coital pain is a disruptive factor (Fig. 9.26) (Graziottin 2000, 2001a, 2004a).

Hyperactivity of the pelvic floor is causally associated with sexual pain disorders, namely dyspareunia and vaginismus (Abramov et al 1994, Glazer et al 1995, Graziottin et al 2004a, 2005a, Harlow et al 2001; Harlow & Stewart 2003, Lamont 1978, McKay et al 2001) and overexertion of the pelvic floor muscles (PFM) may lead to myalgia and 'Kegel' dyspareunia (DeLancey et al 1993).

The pelvic floor is central in understanding how physiological events such as vaginal deliveries may modulate levator ani's sexual competence in a life span perspective (Baessler & Schuessler 2004, Glazener 1997). Pelvic floor disorders are a common denominator in urogenital, proctological and sexual comorbidities (Barlow et al 1997, Cardozo et al 1998, Graziottin et al 2001a, 2004a, Lauman et al 1999, Weiss 2001, Wesselmann et al 1997). Iatrogenic problems, consequent to urogenital surgery, may in parallel affect and impair both a woman's well-being and sexual response (Graziottin 2001b).

Last, but not least, new insights into the role of the hyperactivity of the pelvic floor in adolescence and, possibly, infanthood, as predictors of vulnerability to further sexual pain disorders (vaginismus and dyspareunia) and to vulvar vestibulitis/vulvodynia open a new preventive window for female sexual dysfunctions (FSD) (Chiozza & Graziottin 2004, Graziottin 2005a, Harlow et al 2001). Appropriate management of early hyperactivity of the pelvic floor could hopefully prevent the urogenital and sexual comorbidities that affect so many young lives.

In this book, dedicated to physical therapy for the pelvic floor, FSD is reviewed paying special attention to the genital components of women's sexual response in physiological and pathological conditions. However, the role of the biological and medical factors should always be considered in the appropriate psychosexual and sociocultural context.

THE COMPLEXITY OF WOMEN'S SEXUALITY

Women's sexuality is multifactorial, rooted in biological, psychosexual and context-related factors (Basson et al 2000, 2004, Binik et al 2002, Dennerstein 2004, Dennerstein et al 1999, Levin 2002, Graziottin 2004a, 2004b, Leiblum & Rosen 2000, Klausmann 2002, Plaut et al 2004, Segraves & Balon 2003), correlated to couple dynamics and family and sociocultural issues. It is multisystemic: in men and women, a physiologic response requires the integrity of the hormonal, vascular, nervous, muscular, connective and immune systems; this fact has been too often overlooked in women until recently (Bachmann et al 2002, Goldstein & Berman 1998, Graziottin 2000, 2004b, Graziottin & Brotto 2004, Levin 2002, Meston & Frolich 2000, O'Connell et al 1998, 2004, Pfaus & Everitt 1995).

Three major dimensions – female sexual identity, sexual function and sexual relationship – interact to give women's sexual health its full meaning or its problematic profile (Graziottin 2000, 2004a, Graziottin & Basson 2004). Women's sexuality is discontinuous throughout

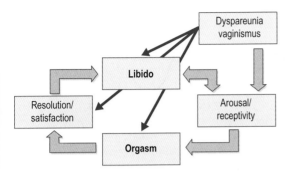

Fig. 9.26 Circular model of female sexual function and the interfering role of sexual pain disorders. This model contributes to the understanding of frequent overlapping of sexual symptoms reported in clinical practice (comorbidity) because different dimensions of sexual response are correlated from a pathophysiological point of view. Potential negative or positive feedback mechanisms operate in sexual function: dyspareunia and/or vaginismus has a direct inhibiting effect on genital arousal and vaginal receptivity and may have an indirect inhibiting effect on orgasm, satisfaction and libido, with close interplay between biological and psychosexual factors. Pelvic floor disorders of the hyperactive type causally related to sexual pain disorders may rapidly affect the sexual response. Modified from Graziottin 2000, with permission.

the life cycle and is dependent on biological (reproductive events) as well as personal, current contextual and relationship variables (Basson et al 2000, 2004).

FSD is age related, progressive and highly prevalent, affecting up to 20–43% of premenopausal women (Lauman et al 1999), and 48% of older women who are still sexually active in the late postmenopause (Dennerstein et al 2003, 2007, Graziottin & Koochaki 2003).

FSD may occur along a continuum from dissatisfaction (with potential integrity of the physiological response but emotional/affective frustration) to dysfunction (with or without pathological modifications), to severe pathology (Basson et al 2000, 2004). Pelvic floor disorders are among the most important and yet neglected medical contributors to FSD (Graziottin 2001a, 2005a, 2005b). However, sexual dissatisfaction, disinterest and even dysfunction may be appropriate for an 'antisexual' context (e.g. a partner affected by male sexual disorder or abusive) and they should not be labelled per se as 'diseases' or dysfunctions requiring medical treatment (Bancroft et al 2003).

FSD may occur with or without significant personal (and interpersonal) distress (Bancroft et al 2003,

Graziottin & Koochaki 2003). Sociocultural factors may further modulate the perception, expression and complaining modality (i.e. the 'wording') of a sexual disorder. The meaning of sexual intimacy is a strong modulator of the sexual response and of the quality of satisfaction a woman experiences besides the simple adequacy of the physical response (Basson 2003, Kaplan 1979, Klausmann 2002, Levine 2003, Plaut et al 2004). The quality of feelings for the partner and the partner's health and sexual problems may further contribute to FSD (Dennerstein et al 2003, Dennerstein 2004). Sexual problems reported by women are not discrete and often co-occur, comorbidity being one of the leading characteristics of FSD (Basson et al 2000, 2004).

Co-morbidity between FSD and medical conditions (e.g. urological, gynaecological proctological, metabolic, cardiovascular and neurological) is increasingly recognized (Graziottin 2000, 2004a, 2004b, 2005b, Wesselmann et al 1997). For example, latent classes analysis of sexual dysfunctions by risk factors in women indicate that urinary tract symptoms have a RR = 4.02 (2.75–5.89) of being associated with arousal disorders and a RR = 7.61 (4.06–14.26) of being associated with sexual pain disorders according to the epidemiological survey of Laumann et al (1999), credited as being the best survey carried out so far. The attention dedicated to pelvic floor related comorbidities – both between FSD and between FSD and medical conditions – in this paper reflects the clinical relevance of this association, especially in the urogynaecological and proctological domain.

CLASSIFICATION OF FSD

Over the past decades, the classification of FSD has undergone intense scrutiny and revisions that mirrors the new understanding of its complex aetiology. Until a decade ago, the classification of FSD, which constitutes the frame of reference for an appropriate diagnosis, was focused almost entirely on its psychological and relational components. Indeed, FSD was included in the broader manual of 'psychiatric' disorders (American Psychiatric Association 1987, 2000). The first and second consensus conferences on FSD (Basson et al 2000, 2004) set out to define FSD with special attention to bringing together the current level of evidence with definitions to fit women's wording and experiences. The latest classification is shown in Box 9.3.

CLINICAL HISTORY

For a more accurate definition of the sexual symptoms, health care providers should also briefly investigate the

Box 9.3: Classification of female sexual disorders (From Basson et al 2004)

WOMEN'S SEXUAL INTEREST/DESIRE DISORDER
- Absent or diminished feelings of sexual interest or desire, absent sexual thoughts or fantasies and a lack of responsive desire. Motivations (here defined as reasons/incentives), for attempting to become sexually aroused are scarce or absent. The lack of interest is considered to be more than that due to a normative lessening with the life cycle and duration of a relationship.

SEXUAL AVERSION DISORDER
- Extreme anxiety and/or disgust at the anticipation of/ or attempt to have any sexual activity

SUBJECTIVE SEXUAL AROUSAL DISORDER
- Absence of or markedly diminished cognitive sexual arousal and sexual pleasure from any type of sexual stimulation. Vaginal lubrication or other signs of physical response still occur.

GENITAL SEXUAL AROUSAL DISORDER
- Complaints of absent or impaired genital sexual arousal. Self-report may include minimal vulvar swelling or vaginal lubrication from any type of sexual stimulation and reduced sexual sensations from caressing genitalia. Subjective sexual excitement still occurs from non-genital sexual stimuli.

COMBINED GENITAL AND SUBJECTIVE AROUSAL DISORDER
- Absence of or markedly diminished subjective sexual excitement and awareness of sexual pleasure from any type of sexual stimulation as well as complaints of absent or impaired genital sexual arousal (vulvar swelling, lubrication).

PERSISTENT SEXUAL AROUSAL DISORDER
- Spontaneous, intrusive and unwanted genital arousal (e.g. tingling, throbbing, pulsating) in the absence of sexual interest and desire. Any awareness of subjective arousal is typically but not invariably unpleasant. The arousal is unrelieved by one or more orgasms and the feelings of arousal persist for hours or days.

WOMEN'S ORGASMIC DISORDER
- Despite the self-report of high sexual arousal/ excitement, there is either lack of orgasm, markedly diminished intensity of orgasmic sensations or marked delay of orgasm from any kind of stimulation.

DYSPAREUNIA
- Persistent or recurrent pain with attempted or complete vaginal entry and/or penile vaginal intercourse.

VAGINISMUS
- The persistent or recurrent difficulties of the woman to allow vaginal entry of a penis, a finger, and/or any object, despite the woman's expressed wish to do so. There is often (phobic) avoidance and anticipation/fear/ experience of pain, along with variable involuntary pelvic muscle contraction. Structural or other physical abnormalities must be ruled out/ addressed.

---

so-called 'descriptors' of the disorders, as defined by the International Consensus Conferences held in 1998 and 2003 (Basson et al 2000, 2004). They include the following.

The aetiology of the disorder

The aetiology of the disorder is further detailed in predisposing, precipitating and maintaining factors (Box 9.4) (Graziottin 2003a, 2003b, Graziottin & Brotto 2004, Graziottin & Leiblum 2005). Each category includes biological, psychosexual and contextual causes.

Biological descriptors include hormonal dysfunctions, PFDs, cardiovascular problems, neurological conditions (particularly pain-related) (Binik 2005, Binik et al 2002), metabolic disorders (diabetes mellitus), affective disorders (depression and anxiety). All the medical conditions that may directly or indirectly affect sexuality through their multisystemic impact and/or the consequences of pharmacological, surgical and/or radiotherapy treatment should be considered in the differential diagnosis of potential contributors to the reported FSD. Loss of sexual hormones, consequent to natural or iatrogenic menopause is a major contributor to FSD (Dennerstein et al 2003, 2005). It can be addressed with appropriate hormonal replacement therapy (Bachmann et al 2002, Graziottin 2000, 2004, Graziottin & Basson 2004). Current medication use and substance abuse should be actively investigated (Segraves & Balon 2003).

Psychosexual descriptors refer to emotional/affective/psychic factors such as negative upbringing/losses/trauma (physical, sexual, emotional) (Basson 2003, Edwards et al 1997, Rellini & Meston 2004), body

Box 9.4: Factors contributing to female sexual dysfunction (modified from Graziottin & Leiblum 2005)

PREDISPOSING FACTORS

Biological

- Endocrine disorders (hypoandrogenism, hypoestrogenism, hyperprolactinaemia)
- Menstrual cycle disorders/premenstrual syndrome
- Recurrent vulvovaginitis and/or cystitis
- Pelvic floor disorders: lifelong or acquired
- Drug treatments affecting hormones or menstrual cycle
- Contraceptive methods inappropriate for the woman and couple in that period of life
- Chronic diseases (diabetes mellitus, cardiovascular, neurological or psychiatric disease etc)
- Disorders associated with premature ovarian failure (POF): genetic, autoimmune
- Benign diseases (e.g. endometriosis) predisposing to iatrogenic menopause and dyspareunia
- Iatrogenic menopause: bilateral oophorectomy, chemotherapy, radiotherapy
- Persistent residual conditions (e.g. dyspareunia/chronic pain associated with endometriosis)

Psychosexual

- Inadequate/delayed psychosexual development
- Borderline personality traits
- Previous negative sexual experiences: sexual coercion, violence, or abuse
- Body image issues/concerns
- Affective disorders (dysthymia, depression, anxiety)
- Inadequate coping strategies
- Inadequate sexual education (attitudes towards contraception and sexually transmitted diseases)
- Dissatisfaction with social/professional role(s)

Contextual

- Ethnic/religious/cultural messages, expectations, and constraints regarding sexuality
- Social ambivalences towards female sexuality, when separated from reproduction or marriage
- Negative social attitudes towards female contraception
- Low socioeconomic status/reduced access to medical care and facilities
- Support network

PRECIPITATING FACTORS

Biological

- Negative reproductive events (unwanted pregnancies, abortion, traumatic delivery with damage of the pelvic floor, child's problems, infertility)
- Postpartum depression
- Vulvovaginitis/sexually transmitted diseases
- Sexual pain disorders
- Age at menopause
  - premature ovarian failure (POF) – menopause before age 40
  - premature menopause – menopause between age 40 and 45
- Biological vs iatrogenic menopause (especially for premature menopause)
- Iatrogenic menopause
  - androgen (besides oestrogen) loss
  - associated disorder/disease
- Extent and severity of menopausal symptoms and impact on well-being
- Current disorders
- Current pharmacological treatment
- Substance abuse (mainly alcohol and opiates)

Psychosexual

- Loss of loving feelings toward partner
- Unpleasant/humiliating sexual encounters or experiences
- Affective disorders (depression, anxiety)
- Relationship of fertility loss to fulfilment of life goals

Contextual

- Relationship discord
- Life-stage stressors (e.g. child's diseases, divorce, separation, partner infidelity)
- Loss or death of close friends or family members
- Lack of access to medical/psychosocial treatment and facilities
- Economic difficulties

MAINTAINING FACTORS

Biological

- Diagnostic omissions: unaddressed predisposing/precipitating biological aetiologies
- Untreated or inadequately treated comorbidities
  - physiatric: pelvic floor disorders
  - urologic: incontinence, lower urinary tract symptoms (LUTS), urogenital prolapse
  - proctologic: constipation, rhagades
  - metabolic: diabetes mellitus
  - psychiatric: depression, anxiety, phobias
- Pharmacological treatments
- Substance abuse
- Multisystemic changes associated with chronic disease or secondary to menopause

Box 9.4: Factors contributing to female sexual dysfunction—cont'd

- – hormonal
- – vascular
- – muscular
- – neurological
- – immunological
- Contraindications to hormone replacement therapy (HRT)
- Inadequacy of hormone replacement therapy in ameliorating menopause-associated biological symptoms

Psychosexual
- Low or loss of sexual self-confidence
- Performance anxiety
- Distress (personal, emotional, occupational, sexual)

- Diminished affection for or attraction to partner
- Unaddressed affective disorders (depression and/or anxiety)
- Negative perception of menopause-associated changes
- Body image concerns and increased body changes (wrinkles, body shape/weight, muscle tone)

Contextual
- Omission of menopause and female sexual dysfunction from provider's diagnostic and therapeutic approach
- Lack of access to adequate care
- Partner's general health or sexual problems or concerns
- Ongoing interpersonal conflict (with partner or others)
- Environmental constraints (lack of privacy, lack of time)

image issues (Graziottin 2006), binge eating disorders affecting self-esteem and self-confidence, attachment dynamics (secure, avoidant, anxious) (Clulow 2001) that may also modulate the level of trust in the relationship, the intensity of the commitment, and the confidence in loving and attitude towards affective and erotic intimacy.

Contextual descriptors include past and current significant relationships (Basson 2003, Leiblum & Rosen 2000), cultural/religious restrictions (Basson et al 2000, 2004), current interpersonal difficulties (Klausmann 2002, Liu 2003), partner's general health issues and/or sexual dysfunctions (Dennerstein et al 1999, 2003, 2004), inadequate stimulation and unsatisfactory sexual and emotional contexts (Levine 2003).

Generalized or situational?

Is the disorder generalized (with every partner and in every situation) or situational, specifically precipitated by partner-related or contextual factors, which should be specified (Basson et al 2000, 2004)? Situational problems usually rule out medical factors that tend to affect the sexual response with a more generalized effect (Graziottin 2004a, 2004b).

Lifelong or acquired?

Has the disorder been lifelong (from the very first sexual experience) or is it acquired after months or years of satisfying sexual intercourse? Asking the woman what in her opinion is causing the current FSD may offer useful insights into the aetiology of the disorder, particularly when it is acquired (Plaut et al 2004);

Level of distress

The level of distress indicates a mild, moderate, or severe impact of the FSD on personal life (Bancroft et al 2003, Dennerstein et al 2005, Graziottin & Koochaki 2003). Sexual distress should be distinguished from non-sexual distress and from depression. The degree of reported distress may have implications for the woman's motivation for therapy and for prognosis.

An interdisciplinary team is the most valuable resource for a patient-centred approach, both for diagnostic accuracy and tailored treatment. Key professional figures include a medical sexologist, gynaecologist, urologist, psychiatrist, endocrinologist, physiatrist, anaesthetist, neurologist, proctologist, dermatologist, psychotherapist (individual and couple), and physical therapist. Physical therapists are emerging as a key resource in addressing PFDs, which are finally receiving the attention they deserve as key biological factors in the aetiology of FSD.

WOMEN'S SEXUAL DESIRE/ INTEREST DISORDER

Hypoactive sexual desire disorder (HSDD) is the sexual dysfunction most frequently reported by women (Dennerstein et al 2003) The complaint of low desire becomes a sexual disorder when it causes severe personal distress to the woman. Population data indicate a prevalence of low desire in 32% of women between 18 and 59 years of age (Laumann et al 1999). A recent European survey of 2467 women, in France, UK, Germany and Italy indicates that the percentage of women with low sexual desire is 19% in the age cohort from 20 to 49 years; 32% in the same age cohort in women who have experienced surgical menopause; 46% in postmenopausal women aged 50 to 70 years with natural menopause; and 48% in the same age cohort, after surgical menopause (Graziottin & Koochaki 2003).

The percentage of women distressed by their loss of desire and having a HSDD was 27% in premenopausal women and 28% after surgical menopause, in the age cohort 20–49 years, respectively; 11% in women with natural menopause; and 14% in those with surgical menopause aged 50 to 70 years (Graziottin & Koochaki 2003). The likelihood of HSDD increases with age, while the distress associated with the loss of desire is inversely correlated with age.

Surgical menopause secondary to bilateral oophorectomy has a specific damaging effect due to the loss of ovarian oestrogens and androgens. Ovaries contribute to more than 50% of total body androgens in the fertile age. A European survey on 1356 women indicated that women with surgical menopause had an odds ratio (OR) of 1.4 (CI = 1.1, 1.9; p = 0.02) of having low desire. Surgically menopausal women were more likely to have HSDD than premenopausal or naturally menopausal women (OR = 2.1; CI = 1.4, 3.4, p = 0.001). Sexual desire scores and sexual arousal, orgasm and sexual pleasure were highly correlated (p < 0.001). Women with HSDD were more likely to be dissatisfied with their sex life and their partner relationship than women with normal desire (p < 0.001) (Dennerstein et al 2005).

The leading biological aetiology of HSDD includes not only hormonal factors (low testosterone, low oestrogens, or high prolactin), but also depression and/or comorbidity with major diseases (see Box 9.4). Premature iatrogenic menopause is the most frequent cause of a biologically determined generalized loss of desire; the younger the woman, the higher the distress this loss causes to her (Dennerstein et al 2005, Graziottin & Basson 2004). Key questions to address women's desire disorders are summarized in Box 9.5. Unaddressed pain associated with sexual pain disorders, and causally related, among others, to hyperactivity of the pelvic floor up to a frank myalgia, is a frequently overlooked predisposing, precipitating and maintaining factor of acquired loss of desire (Graziottin 2000, Graziottin & Brotto 2004, Graziottin et al, 2001a, 2001b, 2004a).

What the clinician should look for

If a possible biological aetiology is suggested by the clinical history, the clinician should assess (Plaut et al 2004) the following.

Box 9.5: Sexual history for hypoactive sexual desire disorders and associated sexual comorbidities. Modified from Graziottin 2004a, with permission

GENERAL WELL-BEING
- How do you feel (physically and mentally)?
- Are you currently sexually active?
- If not, is that a concern for you? If yes, how's your sex life?

SEXUAL FUNCTION
- Have you always suffered from low sexual desire (lifelong) or has it faded recently (acquired)?
- Do you suffer from other sexual symptoms?
- For example, do you experience vaginal dryness?
- Do you have difficulty in getting aroused or lubricated?
- Do you have difficulty reaching orgasm?
- Do you feel pain during or after intercourse?
- Do you suffer from cystitis 24–72 hours after intercourse and/or other urinary symptoms?
- Is there any lifestyle-related factor that may affect your sexual desire (e.g. body weight, alcohol or drug abuse, little sleep, fatigue, professional distress)?
- What, in your opinion, is causing or worsening your sexual disorder? Is it a psychological problem, a past or current negative event (e.g. sexual harassment or abuse), something related to your physical health or your relationship, or something else?

SEXUAL RELATIONSHIP
- Do you have a stable relationship?
- How's your relationship? Are you satisfied with it?
- How is your partner's health (general and sexual)?
- Do you feel that your current sexual problem is more dependent on a physical or couple (loving/intimacy) problem?
- Is your sexual problem present in every context and/or with different partners (generalized), or do you complain of it in specific situations or with a specific partner (situational)?
- What made you aware of it and willing to look for help (e.g. intolerable personal frustration, fear of losing the partner, partner's complaints, new hope for effective treatment, more self-confidence in reporting)?
- Are you personally interested in improving your sex life?

- **Hormonal profile:**
  - total and free testosterone, dihydroepiandrosterone sulfate (DHEAS), prolactin, 17β-estradiol, sex hormone binding globulin (SHBG), with a plasma sample on the fifth or sixth day from the beginning of the menses in fertile women;
  - follicle stimulating hormone (FSH) and all of the above, in perimenopausal women;
  - thyroid stimulating hormone (TSH) when individually indicated.

- **The pelvic floor:** in all its components, with an accurate gynaecological, sexological and/or physiatric examination, particularly when comorbidity with arousal, orgasm and/or sexual pain disorders is reported.

- **Psychosexual factors and affective state:** depression first, with referral to a psychiatrist, sex therapist or couples therapist for a comprehensive diagnosis if indicated (Leiblum & Rosen 2000).

AROUSAL DISORDERS

Central arousal disorders ('I do not feel mentally excited') are comorbid with loss of sexual desire and can only be separated from it with difficulty. Genital arousal disorders with their key subjective symptom, vaginal dryness, are increasingly reported with age. In epidemiological surveys 19–20% of women complain of arousal disorders (Lauman et al 1999). This figure may increase to 39–45% in postmenopausal sexually active patients (Dennerstein et al 2003, 2005).

Mental arousal may be triggered through different pathways: biologically by androgens and oestrogens, psychologically by motivational forces such as intimacy needs, (i.e. the affective needs of love, tenderness, attention, bonding and commitment) (Laan & Everaerd 1995). With successful genital arousal, most women produce increased quantities of vaginal transudate. The neurotransmitter vasoactive intestinal peptide (VIP) stimulates this neurogenic transudate production. Oestrogens are believed to be powerful 'permitting factors' for VIP (Levin 2002). The neurotransmitter nitric oxide (NO) stimulates the neurogenic congestion of the clitoral and vestibular bulb corpora cavernosa. (Levin 2002). Reduction in vaginal lubrication is one of the most common complaints of postmenopausal women. When the plasma oestradiol concentration is below 50 pg/mL (the normal range in fertile women being 100–200 pg/mL) vaginal dryness is increasingly reported (Sarrel 1998). Physiological studies indicate that after menopause the vaginal pH increases from 3.5–4.5 to 6.0–7.39 owing to decreased glycogen production and metabolism to lactic acid, with dramatic modification of the vaginal ecosystem, and an average reduction of vaginal secretions of 50%.

Leading biological aetiologies of arousal disorders include loss of sexual hormones, primarily oestrogen, and PFDs.

- Hyperactivity of the pelvic floor may reduce the introital opening causing dyspareunia. (Unwanted) pain is indeed the strongest reflex inhibitor of genital arousal: genital arousal disorders, and the consequent vaginal dryness, are often comorbid with dyspareunia (Graziottin 2001a, 2004a, 2005b). Psychosexual and relational factors may also concur in this disorder (Box 9.6);

- A hypoactive or damaged pelvic floor (after traumatic deliveries, with macrosomic children or vacuum extraction) (Baessler & Schuessler 2004) may contribute to genital arousal disorder because it reduces the pleasurable sensations the woman (and partner) feel during intercourse (Graziottin 2004a).

What the clinician should look for

When a patient complains of an arousal disorder, the clinician should check (Plaut et al 2004):

- hormonal profile (see above), more so in hypoestrogenic conditions such as longlasting secondary amenorrhoea, puerperium, menopause (especially iatrogenic);

- general and pelvic health, focusing on pelvic floor trophism: vaginal, clitoral, vulvar, connective and muscular (looking for both hypertonic and hypotonic pelvic floor dysfunctions) (Graziottin 2001a, 2004a);

- vaginal pH with a simple stick because vaginal acidity correlates well with oestrogen tissue levels (Graziottin 2004a);

- biological factors, such as vulvar vestibulitis or poor outcome of perineal/genital surgery causing introital and/or pelvic pain (see dyspareunia);

- vascular factors that may impair the genital arousal response (smoking, hypercholesterolaemia, atherosclerosis, hypertension, diabetes mellitus) (Goldstein & Berman 1998);

- relational issues, inhibition and/or erotic illiteracy if a poor quality of mental arousal, poor or absent foreplay are reported; if this is so refer the willing couple to the sexual or couple therapist (Leiblum & Rosen 2000)

Box 9.6: Aetiology of dyspareunia. Modified from Graziottin 2004a, with permission

Many causes may overlap or be associated with coital pain with complex pathophysiological interplay. The relative weight of each cause in the individual woman may change with chronicity of pain and progressive involvement of other pelvic organs.

BIOLOGICAL

Superficial/introital and/or mid-vaginal dyspareunia
- Infectious: vulvitis, vulvar vestibulitis, vaginitis, cystitis
- Inflammatory, with mast cell upregulation
- Hormonal: vulvovaginal atrophy
- Anatomical: fibrous hymen, vaginal agenesis
- Muscular: primary or secondary hyperactivity of levator ani muscle
- Iatrogenic: poor outcome of genital surgery, pelvic radiotherapy
- Neurological: inclusive of neuropathic pain
- Connective and immunological: Sjögren's syndrome
- Vascular

Deep dyspareunia
- Endometriosis
- Pelvic inflammatory disease (PID)
- Pelvic varicocoele
- Chronic pelvic pain and referred pain
- Outcome of pelvic or endovaginal radiotherapy
- Abdominal nerve entrapment syndrome

PSYCHOSEXUAL
- Comorbidity with desire and /or arousal disorders, or vaginismus
- Past sexual harassment and/or abuse
- Affective disorders: depression and anxiety
- Catastrophism as leading psychological coping modality

CONTEXT OR COUPLE RELATED
- Lack of emotional intimacy
- Inadequate foreplay
- Conflicts: verbally, physically or sexually abusive partner
- Poor anatomical compatibility (penis size and/or infantile female genitalia)
- Sexual dissatisfaction and consequent inadequate arousal

ORGASMIC DISORDERS

Orgasmic disorder has been reported in an average of 24% of women during their fertile years in the epidemiological study of Lauman et al (1999). After the menopause, 39% of women complain of orgasmic difficulties, with 20% complaining that their clitoris 'is dead', according to Sarrel & Whitehead (1985).

Orgasm is a sensorimotor reflex that may be triggered by a number of physical and mental stimuli (Mah & Binik 2004).

Genital orgasm requires:

- integrity of the pudendal sensory nerve fibres (S2, S3, S4) and corticomedullary fibres;
- cavernosal structures that engorged and adequately stimulated convey pleasant sensory stimuli to the medullary centre and the brain;
- adequate motor response of the PFMs.

A short medullary reflex may trigger a muscular response characterized by involuntary contraction (three to eight times, in single or repetitive sequences) of the levator ani. The medullary reflex may be eased or blocked, respectively, by corticomedullary fibres that convey both excitatory stimuli when central arousal is maximal and inhibitory ones when arousal is poor. Performance anxiety may activate adrenergic input, which disrupts the arousal response. Inhibitory fibres are mostly serotonergic: this explains the inhibitory effects of selective serotonin reuptake inhibitors (SSRIs) on orgasm in both men and women (Seagraves & Balon 2003). Fear of leaking during intercourse may inhibit coital intimacy and/or orgasm (Barlow et al 1997, Cardozo et al 1998): leakage during coital thrusting is usually associated with stress incontinence, while leakage at orgasm is associated with urge incontinence.

Significant age-associated changes in the content of smooth muscle and connective tissue in the clitoral cavernosa contributing to age-associated clitoral sexual dysfunction causing hypo-anorgasmia, have been demonstrated from the first to the sixth decade of life and beyond by computer-assisted histomorphometric image analysis (Tarcan et al 1999).

What the clinician should look for

Using the information emerging from the clinical history as a starting point, the physician should assess:

- hormonal balance;
- signs and symptoms of vulvar dystrophy and, specifically, of clitoral and vaginal involution (Graziottin 2004a);

- traumatic consequences of female genital mutilation (infibulation);
- signs and symptoms of urge, stress or mixed incontinence, with either a hypotonic or hypertonic pelvic floor (Barlow et al 1997, Cardozo et al 1998);
- iatrogenic influences when potentially orgasm-inhibiting drugs are prescribed.

SEXUAL PAIN DISORDERS

Various degrees of dyspareunia are reported by 15% of coitally active women, and 22.5–33% of postmenopausal women. Vaginismus occurs in 0.5–1% of premenopausal women. However, mild hyperactivity of the pelvic floor, that could coincide with grade I or II of vaginismus according to Lamont (1978) may permit intercourse, causing coital pain (Graziottin 2003b, 2005a).

Vaginal receptiveness is a prerequisite for intercourse, and requires anatomical and functional tissue integrity, both in resting and aroused states. Normal trophism, both mucosal and cutaneous, adequate hormonal impregnation, lack of inflammation, particularly at the introitus, normal tonicity of the perivaginal muscles, vascular, connective and neurological integrity, and normal immune response are all considered necessary to guarantee vaginal 'habitability'. Vaginal receptiveness may be modulated by psychosexual, mental and interpersonal factors, all of which may result in poor arousal with vaginal dryness (Plaut et al 2004).

Fear of penetration, and a general muscular arousal secondary to anxiety may cause a defensive contraction of the perivaginal muscles leading to vaginismus (Reissing et al 2003, 2004, van der Velde et al 2001). This disorder may be the clinical correlate of a primary neurodystonia of the pelvic floor, as recently proven with needle electromyography (Graziottin et al 2004a). It may be so severe as to prevent penetration completely. Vaginismus is the leading cause of unconsummated marriages in women. The defensive pelvic floor contraction may also be secondary to genital pain of whatever cause (Travell & Simons 1983; Wesselmann et al 1997).

Dyspareunia is the common symptom of a variety of coital pain-causing disorders (see Box 9.6). Vulvar vestibulitis is its leading cause in premenopausal women (Abramov et al 1994, Friedrich 1987, Glazer et al 1995, Graziottin 2001a, Graziottin & Brotto 2004, Graziottin et al 2004b). The diagnostic triad is

1. severe pain upon vestibular touch or attempted vaginal entry;
2. exquisite tenderness to cotton-swab palpation of the introital area (mostly at 5 and 7, when looking at the introitus as a clock face);
3. dyspareunia (Friederich 1987).

From the pathophysiological point of view, vulvar vestibulitis involves the upregulation of:

- the immunological system (i.e. of introital mast cells with hyperproduction of both inflammatory molecules and nerve growth factors [NGF]) (Bohm-Starke et al 1999, 2001a, 2001b, Bornstein et al 2002, 2004);
- the pain system, with proliferation of local pain fibres induced by the NGF (Bornstein et al 2002, 2004, Westrom & Willen 1998), which may contribute to neuropathic pain (Graziottin & Brotto 2004, Woolf 1993);
- hyperactivity of the levator ani, which can be antecedent to vulvar vestibulitis (Abramov et al 1994, Graziottin 2005a, Graziottin et al 2004a), or secondary to the introital pain.

In either case, addressing the muscle component is a key part of treatment (Bergeron et al 2001, Glazer et al 1995, McKay et al 2001). Hyperactivity of the pelvic floor may be triggered by non-genital, non-sexual causes, such as urological factors (urge incontinence, when tightening the pelvic floor may be secondary to the aim of reinforcing the ability to control the bladder), or anorectal problems (anismus, haemorrhoids, rhagades). Comorbidity with other sexual dysfunctions – loss of libido, arousal disorders, orgasmic difficulties, and/or sexual pain-related disorders – is frequently reported with persisting/chronic dyspareunia (Graziottin et al 2001b).

What the clinician should look for

The diagnostic work-up should focus on:

- physical examination to define the 'pain map' (Graziottin 2001a, Graziottin & Basson 2004, Graziottin et al 2001c), (any site in the vulva, mid-vagina and deep vagina where pain can be elicited) because location of the pain and its characteristics are the strongest predictors of type of organicity (Meana et al 1997), and including pelvic floor trophism (vaginal pH), muscular tone, strength and performance (Alvarez & Rockwell 2002, Bourcier et al 2004), signs of inflammation (primarily vulvar vestibulitis) (Friedrich 1987, Graziottin & Brotto 2004), poor outcomes of pelvic (Graziottin 2001b) or perineal surgery (primarily episiotomy/episiorraphy) (Glazener 1997), associated urogenital and rectal pain syndromes (Wesselmann et al 1997), myogenic or neurogenic pain (Bohm-Starke 2001a, 2001b, Bornstein et al 2002, 2004) and vascular problems (Goldstein & Berman 1998);
- psychosexual factors, poor arousal and coexisting vaginismus (Leiblum 2000, Pukall et al 2005);

- relationship issues (Reissing et al 2003);

- hormonal profile, if clinically indicated, when dyspareunia is associated with vaginal dryness.

Pain is rarely purely psychogenic, and dyspareunia is no exception. Like all pain syndromes, it usually has one or more biological aetiological factors. Hyperactive PFDs are a constant feature. However, psychosexual and relationship factors, generally lifelong or acquired low libido because of the persisting pain, and lifelong or acquired arousal disorders due to the inhibitory effect of pain, should be addressed in parallel to provide comprehensive, integrated and effective treatment.

ETHICAL, LEGAL AND COUNSELLING RELATED CONSIDERATIONS

The topic of sexuality requires special attention being given to confidentiality and informed consent depending on the profession of the clinician and any local laws that place limits on confidentiality, such as in the reporting of sexual abuse. Although the discussion of sexual matters is often an appropriate part of medical evaluation and treatment, it is also important not to sexualize the clinical setting when it is not necessary. Patients may be confused or embarrassed by comments about their attractiveness, disclosure of intimate personal information by the clinician, or by sex-related questions that are neither clinically relevant nor justifiable. The modesty of the patient should be respected in touching, disrobing and draping procedures (Plaut et al 2004). Key aspects of appropriate counselling attitudes are summarized in Box 9.7.

CONCLUSION

To address the complexity of FSD requires a balanced clinical perspective between biological and psychosexual/relational factors. Apart from counselling the FSD complaint in a competent way when the issue is openly raised by the patient, physicians and physical therapists can contribute to improving the quality of (sexual) life of their patients, by routinely asking them during the

> **Box 9.7:** Talking with patients about sexual issues. From Plaut et al 2004, with permission
>
> - Ask pointed questions and request clarification that will result in sufficiently specific data about the patient's symptoms
> - Be sensitive to the optimal time to ask the most emotionally charged questions
> - Look for and respond to non-verbal cues that may signal discomfort or concern
> - Be sensitive to the impact of emotionally charged words (e.g. rape, abortion)
> - If you are not sure of the patient's sexual orientation, use gender-neutral language in referring to his or her partner
> - Explain and justify your questions and procedures
> - Teach and reassure as you examine
> - Intervene to the extent that you are qualified and comfortable; refer to qualified medical or mental health specialists as necessary

clinical history taking: 'How's your sex life'? so offering an opening for current or future disclosure. The wish is that the new attention to women's right for a better sexual life will significantly help increase the physician's confidence in asking and listening to complaints of FSD and his or her 'clinical impact factor' (i.e his or her ability to appropriately diagnose and effectively treat FSD).

In the tailoring of treatment, the physical therapist has a crucial role, especially in sexual pain disorders, either lifelong or acquired, and in acquired desire, arousal or orgasmic disorders secondary to coital pain. The enthusiasm that many physical therapists have when they can effectively treat or co-treat FSD for which a woman has been doctor-shopping for years are mirrored by the woman's satisfaction in finally feeling listened to, respected in the truth of her coital pain or other sexual complaints, and re-empowered in her body confidence, when she is taught how to command and appropriately relax her key muscles for sex and love.

REFERENCES

Abramov L, Wolman I, David M P 1994 Vaginismus: An important factor in the evaluation and management of vulvar vestibulitis syndrome. Gynecological and Obstetrical Investigations 38:194–197

Alvarez D J, Rockwell P G 2002 Trigger points: diagnosis and management. American Family Physician 65(4):653–660

American Psychiatric Association 1987 Diagnostic and statistical manual of mental disorders, 3rd edn. American Psychiatric Association, Washington DC

American Psychiatric Association 2000 Diagnostic and statistical manual of mental disorders, 4th edn. American Psychiatric Association, Washington DC

Bachmann G, Bancroft J, Braunstein G et al 2002 FAI: the Princeton consensus statement on definition, classification and assessment. Fertility and Sterility 77:660–665

Baessler K, Schuessler B 2004 Pregnancy, childbirth and pelvic floor damage. In: Bourcier A, McGuire E, Abrams P (eds) Pelvic floor disorders. Elsevier Saunders, Philadelphia, p 33–42

Bancroft J, Loftus J, Long J S 2003 Distress about sex: a national survey of women in heterosexual relationships. Archives of Sexual Behaviour 32(3):193–204

Barlow D H, Cardozo L, Francis R M et al 1997 Urogenital ageing and its effect on sexual health in older British women. British Journal of Obstetrics and Gynecology 104:87–91

Basson R 2003 Women's desire deficiencies and avoidance. In: Levine S B, Risen C B, Althof S E (eds) Handbook of clinical sexuality for mental health professionals. Brunner Routledge, New York, p 111–130

Basson R, Berman J, Burnett A et al 2000 Report of the International Consensus Development Conference on female sexual dysfunction: definition and classification. The Journal of Urology 163:889–893

Basson R, Leiblum S, Brotto L et al 2004 Revised definitions of women's sexual dysfunction. Journal of Sexual Medicine 1(1):40–48

Bergeron S, Khalife S, Pagidas K et al 2001 A randomized comparison of group cognitive–behavioural therapy surface electromyographic biofeedback and vestibulectomy in the treatment of dyspareunia resulting from VVS. Pain 91: 297–306

Binik Y M, Reissing E D, Pukall C F et al 2002 The female sexual pain disorders: genital pain or sexual dysfunction? Archives of Sexual Behaviour 31:425–429

Binik Y M 2005 Should dyspareunia be retained as a sexual dysfunction in DSM-V? A painful classification decision. Archives of Sexual Behaviour 34(1):11–21

Bohm-Starke N, Hilliges M, Falconer C et al 1999 Neurochemical characterization of the vestibular nerves in women with vulvar vestibulitis syndrome. Gynecologic and Obstetric Investigation 48:270–275

Bohm-Starke N, Hilliges M, Blomgren B et al 2001a Increased blood flow and erythema in posterior vestibular mucosa in vulvar vestibulitis. American Journal of Obstetrics and Gynecology 98:1067–1074

Bohm-Starke N, Hilliges M, Brodda-Jansen G et al 2001b Psychophysical evidence of nociceptor sensitization in vulvar vestibulitis syndrome. Pain 94:177–183

Bornstein J, Sabo E, Goldschmid N 2002 A mathematical model for the histopathologic diagnosis of vulvar vestibulitis based on a histomorphometric study of innervation and mast cell activation. Journal of Reproductive Medicine 9:742

Bornstein J, Goldschmid N, Sabo E 2004 Hyperinnervation and mast cell activation may be used as a histopathologic diagnostic criteria for vulvar vestibulitis. Gynecologic and Obstetric Investigation 58:171–178

Bourcier A, McGuire E, Abrams P 2004 Pelvic floor disorders. Elsevier Saunders, Philadelphia

Cardozo L, Bachmann G, McClish D et al 1998 Meta-analysis of estrogen therapy in the management of urogenital atrophy in postmenopausal women: second report of the hormones and urogenital therapy committee. Obstetrics and Gynecology 92:722–727

Chiozza M L, Graziottin A 2004 Urge incontinence and female sexual dysfunction: a life span perspective. In: Graziottin A (ed) Female sexual dysfunction: clinical approach. Urodinamica 14(2):133–138

Clulow C (ed) 2001 Adult attachment and couple psychotherapy. Brunner–Routledge, Hove, UK

DeLancey J O, Sampselle C M, Punch M R 1993 Kegel dyspareunia. Obstetrics and Gynecology. 82:658–659

Dennerstein L, Alexander J, Kotz K 2003 The menopause and sexual functioning: A review of population-based studies. Annual Review of Sex Research 14:64–82

Dennerstein L 2004 Mid-aged women's sexual functioning. In: Graziottin A (ed) Female sexual dysfunction: clinical approach. Urodinamica14(2):68–70. Online. Available: http://www.alessandragraziottin.it

Dennerstein L, Lehert P, Koochaki P E et al 2007 Factors associated with women's health experiences: cross-cultural comparison of women aged 20–70 years. Menopause 14(4) (In press)

Dennerstein L, Lehert P, Burger H et al 1999 Factors affecting sexual functioning of women in the midlife years. Climacteric 2:254–262

Edwards L, Mason M, Phillips M et al 1997 Childhood sexual and physical abuse: incidence in patients with vulvodynia. Journal of Reproductive Medicine 42:135–139

Friedrich E G 1987 Vulvar vestibulitis syndrome. Journal of Reproductive Medicine 32:110–114

Glazer H I, Rodke G, Swencionis C et al 1995 Treatment of vulvar vestibulitis syndrome with electromyographic feedback of pelvic floor musculature. Journal of Reproductive Medicine 40:283–290

Glazener C M A 1997 Sexual function after childbirth: women's experiences, persistent morbidity and lack of professional recognition. British Journal of Obstetrics and Gynaecology 104:330–335

Goldstein I, Berman J 1998 Vasculogenic female sexual dysfunction: vaginal engorgement and clitoral erectile insufficiency syndrome. International Journal of Impotence Research 10:S84–S90

Graziottin A 2000 Libido: the biologic scenario. Maturitas 34(suppl 1)S9–S16

Graziottin A 2001a Clinical approach to dyspareunia. Journal of Sex and Marital Therapy 27:489–501

Graziottin A 2001b Sexual function in women with gynecologic cancer: a review. Italian Journal of Gynecology and Obstetrics 2:61–68

Graziottin A, Nicolosi A E, Caliari I 2001a Vulvar vestibulitis and dyspareunia: Addressing the biological etiologic complexity. Poster presented at the International Meeting of the Female Sexual Function Forum, Boston, MA

Graziottin A, Nicolosi A E, Caliari I 2001b Vulvar vestibulitis and dyspareunia: Addressing the psychosexual etiologic complexity. Poster presented at the International Meeting of the Female Sexual Function Forum, Boston, MA

Graziottin A, Nicolosi A E, Caliari I 2001c Vulvar vestibulitis and dyspareunia: The 'pain map' and the medical diagnosis. Poster presented at the International meeting of the Female Sexual Function Forum, Boston, MA

Graziottin A 2003a Etiology and diagnosis of coital pain. Journal of Endocrinological Investigation 26(3):115–121

Graziottin A 2003b The challenge of sexual medicine for women: overcoming cultural and educational limits and gender biases. Journal of Endocrinological Investigation 26(3):139–142

Graziottin A, Koochaki P 2003 Self-reported distress associated with hypoactive sexual desire in women from four European countries. Poster presented at the North American Menopause Society (NAMS) meeting, Miami, Abstract book, 126, p 105

Graziottin A 2004a Sexuality in postmenopause and senium. In: Lauritzen C, Studd J (eds) Current management of the menopause. Martin Duniz, London, p 185–203

Graziottin A 2004b Women's right to a better sexual life. In: Graziottin A (ed) Female sexual dysfunction: clinical approach. Urodinamica 14(2):57–60. Online. Available: http://www.alessandragraziottin.it

Graziottin A, Basson R 2004 Sexual dysfunctions in women with premature menopause. Menopause 11(6):766–777

Graziottin A, Brotto L 2004 Vulvar vestibulitis syndrome: clinical approach. Journal of Sex and Marital Therapy 30:124–139

Graziottin A, Bottanelli M, Bertolasi L 2004a Vaginismus: a clinical and neurophysiological study. In: Graziottin A (ed) Female sexual dysfunction: clinical approach. Urodinamica 14:117–121. Online. Available: http://www.alessandragraziottin.it

Graziottin A, Giovannini N, Bertolasi L et al 2004b Vulvar vestibulitis: pathophysiology and management. Current Sexual Health Report 1:151–156

Graziottin A 2005a Sexual pain disorders in adolescents. In: Genazzani A (ed) Proceedings of the 12th World Congress of Human Reproduction, International Academy of Human Reproduction, Venice, 10–13. CIC Edizioni Internazionali, Roma, p 434–449

Graziottin A 2006 Why deny dyspareunia its sexual meaning? Archives of Sexual Behaviour 34(1):32–34

Graziottin A 2006 Breast cancer and its effects on women's self-image and sexual function. In: Goldstein I, Meston C, Davis S, Traish A (eds) Women's sexual function and dysfunction: study, diagnosis and treatment. Taylor and Francis, UK, p 276–281

Graziottin A, Leiblum S R 2005 Biological and psychosocial pathophysiology of female sexual dysfunction during the menopausal transition. Journal of Sexual Medicine 2(suppl 3):133–145

Harlow B L, Wise L A, Stewart E G 2001 Prevalence and predictors of chronic lower genital tract discomfort. American Journal of Obstetrics and Gynecology 185:545–550

Harlow B L, Steward E G 2003 A population-based assessment of chronic unexplained vulvar pain: Have we underestimated the prevalence of vulvodynia? Journal of the American Medical Women's Association 58:82–88

Kaplan H S 1979 Disorders of sexual desire. Simon and Schuster, New York

Klausmann D 2002 Sexual motivation and the duration of the relationship. Archives of Sexual Behaviour 31:275–287

Laan E, Everaerd W 1995 Determinants of female sexual arousal: psychophysiological theory and data. Annual Review of Sex Research 6:32–76

Lamont J A 1978 Vaginismus. American Journal of Obstetrics and Gynecology 131:632–636

Lauman E O, Gagnon J H, Michaci R T et al 1999 Sexual dysfunction in the United States: prevalence and predictors. JAMA 281(6):537–542

Leiblum S R 2000 Vaginismus: a most perplexing problem. In: Leiblum S R, Rosen R C (eds) Principles and practice of sex therapy, 3rd edn. Guilford, New York, p 181–202

Leiblum S R, Rosen R C (eds) 2000 Principles and practice of sex therapy, 3rd edn. Guilford, New York

Levin R J 2002 The physiology of sexual arousal in the human female: a recreational and procreational synthesis. Archives of Sexual Behaviour 31(5):405–411

Levine S B 2003 The nature of sexual desire. Archives of Sexual Behavior 32(3):279–285

Liu C 2003 Does quality of marital sex decline with duration? Archives of Sexual Behavior 32(1):55–60

Mah K, Binik I M 2004 Female orgasm disorders: a clinical approach. In: Graziottin A (ed) Female sexual dysfunction: a clinical approach. Urodinamica 19(2):99–104. Online. Available: http://www.alessandragraziottin.it

McKay E, Kaufman R, Doctor U et al 2001 Treating vulvar vestibulitis with electromyographic biofeedback of pelvic floor musculature. Journal of Reproductive Medicine 46:337–342

Meana M, Binik Y M, Khalife S et al 1997 Dyspareunia: sexual dysfunction or pain syndrome? Journal of Nervous Mental Diseases 185(9):561–569

Meston C M, Frolich P F 2000 The neurobiology of sexual function. Archives of General Psychiatry 57:1012–1030

O'Connell H E, Anderson C R, Plenter R J, Hutson J M 2004 The clitoris: a unified structure. Histology of the clitoral glans, body, crura and bulbs. In: Graziottin A (guest ed.) Female dysfunction: clinical approach. Urodinamica 14:127–132

O'Connell H E, Hutson J M, Anderson C R et al 1998 Anatomical relationship between urethra and clitoris. Journal of Urology 159:1892–1897

Pfaus J G, Everitt B J 1995 The psychopharmacology of sexual behaviour. In: Bloom F E, Kupfer D (eds) Psycho-pharmacology. Raven Press, New York, p 743–758

Plaut M, Graziottin A, Heaton J 2004 Sexual dysfunction. Health Press, Abingdon, UK

Pukall C, Lahaie M A, Binik Y M 2005 Sexual pain disorders: etiologic factors. In: Goldstein I, Meston C M, Davis S, Traish A (eds) Women's sexual function and dysfunction: study, diagnosis and treatment. Taylor and Francis, UK, p 236–244

Sarrel P M 1998 Ovarian hormones and vaginal blood flow using laser Doppler velocimetry to measure effects in a clinical trial of post-menopausal women. International Journal of Impotence Research 18:S91–S93

Sarrell P W M, Whitehead M I 1985 Sex and the menopause: defining the issues. Maturitas 7:217–224

Seagraves R T, Balon R 2003 Sexual pharmacology: fast facts. WW Norton & Company, New York

Reissing E D, Binik YM, Khalifé S et al 2003 Etiological correlates of vaginismus: sexual and physical abuse, sexual knowledge, sexual self-schema, and relationship adjustment. Journal of Sex and Marital Therapy 29:47–59

Reissing E D, Binik Y M, Khalifé S et al 2004 Vaginal spasm, pain, and behavior: an empirical investigation of the diagnosis of vaginismus. Archives of Sexual Behavior 33:5–17

Rellini A, Meston C M 2004 Sexual abuse and female sexual disorders: Clinical implications. Urodinamica 14(2):80–83

Tarcan T, Park K, Goldstein I et al 1999 Histomorphometric analysis of age related structural changes in human clitoral cavernosal tissue. Journal of Urology 161:940–944

Travell J, Simons D 1983 Myofascial pain and dysfunction: the trigger points manual. Williams & Wilkins, Baltimore, USA

van der Velde J, Laan E, Everaerd W 2001 Vaginismus, a component of a general defensive reaction. An investigation of pelvic floor muscle activity during exposure to emotion-inducing film excerpts in women with and without vaginismus. International Urogynecology Journal and Pelvic Floor Dysfunction 12:328–331

Weiss J M 2001 Pelvic floor myofascial trigger points: manual therapy for interstitial cystitis and the urgency-frequency syndrome. Journal of Urology 166:2226–2231

Wesselmann U, Burnett A L, Heinberg L 1997 The urogenital and rectal pain syndromes. Pain 73(3):269–294

Westrom L V, Willen R 1998 Vestibular nerve fiber proliferation in vulvar vestibulitis syndrome. Obstetrics and Gynecology 91:572–576

Woolf C J 1993 The pathophysiology of peripheral neuropathic pain: abnormal peripheral input and abnormal central processing. Acta Neurochirurgica. Supplementum 58:125–130

TREATMENT

Alessandra Graziottin

INTRODUCTION

There is no effective therapy without accurate and comprehensive diagnosis. This is even more true for female sexual dysfunction (FSD), which usually has a multifactorial aetiology. Biological, psychosexual and context-related factors (Basson et al 2000, 2004), further characterized as predisposing, precipitating and maintaining (Graziottin 2005a, Graziottin & Brotto 2004) may interact to give the FSD that the woman is complaining about its specific individual characteristics.

The accurate diagnosis of FSD is currently a challenge for researchers and clinicians. The temptation of searching for the aetiology, preliminary to finding the optimal treatment, is usually inappropriate, and continuously frustrated by the complexity of female sexuality.

The delay in the medical approach to FSD and the persistent psychological perspective make it difficult to have evidence-based medical treatments of FSD except in the domain of sexual hormones. As a result of diagnostic delays, inadequacies, and gender biases, **no treatment for FSD is currently approved with this specific indication** with the exception of a clitoral device indicated for female arousal disorders (Wilson et al 2001). From the clinical point of view, an integrated diagnostic and treatment approach is therefore necessary to tailor treatment according to the individual and couple's needs at the best of our current scientific and clinical knowledge (Basson et al 2000, 2004, Graziottin 2001a, 2004a, 2004b, Plaut et al 2004).

The available evidence for treatment of FSD will be reviewed. Special focus will be given to the role of the physical therapist in addressing the muscle and pelvic floor-related contributors to FSD.

DIAGNOSTIC KEY POINTS

Key points in the FSD diagnosis, preliminary to a well tailored treatment, should be:

- accurate listening to the complaint's wording, to verbal and non-verbal messages, with:
  - definition of the nature of the disorders;
  - is it lifelong or acquired?
  - is it generalized or situational?
  - is it organic, psychogenic, contextual or, as in most cases, mixed? with definition of key predisposing, precipitating and maintaining factors;
  - how severe is the distress it causes?
  - are there sexual and/or medical (e.g. urogenital, proctological) associated comorbidity – comorbidities may be other types of FSD, but also other medical conditions, such as urological, gynaecological, proctological, metabolic, cardiovascular and neurological diseases – for example, urinary tract symptoms have a relative risk (RR) of:
    - 4.02 (2.75–5.89) of being associated with arousal disorders
    - 7.61 (4.06–14.26) of being associated with sexual pain disorders (Laumann et al 1999)
  - partner's related issues;
  - the personal motivation the woman has (or does not have) to treatment of FSD, which includes the meaning of the symptom for the woman;

- accurate examination of the woman, and particularly of the external genitalia, vagina and pelvic floor (Graziottin 2004a,b, Graziottin et al 2001a,b,c) – careful physical examination should be performed because the biological aetiology of FSD is better diagnosed when attention is paid to vulvovaginal trophism with pH recording; hypo- or hypertonic pelvic floor conditions, with tender and trigger point evaluation; diagnosis of inflammation and infection, with culture examinations when indicated; and the pain-map accurate description (Graziottin et al 2001c) because location of pain and its onset characteristics are the strongest predictors of its biological aetiology (Meana et al 1997).

This is mandatory when genital arousal disorders, sexual pain disorders (vaginismus and dyspareunia) and orgasm disorders are complained of. It may be useful even when sexual desire disorders and/or subjective sexual arousal disorders ('I do not feel mentally excited') are the leading complaints to diagnose biologically rooted comorbidities with other FSD. Comorbidity should be accurately recorded with attention to which sexual disorder came first. On the positive side, the cascade of positive feedback when a treatment is effective may cause a significant improvement in all domains of sexual response as several studies have proven (Alexander et al 2004, Graziottin & Basson 2004, Laan et al 2001, Shifren et al 2000, Simunic et al 2003).

In stable couples, current feelings for the partner (i.e. quality of the relationship, and the quality of the partner's sexuality [inclusive of general and sexual health]) should be investigated as well (Dennerstein et al 1999, 2003, 2007, Klausmann 2002).

The woman's general health should be examined, with special focus on conditions that may directly or indirectly impair the woman's mental and/or genital response (Basson et al 2000, 2004, Graziottin 2000, 2003a, 2004a,b).

PRINCIPLES OF FSD THERAPY

A growing body of evidence implicates hormonal factors in the genesis of FSD (Alexander et al 2004, Graziottin & Basson 2004, Laan et al 2001, Sarrel 1998, Shifren et al 2000, Simunic et al 2003,). Indeed, during a woman's entire reproductive life span, sex hormones exert both organizational and activational effects on sexual behaviour. The action of hormones is mediated by non-genomic and genomic pathways. Current evidence indicates that there is a specific place in the treatment of FSD for pharmacological hormones, for the most part in postmenopausal women (Alexander et al 2004,

Graziottin & Basson 2004, Laan et al 2001, Sarrel 1998, Shifren et al 2000, Simunic et al 2003). Sexual hormones may be delivered by various routes: oral, transdermal, nasal, vaginal, through subcutaneous implants or intrauterine devices. The most important difference between the oral route and those that bypass the first hepatic pass is that the oral treatment induces an increase of sex hormone-binding globulin (SHBG) by as much as 133%, thus significantly reducing free testosterone (Vehkavaara et al 2000). Levels of SHBG seem to be unaffected by hormones delivered via transdermal, nasal, and vaginal routes.

Depending on the aetiological diagnosis of the leading disorder, the therapy should consider one or more of the following leading options.

Libido disorder

Libido and subjective sexual arousal disorder ('I do not feel mentally excited'), often diagnosed in comorbidity, either lifelong or, more frequently, acquired, may benefit from the following.

Medical treatment

Hormones
Androgen The major androgens in women include testosterone (T) and dihydrotestosterone (DHT), dehydroepiandrosterone sulphate (DHEA-S), dehydroepiandrosterone (DHEA), and androstenedione (A) (Bachmann et al 2002). T is the most potent androgen. Plasma T levels range from 0.2 to 0.7 ng/mL (0.6–2.5 nmol/L), with significant fluctuations related to the phase of the menstrual cycle. T is converted to DHT, but can also be aromatized to estradiol (E_2) in target tissues; DHT is the principal ligand to androgen receptors in women as well. Androgens peak in the early 20s, then decline steadily (Burger et al 2000).

T in premenopausal women: evidence concerning the role of hormones, particularly T, in premenopausal women is limited. Very few studies have been done in premenopausal subjects. Goldstat et al (2003) focused their controlled study on a small group of premenopausal women; subjects with lifelong hypoactive sexual desire disorder with T levels in the lower one-third or less of the normal range may significantly benefit from T cream when compared to placebo.

T in postmenopausal women: menopause can be natural or iatrogenic. Iatrogenic menopause may result from surgery, chemotherapy, or radiation therapy. The most common surgical cause of menopause is bilateral oophorectomy, which leads to a sudden 50% fall in circulating T levels (Bachmann et al 2002). Plasma T values

at or below the lowest quartile of the normal range for women in their reproductive years also suggest a diagnosis of androgen insufficiency syndrome. A recent, systematic review of all available data from randomized and placebo-controlled trials of treatment for FSD in postmenopausal women concluded that use of many frequently used treatments is not supported by adequate evidence (Madelska & Cummings 2003). In their review of randomized, controlled trials involving the use of T in oestrogen-replete women, Alexander et al (2004) found general support for the positive effect of T on different dimensions of women's sexuality. One limit of this analysis is that some of the reviewed studies involved supraphysiological doses. In a study by Shifren et al (2000), the total T was raised above the normal range, but the free and bioavailable T remained within the normal range. Sherwin (2002) and more recently Alexander et al (2004) in their reviews of randomized, controlled trials, found that adding androgens to the standard oestrogen replacement had added sexual benefit in different domains, sexual desire first.

Ostrogens and progestogens In naturally postmenopausal women, progesterone or progestogens protect the endometrium. The positive effect of oestrogens on the well-being and sexuality of postmenopausal women may be variably modulated according to the type of progestogens added in the hormonal replacement therapy (Graziottin & Leiblum 2005). Progesterone, the physiological hormone, may have a mildly inhibiting effect on sexual desire. Progestogens, synthetic molecules with progestinic action, have a wide spectrum of actions from strongly antiandrogenic to neutral to androgenic, according to:

- their structure (whether they are derived from 17-OH-progesterone, 19-nortestosterone or 17-alpha-spironolactone) and their consequent varying pattern of interaction with different hormonal receptors (Graziottin & Leiblum 2005, Schindler 1999, Stanczyk 2002) – progestogens may interact with progestinic, oestrogenic, androgenic, glucocorticoid, and mineralcorticoid receptors, so the consequent metabolic and sexual profile differs;

- their variable binding affinity to SHBG, which modulates the quantity of free T available for its biological action;

- the variable inhibition of the type 2,5-alpha-reductase, which activates T into DHT.

To assimilate progestogens in a unique category focusing on a generalized 'class effect' is wrong and may lead to inappropriate conclusions (Graziottin &

Leiblum 2005). The progestogen with the most favourable effect on sexual function in hormonal replacement therapy is norethisterone, with a positive impact on desire, arousal, orgasm, and satisfaction in natural postmenopausal women with an intact uterus. Controlled head-to-head studies are necessary to evaluate the correlation between the pharmacological profile and the clinical effect.

Tibolone Tibolone is a 19-nortestosterone derivate with mild oestrogenic, progestinic and androgenic activity. It lowers SHBG, thus increasing free E_2, T, and DHEA-S levels. It is not available in the USA, but is widely used in Europe. In randomized studies comparing it with placebo, tibolone (2.5 mg/day) alleviated vaginal dryness and dyspareunia, increasing libido, arousal, and sexual satisfaction in postmenopausal women with natural or surgical menopause (Laan et al 2001, Madelska & Cummings 2002).

DHEA-S Studies conducted in elderly women have shown a positive effect of DHEA-S on mental well-being and on motivational aspects of sexuality with a mild relief of climacteric symptoms (Labrie et al 2001, Stomati et al 2000).

Hypoprolactinaemic drugs Prolactin is the most powerful inhibiting hormone when sexual desire is considered, with increasing inhibiting effect with increasing plasma levels. Hypoprolactinaemic drugs are useful to improve sexual desire when the prolactin level is supraphysiological.

Antidepressants Affective disorders, namely depression and anxiety, when associated with sexual desire disorders should be addressed with a mixed approach, both pharmacological and psychodynamic (Alexander & Kotz 2004). Among antidepressants, bupropion seems to have the most positive effect on sexual desire (Clayton et al 2004, Seagraves & Balon 2003). Comorbidity between low testosterone and depression should be considered and appropriately treated.

Pelvic floor rehabilitation A few physicians and medical sexologists recommend careful physical examination of the woman complaining of low desire on the wrong assumption that the disorder is either 'all psychogenic and/or couple dependent' or at best 'hormone-dependent'. Low desire can result from negative feedback from disappointing arousal, coital pain, coital anorgasmia, dissatisfaction (see Fig. 9.26, p. 267). Indeed, low desire may be concomitant to sexual aversion disorders associated with vaginismus (with a variable hyperactivity of the pelvic floor) (Graziottin et al 2004a)

or secondary to sexual pain disorders such as dyspareunia associated with vulvar vestibulitis (Graziottin et al 2001b), in which defensive contraction of levator ani is common (Bergeron et al 2001, Glazer et al 1995, Graziottin et al 2004b, McKay et al 2001).

Antalgic treatment When loss of desire is acquired and secondary to persistent chronic coital pain, antalgic treatment aimed at reducing or eliminating pain (especially if neuropathic) is preliminary to effective normalization of sexual desire (Vincenti & Graziottin 2004).

Psychosexual treatment

Individual psychosexual or behavioural therapy Individual psychosexual or behavioural therapy is the approach of choice if the FSD aetiology includes sexual inhibitions, poor erotic skills, poor body image, low self-confidence or previous abuse (Leiblum & Rosen 2000, Rellini & Meston 2004).

Couple therapy Couple therapy is used when symbiotic dynamics with poor differentiation according to Schnarch (2000) or conflicts and/or destructive dynamics are reported.

Referral

The multisystemic and multifactorial aetiology of FSD requires a professional multidisciplinary team. Appropriate referral is a key part of successful treatment (Box 9.8) (Plaut et al 2004). For example, referral of the partner to the uroandrologist should be recommended when male disorders (premature ejaculation, erectile deficit, libido disorders) emerge as critical co-factors in the aetiology of FSD (i.e. if the partner appears to be the 'symptom inducer' and the woman is the 'symptom carrier' [Kaplan 1979, Plaut et al 2004]).

Acquired libido disorder should be treated on the basis of the leading aetiological factor, especially if it is comorbid with other lifelong or acquired FSD, such as pain disorder, arousal disorder or orgasm disorder (Graziottin et al 2001b), or biological factors such as iatrogenic menopause (Graziottin & Basson 2004).

Arousal disorders

Subjective sexual arousal disorders, either lifelong or acquired, usually in comorbidity with sexual desire disorders, should be treated as mentioned above. Postmenopausal mixed genital and subjective arousal disorders may benefit from systemic hormonal replacement therapy, especially androgens (see above) (Alexander et al 2004, Traish et al 2002).

Box 9.8: Referral resources. Modified from Plaut et al 2004, with permission

- Medical sexologist or gynaecologist trained in sexual medicine: FSD requires appropriate medical diagnosis and treatment
- Urologist or andrologist: when the partner has erectile or ejaculatory dysfunction that requires medical intervention
- Family physician trained in sexual medicine: for sexual dysfunctions in either partner
- Oncologist: when hormonal treatment is considered for patients who have had cancer
- Psychiatrist: when depression and anxiety are associated with FSD
- Sex therapist: to carry out the psychosexual therapy
- Couple therapist: when relationship issues are a primary contributor to the sexual dysfunction
- Individual psychotherapist: when personal psychodynamic issues are inhibiting sexual function
- Physical therapist: when hyper- or hypotonicity of pelvic floor is contributory

Isolated acquired genital arousal disorders may benefit from the following.

Medical treatment

Topical oestrogens   A number of studies suggest that topical vaginal oestrogens may significantly reduce vaginal dryness, increase genital arousal, and reduce dyspareunia (Dessole et al 2004, Rioux et al 2000, Simunic et al 2003). A multicentre, double-blind, randomized, placebo-controlled study (n = 1612 postmenopausal women with urogenital and sexual complaints) indicates that 25 μg of estradiol applied vaginally twice a week for a year may significantly improve six vaginal symptoms and signs: vaginal dryness ($p < 0.0001$), itching/burning ($p < 0.0001$), recurrent vaginitis ($p < 0.0001$), petechiae ($p < 0.0002$), dyspareunia ($p < 0.0001$), and vaginal atrophy ($p < 0.0001$), and five bladder symptoms and signs: dysuria ($p < 0.003$), frequency/nocturia ($p < 0.001$), urinary tract infection ($p < 0.034$), urinary incontinence, urge mostly ($p < 0.002$), and urinary atrophy ($p < 0.001$) (Simunic et al 2003). Furthermore, cystometry performed at baseline and after 12 months indicates that the maximal cystometric capacity increases from 200 mL to 290 mL ($p < 0.023$); the bladder volume at first urgency increases from 140 mL to 180 mL ($p < 0.048$); and bladder volume at strong urgency increases from 130 mL to 170 mL ($p < 0.045$). The comorbidity between urogenital and sexual symptoms in postmenopausal women may therefore be effectively addressed with a topical vaginal treatment that is easy to use and safe both for the endometrium and the breast.

Topical   testosterone   Testosterone propionate powder 1% or 2% in vaseline jelly applied in minimal daily quantity to the clitoris and the vulvar region may improve genital arousal in the external genitalia (Notelovitz 2002). Controlled studies, however, are lacking.

Vasoactive drugs   Evidence on the effectiveness of vasoactive drugs (sildenafil, vardenafil, tadalafil) in addressing genital arousal disorders in women is negative or at best controversial, with one exception (Berman et al 2003). The frequent comorbidity with desire disorders, the frequent couple issues, the difficulty in diagnosing a 'pure' genital arousal disorder and the lack of a personal motivation for a pharmacological treatment of genital arousal disorder may explain the substantial lack of efficacy in comparison to men's genital arousal disorders (i.e. erectile deficit of vascular aetiology).

Clitoral vacuum device   Clitoral vacuum device is the only FDA-approved treatment for genital arousal disorders with a vascular and/or neurogenic aetiology (Wilson et al 2001). It may be useful in women treated for invasive carcinoma of the cervix who have undergone surgery and pelvic radiotherapy.

Pelvic floor rehabilitation   Genital arousal disorders may be secondary to coital pain: unwanted pain is the strongest reflex inhibitor of vaginal congestion and lubrication. Diagnosing and treating the muscular component of coital pain (both in vaginismus and dyspareunia) is a key part of the medical treatment (Bergeron et al 2001, Glazer et al 1995, Graziottin 2004d, McKay et al 2001) and is preliminary to resuming a normal vasocongestive response (Graziottin & Brotto 2004).

Psychosexual treatment

Indications for psychosexual treatment of subjective sexual arousal disorders overlap with those for desire disorders. Co-treatment may therefore effectively address comorbidity. However, treatment of the potential parallel biological aetiology of the genital arousal disorder is mandatory if cure for the reported FSD is to be achieved (Plaut et al 2004). Couple psychotherapy should be proposed when relational dynamics are contributing to maintenance of the sexual problem (Clulow 2001, Leiblum & Rosen 2000).

Orgasm disorders

Orgasm disorders have a prevalent psychogenic aetiology in young women (Mah & Binik 2004). Biological factors – age, menopause-related loss of sexual hormones, pelvic floor disorders, iatrogenic issues (such as antidepressant serotoninergic drugs inhibiting orgasm), and comorbidities (mainly with stress and urge incontinence) – become increasingly important with increasing age (Graziottin 2004a). According to the aetiologic diagnosis, the main therapeutic options include the following.

Medical treatment

Systemic and/or topical hormonal replacement therapy Systemic and/or topical hormonal replacement therapy is discussed above. Testosterone has a special role in the treatment of orgasmic disorders associated with loss of sexual hormones, especially after bilateral oophorectomy (Alexander et al 2004, Sherwin 2002, Shifren et al 2000). It behaves as 'initiator' in the brain and as 'modulator' in the cavernosal bodies, where it works as 'permitting factor' for nitric oxide (NO), in women as well as in men (Graziottin 2004d).

Change of pharmacological treatment inhibiting orgasm (e.g. antidepressants such as selective serotonin reuptake inhibitor [SSRI] or tricyclics) should be considered when feasible from the medical point of view if orgasm inhibition is reported as a side-effect. Bupropion seems to be a better choice (Clayton et al 2004, Segraves & Balon 2003).

Pelvic floor rehabilitation Pelvic floor rehabilitation is of the highest importance for hypotonic conditions of the pelvic floor, as pioneered by Kegel (1952), after delivery (Baessler & Schuessler 2004, Glazener 1997); even more so when incontinence is a strong inhibiting orgasmic factor. Fear of leaking during thrusting in stress incontinence and at orgasm in urge incontinence is an often under-reported and yet powerful disruptor of orgasm potential. Orgasm inhibition may also be secondary to coital pain (Graziottin et al 2001b). Again, accurate diagnosis of comorbidity and appropriate co-treatment with relaxation of the pelvic floor in this latter case is key.

Psychosexual treatment

Individual psychosexual or behavioural therapy Lifelong 'isolated' orgasmic disorders may benefit from a behavioural educational treatment, encouraging self-knowledge and eroticism with the experience of higher arousal sensations, use of vibrators or of a clitoral device up to orgasm (Meston et al 2004). More often, however, the orgasmic disorder is associated with poor arousal with or without performance anxiety. These conditions should therefore be treated together (Leiblum & Rosen 2000).

Couple therapy Lifelong orgasm difficulties may need a couple therapy when sexual inhibitions, poor erotic skills and/or low self-confidence are shared by the couple (Meston et al 2004).

Appropriate behavioural and pharmacological treatment of premature ejaculation should be proposed to the partner when it causes inadequate coital stimulation and increasing erotic dissatisfaction in the female partner.

If all of the sexual response is impaired, with significant comorbidity with desire and arousal disorders, accurate treatment of predisposing, precipitating and maintenance factors, biological, psychosexual and/or contextual, should be proposed (Plaut et al 2004).

Sexual pain disorders

Dyspareunia and vaginismus because of coital pain directly inhibit genital arousal and vaginal receptivity. Indirectly, they may affect orgasm potential, the physical and emotional satisfaction, causing loss of desire up to avoidance of sexual intimacy. Dyspareunia may have many biological aetiologies: the leading cause of coital pain in premenopausal women is vulvar vestibulitis, whereas postmenopausally it is vaginal dryness.

Dyspareunia may benefit from the following (Box 9.9).

Medical treatment

Multimodal therapy Vulvar vestibulitis should be treated with a combined treatment aimed at reducing:

- upregulation of mast cells, both by reducing the agonist stimuli (such as candida infections, microabrasions of the introital mucosa because of intercourse with a dry vagina and/or a contracted pelvic floor, chemicals, allergens etc) that cause degranulation leading to chronic tissue inflammation, and/or with antagonist modulation of its hyper-reactivity, with amitriptyline or aliamides gel (Graziottin & Brotto 2004, Graziottin et al 2004b);

- upregulation of the pain system secondary to proliferation of introital pain fibres (Bohm-Starke et al 1999, 2001a,b, Bornstein et al 2002, 2004) induced by nerve

Box 9.9: Treatment of the medical causes of dyspareunia

INFLAMMATORY AETIOLOGY (UPREGULATION OF MAST CELLS)

Pharmacological modulation of mast cell hyper-reactivity
- Antidepressants: amitriptyline
- Aliamides topical gel

Reduction of agonist factors causing mast cell hyper-reactivity
- Recurrent candida or *Gardnerella vaginitis*
- Microabrasions of the introital mucosa
  - from intercourse with a dry vagina
  - from inappropriate lifestyles
- Allergens/chemical irritants
- Physical agents
- Neurogenic stimuli

MUSCULAR AETIOLOGY (UPREGULATION OF THE MUSCULAR SYSTEM)
- Self-massage and levator ani stretching
- Physical therapy of the levator ani
- Electromyographic biofeed-back
- Type A botulinum toxin

NEUROLOGICAL AETIOLOGY (UPREGULATION OF THE PAIN SYSTEM)

Systemic analgesia
- Amitriptyline
- Gabapentin
- Pregabalin

Local analgesia
- Electroanalgesia
- Ganglion impar block

Surgical therapy
- Vestibulectomy

HORMONAL AETIOLOGY

Hormonal therapy
- Local:
  - vaginal oestrogens
  - testosterone for the vulva
- Systemic:
  - hormonal replacement therapies

*Aliamides is a class of endogenous molecules with an anti-inflammatory activity. The most important is the palmitoiletanolamide, belonging to the class of fatty acid amides, chemically known as N-(2-idrossietil)-esadecanamide. They work through the down-regulation of the hyperactive mast cells. In Italy they are available in the form of vaginal gel and now of pills. They constitute an innovative approach to the vaginal and bladder chronic inflammation, secondary to mast cells' upregulation.

growth factor produced by the upregulated mast cells, and the lowered central pain threshold (Pukall et al 2006) – a thorough understanding of the pathophysiology of pain in its nociceptive and neuropathic component, is mandatory – antalgic treatment should be prescribed: locally, with electroanalgesia (Nappi et al 2003) or, in severe cases, with the ganglion impar block; systemically with tricyclic antidepressant or gabapentin in the most severe cases (Graziottin & Brotto 2004, Vincenti & Graziottin 2004).

- upregulation of the muscular response, with hyperactvity of the pelvic floor (Graziottin et al 2004a), which may precede vulvar vestibulitis when the predisposing factor is vaginismus (Abramov et al 1994, Graziottin et al 2001b) or be acquired in response to genital pain (Graziottin et al 2004a,b) – in controlled studies, electromyographic feedback (Bergeron et al 2001, Glazer et al 1995, McKay et al 2001) has proven to significantly reduce pain of vulvar vestibulitis; self massage, pelvic floor stretching and physical therapy may also reduce the muscular component of coital pain (Graziottin 2004a, Graziottin & Brotto 2004), but high-quality randomized controlled trials are needed to determine the true effect of such interventions; for hyperactivity of the pelvic floor, treatment with type A botulinum toxin has been proposed (Bertolasi 2004, personal communication) – individually tailored combinations of this approach are useful for treating introital dyspareunia with different aetiologies from vulvar vestibulitis.

Deep dyspareunia, secondary to endometriosis, pelvic inflammatory disease (PID), chronic pelvic pain and other less frequent aetiologies requires specialistic treatment that goes beyond the scope of this chapter.

Topical hormones Vaginal oestrogen treatment is mandatory when vaginal dryness is causing postmenopausal dyspareunia, either spontaneous or iatrogenic

(Graziottin 2001a,b, 2004a, Simunic et al 2003). Vulvar treatment with testosterone may be considered when vulvar dystrophy and/or lichen sclerosus contribute to introital dyspareunia.

Psychosexual treatment

Psychosexual and/or behavioural therapy   Psychosexual and/or behavioural therapy is the leading treatment of lifelong vaginismus (Leiblum 2000). It should be offered in parallel with progressive rehabilitation of the pelvic floor and pharmacological treatment to modulate the intense systemic arousal in the subset of intensely phobic patients (Plaut et al 2004). In this latter group, comorbidity with sexual aversion disorder should be investigated and treated first.

Psychosexual and/or behavioural therapy contributes to the multimodal treatment of lifelong dyspareunia, which is reported in one-third of our patients (Graziottin et al 2001b). Anxiety, fear of pain and sexual avoidant behaviours should be addressed as well. The shift from pain to pleasure is key from the sexual point of view. Sensitive and committed psychosexual support to the woman and the couple is mandatory.

WHEN THE PHYSICAL THERAPIST COUNTS

Pelvic floor muscles are critically involved in the physiology and pathophysiology of women's sexual response. The physical therapist should be part of the multidisciplinary team involved in the centre of sexual medicine. He or she should diagnose and address the following.

Hyperactivity/hypertonus of the pelvic floor

The physical therapist should diagnose and address:

- primary pelvic floor hyperactivity in children and adolescents, thus preventing one of the most neglected predisposing factors to dyspareunia and vulvar vestibulitis (Chiozza & Graziottin 2004, Graziottin 2005a, Harlow et al 2001);

- acquired hyperactivity with levator ani myalgia by overexertion (i.e. 'Kegel dyspareunia'; DeLancey et al 1993);

- lifelong hyperactivity of the pelvic floor in vaginismus and lifelong or acquired hyperactivity in dyspareunia of any aetiology (Graziottin 2003a);

- levator ani tender and/or trigger points with referred pain (Alvarez & Rockwell 2002, Travell & Simons 1983);

- levator ani hyperactivity associated with recurrent cystitis, urge incontinence and dyspareunia (Graziottin 2004a);

- systemic postural problems in chronic pelvic pain, dyspareunia and vaginismus;

- chronic pelvic pain and chronic coital pain-associated myalgias and pertinent antalgic treatment (Bourcier et al 2004).

Hypoactivity/hypotonus of the pelvic floor

The physical therapist should diagnose and address:

- pelvic floor damage after delivery;
- hypotonicity worsening after the menopause;
- pelvic floor hypotonus in comorbidity with urogenital and/or proctological disorders (Bourcier et al 2004, Wesselmann et al 1997);

The physical therapist may also help the patient to increase awareness of the levator ani role in sexual receptivity and vaginal sensitivity to increase the woman's and her partner's coital pleasure.

CONCLUSIONS

The complexity of FSD requires a dedicated diagnostic and therapeutic team, sharing a common pathophysiological and psychodynamic cultural scenario with the aim of offering the most integrated understanding of the meaning of the symptoms and the most effective comprehensive treatment.

Pelvic floor muscles are critically involved in the physiology and pathophysiology of a women's sexual response. Physical therapists may therefore greatly contribute to improving women's sexual health. They deserve appreciation and an increasing role in the multimodal treatment of FSD. There is, however, an urgent need for high-quality randomized controlled trials to evaluate the effect of different physical therapy interventions for FSD. A collaboration between physical therapists and sexologists/gynaecologists in future research projects in this important field is highly recommended.

REFERENCES

Abramov L, Wolman I, David M P 1994 Vaginismus: an important factor in the evaluation and management of vulvar vestibulitis syndrome. Gynecological and Obstetrical Investigations 38:194–197

Alexander Leventhal J, Kotz K 2004 Depression, antidepressants and female sexual dysfunction in women: clinical approach In: Graziottin A (ed) Female sexual dysfunction: clinical approach. Urodinamica 14(2):76–79. Online.available at http://www.alessandragraziottin.it

Alexander Leventhal J, Kotz K, Dennerstein L et al 2004 The effects of menopausal hormone therapies on female sexual functioning: Review of double–blind randomized controlled trials. Menopause 11(6 Pt 2):749–765

Alvarez D J, Rockwell PG 2002 Trigger points: diagnosis and management. American Family Physician 65(4):653–660

Bachmann G, Bancroft J, Braunstein G et al 2002 FAI: the Princeton consensus statement on definition, classification and assessment. Fertility and Sterility 77:660–665

Baessler K, Schuessler B 2004 Pregnancy, childbirth and pelvic floor damage. In: Bourcier A, McGuire E, Abrams P (eds) Pelvic Floor Disorders. Elsevier Saunders, Philadelphia, p 33–42

Bancroft J, Loftus J, Long J S 2003 Distress about sex: A national survey of women in heterosexual relationships. Archives of Sexual Behaviour 32(3):193–204

Basson R, Berman J, Burnett A et al 2000 Report of the International Consensus Development Conference on female sexual dysfunction: definition and classification. The Journal of Urology 163:889–893

Basson R, Leiblum S, Brotto L et al 2004 Revised definitions of women's sexual dysfunction. Journal of Sexual Medicine 1(1):40–48

Bergeron S, Khalife S, Pagidas K et al 2001 A randomized comparison of group cognitive-behavioural therapy surface electromyographic biofeedback and vestibulectomy in the treatment of dyspareunia resulting from VVS. Pain 91:297–306

Berman J R, Berman L A, Toler S M et al 2003 Safety and efficacy of sildenafil citrate for the treatment of female sexual arousal disorder: a double-blind, placebo controlled study. The Journal of Urology 170:2333–2338

Bohm-Starke N, Hilliges M, Blomgren B et al 2001a Increased blood flow and erythema in posterior vestibular mucosa in vulvar vestibulitis. American Journal of Obstetrics and Gynecology 98:1067–1074

Bohm-Starke N, Hilliges M, Brodda-Jansen G et al 2001b Psychophysical evidence of nociceptor sensitization in vulvar vestibulitis Syndrome. Pain 94:177–183

Bohm-Starke N, Hilliges M, Falconer C et al 1999 Neurochemical characterization of the vestibular nerves in women with vulvar vestibulitis syndrome. Gynecologic and Obstetric Investigation 48:270–275

Bornstein J, Goldschmid N, Sabo E 2004 Hyperinnervation and mast cell activation may be used as a histopathologic diagnostic criteria for vulvar vestibulitis. Gynecologic Obstetric Investigation 58:171–178

Bornstein J, Sabo E, Goldschmid N 2002 A mathematical model for the histopathologic diagnosis of vulvar vestibulitis based on a histomorphometric study of innervation and mast cell activation. Journal of Reproductive Medicine 9:742

Bourcier A, McGuire E, Abrams P 2004 Pelvic floor disorders. Elsevier Saunders, Philadelphia

Burger H G, Dudley E C, Cui J et al 2000 A prospective longitudinal study of serum testosterone dehydroepiandrosterone sulfate, and sex hormone-binding globulin levels through the menopause transition. The Journal of Clinical Endocrinology and Metabolism 85:2832–2838

Chiozza M L, Graziottin A 2004 Urge incontinence and female sexual dysfunction: a life span perspective. In: Graziottin A (ed) Female sexual dysfunction: clinical approach. Urodinamica14(2):133–138. Online. Available: http://www.alessandragraziottin.it

Clayton A H, Warnock J K, Kornstein S G et al 2004 A placebo-controlled trial of bupropion SR as an antidote for selective serotonin reuptake inhibitor-induced sexual dysfunction. The Journal of Clinical Psychiatry 65:62–67

Clulow C (ed) 2001 Adult attachment and couple psychotherapy. Brunner–Routledge, Hove, UK

DeLancey J O, Sampselle C M, Punch M R 1993 Kegel dyspareunia: levator ani myalgia caused by overexertion. Obstetrics and Gynecology 82:658–659

Dennerstein L, Alexander J, Kotz K 2003 The menopause and sexual functioning: A review of population-based studies. Annual Review of Sex Research 14:64–82

Dennerstein L, Alexander J, Kotz K 2003 The menopause and sexual functioning: A review of population-based studies. Annual Review of Sex Research 14:64–82

Dennerstein L, Lehert P, Koochaki P E et al 2007 Factors associated with women's health experiences: a cross-cultural comparison of women aged 20–70 years. Menopause 14(4) (In press)

Dennerstein L, Lehert P, Burger H et al 1999 Factors affecting sexual functioning of women in the midlife years. Climacteric 2:254–262

Dessole S, Rubattu G, Ambrosini G et al 2004 Efficacy of low-dose intravaginal estriol on urogenital aging in postmenopausal women. Menopause 11(1):49–56

Glazener C M A 1997 Sexual function after childbirth: women's experiences, persistent morbidity and lack of professional recognition. British Journal of Obstetrics and Gynaecology 104: 330–335

Glazer H I, Rodke G, Swencionis C et al 1995 Treatment of vulvar vestibulitis syndrome with electromyographic feedback of pelvic floor musculature. The Journal of Reproductive Medicine 40:283–290

Goldstat R, Briganti E, Tran J et al 2003 Transdermal testosterone therapy improves well-being, mood, and sexual function in premenopausal women. Menopause 10:390–398

Graziottin A 2000 Libido: the biologic scenario. Maturitas 34(suppl 1)S9–S16

Graziottin A 2001a Clinical approach to dyspareunia. Journal of Sex and Marital Therapy 27:489–501

Graziottin A 2001b Sexual function in women with gynecologic cancer: a review. Italian Journal of Gynecology and Obstetrics 2:61–68

Graziottin A 2003a Etiology and diagnosis of coital pain. Journal of Endocrinological Investigation 26(3):115–121

Graziottin A 2003b The challenge of sexual medicine for women: overcoming cultural and educational limits and gender biases. Journal of Endocrinological Investigation 26(3):139–142

Graziottin A 2004a Sexuality in postmenopause and senium. In: Lauritzen C, Studd J (eds) Current management of the menopause. Martin Duniz, London, p 185–203

Graziottin A (ed) 2004b Female sexual dysfunction: clinical approach. Urodinamica 14 (2):57–138 Online.Available: http://www.alessandragraziottin.it

Graziottin A 2004c Women's right to a better sexual life. In: Graziottin A (ed) Female sexual dysfunction: clinical approach. Urodinamica 14(2):57–60 Online. Available: http://www.alessandragraziottin.it

Graziottin A 2004d Sexual arousal: similarities and differences between men and women. The Journal of Men's Health & Gender 1(2–3):215–223

Graziottin A 2004e Sexual pain disorders: clinical approach. In: Graziottin A (ed) Female sexual dysfunction: clinical approach. Urodinamica 14(2):105–111 Online. Available: http://www.alessandragraziottin.it

Graziottin A 2005a Sexual pain disorders in adolescents. Proceedings of the 12th World Congress of Human Reproduction, International Academy of Human Reproduction, Venice, 10–13. In: Genazzani A (ed) CIC Edizioni Internazionali, Roma, p 434–449

Graziottin A 2005b Why deny dyspareunia its sexual meaning? Archives of Sexual Behaviour 34(1):32–34

Graziottin A 2006 Breast cancer and its effects on women's self-image and sexual function. In: Goldstein I, Meston C, Davis S, Traish A (eds) Women's Sexual Function and Dysfunction: Study, Diagnosis and Treatment. Taylor and Francis, UK, p 276–281

Graziottin A, Basson R 2004 Sexual dysfunctions in women with Premature Menopause. Menopause 11(6):766–777

Graziottin A, Bottanelli M, Bertolasi L 2004a Vaginismus: a clinical and neurophysiological study. In: Graziottin A (ed) Female sexual dysfunction: clinical approach. Urodinamica 14:117–121 Online. Available: http://www.alessandragraziottin.it

Graziottin A, Brotto L 2004 Vulvare Vestibulitis Syndrome: clinical approach. Journal of Sex and Marital Therapy 30:124–139

Graziottin A, Giovannini N, Bertolasi L et al 2004b Vulvar vestibulitis: pathophysiology and management. Current Sexual Health Report 1:151–156

Graziottin A, Leiblum S R 2005 Biological and psychosocial pathophysiology of female sexual dysfunction during the menopausal transition. Journal of Sexual Medicine 2(suppl 3):133–145

Graziottin A, Nicolosi A E, Caliari I 2001a Vulvar vestibulitis and dyspareunia: addressing the biological etiologic complexity. Poster presented at the international meeting of the Female Sexual Function Forum, Boston, MA

Graziottin A, Nicolosi A E, Caliari I 2001b Vulvar vestibulitis and dyspareunia: Addressing the psychosexual etiologic complexity. Poster presented at the International meeting of the Female Sexual Function Forum, Boston, MA

Graziottin A, Nicolosi A E, Caliari I 2001c Vulvar vestibulitis and dyspareunia: The 'pain map' and the medical diagnosis. Poster presented at the international meeting of the Female Sexual Function Forum, Boston, MA

Harlow B L, Wise L A, Stewart E G 2001 Prevalence and predictors of chronic lower genital tract discomfort. American Journal of Obstetrics and Gynecology 185:545–550

In: Graziottin A (ed) Female sexual dysfunction: a clinical approach. Urodinamica 19(2):112–116. Online. Available: http://www.alessandragraziottin.it

Kaplan H S 1979 Disorders of sexual desire. Simon and Schuster, New York

Kegel A H 1952 Stress incontinence and genital relaxation: a non-surgical method of increasing the tone of sphincters and their supporting structures. Clinical Symposia 4(2):35–51

Klausmann D 2002 Sexual motivation and the duration of the relationship. Archives of Sexual Behaviour 31:275–287

Laan E, Everaerd W 1995 Determinants of female sexual arousal: psychophysiological theory and data. Annual Review of Sex Research 6:32–76

Laan E, van Lunsen R H W, Everaerd H 2001 The effect of tibolone on vaginal blood flow, sexual desire and arousability in postmenopausal women. Climacteric 4:28–41

Labrie F, Luu-The V, Labrie C et al 2001 DHEA and its transformation into androgens and estrogens in peripheral target tissues: intracrinology. Frontiers in Neuroendocrinology 22(3):185–212

Lauman E O, Gagnon J H, Michaci R T et al 1999 Sexual dysfunction in the United States: prevalence and predictors. JAMA 10;281(6):537–542

Leiblum S R 2000 Vaginismus: a most perplexing problem. In: Leiblum S R, Rosen R C (eds) Principles and practice of sex therapy, 3rd edn. Guilford, New York, p 181–202

Leiblum S R 2004 Sexual arousal problems in women: a clinical perspective. In: Graziottin A (ed) Female Sexual Dysfunction: a clinical approach. Urodinamica 19(2):89–93. Online. Available: http://www.alessandragraziottin.it

Leiblum S R, Rosen R C (eds) 2000 Principles and Practice of Sex Therapy, 3rd edn. Guilford, New York, p 181–202

Liu C 2003 Does quality of marital sex decline with duration? Archives of Sexual Behavior 32(1):55–60

Madelska K, Cummings S 2002 Tibolone for post-menopausal women: systematic review of randomized trials The Journal of Clinical Endocrinological and Metabolism 87(1):16–23

Madelska K, Cummings S 2003 Female sexual dysfunction in postmenopausal women: systematic review of placebo-controlled trials. American Journal of Obstetric and Gynecology 188:286–293

Mah K, Binik I M 2004 Female orgasm disorders: a clinical approach. In Graziottin A (ed) Female sexual dysfunction: a clinical approach. Urodinamica 19(2):99–104 Online. Available: http://www.alessandragraziottin.it

McKay E, Kaufman R, Doctor U et al 2001 Treating vulvar vestibulitis with electromyographic biofeedback of pelvic floor musculature. Journal of Reproductive Medicine 46:337–342

Meana M, Binik Y M, Khalife S et al 1997 Dyspareunia: sexual dysfunction or pain syndrome? Journal of Nervous Mental Diseases 185(9):561–569

Meston C M, Levin R J, Sipski M L, Hull E M, Heiman J R 2004 Women's orgasm. Annu Rev Sex Res 15:173–257. Review

Nappi R E, Federghini F, Abbiati L et al 2003 Electrical stimulation (ES) in the management of sexual pain disorders. Journal of Sex and Marital Therapy 29:103–110

Notelovitz M 2002 A practical approach to post-menopausal Hormone Therapy (ob/gyn, special edn), Mac Mahon, New York

Plaut M, Graziottin A, Heaton J 2004 Sexual dysfunction. Health Press, Abingdon, UK

Pukall C, Lahaie M A, Binik Y M 2006 Sexual pain disorders: etiologic factors. In: Goldstein I, Meston C M, Davis S, Traish A (eds) Women's Sexual function and dysfunction: study, diagnosis and treatment. Taylor and Francis, p 236–244

Rellini A, Meston C M 2004 Sexual abuse and female sexual disorders: clinical implications. In Graziottin A (ed) Female sexual dysfunction: a clinical approach. Urodinamica19(2):80–83. Online. Available: http://www.alessandragraziottin.it

Rioux J E, Devlin M C, Gelfand M M et al 2000 17 beta estradiol vaginal tablet versus conjiugated equine estrogen vaginal cream to relieve menopausal atrophic vaginitis. Menopause 7(3):156–161

Sarrel P M 1998 Ovarian hormones and vaginal blood flow using laser Doppler velocimetry to measure effects in a clinical trial of post–menopausal women. International Journal of Impotence Research 18:S91–S93

Schindler A E 1999 Role of progestins in the premenopausal climacteric. Gynecological Endocrinology 13(suppl 6):35–40

Schnarch D 2000 Desire problems: a systemic perspective. In: Leiblum S R, Rosen R C (eds) Principles and Practice of Sex Therapy, 3rd edn. Guilford, New York, p 17–56

Seagraves R T, Balon R 2003 Sexual pharmacology: fast facts. WW Norton & Company, New York

Sherwin B B 2002 Randomized clinical trials of combined estrogen–androgen preparations: effects on sexual functioning. Fertility and Sterility 77(Suppl 4):S49–S54

Shifren J L, Braunstein G D, Simon J A et al 2000 Transdermal testosterone treatment in women with impaired sexual function after oophorectomy. New England Journal of Medicine 343:682–688

Simunic V, Banovic I, Ciglar S et al 2003 Local estrogen treatment in patients with urogenital symptoms. International Journal of Gynaecology and Obstetrics 82:187–197

Stanzczyk F Z 2002 Pharmacokinetics and potency of progestins used for hormone replacement therapy and contraception. Reviews in Endocrine & Metabolic Disorders 3:211–224

Stomati M, Monteleone P, Casarosa E et al 2000 Six-month oral dehydroepiandrosterone suplementation in early and late postmenopause. Gynecological Endocrinology 14:342–363

Traish A M, Kim N, Min K et al 2002 Role of androgens in female genital sexual arousal: receptor expression, structure, and function. Fertility and Sterility 77(suppl 4):S11–S18

Travell J, Simons D 1983 Myofascial pain and dysfunction The trigger points manual, vol. 1. Williams & Wilkins, Baltimore, USA

Vehkavaara S, Hakala-Ala-Pietila T, Virkamaki A et al 2000 Differential effects of oral and transdermal estrogen replacement therapy on endothelial function in postmenopausal women. Circulation 102:2687–2693

Vincenti E, Graziottin A 2004 Neuropathic pain in vulvar vestibulitis: diagnosis and treatment.

Wesselmann U, Burnett A L, Heinberg L 1997 The urogenital and rectal pain syndromes. Pain 73(3):269–294

Wilson S K, Delk J R, Billups K L 2001 Treating symptoms of female sexual arousal disorder with the Eros clitoral therapy device. The Journal of Gender Specific Medicine 4(2):54–58

Male sexual dysfunction

Grace Dorey

INTRODUCTION

Sexual function in normal men is dependent on satisfactory libido, erectile function, ejaculation and orgasm. Sexual dysfunction occurs when there is a problem in any of these events. Sexual dysfunction embraces low libido, erectile dysfunction, premature ejaculation, retrograde ejaculation, retarded ejaculation, anorgasmia, anejaculation, and sexual pain.

LOW LIBIDO

Definition

A low libido can be defined as 'a reduced sexual urge'. As men age, there is a partial androgen decline.

Classification of different forms

Men can be classified as having low or absent libido.

Prevalence

The exact prevalence of men who have low libido remains unknown. It is estimated that at 40 years of age, there will be a 10% decline of total testosterone every decade, though the mechanisms are not fully understood (1st Latin American Erectile Dysfunction Consensus Meeting 2003a).

Aetiology

The cause of diminished libido is a result of ageing and a gradual decline in androgen production. The testis produces 95–98% of androgen with the adrenal glands producing the remaining 2–5% (1st Latin American Erectile Dysfunction Consensus Meeting 2003a).

ERECTILE DYSFUNCTION

Erectile dysfunction is a common condition linked to increasing age and age-related diseases. Men with erectile dysfunction suffer from depression and low self-esteem and experience difficulties establishing and maintaining relationships.

Definition

Erectile dysfunction is defined as 'the inability to achieve or maintain an erection sufficient for satisfactory sexual performance (for both partners)' (National Institutes of Health (NIH) Consensus Development Conference in 1993).

Classification of different forms

The severity of erectile dysfunction has been classified as mild, moderate or severe. Men who achieve satisfactory sexual performance 7–8 attempts out of 10 are classified as having mild erectile dysfunction, those who achieve 4–6 out of 10 are classified moderate, and those who achieve 0–3 out of 10 are classified severe (Albaugh & Lewis 1999).

Prevalence

The exact prevalence of erectile dysfunction is unknown. It is common and strongly age-related (Feldman et al 1994) affecting more than 20% of men under 40 years of age, more than 50% of men over 40 years of age, and more than 66% of men over 70 years of age (Feldman et al 1994, Heruti et al 2004). It may affect 10% of healthy men and significantly greater numbers of men with existing comorbidities such as hypertension (15%), diabetes mellitus (28%) and heart disease (39%) (Feldman et al 1994, Wagner et al 1996). The number of men with erectile dysfunction is predicted to rise with increased life expectancy and with a growing population of elderly people.

Aetiology

The causes of erectile dyfunction are listed in Table 9.15.

Anatomy of the penis

The internal structure of the penis consists of three cylindrical bodies: dorsally, the two corpora cavernosa communicate with each other for three-quarters of their length and ventrally the corpus spongiosum surrounds the penile portion of the urethra (Fig. 9.27). The proximal end of the corpus spongiosum forms a bulb attached to the urogenital diaphragm and at the distal end expands to form the glans penis (Kirby et al 1999). The tunica albuginea, which is composed of two layers of elastic and collagen fibres, surrounds the erectile bodies.

The erectile tissue in the corpora cavernosa and the corpus spongiosum is comprised of vascular lacunar spaces, which are surrounded by smooth muscle (Fig. 9.28). The lacunar spaces derive blood from the helicine arteries, which open directly into these sinusoids. Subtunical veins between the inner and outer tunica albuginea form a network, which drains blood from the erectile tissue.

Neurophysiology of penile erection

From a neurophysiological aspect, erection can be classified into three types (Brock & Lue 1993).

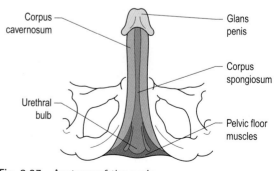

Fig. 9.27   Anatomy of the penis.

Table 9.15   Risk factors for erectile dysfunction

Risk factor	Possible components	Reference
Psychological	Marital conflict Depression Poor body image Performance related Bereavement	Feldman et al (1994)
Vascular	Arterial Venous	Feldman et al (1994)
Neurological	Spinal cord trauma Multiple sclerosis Spinal tumour Parkinson's disease	Feldman et al (1994)
Endocrinological	Hormonal deficiency	Feldman et al (1994)
Diabetic	Peripheral neuropathy Hypertension Renal failure	Benet & Melman (1995)
Drug-related	Some antihypertensives Some psychotropics Hormonal agents	Benet & Melman (1995)
Surgical trauma	Transurethral and radical prostatectomy Pelvic surgery Radiotherapy	Lewis & Mills (1999)
Lower urinary tract symptoms (LUTS)	Severity of LUTS, particularly incontinence	Frankel et al (1998)
Prostatic	Benign prostatic hyperplasia	Baniel et al (2000)
Lifestyle related	Trauma to the perineum Bicycling Nicotine abuse Drug abuse Alcohol abuse	Bortolotti et al (1997) Andersen & Bovim (1997) Rosen et al (1991) Lewis & Mills (1999) Fabra & Porst (1999)
Weak pelvic floor musculature	Weak pelvic floor muscles Ageing	Dorey et al (2004) Colpi et al (1999)

Reflexogenic erection Reflexogenic erection originates from tactile stimulation to the genitalia. Impulses reach the spinal erection centre via sacral sensory nerves (S2–S4) and thoracic nerves (T10–L2) and some follow the ascending tract culminating in sensory perception, whereas others activate the autonomic nuclei of the efferent nerves that induce the erection process.

Psychogenic erection Psychogenic erection originates from audiovisual stimuli or fantasy. Signals descend to the spinal erection centre to activate the erection process.

Nocturnal erection Nocturnal erection occurs mostly during the rapid eye movement stage of sleep. Most men experience three to five erections lasting up to 30 minutes in a normal night's sleep (Fisher et al 1965). Central impulses descend the spinal cord (through an unknown mechanism) to activate the erection process.

Pathophysiology of penile erection

Penile erection occurs following a series of integrated vascular processes culminating in the accumulation of

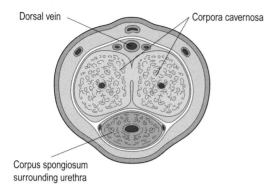

Fig. 9.28   Cross-section of the penis.

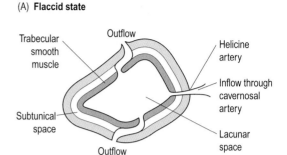

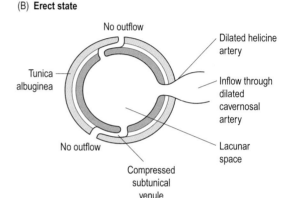

Fig. 9.29   Veno-occlusive mechanism of penile erection.

blood under pressure and end-organ rigidity (Moncada Iribarren & Sáenz de Tejada 1999). This vascular process can be divided into six phases:

- **Flaccidity**: A state of low flow of blood and low pressure exists in the penis in the flaccid state (Fig. 9.29a). The ischiocavernosus and bulbocavernosus muscles are relaxed.

- **Filling phase**: when the erection mechanism is initiated, the parasympathetic nervous system provides excitatory input to the penis from efferent segments S2–S4 of the sacral spinal cord; the penile smooth arterial muscle relaxes and the cavernosal and helicine arteries dilate enabling blood to flow into the lacunar spaces.

- **Tumescence**: the venous outflow is reduced by compression of the subtunical venules against the tunica albuginea (corporal veno-occlusive mechanism) causing the penis to expand and elongate but with a scant increase in intracavernous pressure.

- **Full erection**: the intracavernous pressure rapidly increases to produce full penile erection.

- **Rigidity**: the intracavernous pressure rises above diastolic pressure and blood inflow occurs with the systolic phase of the pulse enabling complete rigidity to occur. Contraction or reflex contraction of the ischiocavernosus and bulbocavernosus muscles produce changes in the intracavernous pressure. When full rigidity is achieved, no further arterial flow occurs (Fig. 9.29B).

- **Detumescence**: the sympathetic nervous system is responsible for detumescence via thoracolumbar segments (T10–T12, L1–L2) in the spinal cord. Contraction of the smooth muscle of the penis and contraction of the penile arteries lead to a decrease of blood in the

lacunar spaces and contraction of the smooth trabecular muscle leads to a collapse of the lacunar spaces and detumescence.

Pathophysiology of erectile dysfunction

Three types of erectile dysfunction are acknowledged: psychogenic, organic and mixed. They may be primary or secondary after a period of normal erectile function (1st Latin American Erectile Dysfunction Consensus Meeting 2003b). In organic erectile dysfunction, the events leading to full erection do not happen due to insufficient blood reaching the penis or blood escaping from the penis.

Role of the pelvic floor muscles

The ischiocavernosus and bulbocavernosus muscles are active during penile erection (Fig. 9.30).

Contractions of the ischiocavernosus muscles increase intracavernous pressure and influence penile rigidity. The area of the corpora cavernosum compressed by the ischiocavernosus muscle ranges from 35.6 to 55.9% (Claes et al 1996). The middle fibres of the bulbocaver-

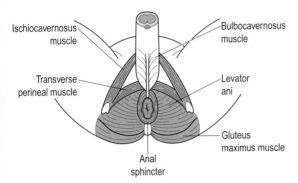

Ischiocavernosus muscle

Bulbocavernosus muscle

Transverse perineal muscle

Levator ani

Gluteus maximus muscle

Anal sphincter

Fig. 9.30 Superficial pelvic floor muscles.

nosus muscle assist in erection of the corpus spongiosum penis by compressing the erectile tissue of the bulb of the penis. The anterior fibres spread out over the side of the corpus cavernosum and are attached to the fascia covering the dorsal vessels of the penis and contribute to erection by compressing the deep dorsal vein of the penis, thus preventing the outflow of blood from the penis.

Weak pelvic floor muscles compromise penile erection (Colpi et al 1999, Dorey et al 2004).

ORGASMIC AND EJACULATORY DISORDERS

The final phase of sexual response in men culminates in orgasm and ejaculation. Although erection and ejaculation are coordinated, they are produced by different mechanisms.

Classification of different forms

Orgasmic and ejaculatory disorders may be classified as anejaculation, anorgasmia, premature ejaculation, retrograde ejaculation and delayed ejaculation (Hendry et al 2000). Ejaculatory disorders such as anejaculation, delayed ejaculation and premature ejaculation may lead to complete or partial loss of the ejaculate needed for impregnation of the female partner.

Anejaculation

Definition   Anejaculation is defined as 'the absence of ejaculation during orgasm' (Hendry et al 2000).

Classification of different forms   Anejaculation may be congenital or acquired and/or psychological (1st Latin American Erectile Dysfunction Consensus Meeting 2003c).

Prevalence   The prevalence of anejaculation is unknown.

Aetiology   Ejaculatory dysfunction can be due to congenital abnormalities, surgical trauma, genital infection, stones in the ejaculatory duct, paraplegia, dilatation of the seminal vesicles, or functional (Hendry et al 2000). Functional ejaculatory dysfunction includes congenital anorgasmia, where an excessively strict upbringing may produce an inability to achieve orgasm, premature ejaculation and the side-effects of some antihypertensive and psychotropic drugs.

Anorgasmia

Definition   Anorgasmia is defined as 'the inability to achieve orgasm during conscious sexual activity, although nocturnal emission may occur' (Hendry et al 2000).

Classification of different forms   Anorgasmia may be congenital, acquired and/or psychological (Hendry 1999).

Prevalence   The exact prevalence of anorgasmia is unknown. However, 37% of men reported anorgasmia after radical prostatectomy, and a further 37% reported a decreased intensity of orgasm (Barnas et al 2004).

Aetiology   There are a number of causes of anorgasmia. These range from congenital abnormalities, surgical trauma following imperforate anus, para-aortic lymphadenectomy or prostate surgery, genital infections such as gonorrhoea or non-specific urethritis, spinal cord injury, antidepressants, antipsychotics and polycystic kidney associated with dilatation of the seminal vesicles (Hendry 1999).

Retrograde ejaculation

Definition   Retrograde ejaculation is defined as 'backward passage of semen into the bladder after emission usually due to failure of closure of the bladder neck mechanism, demonstrated by presence of spermatozoa in the urine after orgasm' (Hendry et al 2000).

Classification of different forms   Retrograde ejaculation can be congential or acquired and/or psychological (1st Latin American Erectile Dysfunction Consensus Meeting 2003c).

Prevalence   The prevalence of retrograde ejaculation is unknown.

Aetiology Retrograde ejaculation can be due to damage of the bladder neck during prostate surgery, bladder neck disorder from alpha-adrenergic, neuroleptic or antidepressant blocking agents, diabetes mellitus, and some neuropathies (1st Latin American Erectile Dysfunction Consensus Meeting 2003c).

Retarded ejaculation

Retarded ejaculation is defined as 'undue delay in reaching a climax during sexual activity' (Hendry et al 2000).

Prevalence The prevalence of retarded ejaculation is unknown.

Classification of different forms Retarded ejaculation can be drug related or psychological (Hendry et al 2000).

Aetiology Retarded ejaculation can be due to emotional suppression, an inability to relax, relationship difficulties, medications, societal and religious attitudes, and the use of alcohol and recreational drugs (1st Latin American Erectile Dysfunction Consensus Meeting 2003c).

Role of the pelvic floor muscles During sexual activity, rhythmic contractions of the bulbocavernosus muscle along with the other pelvic floor muscles result in ejaculation (Gerstenberg et al 1990). The external urethral sphincter and deep pelvic floor muscles relax rhythmically to allow the ejaculate to pass through the urethra. An ability to relax may compromise this process.

Premature ejaculation

Premature ejaculation is one of the commonest forms of sexual dysfunction (Rosen 2000). It is characterized by a lack of ejaculatory control and is associated with significant effects on sexual functioning and satisfaction (Rowland et al 2004).

Definition Premature ejaculation has been defined as 'recurrent ejaculation that occurs with minimal stimulation and earlier than desired, before or soon after penetration, which causes bother or distress, and upon which the sufferer has little or no control' (World Health Organization 1992). It is also defined as 'the inability to delay ejaculation sufficiently to enjoy lovemaking. Persistent or recurrent occurrence of ejaculation with minimal sexual stimulation before, on, or shortly after penetration and before the person wishes it' (Hendry et al 2000).

Premature ejaculation is typically defined by three characteristics: short latency to ejaculation, lack of self-efficacy regarding the rapid ejaculation, and distress or dissatisfaction with the condition (Rowland 2003). In some men ejaculation occurs before or within 1 minute of the beginning of intercourse (Waldinger et al 1998). Rowland et al (2001) believed that the latency for men with premature ejaculation varied from 1 to 5 minutes. However, a study investigating the ejaculatory time of 'normal' men in different countries showed that the average time to ejaculation varies between 7 and 14 minutes (Montorsi 2005). Therefore, the definition of premature ejaculation should not be counted in minutes but acknowledge three core components: short ejaculatory time, lack of control over ejaculation and lack of sexual satisfaction (Montorsi 2005). It may occur in the absence of sufficient erection and the problem is not the result of prolonged abstinence from sexual activity.

Classification of different forms There are several different subtypes of biogenic and psychogenic premature ejaculation according to aetiological features (Metz & Pryor 2000). Physiological types of premature ejaculation are due to neurological constitution, acute physical illness, physical injury, and pharmacological side-effects. Psychological types are due to psychological constitution, acute psychological distress, relationship distress, and deficient psychosexual skills. Premature ejaculation may be labelled psychogenic when the physical cause is unknown.

Prevalence The prevalence of premature ejaculation is 16.3 to 32.5% (Rowland et al 2004). There is no evidence that ejaculation latency increases with age. In a stopwatch study of 110 men aged 18 to 65 years, 76% reported their ejaculation to be as rapid at their first sexual contacts with 23% reporting increasing rapidity and only 1% reporting a delay (Waldinger et al 1998).

Aetiology The aetiology of premature ejaculation is unknown, but psychological, behavioural and biogenic components are likely (Montague et al 2004). There may be an organic basis for some forms. The causes can be congenital or acquired and/or psychological (1st Latin American Erectile Dysfunction Consensus Meeting 2003).

Pathophysiology Data suggest that men with premature ejaculation have hypersensitivity and hyperexcitability of the glans penis and the dorsal nerve (Xin et al 1996, 1997).

Role of pelvic floor muscles During sexual activity, rhythmic contractions of the bulbocavernosus muscle along with the other pelvic floor muscles result in ejaculation (Gerstenberg et al 1990). Contraction of the pelvic floor muscles combined with intermittent relaxation of the external urinary sphincter and urogenital diaphragm allows ejaculation (Krane et al 1989). The bladder neck sphincter under involuntary control remains closed.

It is hypothesized that weak pelvic floor musculature affords little control to delay ejaculation and that the voluntary use of the pelvic floor muscles could delay ejaculation.

SEXUAL PAIN

Sexual pain is any pain that affects the ability to gain and maintain an erection and achieve orgasm and ejaculation.

REFERENCES

1st Latin American Erectile Dysfunction Consensus Meeting 2003a Androgen deficiency in the aging male. International Journal of Impotence Research 15(suppl 7):S12–S15

1st Latin American Erectile Dysfunction Consensus Meeting 2003b Anatomy and physiology of erection: pathophysiology of erectile dysfunction. International Journal of Impotence Research 15(suppl 7):S5–S8

1st Latin American Erectile Dysfunction Consensus Meeting 2003c Psychogenic erectile dysfunction and ejaculation disorders. International Journal of Impotence Research 15(suppl 7):S16–S21

Albaugh J, Lewis J H 1999 Insights into the management of erectile dysfunction: part I. Urologic Nursing 19(4):241–247

Andersen K V, Bovim G 1997 Impotence and nerve entrapment in long distance amateur cyclists. Acta Neurology Scandinavica 95(4):233–240

Baniel J, Israilov S, Shmueli J et al 2000 Sexual function in 131 patients with benign prostatic hyperplasia before prostatectomy. European Urology 38(1):53–58

Barnas JL, Pierpaoli S, Ladd P et al 2004 The prevalence and nature of orgasmic dysfunction after radical prostatectomy. BJU International 94(4):603–605

Benet H E, Melman A 1995 The epidemiology of erectile dysfunction. Urologic Clinics of North America 22(4):699–709

Bortolotti A, Parazzini F, Colli E et al 1997 The epidemiology of erectile dysfunction and its risk factors. International Journal of Andrology 20(6):323–334

Brock G B, Lue T F 1993 Drug-induced male sexual dysfunction: an update. Drug Safety 8(6):414–426

Claes H I M, Vandenbroucke H B, Baert L V 1996 Pelvic floor exercise in the treatment of impotence. The Journal of Urology 157(suppl 4):786

Colpi G M, Negri L, Nappi R E et al 1999 Perineal floor efficiency in sexually potent and impotent men. International Journal of Impotence Research 11(3):153–157

Dorey G, Speakman M, Feneley R et al 2004 Randomised controlled trial of pelvic floor muscle exercises and manometric biofeedback for erectile dysfunction. British Journal of General Practice 54(508):819–825

Fabra M, Porst H 1999 Bulbocavernosus-reflex latencies and pudendal nerve SSEP compared to penile vascular testing in 669 patients with erectile failure and sexual dysfunction. International Journal of Impotence Research 11(3):167–175

Feldman H A, Goldstein I, Hatzichristou D G et al 1994 Impotence and its medical and psychological correlates: results of the Massachusetts Male Ageing Study. The Journal of Urology 151:54–61

Fisher C, Gross J, Zuch J 1965 Cycle of penile erections synchronous with dreaming (REM) sleep. Archives of General Psychiatry 12:29–45

Frankel S J, Donovan J L, Peters T I et al 1998 Sexual dysfunction in men with lower urinary tract symptoms. Journal of Clinical Epidemiology 51(8):677–685

Gerstenberg T C, Levin R J, Wagner G 1990 Erection and ejaculation in man. Assessment of the electromyographic activity of the bulbocavernosus and ischiocavernosus muscles. British Journal of Urology 65:395–402

Hendry WF 1999 Causes and treatment of ejaculatory disorders. In: Carson C C, Kirby R S, Goldstein I (eds) Textbook of erectile dysfunction. Isis Medical Media, Oxford, p 569–581

Hendry W F, Althof S E, Benson G S et al 2000 Male orgasmic and ejaculatory disorders. In: Jardin A, Wagner G, Khoury S et al (eds) Erectile dysfunction. Health Publication, Plymouth, UK p 479–506

Heruti R, Shochat T, Tekes-Manova D et al 2004 Prevalence of erectile dysfunction among young adults; results of a large-scale survey. Journal of Sexual Medicine 1:284–291

Kirby R, Carson C, Goldstein I 1999 Anatomy, physiology and pathophysiology. In: Kirby R (ed) Erectile dysfunction: a clinical guide. Isis Medical Media, Oxford, p 11–28

Krane R J, Goldstein I, Saenz de Tejada I 1989 Impotence. New England Journal of Medicine 321(24):1648–1659

Lewis R W, Mills T M 1999 Risk factors for impotence. In: Carson C C, Kirby R S, Goldstein I (eds) Textbook of erectile dysfunction. Isis Medical Media, Oxford, p 141–148

Metz M E, Pryor J L 2000 Premature ejaculation: a psychophysiological approach for assessment and management. Journal of Sex and Marital Therapy 26(4):293–320

Moncada Iribarren I, Sáenz de Tejada I 1999 Vascular physiology of penile erection. In: Carson C C, Kirby R S, Goldstein I (eds) Textbook of erectile dysfunction. Isis Medical Media, Oxford, p 51–57

Montague D L, Jarow J, Broderick G A et al 2004 American Urological Association guidelines on pharmacologic management of premature ejaculation

Montorsi F 2005 Prevalence of premature ejaculation: a global and regional perspective. The Journal of Sexual Medicine 2(2):96–102

National Institutes of Health Consensus Development Panel on Impotence 1993 Impotence. JAMA 270(1):83–90

Rosen M P, Greenfield A J, Walker T G et al 1991 Cigarette smoking: an independent risk factor for atherosclerosis in the hypogastric-cavernous arterial bed of men with arteriogenic impotence. The Journal of Urology 145(4):759–763

Rosen R C 2000 Prevalence and risk factors of sexual dysfunction in men and women Current Psychiatry Reports 2:189–195

Rowland 2003 The treatment of premature ejaculation: selecting outcomes to determine efficacy. International Society for Sexual and Impotence Research Newsbulletin 10:26–28

Rowland D L, Cooper S E, Schneider M 2001 Defining premature ejaculation for experimental and clinical investigations. Archives of Sexual Behavior 30(3):235–253

Rowland D, Perelman M, Althof S et al 2004 Self-reported premature ejaculation and aspects of sexual functioning and satisfaction. Journal of Sexual Medicine 1(2):225–232

Sackett DL 1986 How are we to determine whether dietary interventions do more good than harm to hypertensive patients? Canadian Journal of Physiology and Pharmacology 64(6):781–783

Wagner T H, Patrick D L, McKenna S P et al 1996 Cross-cultural development of a quality of life measure for men with erection difficulties. Quality of Life Research 5:443–449

Waldinger M D, Hengeveld M W, Zwinderman A H et al 1998 An empirical operationalization study of DSM-IV diagnostic criteria for premature ejaculation. International Journal of Psychiatric Practice 2:287

World Health Organization 1992 International statistical classification of diseases and related health problems. 1989 Revision. World Health Organization, Geneva

Xin Z C, Choi Y D, Rha K H et al 1997 Somatosensory evoked potentials in patients with primary premature ejaculation. The Journal of Urology 158(2):451–455

Xin Z C, Chung W S, Choi Y D et al 1996 Penile sensitivity in patients with primary premature ejaculation. The Journal of Urology 156(3):979–981

TREATMENT

Grace Dorey

The treatment of male sexual dysfunction by physical therapists has been based on the evidence from a few trials. These trials were limited to the treatment of erectile dysfunction and premature ejaculation.

ERECTILE DYSFUNCTION

A literature review was undertaken to ascertain if physical therapy had merit as a conservative treatment for erectile dysfunction.

Literature search strategy

A search of the following computerized databases from 1980 to 2005 was undertaken: Medline, AAMED (Allied and Alternative Medicine), CINAHL, EMBASE – Rehabilitation and Physical Medicine and The Cochrane Library Database. The keywords chosen were erectile dysfunction, impotence, conservative treatment, physical therapy, physical therapy, pelvic floor exercises, biofeedback, electrical stimulation and electrotherapy. A manual search was undertaken of identified manuscripts reporting on research studies gained from the references of this literature.

Selection criteria

A study was included if the trial reported the results of physical therapy for men with erectile dysfunction and the outcome measures were reliable and relevant to the problem under investigation (Table 9.16).

Methodological quality

Methodological rigor was assessed by a PEDro quality score (Table 9.17).

Evidence for the effect

Only two randomized controlled trials (RCTs) provided evidence that pelvic floor muscle exercises (PFME) cured or improved erectile function (Dorey et al 2004, Sommer et al 2002). The trial by Sommer et al (2002) scored 7/10 using a PEDro quality score and the trial by Dorey et al (2004) scored 8/10 (see Table 9.17).

Five trials that were either non-randomized or uncontrolled provided weak evidence (Claes & Baert 1993, Claes et al 1995, Colpi et al, 1994, Mamberti-Dias & Bonierbale-Branchereau 1991, Van Kampen et al 2003). Two non-randomized uncontrolled trials solely used electrical stimulation and provided only weak evidence (Derouet et al 1998, Stief et al 1996).

The trial by Sommer et al (2002) used a large sample size of 124 men with venogenic erectile dysfunction. Men were randomized into three groups with one group receiving PFME, one group receiving Viagra and one group receiving a placebo. At 3 months the PFME group improved more than the Viagra group and significantly more than the placebo group. In the trial by Dorey et al (2004) 55 men were randomized into two groups with one group receiving PFME and one group receiving lifestyle changes. At 3 months the PFME group improved significantly compared to the control group. The control group were then given PFME and they improved significantly when compared to their erectile function at baseline. Both groups continued home exercises for a further 3 months.

Effect size

The two randomized controlled trials both showed significantly improved erectile function with PFME.

Dorey et al (2004) found at 3 months using the erectile function domain of the International Index of Erectile Function (IIEF) that the PFME group improved significantly ($p = 0.001$) compared with the control group ($p = 0.658$) (Fig. 9.31). At 3 months, when the control group were given PFME they improved erectile function significantly ($p < 0.001$). This trial also found that anal pressure in the intervention group significantly improved after 3 months PFME ($p < 0.001$) when compared to the control group.

Sommer et al (2002) found that the group of men who performed PFME improved more than the group of men receiving oral phosphodiesterase type 5 (PDE5) inhibi-

Table 9.16   Literature review of physical therapy for erectile dysfunction

Study	Mamberti-Dias & Bonierbale-Branchereau 1991
Design	Not random No control
n	210 men with erectile dysfunction Some with venous leakage Some psychological
Diagnosis	Some with venous leakage Some psychological erectile dysfunction
Training protocol	PFME & electrical stimulation sacral & penile or perineal electrode 5–25 Hz then 50–400 Hz intermittent Visual stimulation and penile temperature 15 treatments
Drop-out	Drop-outs not given
Adherence	Adherence not given
Results	**At 3 months** 111 (53%) cured 44 (21%) improved 55 (26%) failed 67% attained 4/10 to 8/10 ISMR (index of subjective mean rigidity) Subjective outcome
Study	Claes & Baert 1993
Design	Randomized No control
n	150 men with venogenic erectile dysfunction Age 23–64 Median age 48.7 *Group 1* 72 surgery *Group 2* 78 PFME
Diagnosis	Venogenic erectile dysfunction
Training protocol	*Group 1* Surgery deep dorsal vein *Group 2* Patient education 5-weekly PFME Home exercises Digital anal assessment baseline, 4 and 12 months 40 mg papaverine + needle EMG ischiocavernosus muscle + maximum PFM contraction
Drop-out	Drop-outs not given
Adherence	Adherence not given

Table 9.16   Literature review of physical therapy for erectile dysfunction—cont'd

Results	**At 4 months**
	Group 1
	44 (61%) cured
	17 (23.6%) improved
	11 (15.2%) failed
	Group 2
	36 (46%) cured
	22 (28%) improved
	20 (25.6%) failed
	At 12 months
	Group 1
	30 (42%) cured
	23 (32%) improved
	Group 2
	33 (42%) cured
	24 (31%) improved
	45 (58%) refused surgery
	Subjective and objective outcomes
Study	Colpi et al 1994
Design	Not random
	Controlled
n	59 men
	Age 20–63
	Mean age 39
	Group 1 33 men: PFME and biofeedback
	Group 2 26 men: controls
Diagnosis	Venogenic erectile dysfunction
Training protocol	30 of 59 deep dorsal vein surgery
	30 of 59 psychological therapy
	No information which?
	No information on type of biofeedback
Drop-out	Drop-outs not given
Adherence	Adherence not given
Results	**At 11 months**
	Group 1
	21 (63%) cured or improved
	Group 2
	4 (15%) cured or improved
	9 refused surgery
	Subjective outcome
Study	Claes et al 1995
Design	Not random
	No control
n	122 men with venogenic erectile dysfunction

Table 9.16   Literature review of physical therapy for erectile dysfunction—cont'd

Diagnosis	Venogenic erectile dysfunction
Training protocol	Patient education PFME EMG or pressure biofeedback ES with anal or surface electrode, symmetrical biphasic low frequency 50 Hz pulse 100 μs 6 s stimulation 12 s rest maximum intensity
Drop-out	14/122 drop-outs (11.5%)
Adherence	88.5% adhered
Results	**At 4 months** 53 (43%) cured 37 (30%) improved 32 (26.2%) failed including 14 drop-outs **At 12 months** 44 (36%) cured 41 (33.6%) improved 37 (30.3%) failed including 14 drop-outs 65 (53.4%) refused surgery Subjective outcome
Study	Stief et al 1996
Design	Not random Controlled
n	22 men with erectile dysfunction who were vasoresponders
Diagnosis	Venogenic erectile dysfunction
Training protocol	Transcutaneous ES to smooth muscle corpus cavernosum Low-frequency symmetrical trapezoidal 100–200 μs 12 mA alternating 10–20 Hz & 20–35 Hz 5 s stimulation 2–5 days for 20 min
Drop-out	Drop-outs not given
Adherence	Adherence not given
Results	**At 5 days** 5 (23%) cured 3 (13.6%) responded to vasoactive drugs 14 (63%) failed Subjective outcome
Study	Derouet et al 1998
Design	Not random No control
n	48 men with erectile dysfunction
Diagnosis	Erectile dysfunction
Training protocol	Transcutaneous ES penile or perineal electrodes bipolar pulsed 85 μs 30 Hz 20–120 mA 3-s stimulation 6-s rest 20 min daily for 3 months
Drop-out	10/48 drop-outs (20.8%)

Table 9.16 Literature review of physical therapy for erectile dysfunction—cont'd

Adherence	79.2% adhered
Results	**At 3 months** 5 (10.4%) cured 20 (41.6%) improved 23 (47%) failed including 10 drop-outs Subjective improvement
Study	Sommer et al 2002
Design	Randomized Controlled PEDro score 7/10
n	124 men with venogenic erectile dysfunction Aged 21–72 Mean age 43.7 *Group 1*: 40 men *Group 2*: 36 men *Group 3*: 28 men
Diagnosis	Venogenic erectile dysfunction
Training protocol	*Group 1*: 3 weekly PFME *Group 2*: oral PDE5 inhibitor *Group 3*: placebo At baseline, 4 weeks and 3 months: KEED erectile dysfunction questionnaire, IIEF Q 3 and 4, GAQ At baseline and 3 months: caversonography
Drop-out	Drop-outs not given
Adherence	Adherence not given
Results	**At 3 months** *Group 1* 80% improved significantly 46% improved penile rigidity *Group 2* 74% improved *Group 3* 18% improved Subjective and objective
Study	Van Kampen et al 2003
Design	Not random No control
n	51 men with erectile dysfunction with mixed aetiology Age 25–64 Mean age 46
Diagnosis	Erectile dysfunction
Training protocol	Patient education PFME in lying, sitting and standing Anal pressure biofeedback ES anal or surface electrode 50 Hz 200 μs 6 s stimulation 12 s rest once a week for 4 months Home exercise 90 contractions

Table 9.16   Literature review of physical therapy for erectile dysfunction—cont'd

Drop-out	9/51 drop-outs (18%)
Adherence	82% adhered
Results	**At 4 months** 24 (46%) cured 12 (24%) improved 15 (31%) failed including drop-outs Subjective outcome
Study	Dorey et al 2004
Design	Randomized Controlled PEDro score 8/10
n	55 men with erectile dysfunction with mixed aetiology Age 22–78 Mean age 59 Intervention group 28 men PFME + lifestyle changes Control group 27 men lifestyle changes
Diagnosis	Erectile dysfunction
Training protocol	*Intervention group* Patient education 5 weekly PFME and anal pressure biofeedback + home exercises + lifestyle changes *Control group* 5× weekly lifestyle changes At 3 months control group given intervention Outcome measures at 3 and 6 months: IIEF, ED-EQOL, anal manometry, blind assessment
Drop-out	At 3 months 5/55 drop-outs (9%)
Adherence	Adherence at 3 months (91%)
Results	**At 3 months** Erectile function domain of IIEF: intervention group significantly improved (p = 0.001) Control group (p = 0.658) Anal pressure: intervention group significantly improved (p < 0.001) **At 6 months** Blind assessment 22 (40%) normal function including drop-outs 19 (34.5%) improved including drop-outs 14 (25.5%) failed including drop-outs Subjective and objective outcomes

ED-EQOL, Erectile Dysfunction Effect on Quality of Life; ES, electrical stimulation; IIEF, International Index of Erectile Function; KEED, Kölner Erfassungsbogen für Erektile Dysfunktion; PDE5 inhibitor, phosphodiesterase type 5 inhibitor; PFME, pelvic floor muscle exercises.

Table 9.17 PEDro quality score of RCTs in systematic review of physiotherapy for erectile dysfunction

E – Eligibility criteria specified
1 – Subjects randomly allocated to groups
2 – Allocation concealed
3 – Groups similar at baseline
4 – Subjects blinded
5 – Therapist administering treatment blinded
6 – Assessors blinded
7 – Measures of key outcomes obtained from over 85% of subjects
8 – Data analysed by intention to treat
9 – Statistical comparison between groups conducted
10 – Point measures and measures of variability provided

Study	E	1	2	3	4	5	6	7	8	9	10	Total score
Sommer et al 2002	+	+	+	+	–	–	–	+	+	+	+	7/10
Dorey et al 2004	+	+	+	+	–	–	+	+	+	+	+	8/10

+, criterion is clearly satisfied; –, criterion is not satisfied; ?, not clear if the criterion was satisfied. Total score is determined by counting the number of criteria that are satisfied, except that scale item one 'eligibility criteria specified' is not used to generate the total score. Total scores are out of 10.

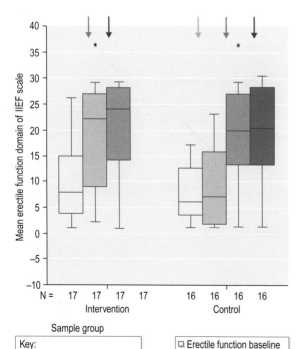

Fig. 9.31 Mean erectile function domain of International Index of Erectile Function (IIEF) scores for both groups at each assessment. (From Dorey et al 2004, with permission. © British Journal of General Practice.)

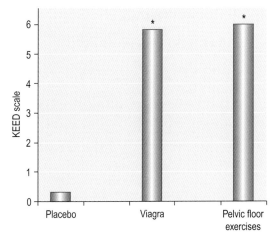

Fig. 9.32 Changes in Kölner Erfassungsbogen für Erektile Dysfunktion (KEED) at 3 months compared to baseline. (From Sommer et al 2002.)

tor (Viagra) and significantly more than the group receiving a placebo (Fig. 9.32).

Clinical significance

Both Sommer et al (2002) and Dorey et al (2004) found that PFME improved erectile function clinically. Sommer found that 46% of men had improved penile rigidity and Dorey found that 40% of men regained normal erectile function, and a further 34.5% improved erectile function.

Methodological quality

The methodological quality was good in the two randomized controlled trials. The sample size was larger in the study by Sommer et al (2002). Sommer et al (2002) studied men with proven venogenic erectile dysfunction. Dorey et al (2004) studied men with a wide range of aetiology. Both used validated subjective outcome measures and unlike the other trials both used objective outcome measures.

The results from the uncontrolled or non-randomized trials should be interpreted with caution due to poor methodology. Only one of these trials used randomization, five of the trials lacked controls, and seven provided only subjective outcomes. The lack of control groups in these trials impinged on the validity of evidence provided. The lack of randomization is an important methodological limitation that fundamentally limits any definitive interpretation and translation of the findings from these trials.

Type of intervention

Only one trial used PFME alone (Sommer et al 2002). This trial provided good results without biofeedback and questions the need for biofeedback. Two trials included biofeedback as the only other modality (Colpi et al 1994, Dorey et al 2004), while two combined PFME with biofeedback and electrical stimulation (Claes et al 1995, Van Kampen et al 2003). It is impossible to determine which modality has caused the effect when three modalities are used.

The amount of PFME varied. Colpi et al (1994) expected men to perform daily home exercises for 30 minutes a day for 9 months as a realistic alternative to surgery. Dorey et al (2004) instructed men to perform 18 strong contractions a day with an emphasis on functional work. No trial mentioned a long-term follow-up or advised a maintenance programme for life, though Claes & Baert (1993), and Claes et al (1995) followed up subjects for 12 months with encouraging results.

Two trials used electrical stimulation alone. Derouet et al (1998) found electrical stimulation to the ischiocavernosus muscle produced a cure rate of only 10.4% while Stief et al (1996) in a controlled trial explored transcutaneous electrical stimulation to the smooth muscle of the penile corpus cavernosum and effected a 23% cure rate. Whatever effect was achieved, both cure rates were low compared to the PFME trials.

Frequency and duration of training

The amount of treatment varied from between five and 20 treatment sessions, though some papers did not provide this information. Sommer et al (2002) treated men in three weekly PFME sessions and monitored the men at 4 weeks and 3 months. Dorey et al (2004) treated men in five weekly PFME sessions and monitored the men at 3 months and at 6 months. In both studies men performed home exercises.

Short- and long-term effects

From the available data, it appears that patients were assessed initially and then at between 3 and 12 months. The exception to this was the trial by Stief et al (1996) where outcomes were assessed after 5 days.

Both Sommer et al (2002) and Dorey et al (2004) used the subjective validated IIEF, which is used extensively for trials using oral medication for erectile dysfunction. Sommer et al (2002) used the validated Kölner Erfassungsbogen für Erektile Dysfunktion (KEED). Dorey et al (2004) used an assessor who was blinded to the subject group to report trial outcomes. Mamberti-Dias & Bonierbale-Branchereau (1991) used an index of subjective mean rigidity (ISMR) and reported an increase from 4 out of 10 to 8 out of 10 mean ISMR.

Most outcomes used patient reported 'cure', 'improved' or 'failure'. 'Cure' was defined as an erection suitable for satisfactory sexual performance with vaginal penetration in all studies. 'Improvement', however, was defined in a number of ways from 'a significant increase of erection quality and performance' (Colpi et al 1994) to 'partial response for those patients who reported some increase in quality (duration or rigidity) of erections but not sufficient for sexual intercourse' (Claes et al 1995).

Three trials used objective outcome measurements. Claes & Baert (1993) injected 40 mg papaverine to achieve penile rigidity and tested with needle electromyography (EMG) while contracting the ischiocavernosus muscle maximally. Sommer et al (2002) used Rigiscan® as an objective measurement of penile rigidity and Dorey et al (2004) used anal manometric biofeedback readings.

Sommer et al (2002) used a quality of life instrument and Dorey et al (2004) used the validated Erectile Dysfunction – Effect on Quality of Life (ED-EQoL) (MacDonagh et al 2002). Dorey et al (2004) found there was poor correlation of the IIEF with the ED-EQoL in the intervention group, but significant correlation in the control group. This finding showed that erectile dysfunction may have impacted on men in different ways and demonstrated a clear reason for the clinical usefulness of a quality of life questionnaire.

The short-term effects were good in all trials of PFME for erectile dysfunction. The two randomized controlled trials have provided good results at 3 months (Dorey et al 2004, Sommer et al 2002) and 6 months (Dorey et al 2004). The results were good at 12 months in the trial by Claes & Baert (1993).

Psychosexual issues

All the trials used a sample of heterosexual men. No study mentioned any cultural factors. The perceptions of sexual activity vary from one man to another and impact on the expectations and the subjective measurement of sexual performance. Not all men wish to practise penetrative sex. There were no studies that identified and addressed the difficulties and needs of homosexual men who practise anal intercourse.

Recommendations based on evidence

PFME should be the first-line treatment for erectile dysfunction (Fig. 9.33). They may be performed in conjunction with other treatment for erectile dysfunction such as oral therapy, vacuum devices, intracavernosus injections, intraurethral medication, constriction bands and counselling.

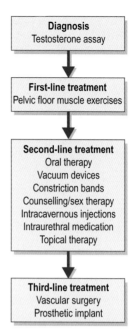

Fig. 9.33 Suggested algorithm for treatment of erectile dysfunction. (From Dorey et al 2004, with permission. © British Journal of General Practice.)

Conservative management for the prevention of erectile dysfunction

There were no publications using preventative conservative treatment. However, if the pelvic floor musculature is poor and PFME can relieve erectile dysfunction, then it seems reasonable to suppose that preventative muscle strengthening may help to prevent erectile dysfunction.

Conclusions

There is good-level evidence that PFME seem to have merit as a treatment for erectile dysfunction. For those patients who appear to have been cured or improved with PFME, it may be prudent to continue these simple exercises for life and possibly avoid a return of erectile dysfunction. However, long-term compliance may be a problem. Following initial pelvic floor training, it may be possible to maintain muscle performance with a minimal exercise programme.

There was no strong evidence that electrical stimulation was effective.

No studies demonstrating preventative conservative treatment were found.

A multicentre randomized controlled trial with larger sample numbers is needed to explore the use of PFME as a first-line treatment for men with erectile dysfunction. Similar trials are also needed to ascertain the role of PFME as prophylaxis for erectile dysfunction.

PREMATURE EJACULATION

A literature review was undertaken to ascertain whether PFME may have merit as a treatment for premature ejaculation.

Literature search strategy

A search of the following computerized databases from 1980 to 2005 was undertaken: Medline, AAMED (Allied and Alternative Medicine), CINAHL, EMBASE – Rehabilitation and Physical Medicine and The Cochrane Library Database. The keywords chosen were premature ejaculation, conservative treatment, physical therapy, physical therapy, pelvic floor muscle exercise, biofeedback, electrical stimulation and electrotherapy. A manual search was also undertaken.

Selection criteria

A study was included if it reported the results of physical therapy for men with premature ejaculation.

Methodological quality

No RCTs were identified.

Results

Only two non-randomized uncontrolled trials was found providing weak evidence (Table 9.18).

Methodology

La Pera & Nicastro (1996) used PFME, pressure biofeedback and electrical stimulation in a non-randomized and uncontrolled trial of 18 patients with a mean age of 34 years (range 20–52 years) to treat premature ejaculation; 15 had experienced the problem for over 5 years. The results showed that 11 patients (61%) were cured and able to control the ejaculatory reflex associated with improved PFM control and seven (39%) had no improvement. The biofeedback readings were not given. This non-randomized, uncontrolled study has shown that there may be merit in strengthening the PFM to control the ejaculatory reflex to prevent premature ejaculation.

In a non-randomized uncontrolled trial, Claes & van Poppel (2005) investigated the action of PFME and electrical stimulation on 29 men with premature ejaculation. After treatment, they found that 19 men (65.5%) showed improvement, which was verified by their partner. At 12 months, most of the men who had improved still showed a positive result.

Methodological quality

The methodology used in these two trials without randomization or the use of a control group and with a small sample size provided only weak evidence. However, results from these trials indicated that this subject is worth further exploration.

Recommendations

RCTs need to be undertaken to investigate PFME for premature ejaculation before any conclusions can be made.

Table 9.18   Trials of physical therapy for premature ejaculation

Study	Design	Subjects	Method	Outcomes
La Pera & Nicastro 1996	Non-randomized No control	18 men with premature ejaculation Aged 20–52 Mean age 34	PFME Pressure biofeedback ES Anal probe 50 Hz 3×/week for 20 sessions	**At 7 weeks** 11 (61%) cured 7 (39%) no improvement Subjective and objective outcomes
Claes & van Poppel 2005	Non-randomized No control	29 men with premature ejaculation Age not disclosed	PFME ES Parameters not given Ejaculatory latency time Method of measurement not given	**After treatment** 19 (65.5%) improved 10 (34.5%) failed to improve **At 12 months** Most of the 19 who improved still showed a positive response

ES, electrical stimulation; PFME, pelvic floor muscle exercises.

REFERENCES

Claes H, Baert L 1993 Pelvic floor exercise versus surgery in the treatment of impotence. British Journal of Urology 71:52–57

Claes H, Van Kampen M, Lysens R et al 1995 Pelvic floor exercises in the treatment of impotence. European Journal of Physical Medicine Rehabilitation 5:135–140

Claes HI, van Poppel H 2005 Pelvic floor exercise in the treatment of premature ejaculation. The Journal of Sexual Medicine 2(suppl 1):9

Colpi GM, Negri L, Scroppo FI et al 1994 Perineal floor rehabilitation: a new treatment for venogenic impotence. Journal of Endocrinological Investigation 17:34

Derouet H, Nolden W, Jost W H et al 1998 Treatment of erectile dysfunction by an external ischiocavernosus muscle stimulator. European Urology 34(4)355–359

Dorey G, Speakman M, Feneley R et al 2004 Randomised controlled trial of pelvic floor muscle exercises and manometric biofeedback for erectile dysfunction. British Journal of General Practice 54(508):819–825

La Pera G, Nicastro A 1996 A new treatment for premature ejaculation: the rehabilitation of the pelvic floor. Journal of Sex and Marital Therapy 22(1):22–26

MacDonagh R, Ewings P, Porter T 2002 The effect of erectile dysfunction on quality of life: psychometric testing of a new quality of life measure for patients with erectile dysfunction. The Journal of Urology 167:212–217

Mamberti-Dias A, Bonierbale-Branchereau M 1991 Therapy for dysfunctioning erections: four years later, how do things stand? Sexologique 1:24–25

Sackett DL 1986 How are we to determine whether dietary interventions do more good than harm to hypertensive patients? Canadian Journal of Physiology and Pharmacology 64(6):781–783

Sommer F, Raible A, Bondarenko B et al 2002 A conservative treatment option of curing venous leakage in impotent men. European Urology 1(suppl 1):153

Stief C G, Weller E, Noack T et al 1996 Functional electromyostimulation of the penile corpus cavernosum (FEMCC). Initial results of a new therapeutic option of erectile dysfunction. Der Urologe Ausg A 35(4):321–325

Van Kampen M, De Weerdt W, Claes H et al 2003 Treatment of erectile dysfunction by perineal exercises, electromyographic biofeedback and electrical stimulation. Physiotherapy 83(6):536–543

Fecal incontinence

INTRODUCTION

Ylva Sahlin and Espen Berner

Fecal incontinence is defined as the involuntary passage of gas or stool from the anal canal. The condition may seriously affect quality of life (QoL) (Bravo Gutierrez et al 2004). Patients have described their lack of bowel control as the loss of adulthood (Rozmovits & Ziebland, 2004). When handling patients with fecal incontinence health care workers should be aware of the adverse psychological effects of the condition. Embarrassment, social isolation, depression and reduced QoL characterize patients with fecal incontinence.

There is a lack of knowledge about the problems of fecal incontinence both among people in general and among health care workers. Physicians too often ignore symptoms, hence necessary treatment is not initiated. Patients often hesitate discussing the condition of fecal incontinence. Only one-third of patients affected seek medical advice (Johanson & Lafferty 1996, Kantalar et al 2002). Many patients are unaware that the condition can often be treated. Patients tend to suffer in silence because fecal incontinence is a taboo subject.

DEFINITION AND CLASSIFICATION

Fecal incontinence is described as the unintentional loss of rectal contents. There is no validated consensus definition for the condition. The main diversity in definition is whether the loss of gas should be considered as an aspect of fecal incontinence. It is therefore difficult to compare results from the studies done in this field. This is especially a problem when trying to estimate prevalence. How common is this condition? There is a need for a standard definition of fecal incontinence based on severity and frequency.

Examination for fecal incontinence should include a general physical examination and supplementary investigation procedures. Endoanal ultrasound, rectoanal endoscopy, anal manometry and pudendal nerve terminal motor latency (PNTML) show no correlation with the quantity and quality of symptoms and no objective measures correlate with severity. Grading is therefore best described using patient-reported symptoms. There is no official method for collecting data. One can either use a retrospective questionnaire or an incontinence diary.

Table 9.19   St Marks Incontinence Score

Type of incontinence	Never No episodes past 4 weeks	Rarely 1 episode past 4 weeks	Sometimes >1 episode past 4 weeks	Weekly 1 or more episodes a week	Daily 1 or more episodes a day
Solid stool	0	1	2	3	4
Liquid stool	0	1	2	3	4
Gas	0	1	2	3	4
Alterations in lifestyle	0	1	2	3	4

	No	Yes
Need to wear pad or plug	0	2
Taking constipating medicines	0	2
Lack of ability to defer defecations for 15 minutes	0	4

Add one score from each row:
Minimum score = 0 = perfect continence, maximum score = 24 = totally incontinent.

Fecal incontinence is in general graded from 1 to 4 using the Parks incontinence scoring system (Browning & Parks, 1983):

- Grade 1 – normal: complete continence.
- Grade 2 – mild incontinence: the loss of gas and minor staining.
- Grade 3 – moderate incontinence: the loss of gas and liquid stool.
- Grade 4 – severe incontinence: complete incontinence of gas, liquid and solid stool.

Several medical units use a modified edition of this scoring system in their studies of fecal incontinence. Still, this system gives no information about the frequency of bowel accidents, which is important in evaluating patients and treatment. Other frequently used grading systems of fecal incontinence have emerged in the absence of a uniform classification (Jorge & Wexner, 1993, Pescatori et al 1993, Rockwood et al 1999, Vaizey et al 1999). The Wexner Incontinence Grading Scale and St Marks Incontinence Score are most often used (Table 9.19). These grading scales give a fine description of the severity of symptoms and are easy to use in a clinical context.

The Fecal Incontinence Quality of Life Scale (FIQL) developed by Rockwood et al (2000) is a specific QoL questionnaire for fecal incontinence and is a useful instrument in evaluating patients with fecal incontinence (Halverson & Hull, 2002).

Box 9.10: Categories of fecal incontinence

PASSIVE INCONTINENCE
- Passive incontinence is unconscious loss of stool
- The patient feels nothing before leakage

URGE INCONTINENCE
- Urge incontinence is the inability to control a perceived impending bowel movement.

ICD-10, The International Classification of Diseases by the World Health Organization (2005) classifies fecal incontinence as R15: 'A symptom or sign associated with gastrointestinal disorders'. Fecal incontinence is in this respect not a specific disease, but rather a symptom resulting from one ore more disorders that impair continence by various mechanisms. There is no further classification of the condition in the ICD-10. This illustrates the lack of acknowledgement of fecal incontinence as a disorder of its own. Based on aetiology and patient-reported symptoms, the condition should be placed into two categories: passive and urge incontinence (Box 9.10).

Fecal incontinence in children includes both encopresis and soiling. Encopresis is the expulsion of a normal bowel movement in inappropriate places by a child aged 4 years or older. Soiling is the involuntary leakage of small amounts of stool.

Prevalence and risk factors

The prevalence of fecal incontinence varies with age, sex, general health status and physical debilities. Data on prevalence are mostly based upon epidemiological studies. The results are diverse due to the variety of populations studied and the diversity in definitions of fecal incontinence. In broad community-based studies the prevalence of fecal incontinence is estimated to 2–18% in the population studied (Macmillan et al 2004, Madoff et al 2004, Nelson et al 1995).

Younger female patients dominate clinical management studies of fecal incontinence. Nelson et al (1995) have explained this by a higher incidence in young females. Obstetric trauma causing an injury to the anal sphincter muscles and the pudendal nerves is described as the primary risk factor. Injury to the anal sphincter muscles occurs in 0.5–2.5% of all vaginal deliveries (Sultan et al 1999). Risk factors are primiparous women, large birth weight and instrumental deliveries, especially when forceps are used. Most sphincter injuries are surgically reconstructed immediately after delivery. However, more than one-third of all patients with sphincter disruption develop symptoms of fecal incontinence despite primary repair (Gjessing et al 1998). The physical postpartum examination underestimates the frequency of sphincter disruption. Many women live on with occult defects causing fecal incontinence or predisposing to fecal incontinence later in life.

Irritable bowel syndrome is also a risk factor for developing fecal incontinence. It tends to be more common among women and is correlated to postpartum fecal incontinence (Drossman 1989). In addition, young adult women are probably more active in seeking medical treatment and more willing to report symptoms than men (Nelson et al 1995). There seems to be a referral bias in the reporting of symptoms of fecal incontinence.

Studies have shown that the prevalence of fecal incontinence among the elderly in institutions is extraordinarily high. In populations of long-term hospitalized patients and patients in nursing homes the prevalence is close to 50% (Borrie & Davidson 1992, Nelson et al 1998). Fecal incontinence is in fact often the main reason for nursing home admissions. Long-term hospitalized patients have in general poorer health status and often suffer from physical disabilities; both related to fecal incontinence. Patients who are in need of physical help either to get to the toilet or evacuate stool must alter their normal bowel habits. On occasions they have to postpone toilet visits due to lack of help at desired moments of defecation. Being unable to follow their own toilet habits may contribute to fecal incontinence. In addition they often have other medical problems and

often use a variety of drugs that may further impair their fecal continence. Age above 65 years seems to be an independent risk factor (Nelson et al 1995) and cognitive dysfunction is associated with a high prevalence (Porell et al 1998). Without the conscious desire to maintain continence the ability to maintain normal bowel habits declines. In the Wisconsin nursing homes' study Nelson et al (1998) found that urinary incontinence was the factor that most commonly correlated to fecal incontinence. In this study there was no difference in prevalence of fecal incontinence between the sexes. The mean age of this population was 84 years. Several epidemiological studies also show a high prevalence among ageing men. High age seems to wipe out the difference in prevalence between the sexes (Tariq et al 2003).

Diarrhoea is associated with fecal incontinence. This is mainly caused by volume and liquid overflow and rapid stool transport. Patients with Crohn's disease, ulcerative colitis and diseases of other intestinal disorders have a higher incidence of fecal incontinence (Leigh & Turnberg 1982). Diabetes mellitus, multiple sclerosis, Parkinson's disease, stroke and spinal cord injury may cause diarrhoea or constipation, which trigger incontinence (Wald 1995). Surgical procedures of the anal canal such as lateral internal sphincterotomy, anal dilatation and fistulotomy may also result in fecal incontinence (Lindsey et al 2004). In addition, certain congenital anomalies are associated with continued fecal incontinence despite surgical corrections.

As there are no high-quality data based on randomized clinical trials (RCTs) for any risk factors for fecal incontinence there is a need for prospective epidemiological studies to determine prevalence and aetiology.

PATHOPHYSIOLOGY

Passage of rectal contents occurs when the pressure in the rectum overcomes the pressure in the anal canal. Incontinence results when the normal anatomy or physiology that maintains the structure and function of the anorectal unit is impaired. Fecal incontinence is rarely related to only one single factor. Rao & Patel (1997) found more than one pathogenic abnormality in over 80% of patients; there seems to be a cumulative multifactorial process leading to fecal incontinence.

The development of fecal incontinence occurs by three mechanisms:

- mechanical weakening and disruption;
- neuropathy; or
- intestinal disorders.

The anal sphincter consists of two muscles: the internal (IAS) and external anal sphincter (EAS). The smooth

IAS muscle contributes to about 60–80% of anal pressure at rest. The striated EAS also contributes to the pressure at rest by a constant tonus, which is characteristic of the striated muscles of the pelvic floor. The EAS controls voluntary anal continence.

In general, passive incontinence is associated with IAS dysfunction whereas urge incontinence is associated with EAS dysfunction. Often there is a combined injury and the symptoms overlap. Obstetric trauma is the most common cause of anal sphincter disruption (Kamm 1994). Many patients with sphincter injury may be asymptomatic for a long period of time after delivery and first become incontinent at menopause. This demonstrates that the cause is multifactorial. An age-related change and weakening of the pelvic floor may predispose to fecal incontinence (Nygaard et al 1997). It is a common opinion that ageing causes a physiological decrease in sphincter pressure.

The structural condition of the pelvic floor muscles is important in maintaining continence. The EAS is on the posterior side of the rectum followed proximally by the medial fibres of the pubococcygeus muscle. This posterior muscle sling is called puborectalis. The puborectalis muscle is crucial in maintaining the anorectal angle. The axis of the anus is at rest about 90° to the axis of the rectum. An injury to or weakening of the muscles of the pelvic floor may open the anorectal angle and an obtuse anorectal angle may impair continence. The significance of the anorectal angle in fecal continence is not entirely known (Womack et al 1988).

The pudendal nerves are the main nerves of the anorectum and the EAS. They arise from the sacral nerves S2–S4 and serve both sensory and motor functions. An injury to the pudendal nerve impairs innervation of the anorectum and perineum, causes weakening of the sphincter muscle, and may result in passive incontinence. An injured pudendal nerve causes a block in the rectoanal contractile reflex. This reflex is vital in inhibiting discharge of rectal contents during bowel movement. Rectal distension and a decrease in rectoanal pressure initiate a contractile response of the EAS mediated by the pudendal nerve. Neuropathy following neurological diseases, spinal cord injury, surgery or excessive straining results in altered bowel control for the same reason. Intact sensation provides warning of imminent defecation and discriminates between flatus, liquid and solid stool.

Consistency and volume of stool are important in the pathophysiology of fecal incontinence. In healthy individuals the colon absorbs liquid and passes only one-tenth of its contents further to the rectum. The rectum functions as a reservoir of stool. It can obtain large quantities without increasing its pressure. Impaired compliance of the rectum reduces this capacity and patients may develop fecal incontinence. This mechanism is seen in patients with colitis or radiation proctitis. Continence mechanisms are designed anatomically and physiologically to eliminate formed stool. If these mechanisms are impaired the anorectum and sphincter muscles become stressed. An overflow may produce urgency and incontinence.

Constipation may also lead to fecal incontinence, in particular an urge incontinence of the overflow type. The mechanism is decreased anorectal sensation and reduced sphincter pressure (Wrenn 1989). Constipation is associated with repeated straining to discharge rectal contents. Lasting many years, constipation may lead to descent of the pelvic floor, damage to the EAS due to repeated stretch injury, and progressive denervation of the muscles (Lubowsky et al 1988). Whether this causes fecal incontinence depends on the general state of the pelvic floor and strength of the sphincter muscles.

The pathophysiology of fecal incontinence is complex and multifactorial. Clinicians should consider a full anorectal investigation of adult patients before treating it. This is especially important before surgical treatment. Physical investigation often reveals the aetiology. Anorectal ultrasound and endoscopy are the most vital complementary tools in the physical examination. PNTML and anal manometry should be considered but give less clinical information.

CONSERVATIVE TREATMENT

Numerous medical conditions may cause fecal incontinence. Muscle injuries to the anal sphincter complex caused by childbirth, anorectal surgery, anorectal trauma, inflammatory processes or tumours are typical causes of disruption of the muscles of the anal canal. Neurological conditions causing degeneration of the pelvic floor muscles and the sphincter complex may be caused by childbirth, spinal cord injuries or congenital abnormalities such as spina bifida or myelomeningocele. Neurological conditions such as dementia, multiple sclerosis and brain tumours may lead to general dysfunction of the pelvic floor, consequently affecting fecal continence. Diarrhoea and constipation occasionally cause fecal incontinence; in such cases it is obvious that the goal of the treatment must be treating the diarrhoea or constipation and not the pelvic floor.

The primary treatment for fecal incontinence is conservative. The treatment has to be multifactorial. Strengthening of the pelvic floor muscles, increasing sensibility of the rectal ampulla, keeping the rectal ampulla empty and finally changing the consistence of the stool are factors that may lead to improved fecal continence. The aim of the treatment should be to diminish the frequency of incontinence episodes and to change the quality of the stool; gas incontinence and soiling is not as distressing as incontinence of loose or solid stool.

A systematic review of RCTs assessing the effect of biofeedback and physical therapy modalities in general to treat fecal incontinence is given on p. 310.

MEDICAL TREATMENT

Mild incontinence is often cured by dietary changes, avoiding food that may cause diarrhoea. This is often combined with bowel habit training. Bulking agents increase the volume of the stool and improve stool evacuation, resulting in an empty rectal ampulla, consequently improving continence. This can also be achieved using routine enemas. Loperamide is an antidiarrhoeal drug and a useful measure for reducing incontinence (Madoff et al 2004).

SURGERY

Surgical treatment is the treatment of choice for severe fecal incontinence. An established injury to the anal sphincter is treated with an overlapping sphincteroplasty. The success rates for this type of surgery vary between 60 and 80% (Wexner & Marchetti 1991). However, several studies have shown that the results after sphincteroplasty deteriorate substantially over time (Halverson & Hull, 2002, Malouf et al 2000,

Rothelbarth et al 2000). Whether biofeedback and pelvic floor exercises are profitable additional therapies for improving the long-term results is still uncertain. Unpublished data show promising results.

Severe incontinence due to spinal cord injuries or other neurological disorders may be helped with a colostomy, which has been shown to improve quality of life for patients (Kelly et al 1999, Rosito et al 2002).

Sacral nerve stimulation is an option for patients with functional but not anatomical deficits of the anal sphincter muscle. An electrode is placed through the sacral foramen to stimulate the sacral nerve segment S3. The results so far are promising with a high success rate and little morbidity. The long-term results for this treatment are still unknown (Jarret et al 2004).

CLINICAL RECOMMENDATIONS

Fecal incontinence is an embarrassing and often debilitating disorder. Its prevalence increases with age and it is more frequent among women. Obstetric sphincter rupture is the most common cause in the young female adult population. Knowledge of the treatment measures available is not widely known among health care takers or by patients. Therefore many patients remain untreated though most conditions are treatable. Conservative treatment including dietary restrictions and medical treatment are often successful for mild incontinence. The role of biofeedback treatment and pelvic floor exercises remains unclear. Surgery is the treatment of choice for severe incontinence.

REFERENCES

Borrie M J, Davidson H A 1992 Incontinence in institutions: cost and contributing factors. CMAJ 147:322–328

Bravo Gutierrez A, Madoff R D, Lowry A C et al 2004 Long-term results of anterior sphincteroplasty. Diseases of the Colon and Rectum 47(5):727–732

Browning G, Parks A 1983 Postnatal repair for the neurological faecal incontinence: correlation of clinical results and anal canal pressure. The British Journal of Surgery 70:101–104

Drossman D A 1989 What can be done to control incontinence associated with the irritable bowel syndrome? The American Journal of Gastroenterology 84:355–357

Gjessing H, Backe B, Sahlin Y 1998 Third degree obstetric tears; outcome after primary delivery. Acta Obstetricia et Gynecologica Scandinavica 77(7):736–740

Halverson A L, Hull T L 2002 Long-term outcome of overlapping anal sphincter repair. Diseases of the Colon and Rectum 45:345–348

Jarrett M E, Mowatt G, Glazener C M et al 2004 Systemic review of sacral nerve stimulation for faecal incontinence and constipation. The British Journal of Surgery 91:1559–1569

Johanson J F, Lafferty J 1996 Epidemiology of fecal incontinence: the silent affliction. The American Journal of Gastroenterology 91:33–36

Jorge J M, Wexner S D 1993 Etiology and management of fecal incontinence. Diseases of the Colon and Rectum 36:77–97

Kamm M A 1994 Obstetric damage and faecal incontinence. Lancet 344:730–733

Kantalar J S, Howell S, Talley N J 2002 Prevalence of faecal incontinence and associated risk factors; an underdiagnosed problem in the Australian community? The Medical Journal of Australia 176:54–57

Kelly S R, Shashidharan M, Borwell B et al 1999 The role of intestinal stoma in patients with spinal cord injury. Spinal Cord 37:211–214

Leigh R J, Turnberg L A 1982 Faecal incontinence: the unvoiced symptom. Lancet 1:1349–1351

Lindsey, I, Jones O M, Smilgin-Humphreys M M et al 2004 Patterns of fecal incontinence after anal surgery. Diseases of the Colon and Rectum 47(10):1643–1649

Lubowsky D Z, Swash M, Nicholls R J et al 1988 Increase in pudendal nerve terminal motor latency with defaecation straining. The British Journal of Surgery 75(11):1095–1097

Macmillan A K, Merrie A E, Marshall R J et al 2004 The prevalence of fecal incontinence in community-dwelling adults: a systematic review of the literature. Diseases of the Colon and Rectum 47(8):1341–1349

Madoff R D, Parker S C, Varma M G et al 2004 Faecal incontinence in adults. Lancet 364:621–632

Malouf, A J, Norton C S, Engel A F et al 2000 Long term results of overlapping anterior anal-sphincter repair for obstetric trauma. Lancet 355:260–265

Nelson R, Furner S, Jesudason V et al 1998 Fecal incontinence in Wisconsin nursing homes: prevalence and associations. Diseases of the Colon and Rectum 41(10):1226–2129

Nelson R, Norton N, Cautley E et al 1995 Community-based prevalence of anal incontinence. JAMA 274(7):559–561

Nygaard I E, Rao S S, Dawson J D 1997 Anal incontinence after anal sphincter disruption: a 30-year retrospective cohort study. Obstetrics and Gynecology 89(6):896–901

Pescatori M, Anastasio G, Bottini C et al 1993 New grading system and scoring for anal incontinence. Evaluation of 335 patients. Diseases of the Colon and Rectum 36:482–487

Porell F, Caro F G, Silva A et al 1998 A longitudinal analysis of nursing home outcomes. Health Services Research 33(4 pt 1):835–865

Rao S S C, Patel R S 1997 How useful are manometric tests of anorectal function in the management of defecation disorders? The American Journal of Gastroenterology 92:469–475

Rockwood T H, Church J M, Fleshman J W et al 2000 Fecal incontinence quality of life scale. Diseases of the Colon and Rectum 43:9–17

Rockwood T H, Church J M, Fleshman J W et al 1999 Patient and surgeon ranking of the severity of symptoms associated with fecal incontinence. Diseases of the Colon and Rectum 42:1525–1532

Rosito O, Nino-Murcia M, Wolfe V A et al 2002 The effects of colostomy on the quality of life in patients with spinal cord injury: a retrospective analysis. The Journal of Spinal Cord Medicine 25(3):174–183

Rothelbarth J, Bemelman W A, Meijerink W J et al 2000 Long-term results of anterior anal sphincter repair for fecal incontinence due to obstetric injury. Digestive Surgery 17(4):390–394

Rozmovits L, Ziebland S 2004 Expressions of loss of the narratives of people with colocectal cancer. Qualitative Health Research 14:187–203

Sultan A H, Monga A K, Kumar D et al 1999 Primary repair of obstetric anal sphincter rupture using the overlap technique. British Journal of Obstetrics and Gynaecology 106:318–323

Tariq S H, Morley J E, Prather C M 2003 Fecal incontinence in the elderly patient. The American Journal of Medicine 115:217–227

Vaizey C J, Carapeti E, Cahill J A et al 1999 Prospective comparison of faecal incontinence grading systems. Gut 44:77–80

Wald A 1995 Systemic diseases causing disorders of defecation and continence. Seminars in Gastrointestinal Disease 6:194–202

Wexner S D, Marchetti G 1991 The role of sphincteroplasty for fecal incontinence reevaluated: a prospective physiologic and functional review. Diseases of the Colon and Rectum 34:22–30

Whitehead W E, Burgio KL, Engel BT 1985 Biofeedback treatment of fecal incontinence in geriatric patients. Journal of the American Geriatrics Society 33:320–324

Womack N R, Morrison J F, Williams N S 1988 Prospective study of effects of postnatal repair in neurogenic faecal incontinence. The British Journal of Surgery 75:48–52

World Health Organization 2005 The international classification of diseases. World Health Organization, Geneva

Wrenn K 1989 Fecal impaction. The New England Journal of Medicine 321:658–662

PHYSICAL THERAPY FOR FECAL INCONTINENCE

Siv Mørkved

The treatment of fecal incontinence by physical therapists has mainly focused on activation and strengthening of the pelvic floor muscles (PFM). Different interventions have been used; PFM training (PFMT) with and without the use of biofeedback, and electrical stimulation (ES). Similar treatment modalities have been conducted by nurses, and it is therefore difficult to distinguish between studies including treatment by nurses and by physical therapists. Two Cochrane reviews addressing conservative treatment of fecal incontinence (Hosker et al 2000, Norton et al 2000), and one addressing physical therapies for prevention of urinary and fecal incontinence in adults (Hay-Smith et al 2002) have been published. All three reviews conclude that the limited numbers of trials do not allow a reliable assessment of the possible role of the different interventions in the prevention and treatment of fecal incontinence. However, several new studies have been published. Therefore a literature review was undertaken to ascertain whether PFMT with and without the use of biofeedback or ES have merit as conservative treatments for fecal incontinence.

LITERATURE SEARCH STRATEGY

A search of the following computerized databases from 1999 to 2005 was undertaken: Medline, CINAHL, EMBASE, The Cochrane Library Database. The search strategy recommended by the International Continence Society was used. A manual search was undertaken of identified manuscripts reporting on research studies gained from the references of this literature. Only randomized or quasi-randomized trials with sufficient data to allow statistical analyses were included. A study was included if the trial reported the results of physical therapy (PFMT with or without the use of additional biofeedback and/or ES) for adults with fecal incontinence and where symptoms of fecal incontinence was a predefined outcome measure. We found eight studies meeting the inclusion criteria (Table 9.20). In addition, two studies with different clinically relevant interventions, but not totally meeting the inclusion criteria are discussed below (Miner et al 1990, Schnelle et al 2002).

METHODOLOGICAL QUALITY

Methodological rigor was assessed from a hierarchy of evidence following the PEDro method score. The

Table 9.20 Randomized controlled trials on conservative treatment (PFMT with or without biofeedback, ES) in the treatment of fecal incontinence

Study	Fynes et al 1999
Design	2-arm RCT: vaginal BF + home PFMT, anal BF + ES + home PFMT
n	40 women, mean age 32 (range 18–48)
Diagnosis	FI caused by obstetric anal sphincter injury
Training protocol	1. Vaginal BF: 12 weeks with one weekly 30-min session (20 short max contractions of 6–8 s,10 s rest between + long contractions 30 s) + home training (standard Kegel PFMT–instructions not reported). 2. Anal BF: 12 weeks with one weekly session of audiovisual EMG feedback and ES + home training (standard Kegel PFMT–instructions not reported)
Drop-out Adherence	1/40 No ITT analysis Adherence not reported
Results	After the 12-week intervention: sign. difference in favour of the group training with anal BF + ES in the number of people who became asymptomatic (OR 4.54 95% CI 1.30 to 1.83) or improved in their continence status (OR 12.38 95% 2.67 to 57.46)
Study	Glazener et al 2001 and 2005
Design	2-arm RCT: advice on PFMT + visits by nurse (n = 371), standard care (n = 376)
n	747 women with urinary incontinence 3 months postnatally, at three centres
Diagnosis	Self-reported symptoms of FI 3 months postnatally
Training protocol	Advice on PFMT at 5, 7, and 9 months after delivery (8–10 sessions each day of 80–100 fast and slow contractions + bladder training if appropriate
Drop-out Adherence	Lost to follow-up 12 months: 25% in TG, 35% in CG 6 years: 29% in TG, 33% in CG Adherence reported ITT analysis
Results	FI at baseline: TG 57/371 (16%), CG 54/376 (15%) FI at 12 months postnatally: TG 12/273 (4%) CG 25/237 (10%) p = 0.012 (sign) FI at 6-year follow-up: TG 32/261 (12%), CG 32/248 (13%) NS
Study	Norton et al 2003
Design	4-arm RCT: standard care (advice) (n = 29), advice + instruction on sphincter exercises + home training (n = 32), hospital-based computer-assisted sphincter pressure BF (n = 44), hospital biofeedback + use of a home EMG BF (n = 35)
n	171 patients (male/female) with FI at a specialized colorectal hospital, mean age 56 years (range 26–85), 1-year follow-up 106/160
Diagnosis	Any self-reported symptom of FI
Training protocol	1. Standard care (advice) 2. Advice + instruction on sphincter exercises + home training: 50 maximal voluntary sustained sphincter contractions and 50 fast-twitch contractions per day 3. Hospital-based computer-assisted sphincter pressure BF to improve rectal sensitivity and muscle strength and endurance 4. Hospital BF + use of a home intra-anal EMG BF device. Median five sessions (1–9) over a period of 3–6 months

Table 9.20 Randomized controlled trials on conservative treatment (PFMT with or without biofeedback, ES) in the treatment of fecal incontinence—cont'd

Drop-out Adherence	9.4% drop-out 5 withdrawal, 10 did not return questionnaires Adherence not reported 34% did not attend 1-year follow-up
Results	Immediately after the intervention period: NS difference between groups in symptom change or QoL (SF-36 and unpublished disease specific) Combination of groups: 60% reduction in FI (sign) 4.6% cured QoL sign improved in all domains 1-year follow-up: NS difference between groups Combination of groups: virtually all parameters remained sign. improved from pre-treatment values
Study	Solomon et al 2003
Design	3-arm RCT: BF with anal manometry (n = 39), BF with transanal ultrasound (n = 40), PFMT with feedback from digital examination (n =41)
n	120 patients (male/female) with mild to moderate FI
Diagnosis	Self-reported symptoms of mild to moderate FI with at least mild neuropathy and no anatomical defect in the external sphincter
Training protocol	Sessions of 30 min once a month in 5 months Home exercises twice daily: 10 sessions of 10×5 s sphincter contractions
Drop-out Adherence	15% drop-out Adherence reported ITT analysis
Results	NS difference between groups in any outcome measure Combination of groups: 70% improvement in symptom severity (sign.), 69% improvement in QoL (direct questioning of objectives) (sign.)
Study	Davis et al 2004
Design	2-arm RCT: sphincter repair (n = 17), sphincter repair + BF (n = 14)
n	43 women with FI referred to a colorectal unit undergoing sphincter repair operation, mean age 60.48 (11.92)
Diagnosis	Persistent leakage of liquid or solid stool over at least the previous 12 months
Training protocol	Sphincter repair + anal BF starting 3 months after surgery. 1 h/week for 6 weeks (5 series of maximal long contractions 10 s, submaximal contractions 5 s and series of fast contractions) + daily home training twice daily and in functional situations
Drop-out Adherence	5 withdrawals 2 excluded from analyses Adherence not reported
Results	At 6 and 12 months after surgery: NS difference in improved FI between groups (93% in BF group, 65% in CG) At 6 months one patient in each group achieved complete continence Lower embarrassment QoL (disease-specific) score in BF group Improvement in mean resting and squeeze pressures in BF group at 6 months and still above preoperative levels at 12 months, NS In CG mean pressures reduced sign. between 6 and 12 months

Table 9.20 Randomized controlled trials on conservative treatment (PFMT with or without biofeedback, ES) in the treatment of fecal incontinence—cont'd

Study	Mahony et al 2004
Design	2-arm RCT: intra-anal BF + home exercises daily (n = 26), intra-anal BF + ES + home exercises daily (n = 28)
n	60 women with symptoms of FI at 12 weeks after vaginal delivery, mean age 1. 35 (23–39) 2. 32 (22–42)
Diagnosis	Symptoms of impaired fecal continence
Training protocol	12 week intervention: 1. Intra-anal BF. 10 min: 3 rapid maximal contractions in 5 s and rest 8 s alternating with slow contractions of 5 s and 8 s rest 2. Intra-anal BF + intra-anal neuromuscular electrical stimulation. Standard frequency of 35 Hz with 20% ramp modulation time. 20 min with 5 s stimulation and 8 s rest. Intensity that elicited external anal sphincter contractions
Drop-out Adherence	10% drop-out Adherence reported
Results	Immediately after the intervention period: NS difference between groups in symptoms of FI and other outcome measures Combination of groups (sign. change): improvement in FI 85%, cure FI 26%, improvement in anal squeeze pressure improvement QoL (disease-specific FIQL)
Study	Österberg et al 2004
Design	2-arm RCT: anterior levatorplasty, anal plug ES of the pelvic floor
n	59/70 male and female, median age 68 (range 52–80), median age 64 (range 43–81)
Diagnosis	Incontinence of idiopatic (neurogenic) origin, persisting after dietary advice
Training protocol	Levatorplasty, median hospital stay 3 (range 2–7) days Anal plug ES median 4 (range 2–7) weeks (12 sessions of 20 min). MS210, frequency was 25 Hz, duration 1.5 s, with pulse-train interval of 3 s
Drop-out Adherence	11 drop-outs Adherence not reported No ITT analysis
Results	At 3 months: sign. higher proportion of patients with improved Miller's incontinence score, and physical and social handicap in the levatorplasty group At 12 months: NS difference in incontinence score, sign. difference in physical and social handicap At 24 months: NS difference in incontinence score, sign. difference in physical and social handicap NS improvement in objective indices of sphincter function (manometric evaluation)

BF, biofeedback; CG, control group; CI, confidence interval, ES, electrical stimulation; FI, fecal incontinence; ITT, intention to treat; NS, not statistically significant; OR, odds ratio; PFMT, pelvic floor muscle training; QoL, quality of life; RCT, randomized clinical trial; TG, training group; Sign, statistically significant.

methodological quality based on PEDro method score varies between 5/10 and 8/10. This reflects a fairly good quality, accepting that the two criteria related to blinding of therapist and patient are almost impossible to meet in this kind of trial (Table 9.21).

EFFECT SIZE

It is difficult to compare effect size due to different study populations and different outcome measures in all included studies. All interventions used in the presented studies have an effect on reduction of symptoms of fecal incontinence. Most studies measure self-reported symptoms (see Table 9.20), and distinctions between incontinence of gas, fluid or solid stool are not made. Nevertheless, no statistically significant differences between interventions have been found, except for two studies. In one study a combination of anal biofeedback and ES was more effective than vaginal biofeedback in reducing fecal incontinence (Fynes et al 1999). However, the PFMT protocols in the two groups were not similar. It is therefore questionable if the difference in outcome is attributable to ES and the placement of the biofeedback advice. The other study showed that fecal incontinence was less common in postpartum women following a PFMT programme than in women randomized to standard care (Glazener et al 2001). Only women with postnatal urinary incontinence were included, and fecal incontinence was a secondary outcome measure.

CLINICAL SIGNIFICANCE

All studies reported clinically significant effects of the interventions, addressing a significant reduction in symptoms or episodes of fecal incontinence after intervention. No adverse effects of the interventions were reported. However, no specific intervention can yet be recommended as preferable.

Table 9.21 PEDro quality score of RCTs in systematic review

E – Eligibility criteria specified
1 – Subjects randomly allocated to groups
2 – Allocation concealed
3 – Groups similar at baseline
4 – Subjects blinded
5 – Therapist administering treatment blinded
6 – Assessors blinded
7 – Measures of key outcomes obtained from over 85% of subjects
8 – Data analysed by intention to treat
9 – Comparison between groups conducted
10 – Point measures and measures of variability provided

Study	E	1	2	3	4	5	6	7	8	9	10	Total score
Fynes et al 1999	+	+	−	+	−	−	+	+	−	+	+	6/10
Glazener et al 2001 & 2005	+	+	+	+	−	−	−	−	+	+	+	6/10
Norton et al 2003	+	+	+	+	−	−	−	+	+	+	+	7/10
Solomon et al 2003	+	+	+	+	−	−	+	+	+	+	+	8/10
Davis et al 2004	+	+	+	+	−	−	+	+	+	+	+	8/10
Mahony et al 2004	+	+	+	+	−	−	+	+	−	+	+	7/10
Österberg et al 2004	+	+	?	+	−	−	−	+	−	+	+	5/10

+, criterion is clearly satisfied; −, criterion is not satisfied; ?, not clear if the criterion was satisfied. Total score is determined by counting the number of criteria that are satisfied, except that E (eligibility criteria specified) is not used to generate the total score. Total scores are out of 10.

TYPE OF INTERVENTION

In all studies the interventions included PFMT, but following several different training protocols. The studies compared PFMT with (Davis et al 2004, Fynes et al 1999, Mahony et al 2004, Norton et al 2003) or without (Glazener et al 2001, Mahony et al 2004, Norton et al 2003) the use of biofeedback or ES (Fynes et al 1999, Mahony et al 2004). In two studies (Glazener et al 2001, Norton et al 2003) a control group received standard care (advise), and in another study (Österberg et al 2004) the effect of ES was compared to levatorplasty. All biofeedback studies, except one, included anal biofeedback. Anal ES was also used.

In a controlled study by Miner et al (1990) (not meeting the inclusion criteria and not included in the table) active sensory retraining reduced the sensory threshold, corrected any sensory delay, and reduced the frequency of incontinence. In another study by Schnelle et al (2002) (not meeting the inclusion criteria and not included in the table) an intervention including incontinence care and general exercises resulted in reduced frequency of fecal incontinence in patients in a nursing home.

FREQUENCY AND DURATION OF TRAINING

In the studies including PFMT the frequency and duration varied from weekly sessions for 6 weeks (Davis et al 2004) to 1–9 sessions over a period of 3–6 months (Norton et al 2003). Additional daily home training was emphasized in most studies. Both short and long contractions of the PFM were parts of the training protocols. However, the duration of the contractions classified as fast- and slow-twitch contractions differed between studies. The rationale behind the training protocols was poorly described in most studies. In addition, there was a lack of assessment of adherence to the training protocol in several publications. This fact makes it difficult to discuss the real effect of the intervention.

SHORT- AND LONG-TERM EFFECTS

Three studies reported short-term effects (effect immediately after cessation of the training protocol) (Fynes et al 1999, Glazener et al 2001, Mahony et al 2004), and two studies reported longer term effects (9–12 months after cessation of the training protocol) (Davis et al 2004, Norton et al 2003), while one study reported effects from a 6-year follow-up (Glazener et al 2005). The effects of the intervention seem to be still present at the 1 year follow-up studies, but not in the 6-year follow-up study.

RECOMMENDATIONS BASED ON EVIDENCE

According to the results of the present review PFMT with and without biofeedback and also ES seem to be effective in reducing fecal incontinence in different study populations. However, the results of one trial showed that exercises and biofeedback did not enhance the effect of standard nursing support and advice (diet, fluids, techniques to improve evacuation, a bowel training programme, titration of dose of anti-diarrhoeal medication if previously prescribed, and practical management). These results indicate that the reported beneficial effects of other interventions may be associated with the relationship with the therapist and advice given. It is open to discussion whether these results may be generalized to other study populations with different underlying pathophysiology.

Another aspect is that the training protocols used in several studies do not follow recommendations from exercise science (American College of Sports Medicine 1990), highlighting intensity and frequency of training. Nevertheless, PFMT with and without the use of biofeedback has been shown to be effective in several studies. Anal biofeedback may be more effective than vaginal biofeedback. There is still a question whether biofeedback has an additional effect compared to PFMT without biofeedback. Based on the current knowledge no first-choice treatment can be determined.

Both in clinical practice and in research, distinctions should be made between incontinence of gas, fluid or solid stool.

Clinicians have to take into account that the pathophysiology of fecal incontinence is complex and multifactorial. Thus, interventions should most likely be multifactorial, aiming at reducing the frequency of incontinence episodes, improving rectal sensibility and changing the quality of the stool. To enhance the quality of the PFMT protocols recommendations for strength training from exercise science should be applied.

There is a need for further long-term follow-up studies with improved experimental design and an adequate sample size that allow meaningful analysis. In addition, the intervention used to treat fecal incontinence should be of the highest quality related to the aims of the intervention.

REFERENCES

American College of Sports Medicine 1990 Position stand. The recommended quantity and quality of exercise for developing and maintaining cardiorespiratory and muscular fitness in healthy adults. Medical Science in Sports and Exercise 22:265–274

Davis K J, Kumar D, Poloniecki 2004 Adjuvant biofeedback following anal sphincter repair: a randomized study. Alimentary Pharmacology & Therapeutics 20:539–549

Fynes M M, Marshall K, Cassidy M et al 1999 A prospective, randomized study comparing the effect of augmented biofeedback with sensory biofeedback alone on fecal incontinence after obstetric trauma. Diseases of the Colon & Rectum 42:753–761

Glazener C M A, Herbison G P, Wilson P D et al 2001 Conservative management of persistent postnatal urinary and faecal incontinence: randomised controlled trial. BMJ 323:1–5

Glazener C M A, Herbison G P, MacArthur C et al 2005 Randomised controlled trial of conservative management of postnatal urinary and faecal incontinence; six year follow up. BMJ 330:337–339

Hay-Smith J, Herbison P, Mørkved S 2002 Physical therapies for prevention of urinary and faecal incontinence in adults. Cochrane Database of Systematic Reviews 2:CD003191

Hosker G, Norton C, Brazzelli M 2000 Electrical stimulation for faecal incontinence in adults. Cochrane Database of Systematic Reviews 2:CD001310

Mahony R T, Malone P A, Nalty J et al 2004 Randomized clinical trial of intra-anal electromyographic biofeedback physiotherapy with intra-anal electrical stimulation of the anal sphincter in the early treatment of postpartum fecal incontinence. American Journal of Obstetrics and Gynecology 191:885–890

Miner P B, Donnelly T C, Read N W 1990 Investigation of mode of action of biofeedback in treatment of fecal ioncontinence. Digestive Diseases and Sciences 35:1291–1298

Norton C, Hosker G, Brazzelli M 2000 Effectiveness of biofeedback and/or sphincter exercises for the treatment of faecal incontinence in adults. Cochrane Database of Systematic Reviews 2:CD002111

Norton C, Chelvanayagam S, Wilson-Barnett J et al 2003 Randomized controlled trial of biofeedback for fecal incontinence. Gastroenterology 125:1320–1329

Solomon M J, Pager C K, Rex J et al 2003 Randomized controlled trial of biofeedback with anal manometry, transanal ultrasound, or pelvic floor retraining with digital guidance alone in the treatment of mild to moderate fecal incontinence. Diseases of the Colon and Rectum 46:703–710

Schnelle J F, Alessi C A, Simmons S F et al 2002 Translating clinical research into practice: a randomized controlled trial of exercise and incontinence care with nursing home residents. The Journal of the American Geriatric Society 50:1476–1483

Österberg A, Edebol Eeg-Olofsson K, Hållden M et al 2004 Randomized clinical trial comparing conservative and surgical treatment of neurogenic faecal incontinence. British Journal of Surgery 91:1131–1137

Chapter 10

Evidence for pelvic floor physical therapy for urinary incontinence during pregnancy and after childbirth

Siv Mørkved

Urinary incontinence during pregnancy and after childbirth

Pregnancy and delivery have been considered main aetiological factors in the development of urinary incontinence. There has been considerable debate as to whether this is due to pregnancy itself or to the act of childbirth (MacLennan et al 2000), and the evidence is contradictory (Hunskaar et al 2002, King & Freeman 1998, Koelbl et al 2002).

DEFINITIONS, CLASSIFICATIONS AND PREVALENCE

Definitions and classifications are given in Chapter 9.

Prevalence estimates of any stress urinary incontinence (SUI) during pregnancy and after childbirth varies between 6 (Stanton et al 1980) and 67% (Francis 1960), and 2–3 months after delivery between 3 (Viktrup et al 1993) and 38% (Mørkved & Bø 1999). The variation may be explained by the different populations investigated (nulliparous, parous), the use of different definitions of incontinence (self-report, urodynamically proven, according to new or old definitions from the International Continence Society), and the registration of incontinence at different stages of pregnancy or postpartum.

AETIOLOGY

Most data regarding risk factors for the development of urinary incontinence have been derived from cross-sectional studies of volunteer and clinical subjects (Hunskaar et al 2002). Risk factors such as smoking, obesity, menopause, restricted mobility, chronic cough, chronic straining for constipation and urogenital surgery have not been as rigorously studied as parity and age (Hunskaar et al 2002). However, there are problems related to reports of risk factors and causal relationships because on many occasions the study designs used are not appropriate to answer such questions.

Urinary incontinence and SUI are strongly associated with vaginal childbirth in many epidemiological studies. Several studies, both epidemiological and clinical, have shown that the prevalence of SUI increases during pregnancy and declines after delivery (Allen et al 1990, Mason et al 1999, Stanton et al 1980, Thorp et al 1999, Viktrup et al 1992,). This indicates that the increased pressure from the growing uterus on the bladder may cause temporary leakage during pregnancy. Conflicting hypotheses have been proposed recently suggesting that pregnancy urinary incontinence is not provoked by the mere onset of pregnancy, but by increasing hormonal concentrations or local tissue changes caused by hormones (Hvidman et al 2002). The pregnancy itself and hereditary factors might predispose more than parturition trauma in some women (Demirci et al 2001, Foldspang et al 1999, Iosif 1981a, 1982), but the exact mechanisms remain uncertain. Nevertheless, the prevalence is higher after delivery than before gestation (Foldspang et al 1999, Mason et al 1999, Stanton et al 1980, Thorp et al 1999, Viktrup & Lose 2000).

Different characteristics related to the pregnant women have been analysed to determine risk factors of urinary incontinence. Obesity has been mentioned as a possible risk factor for postpartum SUI (Rasmussen et al 1997, Wilson et al 1996). However, results from other studies showed no relationship between increase in body mass index during pregnancy and experience of urinary incontinence (Chiarelli & Campell 1997, Højberg et al 1999). Coughing and sneezing on a regular basis during pregnancy increased the risk of experiencing incontinence (Chiarelli & Campell 1997). Initial strength of the pelvic floor muscles (PFM) is another factor that may influence continence status during pregnancy (Mørkved et al 2004) and after delivery (Sampselle et al 1998). Previous urinary incontinence is a significant risk factor (Beck & Hsu 1965, Eason et al 2004, Farrell et al 2001, Hvidman et al 2002), and the results of a 15-year follow-up study support the view that SUI arising during pregnancy increases the risk of SUI developing in the future (Dolan et al 2003).

The association between urinary incontinence and obstetric factors as parity, mode of delivery and weight of the baby have been addressed in several studies. Statistically significant associations between any incontinence and a birth weight of 4000 g or greater has been observed (Højberg et al 1999, Rortveit et al 2003b), but others have reported conflicting results (Farrell et al 2001, Viktrup et al 1992).

The first vaginal delivery seems to be a major risk for developing urinary incontinence (Burgio et al 1996, Højberg et al 1999, Iosif 1981a). Increased prevalence of urinary incontinence has been associated with increased parity (Mason et al 1999), and with women having more than four children (Groutz et al 1999, Thomas et al 1980, Wilson et al 1996). A linear correlation has been found between increased parity and increased frequency of incontinence (Jolleys 1988, Marshall et al 1998, Nygaard 1990). In contrast, no correlation between parity and urinary incontinence has also been reported, and a higher prevalence of urinary incontinence among white compared to black women (Burgio et al 1996).

Vaginal delivery has been found to be an adverse risk factor for postpartum urinary incontinence (Mason et al 1999, Wilson et al 1996). No multivariate association for forceps delivery or vacuum extraction delivery, episiotomy, or perineal suturing was found in a large cross-sectional study (Foldspang et al 1999), but epidural anesthesia has been associated with SUI (Rørtveit et al 2003b). Elective caesarean section appears to be protective, though not completely (Eason et al 2004, Farrell et al 2001, Mason et al 1999, Rørtveit et al 2003a, Wilson et al 1996), but confounding factors may exist. Anatomical structures (the size of the mother's pelvis, muscles, connective tissue) may be one reason for offering some women caesarean section. The same anatomical characteristics may also protect against urinary incontinence after delivery.

According to Brubaker (1998) no method of obstetric perineal management has been demonstrated to reduce the risk for incontinence. There is therefore still a need for strategies to treat and rehabilitate pelvic floor damage related to pregnancy and delivery.

PATHOPHYSIOLOGY

The underlying causes of lower urinary tract symptoms during pregnancy remain uncertain (Cardozo & Cutner 1997). Two different pathological processes may cause the symptom of SUI in pregnancy and during the post-partum period (Cardozo & Cutner 1997). Vaginal delivery may initiate damage to the continence mechanism by direct injury to the PFM, damage to their motor innervations, or both (Koelbl et al 2002). Additional denervations may occur with ageing, resulting in a functional disability many years after the initial trauma. Stress urinary incontinence after childbirth has been explained as a consequence of peripheral nerve damage (Allen & Warell 1987, Allen et al 1990, Snooks et al 1984,

1990). Rupture of muscle fibres and connective tissue and over stretching of supporting ligaments and fascias during pregnancy and delivery are other risk factors (Landon et al 1990, Sayer et al 1990).

The mechanisms behind pelvic floor damage leading to SUI are often divided into two broad categories: denervation injury and support/anatomic injury. Both types of injury may have consequences for the role of the PFM as continence mechanisms (DeLancey 1988, Sultan et al 1994a). In addition, pathological processes in the intrinsic continence mechanisms causing detrusor instability or low urethral pressure during pregnancy may cause the symptom of urinary incontinence (Cardozo & Cutner 1997). Possible mechanisms causing perinatal urinary incontinence will be presented in more detail in the following sections.

Denervation injury. In several studies, manometric and neurophysiological assessments have given evidence of weakness in the pelvic floor, and this weakness is due to partial denervation of the pelvic floor striated muscles (Allen et al 1990, Snooks et al 1984, 1990). In many women, pudendal neuropathy due to vaginal delivery persists and may become worse with time (Snooks et al 1990). However, the results of a 15 year follow up study showed that although pelvic floor reinnervation progressed after the postnatal period, the absence of an adequate marker for pelvic floor denervation makes it of uncertain clinical significance (Dolan et al 2003). It has been found that during the first year postpartum, vaginal surface electromyography, pressure and palpation measurements were reduced in primiparous women with traumatic delivery (Gunnarson & Mattiasson 2002). The difference between women with traumatic and non-traumatic deliveries was significant at 4 and 8 months postpartum for electromyography and pressure measurements and at 8 months for palpation. In addition, the risk of developing symptoms from the lower urinary tract during the first year postpartum was increased in women with traumatic delivery (41%) compared to women with non-traumatic delivery (25%) (Gunnarson & Mattiasson 2002). Women older than 30 years and with a traumatic delivery had more than double the risk for lower urinary tract dysfunction than those under the age of 30 did (Gunnarson & Mattiasson 2002).

Comparison of antepartum and postpartum pudendal nerve conduction has shown that the causative factor of denervation acts during the period of delivery, and specifically during the second stage of labour, whereas throughout pregnancy the nerve conduction is minimally affected (Sultan et al 1994b, Tetzschner et al 1997). There is a relationship between denervation and the period of maximal distension of the soft tissues of the birth canal, including the muscles of the pelvic floor

(Józwik & Józwik 2001). The injury seems to be neurogenic rather than muscular; this may be due to the differences in the vulnerability of nerves and skeletal muscles to withstand distension. Nerves of the PFM can be elongated by 6–22% of their initial length before damage occurs (Jünemann & Thüroff 1994). In contrast, human skeletal muscles are known to sustain distension up to 200% of their initial length (Åstrand & Rodahl 1986).

Support/anatomical injury (PFM/ligaments/fascias)

The hormonal (oestrogen, progesterone, endocrine corticoids, relaxin) changes during pregnancy influence the ligaments and smooth muscles, and may lead to increased joint mobility and increased mobility in pelvic organs that are stabilized by ligaments (Calguneri et al 1982).

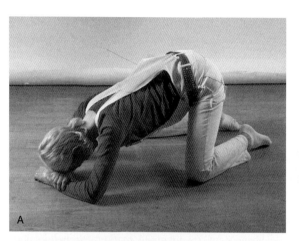

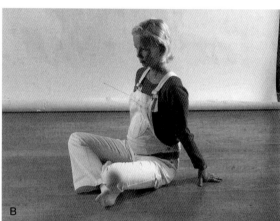

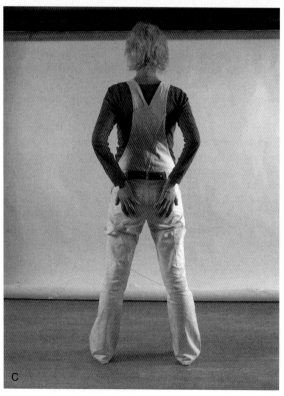

Fig. 10.1A–C Examples of positions for pelvic floor muscle training.

Joint hypermobility has been proposed as a marker for connective tissue weakness and subsequent development of prolapse and genuine SUI (GSUI) (Norton et al 1995). However, descriptive data from studies on pregnant women do not support this proposal (Chaliha et al 1999, Farrell et al 2001, Reilly et al 2002). Nevertheless, weak pelvic floor collagen may be important in the genesis of GSUI (Keane et al 1997) and this may be sig-

nificantly relevant during pregnancy where connective tissue is weaker than in a non-pregnant situation (Landon et al 1990). Reduced tensile strength in pregnant fascia has been found, which may account for the development of SUI in pregnancy (Landon et al 1990). Normally, the fascia regain their previous strength after delivery, but in cases of permanent SUI the occurrence of overstretching may cause irreversible damage.

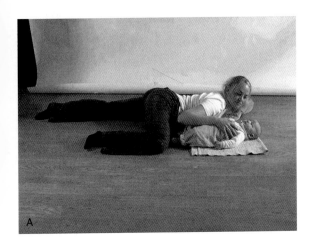

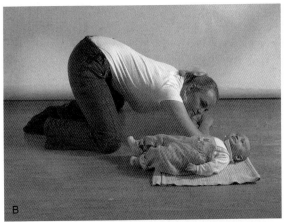

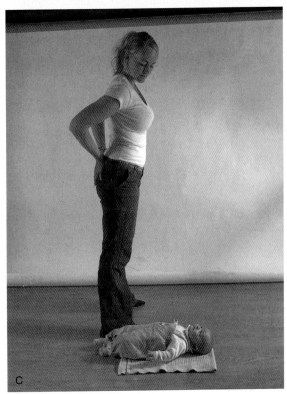

Fig. 10.2A–C Examples of positions for pelvic floor muscle training.

Histomorphological studies of the PFM in female cadavers have shown changes in the PFM related to vaginal childbirth and age (Dimpfl et al 1998). Rupture of muscle fibres and connective tissue because of overstretching during vaginal delivery has been extensively studied (Landon et al 1990, Sayer et al 1990, Sultan et al 1993), and SUI may be due to a combination of muscular and fascial damage (Sayer et al 1990).

Stretching of supporting structures as a result of pregnancy and delivery may lead to changes in the position of the bladder neck, and damage and weakening of the urethral sphincter mechanisms. Increased bladder neck mobility might indicate loss of urethral support (Cutner et al 1990). Meyer et al (1998a) studied bladder neck mobility and urinary sphincter function in pregnant and non-pregnant women. Although they found no significant changes in bladder neck mobility, pregnancy resulted in decreased maximal urethral closure pressure, decreased pressure transmission ratio values, and a backward displacement of the bladder neck. Compared with continent pregnant women, pregnant women with SUI also had a diminished urinary sphincter function.

Several studies have reported altered urethral support in some women after vaginal delivery. The effects of delivery on urinary continence mechanisms have been studied by comparing nulliparous continent women to women who had normal and instrumented deliveries (Meyer et al 1996, 1998b). Delivery induced no modifications of bladder neck position at rest, but was responsible for a lower bladder neck position during the Valsalva manoeuvre in the standing position (Meyer et al 1996, 1998b). Women with previous forceps deliveries and women with SUI had a significantly lower bladder neck than nulliparous continent women (Meyer et al 1996, 1998b). It has been found that vesical neck mobility during Valsalva manoeuvre was increased after childbirth, and that the bladder neck was positioned lower in women who had a vaginal delivery than those who had elective caesareans or were nulligravid (Peschers et al 1996). In one study, women with postpartum SUI had significantly greater antenatal bladder neck mobility than continent women (King & Freeman 1998). Results from another study reported quantifiable differences in vesical neck mobility during a cough and Valsalva manoeuvre in continent women, but not in primiparous stress incontinent women (Howard et al 2000). In another study, vaginal delivery was found to affect bladder neck mobility and its position more negatively than caesarean section, and bladder neck mobility was associated with GSUI. However, the GSUI rate was not significantly different between the groups of women delivered vaginally or by caesarean section (Demirci et al 2001).

Reduced PFM strength in the first week after delivery was found in women after they gave birth vaginally, but not in women after caesarean delivery (Peschers et al 1997); 6–10 weeks later, palpation and vesical neck elevation measured by perineal ultrasound did not show any significant differences to antepartum values. However, perineometric intravaginal pressure measurements remained significantly lower in primiparous women, but not in multiparous women regardless of mode of delivery. Mørkved et al (2003) found that PFM strength (vaginal squeeze pressure) was lower after delivery than during pregnancy. The reduction in muscle strength was greater in a control group than in a group following an intensive pelvic floor training programme during pregnancy (Mørkved et al 2003). In women with onset of incontinence after delivery, transvaginal ultrasound images showed a more pronounced loss of volume in the striated rhabdosphincter muscle after delivery than in continent women (Toozs-Hobson et al 1997).

Magnetic resonance imaging was used to study the levator ani muscle recovery following vaginal delivery, and displacement of the perineum toward the sacrum was shown to persist for up to 6 months after vaginal delivery (Tunn et al 1999). However, there were remarkable variations in levator ani structure changes among different individuals (Tunn et al 1999).

Other considerations

Pregnancy and delivery introduce major anatomical and physiological changes to the urinary tract that may result in alterations in urinary tract function, most commonly manifested by development of urinary symptoms (Chaliha & Stanton 2002). Urodynamic studies during pregnancy and after delivery have been carried out to study potential causes of urinary incontinence.

A high prevalence of detrusor instability has been found during pregnancy, and the detrusor instability has been shown to be significantly higher during pregnancy than after delivery (Cardozo & Cutner 1997, Nel et al 2001). However, in another study neither pregnancy nor delivery resulted in any consistent effects on objective bladder function, and postpartum urodynamic measurements were not related to either obstetric or neonatal variables, but were dependent on antenatal values (Chaliha et al 1999a, b).

Urethral pressure changes during pregnancy and postpartum were reported by Iosif et al (1981b). In continent women there were progressive increases in bladder pressure, maximum urethral closure pressure, urethral pressure, functional urethral length and urethral length with increasing gestation. After delivery, the measurement of these variables returned to early pregnancy values. A group of incontinent women had the same increase in bladder pressure, but no similar increases in maximum urethral closure pressure and functional urethral length (Iosif et al 1981b). Cardozo & Cutner (1997) and van Geelen et al (1982) report similar results. In addition, differences between continent and incontinent women in the transmission of intra-abdominal pressure to the urethra during early pregnancy have been reported (Cardozo & Cutner 1997). These findings indicate that because of the raised bladder pressures that occur during pregnancy, increases in urethral variables are necessary to maintain continence. However, according to Homma et al (2002) urodynamic measurements are prone to artefacts, and the limitations on the accuracy and the interchangeability of study results should be kept in mind during interpretation.

The PFM comprise one factor that may be a target for intervention that aims at preventing symptoms following injury to the pelvic floor. As early as in 1948, the American gynaecologist Arthur Kegel emphasized the value of PFM exercise in restoring function after childbirth. He claimed that genital relaxation after delivery is due to nerve injury, overstretching of muscles and tearing of fascias and that the method of restoring the condition is 'tightening' of the PFM. Kegel (1948) reported that Hippocrates tried 'oil injections, hot douches and salves' to restore the PFM after birth and that Saranus attempted support with the hand to exercise the PFM. In addition, information was given concerning observations of unusually firm perinea in South African tribes due to the practice of the midwives who made women contract the PFM around their distended fingers after birth (Kegel 1948). As a consequence of Kegel's (1951) studies, women in most industrialized countries have been encouraged to engage in PFM exercise during pregnancy and after delivery to strengthen the pelvic floor and to prevent and treat urinary incontinence. Despite the lapse of some 50 years since this practice was introduced, the effects of such exercises have until recently been only sparsely documented (Hay-Smith et al 2002).

One Cochrane review addressing physical therapies for prevention of urinary and fecal incontinence in adults (Hay-Smith et al 2002) has been published. The review concluded that the limited number of trials does not allow a reliable assessment of the possible role of the different interventions in the prevention of urinary incontinence. However, several new studies have now been published. Therefore literature reviews were undertaken to ascertain if PFM training (PFMT) with and without the use of biofeedback or electrical stimulation have merit as prevention and/or treatment for urinary incontinence.

Evidence for pelvic floor physical therapy for urinary incontinence during pregnancy

LITERATURE SEARCH STRATEGY

A search of the following computerized databases from 1985 to 2005 was undertaken: Medline, CINAHL, EMBASE, The Cochrane Library Database. The search strategy recommended by the International Continence Society was used. A manual search was undertaken of identified manuscripts reporting on research studies gained from the references of this literature. Only controlled trials with sufficient data to allow statistical analyses were included; abstracts were excluded. A study was included if the trial reported the results of physical therapy (PFMT with or without the use of additional biofeedback and/or electrical stimulation). We found three studies meeting the inclusion criteria (Table 10.1).

METHODOLOGICAL QUALITY

Methodological rigor was assessed from a hierarchy of evidence following the Pedro method score. The methodological quality based on Pedro method score varies between 7 and 8 out of 10 (Table 10.2). This reflects a high quality, accepting that the two criteria related to blinding of the therapist and patient are almost impossible to meet in this kind of trial.

Table 10.1 Studies assessing the effect of pelvic floor muscle exercises during pregnancy to prevent/treat urinary incontinence

Study	Mørkved et al 2003
Design	2-arm RCT: control (n = 144), customary information from general practitioner/midwife; intervention (n = 145), 12 weeks of intensive PFMT
n	n = 289 primigravid women recruited at 20 weeks gestation; some women had existing UI; three outpatient physiotherapy clinics in Trondheim, Norway
Diagnosis	Self-report of stress incontinence Symptom questionnaire
Training protocol	Control: customary information from general practitioner/midwife. Not discouraged from PFMT. Correct VPFMC checked at enrolment. Intervention: 12 weeks of intensive PFMT (in a group) led by physiotherapist, with additional daily home exercises between 20 and 36 weeks gestation. Correct VPFMC checked before training
Drop-outs/adherence	10 withdrawals (6 PFMT and 4 controls) Adverse events not stated ITT analysis
Results [numbers and percentage (%)]	**Self-reported UI at 36 weeks pregnancy** Control: 74/153 (48%) Intervention: 48/148 (32%) RR (95% CI): 0.67 (0.50–0.89) p = 0.007 **PFM strength (cmH$_2$O) (mean, SD):** Control: 34.4 (32.6, 37.1) Intervention: 39.9 (37.1, 42.7) p = 0.008 **UI at 3 months postpartum** Control: 49/153 (32%) Intervention: 29/148 (19.6%) RR (95% CI): 0.61 (0.40–0.90) p = 0.018 **PFM strength (mean, SD)** Control: 25.6 (23.2, 27.9) Intervention: 29.5 (26.8, 32.2) p = 0.048
Study	Reilly et al 2002
Design	2-arm RCT: control (n = 129), routine antenatal care (verbal advice); intervention (n = 139), individual PFMT with physiotherapist
n	n = 268 primigravid women with bladder neck mobility (on ultrasound) recruited at 20 weeks gestation Single centre, England
Diagnosis	Self-report of stress incontinence – Symptom questionnaire Bladder neck mobility measured by ultrasound
Training protocol	Control: routine antenatal care (verbal advice) Intervention: individual PFMT with physiotherapist at monthly intervals from 20 weeks until delivery; three sets of 8 contractions (each held for 6 s) repeated twice daily; instructed to contract the PFM when coughing or sneezing
Drop-outs/adherence	Data reported for 230/268 women, 38 withdrawals or losses to follow-up 51% of the women in the control group did unsupervised PFMT Adverse events not stated ITT analysis

Table 10.1   Studies assessing the effect of pelvic floor muscle exercises during pregnancy to prevent/treat urinary incontinence—cont'd

Results [numbers and percentage (%)]	**SUI at 3 months' postpartum** Control: 36/110 (32.7%) Intervention: 23/120 (19.2%) RR (95% CI): 0.59 (0.37–0.92) p = 0.023 Quality of life: higher score in the exercise group p = 0.004 Pad test: no significant difference Bladder neck mobility: no significant difference PFM strength: no significant difference
Study	Sampselle et al 1998
Design	2-arm RCT: control (n = 38), routine care; intervention (n = 34): a tailored PFMT programme
n	n = 72 primigravid women recruited at 20 weeks' gestation, mean age 27.2 (SD 5.5) Groups comparable at baseline (including incontinence severity and maximum VPFMC strength) Single centre, USA
Diagnosis	Self-report of stress incontinence Standing stress test

Training protocol	Control: routine care with no systematic review
	Tailored PFMT programme: beginning with muscle identification progressing to strengthening. 30
	    contractions per day at max or near max intensity from 20 weeks of pregnancy. Correct
	    voluntary PFM contraction checked

Drop-outs/adherence	26/72 (36%) withdrawals Unsupervised PFMT reported by 20% of control group Adverse events not stated Self-reported adherence. Partial ITT analysis
Results [numbers and percentage (%)]	**Change in mean UI symptom score** 35-week pregnancy: control 0.20, intervention −0.02, p = 0.07 6 weeks' postpartum: control 0.25, intervention −0.06, p = 0.03 6 months' postpartum: control 0.15, intervention −0.11, p = 0.05 12 months' postpartum: control 0.06, intervention −0.00, p = 0.74 PFM strength: no significant difference (low numbers)

PFMT, pelvic floor muscle training; VPFMC, voluntary pelvic floor muscle contraction; UI, urinary incontinence.

EFFECT SIZE

Studies by Reilly et al (2002) and Mørkved et al (2003) used similar interventions and partly also similar outcome measures. These two studies showed the largest effect size. However, the study by Sampselle et al (1998) concluded that the group performing PFMT had less urinary incontinence at 35 weeks of pregnancy and 6 weeks and 6 months after delivery, but found no difference between groups at 12 months after delivery.

CLINICAL SIGNIFICANCE

All studies included primigravid women recruited at 20 weeks of pregnancy. One study was a pure prevention study, including only women at risk of developing urinary incontinence (with bladder neck mobility) and no previous urinary incontinence. All studies reported clinically significant effects of the interventions, addressing a significant reduction in symptoms or episodes of urinary incontinence after intervention.

Table 10.2 Studies assessing the effect of pelvic floor muscle exercises during pregnancy to prevent/treat urinary incontinence: PEDro quality score of RCTs in systematic review

E – Eligibility criteria specified
1 – Subjects randomly allocated to groups
2 – Allocation concealed
3 – Groups similar at baseline
4 – Subjects blinded
5 – Therapist administering treatment blinded
6 – Assessors blinded
7 – Measures of key outcomes obtained from over 85% of subjects
8 – Data analysed by intention to treat
9 – Comparison between groups conducted
10 – Point measures and measures of variability provided

Study	E	1	2	3	4	5	6	7	8	9	0	Total score
Mørkved et al 2003	+	+	+	+	–	–	+	+	+	+	+	8/10
Reilly et al 2002	+	+	+	+	–	–	+	+	+	+	+	8/10
Sampselle et al 1998	+	+	+	+	–	–	+	–	+	+	+	7/10

+, criterion is clearly satisfied; –, criterion is not satisfied; ?, not clear if the criterion was satisfied. Total score is determined by counting the number of criteria that are satisfied, except that scale item one (eligibility criteria specified) is not used to generate the total score. Total scores are out of 10.

TYPE OF INTERVENTION

No adverse effects of the interventions were reported.

In all three studies the interventions included PFM strength training, with some differences regarding the number of contractions suggested per day. The training protocols in the studies by Reilly et al (2002) and Mørkved et al (2003) addressed close follow-up (monthly and weekly) by a physiotherapist.

FREQUENCY AND DURATION OF TRAINING

The frequency and duration of PFMT are comparable in the studies, starting at 20 weeks of gestation, with 20–30 near-maximal contractions per day during pregnancy.

SHORT- AND LONG-TERM EFFECTS

All studies reported significant short-term effects (effect immediately after cessation of the training protocol).

Sampselle et al (1998) reported long-term effects (12 months after cessation of the training protocol), and found that the effects of the intervention were not present at the 1 year follow-up study.

RECOMMENDATIONS BASED ON EVIDENCE

According to the results of the present review PFMT during pregnancy is effective in reducing urinary incontinence during pregnancy and in the immediate postpartum period. However, the longer term effect is questionable. No adverse effect of the PFMT has been reported. A study by Salvesen & Mørkved (2004) suggests that PFMT during pregnancy can facilitate rather than obstruct labour.

CLINICAL RECOMMENDATIONS

- The same PFMT protocol can be used in pregnant women as recommended for SUI in Chapter 9, p. 184.

Evidence for pelvic floor physical therapy for urinary incontinence after delivery

LITERATURE SEARCH STRATEGY

A search of the following computerized databases from 1985 to 2005 was undertaken: Medline, CINAHL, EMBASE, The Cochrane Library Database. The search strategy recommended by the International Continence Society was used. A manual search was undertaken of identified manuscripts reporting on research studies gained from the references of this literature. Only controlled trials with sufficient data to allow statistical analyses were included, abstracts were excluded. A study was included if the trial reported the results of physical therapy (PFMT with or without the use of additional biofeedback and/or electrical stimulation). We found ten studies meeting the inclusion criteria (Table 10.3).

METHODOLOGICAL QUALITY

Six studies were RCTs: two of these trials have reported results from follow-up studies. One study with an additional 1-year follow-up, had a matched controlled design, while another study had a controlled design. Methodological rigour was assessed from a hierarchy of evidence following the Pedro method score. The methodological quality based on Pedro method score varies between 4 and 8 out of 10 (Table 10.4). This reflects a variability concerning quality. However, it is important to notice that the studies also vary concerning the interventions used, and this issue is in general seldom addressed in reviews.

EFFECT SIZE

It is difficult to compare effect size due to different study populations and different outcome measures in most included studies. All interventions, except for one (Sleep & Grant 1987) used in the presented studies have an effect on reduction in symptoms of urinary incontinence immediately after cessation of the intervention. However, it seems likely that the interventions including close follow-up (monthly and weekly) by a physiotherapist have the best effect.

CLINICAL SIGNIFICANCE

All studies, except one (Sleep & Grant 1987), reported clinically significant effects of the interventions addressing a significant reduction in symptoms or frequency of urinary incontinence after the intervention period. No adverse effects of the interventions were reported.

TYPE OF INTERVENTION

In all studies the interventions included PFMT, though following several different training protocols. Most studies compared PFMT with current standard care, allowing self-managed PFMT but not introducing a control intervention. Only Dumoulin et al (2004) introduced an intervention in the control group (massage), and compared the control intervention with two different combined PFM rehabilitation interventions. The training protocols in the controlled studies by Mørkved & Bø (1997, 2000), Meyer et al (2001), and the RCT by Dumoulin et al (2004) addressed close follow-up (monthly and weekly) by a physiotherapist. No adverse effects of the interventions were reported.

FREQUENCY AND DURATION OF TRAINING

All studies involved PFMT 5 days a week or more. The duration of the PFMT programmes varied between 4 and 8 weeks.

SHORT- AND LONG-TERM EFFECTS

All studies, except one (Sleep & Grant 1987), reported significant short-term effects (effect immediately after cessation of the training protocol). Mørkved & Bø (2000) found that the effect of PFMT was still present 1 year after cessation of the training programme, while Chiarelli et al (2004) and Glazener et al (2005) found no difference in urinary incontinence between groups at 1 and 6 years' follow-up, respectively. Chiarelli et al (2004) reported that continued adherence to PFMT at 12 months was predictive of urinary incontinence at that time.

Table 10.3 Studies assessing the effect of pelvic floor muscle exercises after delivery to prevent/treat urinary incontinence

Study	Chiarelli & Cockburn 2002
Design	2-arm RCT: control (n = 350), usual care; intervention (n = 370), continence promotion
n	720 postnatal women following forceps or ventouse delivery, or delivered a baby ≥ 4000 g, age 15–44 Multicentre (3), Australia
Diagnosis	Self-report (continent or incontinent) Validated survey instrument Urinary diary (3 days)
Training protocol	Control: usual care Intervention: continence promotion: one contact with physiotherapist on postnatal ward and another at 8 weeks postpartum (correct VPFMC checked at second visit). Intervention included individually tailored PFMT, use of transversus abdominus contraction, the 'knack', techniques to minimize perineal descent, postpartum wound management. Written and verbal information
Drop-outs/adherence	Drop-out 6% in each group Adherence to PFMT: control 57.6%, intervention: 83.9% Adverse events not stated ITT analysis
Results (numbers and percentage [%])	**UI 3 months postpartum** Control: 126/328 (38.4%) Intervention: 108/348 (31.0%) (95% CI 0.22–14.6%) p = 0.044 OR of incontinence for the women in the intervention group compared with control group 0.65 (0.46–0.91), p = 0.01
Study	Chiarelli et al 2004
Design	Control (n = 294), usual care Intervention (n = 275), continence promotion
Diagnosis	Telephone interview: Self-report (continent or incontinent)
Drop-outs/adherence	Drop-outs: 30% ITT analysis
Results	**UI 12 months postpartum** NS difference between groups Practice of PFMT at 12 months promotes continence at this time
Study	Dumoulin et al 2004
Design	3-arm RCT: control (n = 20), PFM rehabilitation (n = 21), PFM rehabilitation + training of deep abdominal muscles (n = 23)
n	64 parous women under 45 years, still presenting symptoms of SUI at least once per week 3 months or more after last delivery; recruited during annual gynaecological visit at an obstetric clinic, Canada
Diagnosis	Self-reported urinary incontinence at least once per week
Training protocol	Control: 8 weekly sessions of massage

Table 10.3   Studies assessing the effect of pelvic floor muscle exercises after delivery to prevent/treat urinary incontinence—cont'd

Training protocol —cont'd	PFM rehabilitation: weekly sessions supervised by physiotherapist for 8 weeks: 15-min electrical stimulation (biphasic rectangular form; frequency 50 Hz; pulse with 250 µs; duty cycle, 6 s on and 18 s off for the first 4 weeks and 8 s on and 24 s off for the last 4 weeks; maximal tolerated current intensity) + 25 min PFMT with biofeedback + home training 5 days per week PFM rehabilitation as group 2 + 30 min of deep abdominal muscle training
Drop-outs/adherence	Drop-out rate 6% High adherence ITT analysis No adverse effect reported
Results	**After the intervention period** Objective cure (less than 2 g urine on pad test): Control: 0/19 PFM rehabilitation: 14/20 PFM rehabilitation + training of deep abdominal muscles: 17/23 Significant difference in favour of the PFM rehabilitation groups (p = 0.001) No significant difference between the two PFM rehabilitation groups PFM strength: no significant difference
Study	Glazener et al 2001
Design	2-arm RCT: control (n = 376), no visit; intervention (n = 371), assessment of UI by nurses, with conservative advice on PFM exercises Three centres (Aberdeen, Birmingham, Dunedin)
n	747 women with UI 3 months postnatal, mean age at entry 29.6 (SD 5.0)
Diagnosis	Self-reported persistence of UI
Training protocol	Control: no visit Intervention: assessment of UI by nurses, with conservative advice on PFM exercises (80–100 fast/slow contractions daily) 5, 7, and 9 months after delivery supplemented by bladder training if appropriate at 7 and 9 months
Drop-outs/adherence	Lost to follow-up at 12 months: control 35%, intervention: 25% ITT analysis
Results (numbers and percentage [%])	**Any UI** Control: 169/245 (69%) Intervention: 167/279 (59.9%) p = 0.037 **Severe UI** Control: 78/245 (31.8%) Intervention: 55/279 (19.7%) p = 0.002
Study	Glazener et al 2005 6-year follow-up
Design	Control: n = 253 Intervention: n = 263
n	516, mean age at entry 30.0 (SD 4.7)
Drop-outs/adherence	Lost to follow-up at 6 years: 30% Performing any PFMT: Control: 50% Intervention: 50%

Table 10.3 Studies assessing the effect of pelvic floor muscle exercises after delivery to prevent/treat urinary incontinence—cont'd

Results (numbers and percentage [%])	**Severe UI** Control: 99/253 (39%) Intervention: 100/263 (38%) p = 0.867
Study	Meyer et al 2001
Design	Allocated to 2 groups: control (n = 56), no education; intervention (n = 51), 12 sessions over 6 weeks with physiotherapist
n	107 women after vaginal delivery (previously nulliparous), recruited during pregnancy, mean age 29 years (SD 4) At treatment allocation (2 months' postpartum) 9/56 controls and 16/51 in the pelvic floor re-education group had self-reported SUI Single centre, Switzerland
Diagnosis	Self-reported urinary incontinence Bladder neck position and mobility Urodynamics
Training protocol	Control (n = 56): no pelvic floor re-education offered from 2–10 months' postpartum Intervention (n = 51): 12 sessions over 6 weeks with physiotherapist. PFMT followed by 20 min of biofeedback and 15 min of electrostimulation. Electrostimulation (vaginal electrode, biphasic rectangular waveform, pulse width 200–400 μs, frequency 50 Hz, intensity 5–15 mA, contraction time 6 s, rest time 12 s)
Drop-outs/adherence	No withdrawals or loses to follow-up Adherence not reported Adverse events not stated
Results (numbers and percentage [%])	**SUI 10 months postpartum** Control: 8/56 (32%) Intervention: 6/51 (12%) RR (95% CI): 0.82 (0.31, 2.21) Subjects cured: contro1 1/51(2%) p = 1.0 Intervention: 10/56 (19%) p = 0.02 PFM strength: NS difference Bladder neck position and mobility: NS difference Urodynamic parameters: NS differences
Study	Mørkved & Bø 1997
Design	Prospective matched controlled: control (n = 99), customary written postpartum instructions from the hospital; intervention (n = 99), 8 weeks of intensive PFMT
n	198 postpartum women Criteria for matching: age (±2 years), parity (1, 2, 3, 4 ≥ deliveries) and type of delivery Mean age 28 years (range19–40) Single centre, Norway
Diagnosis	Self-report of SUI Symptom questionnaire Standardized pad test (1 hour) Urodynamics

Table 10.3   Studies assessing the effect of pelvic floor muscle exercises after delivery to prevent/treat urinary incontinence—cont'd

Training protocol	Control: customary written postpartum instructions from the hospital; not discouraged from performing PFM exercises on their own; correct VPFMC checked at enrolment Intervention: 8 weeks of intensive PFMT (in a group) led by physiotherapist with additional daily home exercises between 8 and 16 weeks postpartum; correct VPFMC checked
Drop-outs/adherence	Seven withdrawals in the intervention group 100% in the training group and 65% in the control group reported that they were doing PFMT between 8 and 16 weeks after delivery Adverse events not stated
Results (numbers and percentage [%])	**Self-reported UI at 16 weeks postpartum** Control: 28/99 (28.3%) Intervention: 14/99 (14.1%) p = 0.015 **Standardized pad test** Control: 13/99 (13.1%) Intervention: 3/99 (3.0%) p = 0.009 **PFM strength (cmH$_2$O) improvement** Control: 0.8 (95% CI: 0.3–1.7) Intervention: 5.3 (95% CI: 4.5–6.6) p < 0.01
Study	Mørkved & Bø 2000 1-year follow-up
Design	Control (n = 81), intervention (n = 81)
n	180 women 1-year postpartum. All women, who had participated in a matched controlled trial were contacted per telephone one year after delivery Single centre, Norway
Training protocol	Control: customary written postpartum instructions from the hospital; not discouraged from performing PFM exercises on their own; correct VPFMC checked at enrolment Intervention: 8 weeks of intensive PFMT (in a group) led by physiotherapist with additional home exercises between 8 and 16 weeks postpartum; correct VPFMC checked
Drop-outs/adherence	All longitudinal changes were conducted using a constant sample, including the 81 matched pairs who attended all tests (162/180) 53% in the training group and 24% in the control group reported that they were doing PFMT between 16th week and 1 year postpartum Adverse events not stated
Results (numbers and percentage [%])	**Self-reported UI at 12 months postpartum** Control: 31/81 (38%) Intervention: 14/81 (17%) p = 0.003 **Standardized pad test** Control: 14/81 (13%) Intervention: 5/81 (3%) p < 0.03 **PFM strength improvement** Control: 1.7 (95% CI: 0.8–2.7) Intervention: 4.4 (95% CI: 3.2–5.6) p < 0.001 **Change in PFM strength in women performing PFMT < 3× per week and 3× per week or more** PFMT <3: 1.8 (95% CI: 0.8–2.7) PFMT ≥3: 4.9 (95% CI: 3.7–6.2)

Table 10.3 Studies assessing the effect of pelvic floor muscle exercises after delivery to prevent/treat urinary incontinence—cont'd

Study	Sleep & Grant 1987
Design	2-arm RCT: control (n = 900), current standard care; intervention (n = 900), current standard care + individual sessions PFMT
n	1800 postpartum women recruited within 24 h of vaginal delivery, mean age in control group 26.2 years (SD 5.3) and intervention group 27.1 years (SD 5.3) More women in intervention group had antenatal urinary incontinence (32 vs 29) Single centre, England
Diagnosis	Self-report (continent or incontinent at 3 months)
Training protocol	Controls: current standard antenatal and postnatal care, recommended to do VPFMC as often as remember and mid-stream urine stop 4-week health diary Intervention: as above plus one individual session daily while in hospital with midwifery coordinator, 4-week health diary including additional section recommending a specific PFMT task each week (all tasks related to integrating VPFMC with usual daily activity)
Drop-outs/adherence	Withdrawals at 3 months were 84/900 in control and 107/900 in PFMT group At 3 months' postpartum 58% in the exercise group and 42% in control group reported that they were doing PFMT Adverse events not stated Not ITT analysis
Results (numbers and percentage [%])	**UI 3 months postpartum** Control: 175/793 (22%) Intervention: 180/816 (22%) RR (95% CI): 1(0.83, 1.20)
Study	Wilson & Herbison 1998
Design	2-arm RCT: control (n = 117), customary information from general practitioner/midwife; intervention (n = 113), 12 weeks of intensive PFMT
n	230 women with UI 3 months postpartum, mean age 27.8 (95% CI 27–28.7)
Diagnosis	Self-reported UI Home pad test
Training protocol	Control: standard postnatal PFM exercises Intervention: Instructions by physiotherapist (80–100 fast/slow contractions daily) 3, 4, 6 and 9 months postpartum; use of perineometer to teach awareness of pelvic floor contraction; three groups: 39 women performed only PFM exercises; 36 women trained only with vaginal cones 15 min/day; 38 women used both
Drop-outs/adherence	Women responding on 1-year outcome assessment: Controls: 91/117 Intervention: 54/113
Results (numbers and percentage [%])	**Self-reported UI at 12 months postpartum** Control: 69/91 (76%) Intervention: 27/54 (50%) p = 0.003

ITT, intention to treat analysis; mo, month; NS, non-significant; OR, odds ratio; PC, power calculation; PFM, pelvic floor muscles; PFMT, pelvic floor muscle training; RCT, randomized controlled trial; RR, relative risk; SD, standard deviation; SUI, stress urinary incontinence; UI, urinary incontinence; VPFMC, voluntary pelvic floor muscle contraction; vs, versus; wk, week.

Table 10.4   Studies assessing the effect of pelvic floor muscle exercises after delivery to prevent/treat urinary incontinence: PEDro quality score of RCTs in systematic review

E – Eligibility criteria specified
1 – Subjects randomly allocated to groups
2 – Allocation concealed
3 – Groups similar at baseline
4 – Subjects blinded
5 – Therapist administering treatment blinded
6 – Assessors blinded
7 – Measures of key outcomes obtained from over 85% of subjects
8 – Data analysed by intention to treat
9 – Comparison between groups conducted
10 – Point measures and measures of variability provided

Study	E	1	2	3	4	5	6	7	8	9	0	Total score
Chiarelli & Cockburn 2002	+	+	+	+	−	−	?	+	+	+	+	7/10
Chiarelli et al 2004	+	+	+	+	−	−	?	−	+	+	+	6/10
Dumoulin et al 2004	+	+	+	+	−	−	+	+	+	+	+	8/10
Glazener et al 2001	+	+	+	+	−	−	+	−	+	+	+	7/10
2005	+	+	+	+	−	−	+	−	−	+	+	6/10
Meyer et al 2001	+	?	?	?	−	−	?	+	?	+	+	3/10
Mørkved & Bø 1997	+	−	−	+	−	−	−	+	−	+	+	4/10
2000	+	−	−	+	−	−	−	+	−	+	+	4/10
Sleep & Grant 1987	?	+	?	?	−	−	−	+	−	+	+	4/10
Wilson & Herbison 1998	+	+	+	+	−	−	−	−	−	+	+	5/10

+, criterion is clearly satisfied; −, criterion is not satisfied; ?, not clear if the criterion was satisfied. Total score is determined by counting the number of criteria that are satisfied, except that scale item one (eligibility criteria specified) is not used to generate the total score. Total scores are out of 10.

RECOMMENDATIONS BASED ON EVIDENCE

According to the results of the present review PFMT after delivery is effective in reducing urinary incontinence in the immediate postpartum period. However, the longer term effect is questionable. No adverse effect of the PFMT has been reported.

CLINICAL RECOMMENDATIONS

The same PFMT protocol can be used in pregnant women as recommended for SUI in Chapter 9, p. 189.

REFERENCES

Allen R E, Hosker G L, Smith A R B et al 1990 Pelvic floor damage and childbirth: a neurophysiological study. British Journal of Obstetrics and Gynaecology 90:770–779

Allen R E, Warell D W 1987 The role of pregnancy and childbirth in partial denervation of the pelvic floor. Neurourology and Urodynamics 6:183–184

Åstrand P O, Rodahl K 1986 Textbook of work physiology. McGraw–Hill, New York

Beck R P, Hsu N 1965 Pregnancy, childbirth, and the menopause related to the development of stress incontinence. American Journal of Obstetrics and Gynecology 91:820–823

Brubaker L 1998 Initial assessment: the history in women with pelvic floor problems. Clinical Obstetrics and Gynecology 41:657–662

Burgio K L, Locher J L, Zyczynski H et al 1996 Urinary incontinence during pregnancy in a racially mixed sample: characteristics and predisposing factors. International Urogynecology Journal and Pelvic Floor Dysfunction 7:69–72

Calguneri M, Bird H A, Wright V 1982 Changes in joint laxity occurring during pregnancy. Annals of the Rheumatic Diseases 41:126–128

Cardozo L, Cutner A 1997 Lower urinary tract symptoms in pregnancy. British Journal of Urology 80:14–23

Chaliha C, Bland J M, Monga A 2000 Pregnancy and delivery: a urodynamic viewpoint. British Journal of Obstetrics and Gynaecology 107:1354–1359

Chaliha C, Kalia V, Stanton S et al 1999 Antenatal prediction of postpartum urinary and fecal incontinence. Obstetrics and Gynecology 94:689–694

Chaliha C, Stanton S 2002 Urological problems in pregnancy. BJU International 89(5):469–476

Chaliha C, Sultan A H, Stanton S L 1999 Changes in pelvic floor following childbirth. Fetal and Maternal Review 11:41–54

Chiarelli P, Campell E 1997 Incontinence during pregnancy. Prevalence and opportunities for continence promotion. Australian and New Zealand Journal of Obstetrics and Gynaecology 37:66–73

Chiarelli P, Cockburn J 2002 Promoting urinary continence in women after delivery: randomised controlled trial. BMJ 324:1241–1246

Chiarelli P, Murphy B, Cockburn 2004 Promoting urinary continence in postpartum women: 12-month follow-up data from a randomised controlled trial. International Urogynecology Journal and Pelvic Floor Dysfunction 15:99–105

Cutner A, Cardozo L D, Benness C J et al 1990 Detrusor instability in early pregnancy. Neurourology and Urodynamics 9:328–329

DeLancey J O L 1988 Structural aspects of the extrinsic continence mechanism. Obstetrics and Gynecology 72:296–300

Demirci F, Ozden S, Alpay Z et al 2001 The effects of vaginal delivery and cesarean section on bladder neck mobility and stress urinary incontinence. International Urogynecology Journal and Pelvic Floor Disorders 12:129–133

Dimpfl T, Jaeger C, Mueller-Felber W et al 1998 Myogenic changes of the levator ani muscle in premenopausal women: the impact of vaginal delivery and age. Neurourology and Urodynamics 17:197–205

Dolan L M, Hosker G L, Mallett V T 2003 Stress incontinence and pelvic floor neurophysiology 15 years after the first delivery. British Journal of Obstetrics and Gynaecology 110:1107–1114

Dumoulin C, Lemieux M C, Bourbonnais D et al 2004 Physiotherapy for persistent postnatal stress urinary incontinence: a randomized controlled trial. Obstetrics and Gynecology 104:504–510

Eason E, Labreque M, Marcoux S et al 2004 Effects of carrying a pregnancy and of method of delivery on urinary incontinence: a prospective cohort study. BMC Pregnancy and Childbirth 4:4

Farrell S A, Allen V M, Baskett T F 2001 Parturition and urinary incontinence in primiparas. Obstetrics and Gynecology 97:350–356

Foldspang A, Mommsen S, Djurhuus J C 1999 Prevalent urinary incontinence as a correlate of pregnancy, vaginal childbirth, and obstetric techniques. American Journal of Public Health 89:209–212

Francis W 1960 The onset of stress incontinence. The Journal of Obstetrics and Gynecology of the British Empire 67:899–903

Glazener C M A, Herbison G P, MacArthur C et al 2005 Randomised controlled trial of conservative management of postnatal urinary and faecal incontinence; six year follow up. BMJ 330:337–339

Glazener C M A, Herbison G P, Wilson P D et al 2001 Conservative management of persistent postnatal urinary and faecal incontinence: randomised controlled trial. BMJ 323:593–596

Groutz A, Gordon D, Keidar R et al 1999 Stress urinary incontinence: prevalence among nulliparous compared with primiparous and grand multiparous premenopausal women. Neurourology and Urodynamics 18:419–425

Gunnarsson M, Mattiasson A 2002 Pelvic floor function in primiparous women in early pregnancy and 4–12 months after delivery. In: Gunnarsson M Pelvic floor dysfunction. A vaginal surface EMG study in healthy and incontinent women [thesis]. Faculty of Medicine, Lund University, Sweden

Hay-Smith J, Herbison P, Mørkved S 2002 Physical therapies for prevention of urinary and faecal incontinence in adults (Cochrane Review). In: The Cochrane Library, Issue 4. Update Software, Oxford

Homma Y, Batista J, Bauer S et al 2002 Urodynamics. In: Abrams P, Cardozo L, Khoury S et al (eds) Incontinence, 2nd edn. Plymbridge Distributors, Plymouth, UK, p 317

Højberg K E, Salvig J D, Winslow N A et al 1999 British Journal of Obstetrics and Gynaecology 106:842–850

Howard D, Miller J M, DeLancey J O L et al 2000 Differential effects of cough, valsalva, and continence status on vesical neck movement. Obstetrics and Gynecology 95:535–540

Hvidman L, Foldspang A, Mommsen S et al 2002 Correlates of urinary incontinence in pregnancy. International Urogynecology Journal and Pelvic Floor Dysfunction 13:278–283

Hunskaar S, Burgio K, Diokno A C et al 2002 Epidemiology and natural history of urinary incontinence (UI). In: Abrams P, Cardozo L, Khoury S et al (eds) Incontinence, 2nd edn. Plymbridge Distributors, Plymouth, UK, p 167

Iosif S 1981a Stress incontinence during pregnancy and puerperium. International Journal of Gynaecology and Obstetrics 19:13–20

Iosif S, Ulmsten U 1981b Comparative urodynamic studies of continent and stress incontinent women in pregnancy and in the puerperium. American Journal of Obstetrics and Gynecology 140:645–650

Jolleys J V 1988 Reported prevalence of urinary incontinence in women in a general practice. British Medical Journal 296:1300–1302

Józwik M, Józwik M 2001 Partial denervation of the pelvic floor during term vaginal delivery. International Urogynecology Journal and Pelvic Floor Dysfunction 12:81–82

Jünemann K, Thüroff J 1994 Innervation. In: Schüessler B, Laycock J, Norton P (eds) Pelvic floor re-education. Principles and practice. Springer–Verlag, London, p 22–27

Keane D P, Sims T J, Abrams P 1997 Analysis of collagen status in premenopausal nulliparous women with genuine stress incontinence. British Journal of Obstetrics and Gynaecology 104:994–998

Kegel A H 1948 Progressive resistance exercise in the functional restoration of the perineal muscles. American Journal of Obstetrics and Gynecology 56:238–249

Kegel A H 1951 Physiologic therapy for urinary stress incontinence. JAMA 146:915–917

King J K, Freeman R M 1998 Is antenatal bladder neck mobility a risk factor for postpartum stress incontinence? British Journal of Obstetrics and Gynaecology 105:1300–1307

Koelbl H, Mostwin J, Boiteux J P et al 2002 Pathophysiology. In: Abrams P, Cardozo L, Khoury S et al (eds) Incontinence, 2nd edn. Plymbridge Distributors, Plymouth, UK, p 203

Landon C R, Crofts C E, Smith A R B et al 1990 Mechanical properties of facia during pregnancy: a possible factor in the development of stress incontinence of urine. Contemporary Reviews in Obstetrics and Gynaecology 2:40–46

MacLennan A H, Taylor A W, Wilson D H et al 2000 The prevalence of pelvic floor disorders and their relationship to gender, age, parity and mode of delivery. British Journal of Obstetrics and Gynaecology 107:1460–1470

Marshall K, Thompson K A, Walsh D M et al 1998 Incidence of urinary incontinence and constipation during pregnancy and postpartum: survey of current findings at the Rotunda Lying–in Hospital. British Journal of Obstetrics and Gynaecology 105:400–402

Mason L, Glenn S, Walton I et al 1999 The prevalence of stress incontinence during pregnancy and following delivery. Midwifery 15:120–128

Meyer S, Bachelard O, De Grandi P 1998a Do bladder neck mobility and urethral sphincter function differ during pregnancy compared with during the non-pregnant state? International Urogynecology Journal and Pelvic Floor Dysfunction 9:397–404

Meyer S, De Grandi P, Schreyer A et al 1996 The assessment of bladder neck position and mobility in continent nullipara, multipara, forceps delivered and incontinent women using perineal ultrasound; a future office procedure? International Urogynecology Journal and Pelvic Floor Dysfunction 7:138–146

Meyer S, Hohlfeld P, Achrari C 2001 Pelvic floor education after vaginal delivery. Obstetrics and Gynecology 97:673–677

Meyer S, Schreyer A, De Grandi P et al 1998b The effects of birth on urinary continence mechanisms and other pelvic-floor characteristics. Obstetrics and Gynecology 92:613–618

Mørkved S, Bø K 1997 The effect of postpartum pelvic floor muscle exercise in the prevention and treatment of urinary incontinence. International Urogynecology Journal and Pelvic Floor Dysfunction 8:217–222

Mørkved S, Bø K 1999 Prevalence of urinary incontinence during pregnancy and postpartum. International Urogynecology Journal and Pelvic Floor Dysfunction 10:394–398

Mørkved S, Bø K 2000 Effect of postpartum pelvic floor muscle training in prevention and treatment of urinary incontinence: a one-year follow up. British Journal of Obstetrics and Gynaecology 107:1022–1028

Mørkved S, Bø K, Schei B et al 2003 Pelvic floor muscle training during pregnancy to prevent urinary incontinence – a single blind randomized controlled trial. Obstetrics and Gynecology 101:313–319

Mørkved S, Salvesen K Å, Bø K et al 2004 Pelvic floor muscle strength and thickness in continent and incontinent nulliparous pregnant women. International Urogynecology Journal and Pelvic Floor Dysfunction 15:384–390

Nel J T, Diedericks A, Joubert G et al 2001 A prospective clinical and urodynamic study of bladder function during and after pregnancy. International Urogynecology Journal and Pelvic Floor Dysfunction 12:21–26

Norton P A, Baker J E, Sharp H C et al 1995 Genitourinary prolapse and joint hypermobility in women. Obstetrics and Gynecology 85:225–228

Nygaard I, DeLancey J O L, Arnsdorf L et al 1990 Exercise and incontinence. Obstetrics and Gynecology 5:848–851

Peschers U, Schaer G, Anthuber C et al 1996 Changes in vesical neck mobility following vaginal delivery. Obstetrics and Gynecology 88:1001–1006

Peschers U, Schaer G, DeLancey J O L et al 1997 Levator function before and after childbirth. British Journal of Obstetrics and Gynaecology 104:1004–1008

Rasmussen K L, Krue S, Johansson L E et al 1997 Obesity as a predictor of postpartum urinary symptoms. Acta Obstetricia et Gynecologica Scandinavica 76:359–362

Reilly E T C, Freeman R M, Waterfield M R et al 2002 Prevention of postpartum stress incontinence in primigravidae with increased bladder neck mobility: a randomised controlled trial of antenatal pelvic floor exercises. British Journal of Obstetrics and Gynaecology 109:68–76

Rortveit G, Daltveit A K, Hannestad Y S et al 2003a Urinary incontinence after vaginal delivery or cesarean section. New England Journal of Medicine 348:900–907

Rortveit G, Daltveit A K, Hannestad Y S et al 2003b Vaginal delivery parameters and urinary incontinence: The Norwegian EPINCONT study. Obstetrics and Gynecology 189:1268–1274

Salvesen K Å, Mørkved S 2004 Randomised controlled trial of pelvic floor muscle training during pregnancy. BMJ 329:378–380

Sampselle C M, Miller J M, Mims B L et al 1998 Effect of pelvic muscle exercise on transient incontinence during pregnancy and after birth. Obstetrics and Gynecology 91:406–412

Sayer T R, Dixon J S, Hosker G L et al 1990 A study of periurethral connective tissue in women with stress incontinence of urine. Neurourology and Urodynamics 9:319–320

Sleep J, Grant A 1987 Pelvic floor exercises in postnatal care. Midwifery 3:158–164

Snooks S J, Setchell M, Swash M et al 1984 Injury to innervation of pelvic floor sphincter musculature in childbirth. Lancet 2:546–550

Snooks S J, Swash M, Mathers S E et al 1990 Effect of vaginal delivery on the pelvic floor: a five year follow-up. The British Journal of Surgery 77:1358–1360

Stanton S L, Kerr-Wilson R, Grant Harris V 1980 The incidence of urological symptoms in normal pregnancy. British Journal of Obstetrics and Gynaecology 87:897–900

Sultan A H, Kamm M A, Bartram C I et al 1994a Perineal damage at delivery. Contemporary Reviews in Obstetrics and Gynaecology 6:18–24

Sultan A H, Kamm M A, Hudson C N 1993 Anal sphincter trauma during instrumental delivery. International Journal of Gynaecology and Obstetrics 43:263–270

Sultan A H, Kamm M A, Hudson C N 1994b Pudendal nerve damage during labour: prospective study before and after childbirth. British Journal of Obstetrics and Gynaecology 101:22–28

Tetzschner T, Sørensen M, Lose G et al 1997 Pudendal nerve function during pregnancy and after delivery. International Urogynecology Journal and Pelvic Floor Dysfunction 8:66–68

Thomas T M, Plymat K T, Blannin J et al 1980 Prevalence of urinary incontinence. British Medical Journal 281:1243–1245

Thorp J M, Norton P A, Wall L L et al 1999 Urinary incontinence in pregnancy and the puerperium: a prospective study. American Journal of Obstetrics and Gynecology 181:266–273

Toozs-Hobson P, Athanasiou S, Kullar V et al 1997 Why do women develop incontinence after childbirth? [abstract]. Neurourology and Urodynamics 16:385

Tunn R, DeLancey J O L, Howard D et al 1999 MR imaging of levator ani muscle recovery following vaginal delivery.

International Urogynecology Journal and Pelvic Floor Dysfunction 10:300–307

van Geelen J M, Lemmens W A J G, Eskes T K A B et al 1982 The urethral pressure profile in pregnancy and after delivery in healthy nulliparous women. American Journal of Obstetrics and Gynecology 144:636–649

Viktrup L, Lose G 2000 Lower urinary tract symptoms 5 years after the first delivery. International Urogynecology Journal and Pelvic Floor Dysfunction 11:336–340

Viktrup L, Lose G, Rolff M et al 1992 The symptom of stress incontinence caused by pregnancy or delivery in primiparas. Obstetrics and Gynecology 79:945–949

Viktrup L, Lose G, Rolff M et al 1993 The frequency of urological symptoms during pregnancy and delivery in primiparae. International Urogynecology Journal and Pelvic Floor Dysfunction 4:27–30

Wilson P D, Herbison R M, Herbison J P 1996 Obstetric practice and the prevalence of urinary incontinence three months after delivery. British Journal of Obstetrics and Gynaecology 103:154–161

Wilson P D, Herbison J P 1998 A randomized controlled trial of pelvic floor muscle exercises to treat postnatal urinary incontinence. International Urogynecology Journal 9:257–264

Chapter 11

Evidence for pelvic floor physical therapy for neurological diseases

Marijke Van Kampen

INTRODUCTION

Several neurological disease processes can cause changes in bladder and bowel function and bladder and bowel problems cause much anxiety and may reduce quality of life (Chancellor & Blaivas 1995).

Treatment procedures of neurological patients with genitourinary and bowel problems are largely based on empirical evidence with a limited research base (Chancellor & Blaivas 1995, Harari et al 2004, Leboeuf & Gousse 2004). An assessment of a patient's physical, psychological, cognitive and emotional limitations may influence the treatment strategy. Although many therapeutic options exist, a stepwise approach with initially non-invasive treatment is important considering the course of the disease (Chancellor & Blaivas 1995, Leboeuf & Gousse 2004). The role of pelvic floor physical therapy for bladder and bowel problems in specific neurological diseases has been minimally investigated. Only three randomized controlled studies of pelvic floor physical therapy for patients with stroke and multiple sclerosis (MS) who have urinary incontinence have been published (Tibaek et al 2004, 2005, Vahtera et al 1997). Other neurological pathologies such as spina bifida, syringomyelia, peripheral neuropathies, Parkinson's and Huntington's disease, multiple system atrophy, dementia, spinal cord injuries, disc prolapse and tumours of the spinal cord might be responsible for the development of a neurogenic bladder and bowel dysfunctions. As no studies on evidence for pelvic floor physical therapy in these neurological diseases can be found, this chapter is limited to the treatment of patients with stroke and MS who have genitourinary and/or bowel problems.

Stroke

DEFINITION

Stroke or cerebrovascular accident (CVA) is the clinical manifestation of ischaemia or infarction of brain tissue caused by arterial occlusion, intracerebral and subarachnoid haemorrhage or congenital malformation (Flisser & Blaivas 2004).

INCIDENCE AND PREVALENCE

Each year a typical health authority can expect two new cases of stroke, four recurrent stroke patients and approximately six survivors of stroke living in the community per 1000 men and women (Chancellor & Blaivas 1995).

Urologic and bowel symptoms and urodynamic investigation

Urinary incontinence was reported in 32 to 83% of patients in the early period after stroke. A review of prevalence of incontinence is given by Brittain et al (1998). The natural history of urinary incontinence following stroke is a gradual, spontaneous improvement from 19% at 3 months, 15% at 1 year to 10% at 2 years (Patel et al 2001b). Jorgensen et al (2005) found a prevalence of 17% urinary incontinence among long-term survivors and 7% of control subjects without stroke.

Sakakibara (1996) analysed micturitional histories and urodynamic investigation in 72 stroke patients. A total of 53% of the patients had one or more urinary symptoms within 3 months after stroke: 36% had nocturnal urinary frequency, 29% had urgency incontinence, and 25% difficulty of voiding. Urodynamic investigation shows that initially after stroke, the bladder is often areflexic (Flisser & Blaivas 2004). Detrusor hyperreflexia and urgency incontinence generally follow. Sphincteric incontinence in the recovery phase is normally not a consequence of the stroke, but is almost always a premorbid condition (Flisser & Blaivas 2004).

Fecal incontinence in patients with stroke has been reported in between 23 and 40% of patients on admission and between 7 and 9% 6 months after stroke (Brittain et al 1998, Brocklehurst et al 1985, Nakayama et al 1997).

Initial incontinence is associated with age older than 75 years, visual field defect, dysphagia, motor weakness, severity of stroke, diabetes mellitus, hypertension and comorbidity with other diseases (Gross 2000, Nakayama et al 1997, Patel et al 2001a, Sze et al 2000). Furthermore, urinary incontinence in the acute stage is a predictor of survival and closely associated with severity of disability (Patel et al 2001a). Urinary incontinence emerged as a risk factor for nursing home replacement (Patel et al 2001a, Pettersen et al 2002).

PATHOPHYSIOLOGY

Not all incontinence after stroke is directly related to neurological injury of the micturition pathways. Other mechanisms are general impairment, cognitive deficits and overflow incontinence unrelated to stroke (Flisser & Blaivas 2004). The neurophysiological explanation for detrusor areflexia in the initial phase after stroke is unknown. Detrusor hyperreflexia was noted in lesions of the frontal lobe as well as the basal ganglia. Uninhibited sphincter relaxation is typical for frontal lobe lesions and detrusor sphincter dyssynergia is common in the basal ganglia lesions (Sakakibara et al 1996). The location of the injury, the extent of the damage and the role of the affected area determine the precise urological impact (Flisser & Blaivas 2004).

Physical therapy to strengthen the pelvic floor muscles (PFM) after stroke is aimed at alleviating the problems of urgency, stress and urgency incontinence.

TREATMENT: EVIDENCE FOR EFFECT (PREVENTION AND TREATMENT)

There has been little research into the treatment of urinary and fecal incontinence and constipation in people who have had a stroke. Wikander et al (1998) concluded that incontinence was significantly reduced after a special multidisciplinary programme in comparison with a control group treated with a conventional rehabilitation programme. The special multidisciplinary programme contains physical training (dressing, transfer in hospital and at home with attention to bladder and bowel management), social and cognitive interaction (memory training, problem solving, social inter-action, expression and comprehension). Harari et al (2004) concluded that a single clinical/educational nurse intervention for stroke patients effectively improves bowel dysfunctions up to 6 months later and bowel-modifying lifestyle behaviours up to 12 months later.

The effect of PFM training on incontinence in patients with stroke was evaluated in two randomized control-led studies (RCTs): in fact, it is one RCT study of 26 incontinent women reported in two publications because two different assessment tools were used (Table 11.1). The effect of pelvic floor exercises in women with urinary incontinence after stroke was measured by Quality of life (Qol) parameters (Tibaek et al 2004) and by diary for the frequency of voiding, incontinence epi-sodes and number of pads, 24-hour home pad test and vaginal palpation of PFM (Tibaek et al 2005). The inter-vention included group treatment over 12 weeks com-prising 12–24 standardized pelvic floor exercises. The

control group followed the normal standard programme of rehabilitation without specific treatment of urinary incontinence.

In the first study, the Qol measured with the Short Form 36 Health Survey Questionnaire (SF-36) and Incontinence Impact Questionnaire (IIQ7) did not show significant difference between the two groups after 12 weeks.

In the second study, a significant improvement of frequency of voiding (p = 0.028), 24-hour home pad test (p = 0.013) and endurance of PFM (p = 0.028) was dem-onstrated in the treatment group compared with the control group.

The methodological quality has a score of 6 and 7 out of 10 on the Pedro scale; neither the patients nor the therapist or assessor were blind to the study (Table 11.2). Other limitations of the study are a small sample size (12/14 women in each group). In the first study (Tibaek et al 2004), the instruments to document the effect are

Table 11.1 Randomized controlled studies of physiotherapy for bladder and bowel dysfunctions in neurological patients

Study	Tibaek et al 2004
Design	2-arm RCT: experimental group (E), PFMT; control group(C), no treatment for incontinence
n	26 women (E = 14, C = 12), mean age 60 years (range 56–74) with stroke
Diagnosis	Short Form 36 Health Survey Questionnaire (SF-36) and Incontinence Impact Questionnaire (IIQ7)
Training protocol	E: PFMT: 6-s contraction, 6-s rest, 3-s contraction, 3-s rest, 30-s contraction, 30-s rest; every contraction 4–8× in different positions, group treatment (6–8 patients) 1 h/week during 12 weeks outpatient, vaginal palpation 2–3× over 12 weeks, home exercises 1–2× daily C: no treatment for UI but normal standard programme for rehabilitation
Drop-out	8%
Results	No significant difference between E and C group in SF-36 and IIQ
Study	Tibaek et al 2005
Design	2-arm RCT: experimental group (E) PFMT; control group (C), no treatment for incontinence
n	26 women (E = 14, C = 12), mean age 60 years (range: 56–74) with stroke
Diagnosis	Voiding diary, UI 24-hour pad test, number of pads, digital palpation of pelvic floor muscles
Training protocol	E: PFMT: 6-s contraction, 6-s rest, 3-s contraction, 3-s rest, 30-s contraction, 30-s rest, every contraction 4–8× in different positions, group treatment (6–8 patients) 1 h/week during 12 weeks outpatient, vaginal palpation 2–3× over 12 weeks, home exercises 1–2×/day
Drop-out	8%
Results	Significant difference between E and C group in frequency of voiding (p = 0.028), 24-h home pad test (p = 0.013) and endurance of pelvic floor muscles (p = 0.028)

Table 11.1 Randomized controlled studies of physiotherapy for bladder and bowel dysfunctions in neurological patients—cont'd

Study	Vahtera et al 1997
Design	2-arm RCT: experimental group (E) PFMT and ES; control group (C), no treatment for lower urinary tract dysfunction (LUTS)
n	50 women and 30 men with MS (E = 40, C = 40), mean age 43 years (range: 25–68)
Diagnosis	LUTS by self administered questionnaire, muscle activity by surface EMG BF
Training protocol	E: PFMT – 3-s contraction, 3-s rest (10×) 5-s contraction, 3-s rest (5×) 15-s contraction, 30-s rest (5×), others: 5× in different positions; ES – interferential currents carrier frequency of 2000 Hz treatment frequency of 5–10 Hz, 10–50 Hz and 50 HZ, 10 min of each frequency, 3 min rest; six sessions during 21 days' outpatient; BF, same PFMT after ES during two sessions; home exercises, 20 contractions 3–5×/week during 6 months in sitting and standing position C: no treatment
Drop-out	At 2 months 2/40, at 6 months 3/40 in the E group Not mentioned in control group
Results	Significant difference between E and C group in LUTS (incontinence, nocturia, urge) p < 0.001, Qol (travelling, social shame and need of diapers, muscle activity) p < 0.01

BF, biofeedback; ES, electrical stimulation; LUTS, lower urinary tract symptoms; MS, multiple sclerosis; PFMT, pelvic floor muscle training.

Table 11.2 PEDro quality score of RCTs in systematic review of pelvic floor physiotherapy for neurological diseases

E – Eligibility criteria specified
1 – Subjects randomly allocated to groups
2 – Allocation concealed
3 – Groups similar at baseline
4 – Subjects blinded
5 – Therapist administering treatment blinded
6 – Assessors blinded
7 – Measures of key outcomes obtained from over 85% of subjects
8 – Data analysed by intention to treat
9 – Comparison between groups conducted
10 – Point measures and measures of variability provided

Study	E	1	2	3	4	5	6	7	8	9	0	Total score
Tibaek 2004	+	+	+	+	–	–	–	+	–	+	+	6/10
Tibaek 2005	+	+	+	+	–	–	+	+	–	+	+	7/10
Vahtera 1997	+	+	–	+	–	–	–	–	–	+	+	4/10

+, criterion is clearly satisfied; –, criterion is not satisfied; ?, not clear if the criterion was satisfied. Total score is determined by counting the number of criteria that are satisfied, except that E (eligibility criteria specified) is not used to generate the total score. Total scores are out of 10.

not the optimal choice because the SF-36 gives an indication of general health and the IIQ turned out to be rather insensitive towards women with urgency urinary incontinence. Remarkable is the fact that only 8% of the 339 stroke patients were potential candidates for pelvic floor physical therapy, mostly because of their neurological status (Tibaek et al 2004, 2005).

CLINICAL RECOMMENDATIONS

Clinical recommendations based on current evidence promote pelvic floor exercises to reduce incontinence with special attention to education and improvement of physical functions and social interaction (Tibaek et al 2004, 2005, Wikander et al 1998).

Multiple sclerosis

INTRODUCTION

Definition

MS is caused by inflammatory and demyelinating lesions in the white matter of the brain and spinal cord, leading to a wide variety of neurological deficits (Chancellor & Blaivas 1995).

INCIDENCE AND PREVALENCE

MS has an incidence of approximately 1 new case/10 000 people every year, mostly manifesting between the ages of 20 and 50 years. It is more common in women than men by a ratio of 2 to 1. The prevalence is about 1/1000 in the USA and 2/1000 in North Europe. It is less common in Orientals (Leboeuf & Gousse 2004).

UROLOGICAL AND BOWEL SYMPTOMS

Urological symptoms in MS patients vary greatly from one study to another. Urgency, reported in 24–86% of cases and frequency in 17–82% are the most frequent (Leboeuf & Gousse 2004, Mayo & Chetner 1992). Urgency incontinence is reported in 19–72% while hesitancy and retention occurs in 2–49% (Leboeuf & Gousse 2004, Mayo & Chetner 1992). Constipation occurs in 54% and 29% experience fecal incontinence (Hennessey et al 1999). All these symptoms are rated as the third most important problem in MS after spasticity and incoordination, limiting ability to work (Jawad et al 1999). In men and women with MS not all urological dysfunctions can be presumed to be secondary to MS (Jawad et al 1999). A poor correlation has been found between subjective symptoms and objective urodynamic evaluations (Chancellor & Blaivas 1995).

PATHOPHYSIOLOGY

Damage to the innervation of the lower urinary tract mostly affects the sphincter and the detrusor. Three main types of pattern of urodynamic dysfunction are described:

- detrusor hyperreflexia without bladder outlet obstruction in 26–99% of patients;
- detrusor hyperreflexia with detrusor–external sphincter dyssynergia (DESD) in 23–52%;
- detrusor hypo or areflexia in 6–40% (Chancellor & Blaivas 1995, Gallien et al 1998, Leboeuf & Gousse 2004).

TREATMENT: EVIDENCE FOR EFFECT (PREVENTION AND TREATMENT)

A few authors have investigated physical therapy as a treatment modality in patients with MS but without a control group (De Ridder et al 1999, Klarskov et al 1994, Primus 1992, Skeill & Thorpe 2001, Van Poppel et al 1985) and noted a good subjective improvement in incontinent episodes and pad use after electrical stimulation or biofeedback training. Primus 1992 gave maximal vaginal electrical stimulation to 27 patients with MS and found an initial efficacy of 85%, but a decrease during follow-up to 18% after 3 months. They concluded that long-term treatment is necessary to minimize symptoms in MS. De Ridder et al (1999) offered a practical tool in the selection of patients to predict a good prognosis: pelvic floor physical therapy should be restricted to patients with mild MS, without pelvic floor spasticity or DESD. They designed a digital scoring system for pelvic floor spasticity based on experience:

1. spastic muscle unable to relax even after passive elongation;
2. hypertonic muscle with temporary relaxation after elongation;
3. active relaxation after active contraction.

This digital test has shown inter-examiner reliability (r = 0.90).

Bowel management in patients with MS is empirical with a lack of evidence. Only one study investigated the effect of physical therapy, but without control group. Wiesel et al (2000) offered biofeedback training as treatment to 13 patients with MS complaining of constipation or fecal incontinence. Treatment is more likely to be successful in patients with limited disability and a non-progressive disease course.

Evidence based medicine

Evidence based medicine on MS and pelvic floor physical therapy was limited to one study (see Table 11.1). Vahtera et al (1997) investigated the effect of electrical stimulation (ES) and PFM exercises on lower urinary tract symptoms in patients with MS with near-normal postvoid residual volumes (<100 mL) and mild MS. The control group was not treated or even tested for activity of the pelvic floor. ES with interferential currents in combination with regular PFM exercises significantly improved urgency, frequency, incontinence, nocturia and bladder emptying in comparison with a control group without treatment. ES also significantly improved the maximal strength and endurance of the PFM. Compliance with the PFM exercises was 62.5% after 6 months; others trained irregularly. Three patients relapsed because of bladder symptoms or severe relapses in MS. Men may respond more rapidly to the therapy for incontinence. The symptoms of urgency were relatively easy to reduce in women. The methodological quality of the study was weak. Neither the therapist nor the assessor were blind to the patient and no intention to treat analysis was done (see Table 11.2).

CLINICAL RECOMMENDATIONS

Based on current evidence based on one study ES and PFM exercises in patients with MS decrease urgency, frequency, incontinence, nocturia and improve bladder emptying and PFM activity. Further research will establish the efficacy of these interventions.

CONCLUSION

Conclusions and clinical recommendations on the role of pelvic floor physical therapy for genitourinary and bowel problems in specific neurological diseases such as stroke and MS have to be considered with care because of the lack of good RCTs with a sufficient number of patients.

A significant improvement of incontinence in patients with stroke was demonstrated with a 12-week PFM exercise group treatment while quality of life was the same for both the experimental and control group.

For patients with MS, there was a significant difference in lower urinary tract symptoms and pelvic muscle activity after 3 weeks of ES followed by PFM exercises compared with a control group without specific treatment.

The methodological quality of these three studies is weak to good.

For patients with other neurological disorders, the efficacy of physical therapy has not yet been investigated.

Research on the efficacy and selection criteria for pelvic floor physical therapy is necessary to help prevent urological and bowel complications in neurological patients and improve their quality of life. Future research is being undertaken and studies on patients with stroke, MS and Parkinson's disease are being presented at meetings, but have not yet been published.

REFERENCES

Brittain K, Peet SM, Castleden C M et al 1998 Stroke and incontinence. Stroke 29:524–528

Brocklehurst J C, Andrews K, Richards B et al 1985 Incidence and correlates of incontinence in stroke patients. Journal of the American Geriatrics Society 33:540–542

Chancellor M B, Blaivas J G 1995 Practical neuro-urology. Genitourinary complications in neurologic disease. Butterworth–Heinemann, p 119–137

De Ridder D, Vermeulen C, Ketelaer P et al 1999 Pelvic floor rehabilitation in multiple sclerosis. Acta Neurologica Belgica 99:61–64

Flisser J A, Blaivas J G 2004 Cerebrovascular accidents, intracranial tumors and urologic consequences. In: Corcos J, Schick E Textbook of the neurogenic bladder. Adults and children. Martin Dunitz, London, p 305–313

Gallien P, Robineau S, Nicolas B et al 1998 Vesicourethral dysfunction and urodynamic findings in multiple sclerosis:

a study of 149 cases. Archives of Physical Medicine and Rehabilitation 79: 255–257

Gross J C 2000 Urinary incontinence and stroke outcome. Archives of Physical Medicine and Rehabilitation 81: 22–26

Harari D, Norton C, Lockwood L et al 2004 Treatment of constipation and fecal incontinence in stroke patients. Randomized controlled study. Stroke 35: 2549–2555

Hennessey A, Robertson N P, Swingler R et al 1999 Urinary, faecal and sexual dysfunction in patients with multiple sclerosis. Journal of Neurology 246:1027–1032

Jawad S H, Ward A B, Jones P et al 1999 Study on the relationship between premorbid urinary incontinence and stroke functional outcome. Clinical Rehabilitation 13:447–452

Jorgensen L, Engstad T, Jacobsen B K 2005 Self-reported urinary incontinence in noninstitutionalized long-term stroke survivors: a population-based study. Archives of Physical Medicine and Rehabilitation 86(3):416–420

Klarskov P, Heely E, Nyholdt I et al 1994 Biofeedback treatment of bladder dysfunction in multiple sclerosis: a randomised trial. Scandinavian Journal of Urology and Nephrology 157:61–65

Leboeuf L, Gousse A E 2004 Multiple sclerosis. In: Corcos J, Schick E Textbook of the neurogenic bladder. Adults and children. Martin Dunitz, London p 274–292

Mayo M E, Chetner M P 1992 Lower urinary tract dysfunction in multiple sclerosis. Urology 1:67–70

Nakayama H, Jorgensen H S, Pedersen P M et al 1997 Prevalence and risk factors of incontinence after stroke. The Copenhagen stroke study. Stroke 28:58–62

Patel M, Coshall C, Lawrence E et al 2001a Recovery from poststroke urinary incontinence: associated factors and impact on outcome. Journal of the American Geriatrics Society 49:1229–1233

Patel M, Coshall C, Rudd A G et al 2001b Natural history and effects on 2-year outcomes of urinary incontinence after stroke. Stroke 32:122–127

Pettersen R, Dahl T, Wyller T B 2002 Prediction of long-term functional outcome after stroke rehabilitation. Clinical Rehabilitation 16:149–159

Primus G 1992 Maximal electrical stimulation in neurogenic detrusor hyperactivity: experiences in multiple sclerosis. European Journal of Medicine 1:80–82

Sakakibara R, Hattori T, Yasuda K et al 1996 Micturitional disturbance after acute hemispheric stroke: analysis of the lesion site by CT and MRI. Journal of Neurological Sciences 137:47–56

Skeill D, Thorpe A C 2001 Transcutaneous electrical nerve stimulation in the treatment of neurological patients with urinary symptoms. BJU International 88:899–902

Sze K, Wong E, Or K H et al 2000 Factors predicting stroke disability at discharge: a study of 793 chinese. Archives of Physical Medicine and Rehabilitation 81:876–880

Tibaek S, Gard G, Jensen R 2005 Pelvic floor muscle training is effective in women with urinary incontinence after stroke. A randomised controlled and blinded study. Neurourology and Urodynamics 24(4):348–357

Tibaek S, Jensen R, Lindskov G et al 2004 Can quality of life be improved by pelvic floor muscle training in women with urinary incontinence after ischemic stroke? A randomised controlled and blinded study. International Urogynecology Journal and Pelvic Floor Dysfunction 15:117–123

Vahtera T, Haaranen M, Viramo-Koskela A L et al 1997 Pelvic floor rehabilitation is effective in patients with multiple sclerosis. Clinical Rehabilitation 11:211–219

Van Poppel H, Ketelaer P, Van DeWeerd A 1985 Interferential therapy for detrusor hyperreflexia in multiple sclerosis. Urology 25:607–612

Wiesel P H, Norton C, Roy A J et al 2000 Gut focused behavioural treatment (biofeedback) for constipation and faecal incontinence in multiple sclerosis. Journal of Neurology, Neurosurgery, and Psychiatry 69(2):240–243

Wikander B, Ekelund P, Milsom I 1998 An evaluation of multidisciplinary intervention governed by functional independence measure in incontinent stroke patients. Scandinavian Journal of Rehabilitation Medicine 30:15–21

Chapter 12

Evidence for pelvic floor physical therapy in the elderly

Margaret Sherburn

INTRODUCTION

Population ageing has a great impact on health and societal needs, health systems and disease patterns. In most developed countries of the world populations are ageing, and research into, and the development of age appropriate interventions, is required to meet the growing needs and challenges brought about by population ageing. The major focus of health care for an ageing population must be to ensure an integrated and comprehensive approach to the special needs of older people and their families. This quest for adequate and cost-effective health care for the growing number of older persons has received increased attention from national governments and international organizations. The World Health Organization (WHO) through its Centre for Health Development, Ageing and Health Programme, has initiated studies for the development of community health care models for older and ageing populations. The International Continence Society, in conjunction with the WHO, has also taken an active role in reporting and collating research into the causes and management of incontinence in the elderly through the International Consultation on Incontinence (Abrams et al 2002).

The prevalence of urinary incontinence increases with increasing age, affects women more than men, and is associated with significant personal stress, shame and social stigma (Bogner 2004), with considerable morbidity (Grimby et al 1993) and cost (Fonda 1992). Around one-third of women over 60 years of age are affected (Chiarelli et al 1999). The social and psychological consequences of this problem are such that sufferers reduce their social activity and participation in physical activity, which in turn leads to social isolation and poor health. The incidence of incontinence is expected to increase as populations age and the absolute number of elderly men and women increases worldwide, making incontinence an increasing health problem.

The presence of comorbidities and functional impairments in the elderly can lead practitioners to overlook incontinence and thus preclude its effective treatment. In situations where comorbidities have ceased being life-threatening, continence problems can maintain their lower priority within the frail elderly patient's health management. In particular, with regard to mobility, which decreases with increasing age, it has been shown that there is an association between incontinence and functional impairment, especially mobility impairment (Maggi et al 2001, Thom 1998). However, this association may be complex, and it might be that pre-existing comorbidities can lead to both incontinence and functional impairment independently (Thom 1998). On the other hand, it has been shown that high-intensity muscular training in the frail elderly is effective in reducing functional impairment (Jenkins & Fultz 2005, Fiatarone et al 1994).

There is a strong dose-related response between high-intensity muscular training and strength gains, strength gains and functional improvement (Fiatarone et al 1994, Seynnes et al 2004) and functional improvement and reduced urinary incontinence (Jenkins & Fultz 2005). However, it has not yet been shown whether high-intensity pelvic floor muscle training (PFMT) in the frail elderly is associated with reduced urinary incontinence.

CLASSIFICATION OF INCONTINENCE

Increasing age is not a cause for alteration to the classifications of incontinence. What does change is the prevalence of different types of incontinence. Nocturia, nocturnal polyuria, urgency and urgency incontinence (symptoms of a storage disorder) increase in men and women (Lose et al 2001, Miller 2000, Swithinbank & Abrams 2001), bladder outlet obstruction increases in males (Blanker et al 2000, Diokno et al 1986), and stress urinary incontinence (SUI) decreases relative to other classifications in females (Fonda et al 2002, Simeonova et al 1999).

In addition, in the elderly the underlying causes of incontinence may be unclear due to the presence of comorbidities, which themselves may independently impact on incontinence. Incontinence may be a symptom of for example, Parkinson's disease, multiple sclerosis, diabetes mellitus, dementia or depression, or a side-effect of urinary tract infection, medications, female circumcision or pelvic surgery (Bonita 1998).

Definitions

Definitions of 'elderly' vary within the literature. They depend on the theory of ageing each definition is attempting to explain. A balanced approach to understanding the ageing process can include not only the understanding of the physiological changes that occur, but the social context in which they occur and the attitudinal changes of ageing persons themselves (Stein & Moritz 1999). Health and activity in older age can be therefore a summary of the living circumstances and actions of an individual during a whole life span. This 'life course' conceptual framework considers the influence of modifiable factors of lifestyle, such as not smoking or abusing alcohol, regular exercise, good social supports, and of non-modifiable factors such as economic circumstances and depressive disorders. These factors were shown to be independently predictive of healthy ageing in a 50-year prospective cohort study (Vaillant & Mukamal 2001). Functional status of an individual therefore depends on the interaction of all an individual's life course events and is independent of chronological age (Fig. 12.1).

Chronological age is in fact a very poor indicator of functional status. Individuals of the same age can show a great variability in social, psychological and physical changes. However, as age 65 years is retirement age in many nations, this is the chronological age at which many older age definitions begin. The WHO (Stein &

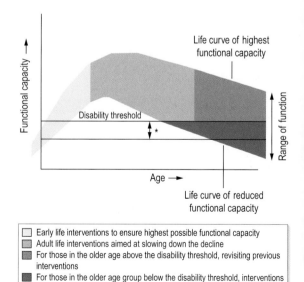

Fig. 12.1 A 'life course' perspective for maintenance of the highest possible level of functional capacity. (From Stein & Moritz 1999, with permission.)

Moritz 1999) uses the 'life course' framework, to define ageing as 'the process of progressive change in the biological, psychological and social structure of individuals' without prescribing any chronological ages associated with this process. When ages are, however, superimposed on this definition, 'mid-life' is defined as beginning at 50 years or after the menopause in women, 'young old' at 60 years and 'very old' at 80+ years (Stein & Moritz 1999).

'Incontinence' as a diagnosis or as a symptom, fits well into the 'life course' model, where comorbidities or life events impact on the course of the disease process or symptoms, and chronological age may not be a significant factor in either symptom presence or severity.

This chapter will focus on incontinence as it relates to the frail or disabled older person. Management of incontinence in young or fit older adults is generally similar to that of young adults, but with due care taken for susceptibility to adverse events, such as altered reaction to medications (Fonda et al 2002). However, frail or disabled older adults have major comorbidities causing functional impairment, such as cognitive, neurological, musculoskeletal, and cardiopulmonary impairments, which will alter incontinence management. Cure for incontinence in the elderly then, as for most other chronic conditions, is the exception rather than the rule. The exclusion of treatable medical conditions, reduction of symptoms and improved quality of life are more achievable and important goals (Ouslander 2000).

PREVALENCE OF INCONTINENCE IN THE ELDERLY

An Australian study reported a prevalence of urinary incontinence of 35% in community-dwelling women aged 70–75 years (Chiarelli et al 1999), which agrees with the prevalence rate of 34% in women who were postmenopausal and over 50 years of age, in a systematic review by Thom (1998). The reported prevalence of urinary incontinence in community-dwelling elderly women in other developed countries is similar: 37.7% in the USA (Herzog et al. 1990), but somewhat lower in the Netherlands at 23.5% (Kok et al 1992), 25–32% in Sweden (Simeonova 1999), and 25% in Norway (Hannestad et al 2000). These differences may be due to different study samples, the type of questionnaires (validated or not), and definitions of incontinence used. The WHO (Stein & Moritz 1999) estimates a prevalence of incontinence of 12% of the total population (i.e. male and female) aged above 75 years in developed countries. For older women reporting daily incontinence prevalence rates have been reported as 14% (Thom 1998) and 18% (Grodstein et al 2003).

Fecal incontinence prevalence rates in the elderly are more difficult to estimate due to a lack of standard definitions of fecal incontinence. Prevalence rates were reported to vary between 5 and 10% in community-dwelling elderly aged over 60 years in The Netherlands (88% response rate) (Teunissen et al 2004). Fecal incontinence rates showed no gender difference, and increased with increasing age for both men and women.

In institutionalized elderly, the prevalence rates of urinary incontinence are even higher and increase to between 50 and 70% in nursing home residents (Sarkar & Ritch 2000). In an Italian study, Aggazzotti et al (2000) found the overall prevalence rate of urinary incontinence in an institutionalized population to be 55%, and higher in institutionalized women (77%) than institutionalized men (60%). These figures increased with:

- increasing age, from 27% in those under 65 years, to 74% in those over 95 years;
- worsening mental status, from 36% if well-orientated to 74% if poorly orientated;
- worsening mobility, from 24% if self-sufficient to 82% if bed-ridden.

Adelmann (2004) in an audit of medical records (n = 910) of community-dwelling elderly poor (aged 65+ years) and of nursing home residents in the same region of the USA, reported a higher rate of urinary incontinence in this low-income population than in the general population. Rates varied between 23% for experiencing urinary incontinence in the previous week, to 42% for experiencing urinary incontinence ever, with prevalence rates for women being significantly higher than for men for all older age groups (65–74 years 34% vs 18%, 75–84 years 45% vs 26%, 85+ years 58% vs 34%). It is interesting to note that the urinary incontinence rates of the community-dwelling group were found to be lower when assessed in a medical setting than when measured by survey self-report.

When considering population differences, there is some disparity in the literature. Duong & Korn (2001) reported higher rates of urgency incontinence in African Americans, whereas Jackson et al (2004) reported higher rates of both stress (OR 4.1, 95% CI 2.5–6.7) and urgency incontinence (OR 3.1, 95% CI 2.0–4.8) in older white Americans. Although an explanation for a population difference is difficult to define, Duong et al question whether it could be related to real or perceived barriers for treatment of urinary incontinence by African Americans, or different causes of urinary incontinence in different populations. Grodstein et al (2003), in the USA Nurses Health Study, surveyed 83 168 professional women aged 50–75 years by mailed questionnaire and found a lower prevalence and severity of urinary incontinence (leaking at least once per month during the previous 12 months) in black (21%), Hispanic (28%) and Asian (26%) women compared with white women (35%), which remained after adjustment for many other risk factors including age, body mass index, parity, comorbidities and functional limitations. Bogner (2004) reported population differences between African and white Americans in the psychological distress caused by urinary incontinence, with black Americans showing higher distress levels, after adjusting for age, gender, education level, activities of daily living (ADL) impairment, mini-mental state examination (MMSE) score and chronic health conditions.

With regards to elderly people seeking assistance for symptoms of incontinence, rates of use of health services have been shown to be consistently low across three nationalities, but higher in one study. Andersson et al (2004) investigated by questionnaire how urinary incontinence affects daily activities and help-seeking behaviours in a Swedish regional population (n = 2129), and found that only 18% of 65–79 year olds requested treatment – those with the worst leakage and level of distress. Hannestad et al (2002) found that only 25% of symptomatic older Norwegian women sought help – again those who were older and with worse symptoms. In the UK, a similar mailed questionnaire to an elderly regional population (n = 915) found that 15% of those with incontinence had used continence services. The most significant factor for continence service usage was being asked about their symptoms by a health professional (OR 15.7, 95% CI 7.3, 33.9). Other significant factors were more severe and bothersome symptoms, and worse general health (Peters et al 2003). These figures were similar to another UK study, in which only 9% of all adults with severe symptoms sought a consultation, which the authors found was associated with an acceptance of incontinence as normal in older women (McGrother et al 2003). However, in an Australian study, 73% of women aged 70–75 years had sought help or advice about their incontinence, and these were women with more severe symptoms (Miller et al 2003).

Although it has been widely stated that having urinary incontinence is a predictor of nursing home admission, few studies confirm this. Holroyd-Leduc & Straus (2004) investigated the relationship of urinary incontinence to key adverse outcomes (death, nursing home admission, functional decline) in 5500 community-dwelling elderly, mean age 77 years (69–103 years), by a baseline interview repeated 2 years later. They concluded that urinary incontinence was not an independent risk factor for these adverse outcomes, but higher

levels of illness severity and functional impairment were.

AETIOLOGY AND PATHOPHYSIOLOGY

Ageing affects the urinary tract in a number of ways, but does not cause incontinence itself (Fonda et al 2002). As prevalence data indicate, not all older people become incontinent. Urogenital symptoms were found to be poorly correlated with age and physical changes on examination in a study of older women who completed a symptom questionnaire before examination at an outpatient clinic (Davila et al 2001). The aetiology of incontinence is a complex interaction of age-related changes and lifestyle factors rather than ageing itself, as described in the 'life course' theory of ageing (see Fig. 12.1, p. 346).

There are differences in causative factors of incontinence in developed and developing countries. In developing countries, problems such as high parity, birthing injuries, circumcision practices and untreated urinary tract infections at a young age lead to incontinence continuing into old age or increase the risk of incontinence developing in older age (Bonita 1998). In developed countries, lifestyle factors such as obesity and lack of exercise leading to a decrease in functional mobility play a larger role (Brown & Miller 2001).

In the elderly, the aetiology of **acute-onset urinary incontinence** can be described according to the DRIP mnemonic:

- D delirium;
- R retention, restricted mobility;
- I infection, inflammation, impaction;
- P polyuria (Timiras & Leary 2003).

Alterantively it can be described according to the DIAPPERS mnemonic:

- D delirium;
- I infection;
- A atrophic urethritis;
- P pharmaceuticals;
- P psychological;
- E excess fluids in/out;
- R restricted mobility;
- S stools/constipation (Fonda et al 2002).

The age-related changes that contribute to **ongoing urinary incontinence** in older adults can be divided into neurogenic and non-neurogenic factors (Corcos & Schick 2001). Neurogenic factors mostly interrupt the central control mechanisms and non-neurogenic factors, the peripheral control mechanisms. Peripheral nerve damage, though neurological, is considered to be non-neurogenic factor because it affects the peripheral control mechansims.

Neurogenic factors

Neurogenic factors are as follows.

1. **Neurological diseases that affect the central control mechanisms**: stroke, brain tumour, Parkinson's disease, multiple sclerosis, diabetes mellitus, cerebral atrophy, dementia, depression (De Ridder et al 1998, Gariballa 2003).

2. **Neurological disorders that affect suprasacral spinal cord pathways**, with deficits affecting both somatic and autonomic nervous systems: multiple sclerosis, dorsal column neuropathies, spinal cord injury (Blok et al 1997) leading to sphincter dyssynergia through upper motor neuron damage, or conversely sphincter underactivity via sympathetic dysfunction (Corcos & Schick 2001).

3. **Progressive sympathetic nervous system activation**: occurs in older age and may be a causal component in urinary tract pathophysiology, though the underlying central nervous system mechanisms mediating this increase in activity are unknown (Esler et al 2002).

Non-neurogenic factors

Non-neurogenic factors contributing to incontinence in the elderly as follows.

- **Peripheral nerve root compression (S2–S4)** from musculoskeletal injury or degeneration, leading to decreased lower limb mobility, impaired sensation and reflexes, and PFM and striated sphincter weakness (Corcos & Schick 2001).

- **Ageing urinary tract:**
    1. **Bladder**: detrusor smooth muscle changes lead to detrusor overactivity or conversely detrusor underactivity, reduced flow rate and risk of post-void residual urine. Yoshida et al (2001, 2004) investigated changes to detrusor neurotransmitters with increasing age. They showed that purinergic neurotransmission increased with age, whereas cholinergic transmission decreased with age, most likely as a result of decreased release of acetylcholine (ACh) from parasympathetic nerves supplying the detrusor and from the urothelium (non-neuronal ACh). The authors suggest that these factors could be contributors to bladder overactivity. Conversely, detrusor compliance can decrease with ageing due to replacement of smooth muscle with fibrous tissue and scarring from radiation, infection or inflammation. Rather than a high vesical pressure leading to a stronger detrusor to overcome this, a slower speed of detrusor contraction and a low flow rate is the result during voiding (Schafer 1999).
    2. **Sphincter integrity**, in both smooth and striated muscle sphincters. In an intraurethral ultrasound investigation, Klauser et al (2004) found that with increasing age, the striated urethral sphincter showed a linear decline in thickness and ability to produce urethral closure pressure. In ageing paraurethral tissue, the connective tissue component has been shown to increase, altering in composition to be more fibrous relative to other components, and show a decrease in the vascularity of the mucosa and urethral nerve supply (Verelst et al 2002). With regard to decreased urethral muscle function, Perucchini et al (2002a) showed a decline in the number of striated muscle fibres, fibre density and total cross-sectional area of striated muscle in a dissection study of the anterior and posterior walls of the urethra in 25 female cadavers aged 15–80 years. A seven-fold variance was seen, however, between the specimens with the most and fewest muscle fibres anteriorly, and localized losses were found in the proximal posterior striated sphincter muscles (Perucchini et al 2002b).
    3. **PFM ageing and atrophic changes**: a full discussion of the effects of ageing and disuse on skeletal muscle is beyond the scope of this chapter and readers are referred to a physiology text for full details (Powers & Howley 2001). Changes in ageing muscle occur in endocrine, neural, enzymatic and energy systems, possibly genetically driven, and result in a decrease in muscle mass by fibre, vascular and mitochondrial degradation and loss. There is a paucity of research on the topic of age-related changes specific to the PFM. Concurrent ageing changes in smooth muscle and connective tissue of the pelvic floor may multiply the dysfunction associated with the sarcopenia of ageing (Powers & Howley 2001, p. 145). The changes in muscle due to disuse and ageing are very similar, so it is difficult to separate these factors in ageing research. Gunnarsson & Mattiason (1999) using surface electromyography (EMG), showed that older women without incontinence did not show as much of a decline in PFM strength, as women with SUI or urgency or mixed incontinence. Their results showed that neuromuscular changes in the pelvic floor are progressive and present for a long time before symptoms appear.

However, Constantinou et al (2002), using magnetic resonance imaging (MRI) showed that older women displaced the pelvic floor significantly less than younger women on voluntary contraction. They stated this could be due to decreased PFM strength, neuronal factors or fat deposition in pelvic spaces, restricting free movement. Dimpfl et al (1998) showed histomorphological changes in the PFM in older women compared to women under 40 years, such as decreased fibre circumference and fibrosis.

4. **Ageing changes and loss of integrity in the fascial supports of the urinary tract**: ageing connective tissue shows evidence of fewer and more immature collagen cross-linkages, resulting in a two- to three-fold reduction in the maximum load to failure, decreased plasticity and elasticity (Frankel & Nordin 1980 p. 101).

- **Obesity**: in a study of postmenopausal women, the odds ratio was found to be 1.5 (95% CI 1.15–1.95) of having symptoms of urinary incontinence with a body mass index (BMI) above 26 (Sherburn et al 2001). If high BMI is paralleled with a decrease in physical activity, renal function is altered and sympathetic nervous system activity is increased, though the implications of this alteration for the urinary system are still unclear (Esler et al 2002).

- **Other aetiologies**:
  1. **Side-effects** of prescription and over-the-counter drugs.
  2. **Social and environmental status**, relating to the availability of a carer and social supports: living at home alone, with partner, living in an adult child's home, residential aged care, nursing home.
  3. **Disturbance of the vasopressin system, or diseases causing a shift in diuresis**: diseases such as diabetes mellitus, congestive heart failure and sleep apnoea cause a shift in diuresis from daytime to night (i.e. nocturnal polyuria [Asplund 2004]).

- **Functional impairment**: of the above risk factors for both urinary and anal incontinence, the single most important factor may be functional impairment (Harari et al 2003). Functional impairment is the difference between environmental demand and functional capability (Eekhof et al 2000), and can be modified by treatable factors such as intercurrent illnesses, medications, nutritional status, vision and hearing status, mobility and dexterity, pain, anxiety and depression (Harari et al 2003). Within functional impairment, strength impairment and lower limb mobility are the critical domains (Jenkins & Fultz

2005) for predicting urinary incontinence. In stroke, functional impairment, particularly needing help to access the toilet, is the strongest independent factor associated with new-onset fecal incontinence after a stroke (Harari et al 2003).

Factors in females

Factors in females are:

- becoming estrogen deficient postmenopausally (Davila et al 2003, Schaffer & Fantl 1996);
- high parity (Simeonova et al 1999);
- certain types of intrapelvic surgery including hysterectomy (Sherburn et al 2001);
- female circumcision (Stein & Moritz 1999).

Becoming estrogen deficient leads to:

- loss of collagen, thinning epithelium in vagina, caused by decreased collagen synthesis (Falconer et al 1996) and increased collagenase activity (Kushner et al 1999);

- decreased vascular plexi in the submucosa of the urethra – this submucosal vascular bed gives passive urethral control and loss can lead to a loss of up to 30% of urethral closure pressure (Corcos & Schick 2001);

- less acidic urethral and vaginal environments (increased pH), leading to changes in the vaginal flora and more risk of colonization with Gram-negative bacteria, which in turn leads to a higher risk of atrophic vaginitis and urinary tract infections. (Bachmann & Nevadunsky 2000, Nilsson et al 1995, Notelovitz 1995, Samsioe 1998).

Factors in males

Factors in males are increased prostatic size in:

- benign prostatic hyperplasia (BPH) (Blanker et al 2000, Madersbacher et al 1999);
- prostatic carcinoma.

In BPH, the outer zones of the prostate progressively atrophy while the inner zones begin to grow again until death. In carcinoma, the outer glandular epithelium enlarges. This leads to:

- impaired urinary flow;
- strangulation of the urethra;
- urinary retention;
- urinary frequency;
- detrusor overactivity;
- incomplete emptying and retrograde filling of the ureters (Timiras & Leary 2003).

Treatment of these disorders by prostatectomy, whether simple, radical or transurethral, carries a risk of urethral vascular bed destruction and nerve damage, even in 'nerve sparing' surgery (Corcos & Schick 2001).

Defecatory dysfunction

Defecatory dysfunction in the elderly has many risk factors, including lifestyle issues such as lack of mobility, inadequate fluid and fibre intake, common medications, and systemic diseases such as diabetes mellitus, neuromuscular diseases and psychiatric disorders. Epidemiological risk factors are increasing age, being female, and low socioeconomic status (Cundiff et al 2000).

Functional obstruction can be caused by pelvic floor dysfunction, including rectocoele, enterocoele, perineal descent and anismus, and disorders of colonic motility (Cundiff et al 2000). In a review into constipation, irritable bowel syndrome and diverticulosis in the ageing gastrointestinal tract, the prevalence of constipation and diverticulosis were found to be greater in the elderly, but the aetiology was unclear. The authors suggest that the ageing changes of increased fibrous connective tissue within the gut wall and a decreased neural supply to the colon are likely causes (Camilleri et al 2000). On high spatial resolution endoanal MRI in normal ageing in continent elderly, Rociu et al (2000) found there was a thinning of the external anal sphincter and longitudinal muscle of the anus, and compensatory thickening of the internal anal sphincter.

EVIDENCE FOR EFFECT OF PFMT IN PREVENTION OF URINARY INCONTINENCE IN THE ELDERLY

The National Library of Medicine, Cinahl, Cochrane and PEDro databases were searched for evidence from randomized controlled trials (RCT) of effectiveness of interventions in the elderly. A PEDro assessment of quality was undertaken for all RCTs cited in this chapter. Clinical Practice Guidelines (AHCQ, USA), and the International Consultation on Incontinence have been used as background sources.

Prevention can occur at three levels (Hay-Smith et al 2002) – primary, secondary and tertiary.

Primary prevention – removing the cause

Primary health care models that aim to educate and alter behaviour may be particularly appropriate at this level. Reducing functional impairment, particularly mobility and strength impairments, from encouraging an active lifestyle in the young old to prescribing walking aids or grab bars in the frail old may be appropriate preventative interventions (Jenkins & Fultz 2005). Vaillant & Mukamal (2001) in their longitudinal study of ageing suggest that 'good' and 'bad' ageing in the 70–80 decade could be predicted by variables assessed before age 50 and addressed at that stage.

Secondary prevention – detecting asymptomatic dysfunction and treat early to prevent symptoms

A Dutch study that investigated the effect of a preventative screening programme for urinary incontinence in 1121 subjects over the age of 75 years from 12 general practices, found that early screening and detection did not result in a measurable effect in reduction of prevalence of urinary incontinence compared to the control group who did not receive the preventative screening. The authors recommended that preventative assessment of the elderly is individually targeted, started before the age of 75 years and offered in the primary health care setting (Eekhof et al 2000). A Canadian study confirmed a need for preventative screening in the 55–74-year age group of women (Tannenbuam & Mayo 2003). A systematic review of physical therapies for prevention of urinary and faecal incontinence (Hay-Smith et al 2002) failed to find evidence for the use of PFM exercises in the prevention of urinary incontinence in adults, but not specifically in older adults. However, the reviewers found that of the 15 trials available for review, 14 included patients with and without incontinence symptoms at recruitment, so were therefore not strictly preventative trials.

Diokno et al (2004) reported the results of an RCT of a preventative behavioural modification programme in a group of continent older women, aged 55 years and over (Tables 12.1 and 12.2). The intervention consisted of a 2-hour classroom presentation, and an individual session 2–4 weeks later to reinforce the home programme, measure PFM strength per vaginum and check bladder training concepts. The main outcome measure of number of incontinent episodes per year measured via a validated questionnaire showed that this programme was significantly effective in maintaining continence in the treatment group compared to the control group (OR 1.97, 95% CI 1.15, 3.38, p = 0.01). In addition, voiding frequency significantly decreased, PFM strength significantly increased, and all improvements remained at 12 months after the intervention.

Table 12.1 Studies assessing the effect of conservative interventions (screening, BMP) for prevention of UI in the elderly

Study	Eekhof et al 2000
Design	2-arm RCT: 1. control (n = 738), no health screening year 1, screening & treatment year 2; 2. intervention (n = 732) screening & treatment for UI years 1 & 2
n	1470 men and women over 75 years of age from GP practices
Outcome variables	Self-report of urine loss more than 2× per month
Intervention protocol	1. No screening. 2. Screening for UI, then appropriate treatment by GP or referral.
Drop-outs/adherence	357/1470 (24%) withdrawals (134 control, 113 intervention) Adverse events stated Not ITT analysis
Results	**Mean (95%CI) UI** 1. Control group Y2 31.1 (27.6, 34.6) p = 0.89 2. Intervention Y1 31.5 (28.0, 35.0) Y2 30.6 (26.3, 34.9) p = 0.68
Study	Diokno et al 2004
Design	2 arm RCT: 1. control (n = 195), no treatment; 2. intervention (n = 164), BMP
n	359 community-dwelling, continent, postmenopausal women 55–80 years
Outcome variables	Incontinence episodes PFM strength Voiding frequency Intervoid interval
Intervention protocol	1. No intervention, 3-monthly phone calls to 12 months 2. 2-hour group education session, individual session 2–4 weeks later, PFMT daily with audiotape, BT if required from baseline evaluation, 3-monthly phone calls to 12 months
Drop-outs/adherence	41/359 withdrawals (18 control, 24 intervention) Adverse events stated
Results	**Intervention vs control** Incontinence episodes same/better OR (p value): 1.86 (0.01) PFM strength ±SE (p value): lift 0.42 ± 0.10 (<0.0001); pressure 0.43 ± 0.11 (0.00) 24-h frequency ±SE (p value): 1.27 ± 0.16 (<0.0001) Intervoid interval ±SE (p value): 0.51 ± 0.09 (<0.0001)

BMP, behavioural modification programme; BT, bladder training; ITT, intention to treat; PFM, pelvic floor muscle; PFMT, pelvic floor muscle training; UI, urinary incontinence.

Table 12.2 Studies assessing the effect of conservative interventions (screening, BMP) for prevention of UI in the elderly: PEDro quality score of RCTs

E – Eligibility criteria specified
1 – Subjects randomly allocated to groups
2 – Allocation concealed
3 – Groups similar at baseline
4 – Subjects blinded
5 – Therapist administering treatment blinded
6 – Assessors blinded
7 – Measures of key outcomes obtained from over 85% of subjects
8 – Data analysed by intention to treat
9 – Comparison between groups conducted
10 – Point measures and measures of variability provided

Study	E	1	2	3	4	5	6	7	8	9	10	Total score
Eekhof et al 2000	+	+	−	+	−	−	?	−	−	+	+	4/10
Diokno et al 2004	+	+	+	+	−	−	−	+	?	+	+	6/10

+, criterion is clearly satisfied; −, criterion is not satisfied; ?, not clear if criterion was satisfied. Total score is determined by counting the number of criteria that are satisfied, except that the scale item 1E (eligibility criteria specified) is not used to generate the total score.

Tertiary prevention – treatment of existing symptoms to prevent progression of disease

In a Cochrane review, Hay-Smith et al (2002) found no studies of the elderly available for inclusion, and concluded that there is little evidence for tertiary prevention. Studies of treatment effects are included below.

A pertinent statistic needs to be mentioned at this point. In 1985, prevalence rates of urinary incontinence in nursing homes were estimated as 50%, and in 2001 as 55% (Palmer 2002). After nearly 20 years of research, preventative measures have not altered these prevalence rates. Much more emphasis on prevention research is needed with findings then implemented.

EVIDENCE FOR EFFECT OF PFMT

In examining the evidence for the effect of treatment of urinary incontinence in the frail elderly, there is little validated research showing long-term efficacy of treatment and few outcome measures have been validated in the elderly population (Fonda et al 1998). Cure or dryness may be achieved using different measures of success than those used for a younger population. 'Independent continence' may be the desired outcome, but 'dependent continence' (dry with the assistance or reminders of a carer) or 'social continence' (dry with the use of appropriate aids and devices) can be achieved with suitable management.

No matter what level of continence is achieved, outcome measures need to be defined. The International Continence Society (ICS) Standardization Committee recommends that outcome measures specific to frail elderly people should be described in the same categories as for all adults as follows:

1. **patient observations and symptoms** (e.g. patient and care giver report of symptom response);
2. **documentation of the symptoms** (e.g. bladder diaries, wet checks, pad weigh tests).
3. **anatomical and functional measures** (e.g. urodynamics, postvoid residual, PFM strength, timed up and go [TUG] test) (Podsiadlo & Richardson 1991);
4. **quality of life** (e.g. condition-specific and generic measurement, validated for elderly populations).
5. socioeconomic measures (e.g. cost, cost–benefit, cost-effectiveness) (Fonda et al 1998).

This Standardization Committee commented that while PFM training 'may be of value in the management of incontinence in the frail elderly . . . there are no validated data on the measurement of PFM strength before and after treatment as a useful outcome measure for frail older patients' (Fonda et al 1998). This situation has changed now as physiotherapists around the world engage in validation and reliability studies of their muscle measurement instruments. However, physiotherapists must be aware of the limitations of their instruments for measuring PFM activity, and continue to submit new and old muscle measurement instruments to testing in the frail elderly population (Bø & Sherburn 2005).

As first-line therapy for conservative management, PFM re-education and lifestyle education by physiotherapists are frequently recommended. A Cochrane review (Hay-Smith et al 2001) concluded that PFMT was an effective treatment for women with SUI and mixed incontinence, but all but two of the studies in this review investigated PFMT in groups of women with a wide range of ages. This review therefore provided no strong evidence for the effectiveness of this intervention in elderly women. When available data regarding conservative management in adults are stratified by age, they do not take into account comorbidities associated with older age. Therefore, for many interventions, it is not known whether age or comorbidities affect the treatment outcomes, or whether the benefits of different interventions are applicable to the elderly. To investigate whether age was a factor in being able to successfully achieve continence after a PFMT programme, Truijen et al (2001) performed a retrospective analysis of 104 women (mean 55 years, 28–79 years) who had achieved continence after PFMT compared to those who had not. After multiple regression analysis, they showed that the possibility of achieving continence after PFMT did not depend on age, but urethral hypermobility, previous surgery for incontinence, high BMI and strong PFM before treatment.

Specific evidence for the management of incontinence related to older men following prostatic surgery is covered in Ch. 14.

SPECIFIC TREATMENTS

Functional activity training

Senescence brings changes that limit muscle mass and strength. However, progressive resistance training has been shown to be effective in improving strength and functional mobility in older populations. Many exercise programmes for elderly populations, however, focus on flexibility and light aerobic exercise with low-dose resistance training, despite growing evidence for progressive resistance training being effective in this population (Fiatarone et al 1994). Skeletal muscle adapts to the demands made on it, and effective conditioning of

any muscle group results from sufficient loading of the muscle, duration and frequency of training, and adherence to a training programme (ACSM 1990). This potential for improvement is often overlooked because of clinicians' tendency to underestimate the plasticity of the muscular system and a fear of worsening a person's comorbidities.

A recent RCT between a flexibility programme and a progressive resistance programme of 10 weeks' duration, both groups being a 1-hour class, twice weekly in a community setting (n = 40, mean age 68 years), found a significant difference on multivariate analysis of variance (MANOVA) between groups on lower and upper limb muscle strength and gait and balance parameters at the end of the programme in favour of the progressive resistance training group (Barrett & Smerdely 2002) (Tables 12.3 and 12.4). Although functional mobility changes were the outcomes measured in this study, rather than measurement of continence status, Jenkins & Fultz (2005) have recently reported a strong association between functional improvement and reduced urinary incontinence.

In a frail nursing home population (n = 190, mean age 88 years, in four nursing homes), Schnelle et al (2002) showed that even a low-intensity functional exercise (rather than PFM exercise) and prompted voiding programme was successful in improving mobility endurance, physical activity, limb strength, and decreasing leakage episodes compared to those who received normal nursing home care, though it raised issues of costs and staffing for such a programme to be maintained in this frail institutionalized population. Subjects were guided, with minimal assistance, through repetitions of sit-to-stand, arm curls and/or arm raises, and walking or wheeling their chairs. Their exercise target goals were reset weekly. Despite the activity dosage in this study being a low intensity, good adherence was maintained by the intervention being instituted with prompted toileting and fluid intake at 2-hourly intervals during the daytime for 8 months.

PFMT alone or within a 'package' of treatment

One recent study only was found investigating PFMT in a frail elderly population (McDowell et al 1999). All other studies that follow show some evidence for the effectiveness of PFMT in an elderly population, but not with the addition of frailty. Whether these results can be extrapolated to a frail population will only be known when the impact of specific comorbidities on incontinence, and of those comorbidities that are most amenable to PFMT, is better understood. It should also be noted that PFMT is only suitable as a

Table 12.3 Studies assessing the effect of functional resistance training, PFMT with or without ES, or ES alone, for the treatment of UI in the elderly

Study	Barrett & Smerdely 2002
Design	2-arm RCT: 1. flexibility exercise group (n = 22); 2. progressive resistance training group (n = 22)
n	44 healthy men and women >60 years
Outcome variables	Quadriceps strength Biceps strength Sit to stand Functional reach Step test 10 m fast walk SF36
Intervention protocol	Both groups: 1-h group exercise 2×/week, for 10 weeks. 1. Stretches, light CV work, low intensity strengthening 2. Warm-up, free weights work, stretches
Drop-out/adherence	4/44 withdrawals (2 from each group) Adverse events stated ITT analysis
Results	**% change difference control vs intervention, (95% CI%), MANOVA p value** Quadriceps strength: 7.7% (3.6, 11.8%), $p < 0.003$ Biceps strength: 15.2% (11.7, 19.2%), $p < 0.003$ Functional reach: 11.7%, (7.1, 16.3%), $p < 0.003$ Step test: 8.6% (3.8, 13.4%), $p < 0.003$ Other measures did not reach significance
Study	Burns et al 1990
Design	3-arm RCT: 1. control (n = 40); 2. PFMT (n = 38); 3. PFMT + BFB (n = 40)
n	135, community-dwelling women, UD proven SUI or mixed UI, >3 losses/week, MMSE >23
Outcome variables	Incontinent episodes sEMG of PFM (μv) Maximal UCP (cmH$_2$O)
Intervention protocol	1. Not stated 2. Home PFMT, fast and slow contractions, weekly clinic visits for 8 weeks 3. Weekly group therapy, BFB with vaginal electrodes, observing screen display of PFMT for 8 weeks
Drop-out/adherence	14/135 for incontinent episodes, 17/135, for sEMG, 48/135 for max UCP scores Adverse events not stated Not ITT analysis
Results	**% change, (p values) ANOVA** Incontinent episodes: Control vs PFMT vs BFB: 9% increase vs 54% decrease vs 61% decrease ($p < 0.001$ control vs other 2 groups) sEMG: Control vs PFMT NS ($p < 1$), BFB significant improvement vs control ($p < 0.007$) and PFMT ($p < 0.005$) MUCP: no differences between all groups for UCPs

Table 12.3 Studies assessing the effect of functional resistance training, PFMT with or without ES, or ES alone, for the treatment of UI in the elderly—cont'd

Study	Fiatarone et al 1994
Design	4-arm RCT: 1. control (n = 25); 2. progressive resistance training (n = 25); 3. training plus nutrient supplementation (n = 25); 4. nutrient supplementation (n = 25)
n	100 aged care facility residents, 70+ years, stable health, walk 6 m, cognitively intact
Outcome variables	Muscle strength Spontaneous activity Gait velocity Body composition Balance, (not reported) Muscle function (overall combination factor, not reported)
Intervention protocol	1. Recreational gentle exercises 2. High-intensity muscle training at 80% of 1 MVC for 10 weeks, three sessions of 45 min/week plus placebo supplement 3. Training plus 240 mL liquid nutritional supplement daily 4. Daily supplement alone
Drop-out/adherence	6/100 withdrawals (3 training, 2 supplement, 1 control) Adverse events stated ITT analysis
Results	**Mean (SE), p value ANOVA, 1 vs 2 vs 3 vs 4** % change in muscle strength (approximate values from graphical report): 13 (12) vs 94 (12) vs 123 (23) vs 8 (14), p = 0.001 **% change spontaneous activity counts:** 2.6 (18.1) vs 51.0 (18.4) vs 17.6 (18.9) vs 6.7 (17.3), p = 0.03 **% change gait velocity:** 7.2 (5.4) vs 8.6 (5.5) vs 14.9 (5.7) vs 5.2 (5.6), p = 0.02 **% change body composition:** 0.5 (0.4) vs 0.4 (0.6) vs 1.8 (0.6) vs 1.5 (0.7), p = 0.19
Study	Fonda et al 1995
Design	2-arm RCT: 1. intervention, conservative continence management (n = 38); 2. delayed intervention (n = 35)
n	73 community-dwelling men and women >60 years with UI of >2 months, stable health
Outcome variables	Bladder diary including: incontinence episodes, deferral >5 min Self-report cure or improvement (not defined) QoL (non-validated questionnaire)
Intervention protocol	1. Delayed treatment for 2 months, then 2. 'Package' of treatment including bladder training, PFMT, continence advice and/or aids for 2 months
Drop-out/adherence	14/73 Adverse events stated Not ITT analysis

Table 12.3 Studies assessing the effect of functional resistance training, PFMT with or without ES, or ES alone, for the treatment of UI in the elderly—cont'd

Results	**Control vs intervention** N (%), Chi square p value. Incontinence >1/day: 64 (87.7%) vs 26 (44.1%). p < 0.001 Deferral: 5 (15.2) vs 23 (39.0), p < 0.01 Self-report cure/improved: 52 (88.1%) QoL: variably significant results for different domains
Study	Schnelle et al 2002
Design	2-arm RCT: 1. control (n = 96) normal care; 2. functional incidental training programme (n = 94)
n	190, institutionalized elderly, incontinent, but not catheterized, able to follow a 1-step command
Outcome variables	Metres walked or wheeled Independent standing 30 s Arm raises, arm curls Voiding frequency Toileting ratio; wetting episodes as ratio of number of daily voids
Intervention protocol	1. Control: normal nursing home continence and functional activity care 2. 2-hourly toilet prompting and functional activity routine, up to 4×/day, 5 days/week, for 32 weeks, including one set of arm exercises when supine
Drop-out/adherence	42/190 withdrawals (22 control, 20 intervention) Adverse events stated Partial ITT analysis
Results	**Repeated measures ANOVA for group by time differences, paired t-tests, p values** All measures were significantly improved at either 0.05 or 0.01 level. Control group declined on walking, wheeling and standing measures; significant differences on these measures represent prevention of decline
Study	Spruijt et al 2003
Design	2-arm RCT: 1. control (n = 11), daily home PFMT after correct performance; 2. intervention (n = 24), alternate days in clinic electrical stimulation
n	37 community-dwelling women over 65 years with UI >3 months
Outcome variables	48-h pad test leakage (g) PFM strength, manometry (mmHg) DI on urodynamics (>15 cmH$_2$O) Subjective improvement
Intervention protocol	1. Daily PFMT at home for 8 weeks 2. Stimulation at 50 Hz (stress UI) or 20 Hz (mixed or urge UI), for 2 s, duty cycle 1–2 s, at tolerable comfort (0–100 mA) for 30 min, 3×/week for 8 weeks
Drop-out/adherence	2/37 (1 from each group) Adverse events stated
Results	**Control vs intervention % change (p value)** 48-h pad test: 36.4 vs 29.2 (0.08) PFM strength: 70.8 vs 44.4 (0.25) DI: 22.2 vs 28.6 (0.85) Subjective improvement: 45.8 vs 45.4 (0.89)

Table 12.3 Studies assessing the effect of functional resistance training, PFMT with or without ES, or ES alone, for the treatment of UI in the elderly—cont'd

Study	Wells et al 1991
Design	2-arm RCT: 1. control (n = 75); α-adrenergic agonist (PPA); 2. intervention PFMT (n = 82)
n	157 community-dwelling women, 55–90 years with urodynamic SUI
Outcome variables	Self-report UI status Leakage episodes PFM strength, digital examination PFM EMG (μv) Cough stress test, standing and lying Adherence, exercise diary
Intervention protocol	1. PPA: 50 mg daily for 2 weeks increasing to twice daily for 2 weeks 2. PFMT: 90–160 contractions, held 10 s, relax 10 s, daily for 6 months, monthly clinic visits
Drop-out/adherence	39/157 (11 from PPA, 28 from PFMT) (p < 0.01) Adverse events stated Not ITT analysis
Results	**Control: intervention (p value)** PFM digital strength 1.54: 1.26 (0.05) Leakage episodes: no difference Cough stress test standing and lying: no difference PFM EMG endurance time and peak, mean endurance, mean fast contractions: no difference

ANOVA, analysis of variance; BFB, biofeedback; DI, detrusor instability; ES, electrical stimulation; ITT, intention to treat; MANOVA, multivariate analysis of variance; MMSE, mini-mental state examination; MUCP, maximum urethral closure pressure; MVC, maximal voluntary contraction; PFM, pelvic floor muscle; PFMT, pelvic floor muscle training; PPA, phenylpropanolamine; QoL, quality of life; sEMG, surface electromyography; SUI, stress urinary incontinence; UI, urinary incontinence.

treatment for those who have the cognitive ability to undertake and adhere to an exercise and/or bladder training programme.

In the prospective RCT by McDowell et al (1999), a crossover design of homebound elderly with high levels of comorbidities (n = 105, mean age 77 years), the authors found a statistically and clinically significant decrease in both urge and stress accidents (74% reduction) as recorded on bladder diaries immediately after 8 weeks of PFMT with biofeedback. Exercise adherence was the best predictor of success in this study. These results however are short term due to the crossover design of the study, and are limited by the lack of intention-to-treat analysis and a 19% drop-out rate. Weinberger et al (1999), however, reported that elderly incontinent women (mean age 76 ± 8 years) derive long-term clinical benefit from non-surgical incontinence therapy (mailed questionnaire follow-up at 21 ± 8 months post-intervention), and that the overall likelihood of improvement was greatest in participants with the most severe incontinence at baseline. They included PFMT with or without biofeedback, bladder training, education and lifestyle management, oestrogen replacement, functional electrical stimulation and pharmacological therapy in their 'package' of interventions. At follow-up, participants reported that PFMT, delayed voiding and caffeine restriction were the most effective interventions within the 'package'.

A review of other studies that used PFMT as an intervention (Berghmans et al 1998), found improvement in incontinence symptoms with PFMT, but to a varying extent. Therefore the evidence for the effectiveness of PFMT in the elderly is not strong. Variations in the size and significance of this effect are due to variations in the training protocol, methods and instruments for measuring the change in muscle, inadequate power in the study, and whether the 'control' group of the study was also an active treatment.

Table 12.4   Studies assessing the effect of functional resistance training, PFMT with or without ES, or electrical stimulation alone, for the treatment of UI in the elderly: PEDro quality score of RCTs

E – Eligibility criteria specified
1 – Subjects randomly allocated to groups
2 – Allocation concealed
3 – Groups similar at baseline
4 – Subjects blinded
5 – Therapist administering treatment blinded
6 – Assessors blinded
7 – Measures of key outcomes obtained from over 85% of subjects
8 – Data analysed by intention to treat
9 – Comparison between groups conducted
10 – Point measures and measures of variability provided

Study	E	1	2	3	4	5	6	7	8	9	10	Total score
Barrett & Smerdely 2002	+	+	+	+	−	−	+	+	+	+	+	8/10
Burns et al 1990	+	+	−	+	−	−	+	+	−	+	+	6/10
Fiatarone et al 1994	+	+	−	+	−	−	+	+	+	+	+	7/10
Fonda et al 1995	+	+	+	−	−	−	−	−	−	+	−	3/10
Schnelle et al 2002	+	+	−	+	−	−	+	+	−	+	+	6/10
Spruijt et al 2003	+	+	?	+	−	−	?	+	−	+	−	4/10
Wells et al 1991	+	+	−	+	−	−	−	−	−	+	−	3/10

+, criterion is clearly satisfied; −, criterion is not satisfied; ?, not clear if criterion was satisfied. Total score is determined by counting the number of criteria that are satisfied, except that the scale item 1E (eligibility criteria specified) is not used to generate the total score.

In 1990, Burns et al undertook a RCT to compare PFMT with or without EMG biofeedback to a control group, in a population of community-dwelling older women (n = 118, mean 62 years) with urodynamically proven SUI. The exercise protocol was maintained at home for 8 weeks with weekly visits for evaluation of progress or biofeedback training. Their results showed significant decrease in the number of leakage episodes for both intervention groups compared to the control group (F[2,118] = 15.60, p = 0.001), with the addition of EMG biofeedback significantly improving EMG readings for 'fast' contractions but not for those held for 3 seconds.

Wells et al (1991) compared PFMT to an α-adrenergic agonist in an RCT of 157 women between 55 and 90 years (mean 66 years). The exercise group performed daily muscle awareness, strength and functional protocol for 6 months (drop-outs 34%) while the pharmacological group took the medication for up to 4 weeks (drop-outs 15%). Muscle strength was measured on a five-point scale by digital vaginal testing and by intravaginal EMG (μv), by non-blinded assessors. Both pharmacology and PFMT improved incontinence similarly, but PFM strength was found to be significantly better for the exercise group. The authors suggest that those participants who performed higher levels of exercise (>80 contractions/day) produced better, though not significant, results on continence measures, and that further investigation into exercise adherence was required.

When vaginal electrical stimulation was compared to PFMT in a study of elderly women of mean age 73 (65–92 years) by Spruijt et al (2003), it was found that while the effectiveness of alternate day electrical stimulation was similar to daily PFMT over 8 weeks in the small numbers (n = 37) enrolled in the study, electrical stimulation had too high an emotional and physical cost in this elderly group for the study to continue.

Bladder or behavioural training

Much has been written about the effects of bladder or behavioural training in the elderly, because this intervention lends itself well to modification according to the cognitive ability of the patient, and is a common intervention for managing incontinence in aged care facilities. Bladder training can be modified to become habit retraining, prompted voiding or timed voiding depending on the level of continence being aimed for (i.e. dependent continence or social continence). It has been the subject of four Cochrane reviews (Eustice et al 2000, Ostaszkiewicz et al 2004a, 2004b, Wallace et al 2000) and its effect has been compared to other forms of treatment, including pharmacology and PFMT (Tables 12.5 and 12.6). However, although there is evidence for bladder training being an effective treatment in the elderly, it is not strong (Wallace et al 2000). This may be because it is a 'package' of interventions and each technique (mental distraction, delayed/prompted/timed voiding, relaxation, PFMT, physiological stimuli including perineal pressure) has its own level of effectiveness and needs to be investigated separately. On the other hand, it may be that the success of bladder training is due as much to the PFMT component, for which there is moderate to strong evidence for effectiveness, as the behavioural components.

To test the relative effectiveness of components of behavioural interventions, Wyman et al (1998) compared bladder training, PFMT and a combination 'package' in 204 older, but not frail, women (mean age 61 ± 10 years) who had stress, urgency or mixed incontinence. The participants undertook 12 weeks of intervention with a follow-up 3 months later. Although this study had adequate power to detect differences in the three treatment groups, at 3-month follow-up, no differences were observed. The authors conclude that specific treatment might not be as important as having a structured intervention programme with frequent patient contact. Other possibilities might be that by including three diagnoses within this study, the treatment undertaken by any subject was not the most suitable for the diagnosis, or that as PFMT was a common intervention in all treatment groups, all groups improved equally because of the PFMT component. However, the training intensity of the PFMT in this study was not high enough to cause a change in muscle strength.

Burgio et al (1998) on the other hand found that bladder training was more effective than anticholinergic medication or placebo in an RCT of 198 women aged 68 ± 8 years with either urgency or mixed incontinence, after 8 weeks of intervention. Behavioural training resulted in an 81% reduction in the number of incontinent episodes per week, compared to 69% in the drug treatment group and 40% in the placebo group. Once again, the bladder training protocol in this study included PFMT three times daily, the 'knack', as well as behavioural training. Szonyi et al (1995) compared anticholinergic medication combined with bladder training to bladder training alone in a randomized double-blind, placebo controlled trial in 57 older (mean age 82 ± 6 years) women with symptoms of overactive bladder. They concluded that the combination of medication with bladder training was superior to bladder training alone in this elderly cohort as measured by reduced urinary frequency over 14 days, leakage episodes and subjective evaluation. Fantl et al (1991) in an earlier study comparing bladder training for the two different diagnoses of overactive bladder and sphincter incompetence, reported results of 57% reduction in leakage episodes for both diagnostic groups, and Subak et al (2002) reported a 50% reduction in leakage episodes per week for bladder training compared to 15% reduction for a no-treatment control group, and that this was maintained 6 months after the 6-week intervention.

In the frail elderly population, behavioural training in the form of habit retraining and prompted voiding is common practice in residential aged-care facilities. A Cochrane review of prompted voiding found that there was suggestive evidence of short-term benefit from prompted voiding as shown by a decrease in leakage episodes and an increase in self-initiated voiding (Eustice et al 2000), but not sufficiently strong evidence to reach firm conclusions for practice. The Cochrane reviews on habit retraining and timed voiding concluded that the research available is not of high enough quality to judge the impact of either intervention on urinary incontinence (Ostaszkiewicz et al 2004a, 2004b).

Despite mostly positive evidence for conservative management, a recent observational study (Gnanadesigan et al 2004) using medical record review and interview of a random group of vulnerable older community-dwelling patients who were at risk of functional decline or death found that the quality of care provided to these patients by their primary care providers was inadequate. Primary care doctors prescribed drug treatment for 50% of these patients, but prescribed 'behavioural' treatments to only 13% of this group. There is clearly much to be done to disseminate the research findings for conservative management of incontinence in the frail elderly, and to undertake more high-quality studies in homogeneous elderly populations.

CLINICAL RECOMMENDATIONS

Assess and treat acute-onset incontinence immediately, following the DRIP or DIAPPERS mnemonics. Refer on

Table 12.5 Studies assessing the effect of bladder training for the treatment of UI in the elderly

Author	Burgio et al 1998
Design	3-arm RCT: 1. control (n = 62); 2. drug treatment (oxybutynin) (n = 65); 3. biofeedback assisted behavioural treatment (n = 63)
n	190 community-dwelling women aged 55–92 years with urgency UI or mixed UI predominantly urge symptoms, for >3 months, >2 accidents/week
Outcome variables	Bladder diaries for: Incontinence episodes % change from baseline Satisfaction with treatment
Intervention protocol	All groups: 4 clinic visits at 2-week intervals for 8 weeks 1 & 2: Both groups managed as a double-blind drug protocol, clinic visits for dosage changes, adverse effects and bladder diary review 3. Clinic 1, PFM BFB; clinic 2, deferral techniques; clinic 3, further BFB with increased fluid volumes, clinic 4, review, home practice schedules
Drop-out/adherence	28/190 (9 control, 10 drug, 2 behavioural) Adverse events stated ITT analysis
Results	**Accidents/week Group 1 vs 2 vs 3 mean (SD), p value ANOVA** 2.8(4.7) vs 5.7(9.8) vs 8.2(11.6), p = 0.005. **% change from baseline Group 1 vs 2 vs 3 (p values)** 39.4 vs 68.5 vs 80.7 (p = 0.04, 3 vs 2, p < 0.001 3 vs 1) **% treatment satisfaction Group 1 vs 2 vs 3 (p values)** 43.1% vs 54.7% vs 96.5% (p < 0.001, 3 vs 2, 3 vs 1)
Author	Fantl et al 1991
Design	2-arm RCT, stratified sample, stable and unstable detrusor groups: 1. control (n = 63); 2. bladder training (n = 60)
n	131 community-dwelling women >55 years, with urodynamically proven incontinence, medically stable, functionally independent
Outcome variables	Leakage episodes per week Pad weigh test Daytime frequency Night time frequency IIQ
Intervention protocol	6-week intervention with 6-month non-intervention period 1. No intervention after initial evaluation 2. Bladder training and education, 6-weekly clinic visits plus home programme
Drop-out/adherence	20/131, 8 (6%) during treatment phase (3 control, 5 treatment) 12/123 in 6-month follow-up Adverse events stated Not ITT analysis
Results	**Mean (SD), p value (χ^2), 1 vs 2 at 6 weeks** Leakage episodes per week, non-stratified: 19(17) vs 9(11), p = 0.001, stratified: no differences Pad weigh test, non-stratified: 47(87) vs 17(36), p = 0.0004 Daytime frequency, non-stratified: 57(27) vs 52(14), p < 0.05 Night time frequency, stable detrusor only: 8(6) vs 5(4), p < 0.05 IIQ score: 0.48(0.59) vs 0.23(0.28), p = 0.001

Table 12.5 Studies assessing the effect of bladder training for the treatment of UI in the elderly—cont'd

Author	Subak et al 2002
Design	2-arm RCT, crossover design: 1. control (n = 75); 2. behavioural therapy (bladder training) (n = 77)
n	152 community-dwelling women, >55 years, reporting >1 episode of incontinence per week, medically stable, functionally independent
Outcome variables	Leakage episodes per week Daytime frequency Night time frequency Treatment satisfaction
Intervention protocol	6-week intervention 1. Control, no treatment, completed urinary diary weekly 2. 6-weekly clinic visits, education, bladder training & PFME
Drop-out/adherence	29/152, (18 control, 11 intervention) Adverse events not stated Not ITT analysis
Results	**Mean (SD), p value (χ^2), 1 vs 2 at 6 weeks** Leakage episodes: 11.0 (17.4) vs 5.2 (6.8), p = 0.001 Daytime frequency: 53.8 (22.7) vs 45.1(11.8), no difference Night time frequency: 6.7 (4.1) vs 9.5 (5.2), no difference Treatment satisfaction: % change: 33% great help, 26% moderately helpful, 29% slightly helpful, 12% not helpful
Author	Szonyi et al 1995
Design	2-arm RCT: 1. bladder training with placebo drug (n = 29); 2. bladder training with oxybutynin (n = 28)
n	57 community-dwelling frail elderly, >70 years, medically stable, with symptoms of urge, urge incontinence and frequency
Outcome variables	First 14 days compared to last 14 days: daytime frequency, nocturia, leakage episodes, day leakage episodes, night subjective response
Intervention protocol	After 2 weeks pre-trial recording a bladder diary 1. Bladder training (deferral techniques only reported) 2. Bladder training with oxybutynin For a 6-week active protocol
Drop-out/adherence	3/60, failed to attend first appointment Adverse events stated ITT analysis
Results	**Median change (95% CI of difference in change), p value (Mann–Whitney U) 1 : 2** Daytime frequency: median change not reported, (−6.0: −27.0), p = 0.0025 Nocturia: −6 (−5: 7.0), no difference Daytime leakage episodes: −9 (−11.0: 3.0), no difference Night leakage episodes: −1 (−3.0: 2.0), no difference Subjective response: (no change: all benefit categories of slight significant, cure) 1 vs 2 (% improvement), p value At 4 weeks: 16/29 (55%) vs 24/28 (86%), p = 0.02 At 6 weeks: 17/29 (59%) vs 20/28 (71%), p = 0.4 At 8 weeks: 16/29 (55%) vs 22/28 (79%), p = 0.09

Table 12.5   Studies assessing the effect of bladder training for the treatment of UI in the elderly—cont'd

Author	Wyman et al 1998
Design	3-arm RCT: 1. bladder training (n = 68); 2. BFB-assisted PFMT (n = 69); 3. combination therapy (n = 67)
n	204 community-dwelling women, 45+ years, >1 leakage episode/week, medically stable, can perform PFM contraction, UD, diagnosed SUI, OAB or both
Outcome variables	Adherence to programme Leakage episodes per week QoL, IIQ & UDI-R Treatment satisfaction Measured at end of intervention and at 3-month follow-up
Intervention protocol	12-week programme of behavioural training, monitoring voiding behaviour 1. Progressive voiding schedule for 6 weeks, weekly clinic visits, using deferral techniques to maintain schedule, then maintained for next 6 weeks 2. PFMT graded home programme with audio practice tapes and 4 clinic visits for BFB 3. Bladder training first, then PFMT added after 3 weeks
Drop-out/adherence	9/204 during intervention, 16/195 at 3-month follow-up, (not stated from which groups) Adverse events reported Not ITT analysis
Results	Adherence % bladder training Group 1 vs 3; 85% vs 81% (NS) PFMT Group 2 vs 3; 84% vs 78% (NS) Leakage episodes/week mean (SD), p values Group 1 vs 2 vs 3 at end of intervention: 10.6 (16.3) vs 9.6 (10.8) vs 6.8 (10.7), p = 0.004 (3 vs other groups) UDI overall mean (SD), p values. Group 1 vs 2 vs 3 at end of intervention: 95.5 (54.8) vs 90/8 (52.0) vs 64.4 (48.6), NS IIQ-R: NS Treatment satisfaction n (%), p values Group 1 vs 2 vs 3 at end of intervention: 25(38%) vs 19(30%) vs 32(52%),p = 0.01 (3 vs other groups)

ANOVA, analysis of variance; BFB, biofeedback; IIQ, incontinence impact questionnaire; ITT, intention to treat; NS, not significant; OAB, overactive bladder; PFMT, pelvic floor muscle training; QoL, quality of life; SUI, stress urinary incontinence; UDI, Urogenital Distress Inventory; UI, urinary incontinence; UD, unstable destrusor.

to appropriate medical personnel for this. No patient should receive physical therapy treatment until these transient causes of incontinence have been addressed. Follow the local authority clinical guidelines when assessing a patient in an aged-care facility.

Physical therapy assessment

- Take a complete subjective examination to determine causative factors and their possible interaction. This may include information from care givers as well as the patient, regarding cognition, musculoskeletal

problems, activities of daily living (ADL), pain and neurological symptoms.

- Complete a subjective and objective continence and pelvic floor assessment, (including per vaginum examination where appropriate) following the guidelines in Ch. 6. Include assessment of bowel function.

- Undertake appropriate assessment measures that can also be used as outcome measures, including a bladder diary, pad weigh test, PFM strength

Table 12.6 Studies assessing the effect of bladder training for the treatment of UI in the elderly: PEDro quality score of RCTs

E – Eligibility criteria specified
1 – Subjects randomly allocated to groups
2 – Allocation concealed
3 – Groups similar at baseline
4 – Subjects blinded
5 – Therapist administering treatment blinded
6 – Assessors blinded
7 – Measures of key outcomes obtained from over 85% of subjects
8 – Data analysed by intention to treat
9 – Comparison between groups conducted
10 – Point measures and measures of variability provided

Study	E	1	2	3	4	5	6	7	8	9	10	Total score
Burgio et al 1998	+	+	−	+	−	−	−	+	+	+	+	6/10
Fantl et al 1991	+	+	−	+	−	−	−	+	−	+	+	5/10
Subak et al 2002	+	+	+	+	−	−	+	+	−	+	+	7/10
Szonyi et al 1995	−	+	−	+	−	−	−	+	+	+	+	6/10
Wyman et al 1998	+	+	−	+	−	−	−	+	−	+	+	5/10

+, criterion is clearly satisfied; −, criterion is not satisfied; ?, not clear if criterion was satisfied. Total score is determined by counting the number of criteria that are satisfied, except that the scale item 1E (eligibility criteria specified) is not used to generate the total score.

measure(s), functional mobility tests such as timed-up-and-go (TUG) test, and quality of life measures.

Physical therapy treatment/management

- Institute general balance exercises, and lower limb strength training (sit to stand, walking and stair climbing training) to address functional impairment. Prescribe, apply, and train in the use of appropriate gait aids or other assistive devices such as 'grab rails'. Refer to appropriate professionals to address factors such as vision, hearing or podiatry deficits, which in themselves may contribute to the functional impairment.

- Educate, and initiate lifestyle interventions as appropriate (e.g. night lights for toileting, commode in bedroom, 'Velcro' or other easy-to-use fastening for pants, raised toilet seat, reminders to void, adjust-ment of bed and chair heights for ease of getting up, education regarding the most suitable pads or other containment devices and mechanism of accessing these through national or local funding schemes). Where appropriate, include education about postural changes such as taking a recumbent position during the afternoon to assist with nocturnal polyuria management.

- PFMT with cognitively intact patients, specifically a progressive resistance protocol and functional use of PFM during activities ('the knack') (Fig. 12.2). Although there are no studies to support the use of electrical stimulation in the elderly, if appropriate, include electrical stimulation to assist a strengthening programme for marked weakness or poor sensation of PFM. Begin electrical stimulation with low intensity, taking care to monitor the condition of atrophic mucosa or skin.

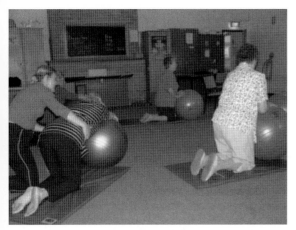

Fig. 12.2 Pelvic floor muscle training in a class situation enhances functional training, motivation and adherence.

- Institute bladder training where required, including education about ideal bladder habits and hygiene. Include in this the amount and type of fluid and fibre intake, redistribution of fluid and food intake during the day, relaxation and deferral techniques, toilet positioning to facilitate complete emptying, timed or prompted voiding. If appropriate, use neuromodulation for symptoms of urgency, with either vaginal or external electrodes, taking care to monitor the condition of atrophic mucosa or skin.

- Include PFM exercises and education about good bladder habits in all general exercise classes for older people, whether in community or residential aged-care facilities.

REFERENCES

Abrams P, Cardozo L, Khoury S et al (eds) 2002 Incontinence, 2nd edn. Plymbridge Distributors, Plymouth, UK

ACSM (American College of Sports Medicine) Position Stand 1990 The recommended quantity and quality of exercise for developing and maintaining cardiorespiratory and muscular fitness in healthy adults. Medicine and Science in Sports and Exercise 22(2):265–274

Adelmann P K 2004 Prevalence and detection of urinary incontinence among older Medicaid recipients. Journal of Health Care for the Poor and Underserved 15:99–112

Aggazzotti G, Pesce F, Grassi D et al 2000 Prevalence of urinary incontinence among institutionalised patients: a cross-sectional epidemiological study in a midsized city in northern Italy. Urology 56:245–249

Andersson G, Johansson J E, Garpenholt O et al 2004 Urinary incontinence – prevalence, impact on daily living and desire for treatment: a population-based study. Scandinavian Journal of Urology and Nephrology 38(2):125–130

Asplund R 2004 Nocturia, nocturnal polyuria, and sleep quality in the elderly. Journal of Psychosomatic Research 56(5):517–525

Bachmann G A, Nevadunsky N S 2000 Diagnosis and treatment of atrophic vaginitis. American Family Physician 61(10):3090–3096

Barrett C, Smerdely P 2002 A comparison of community-based resistance exercise and flexibility exercise for seniors Australian Journal of Physiotherapy 48:215–219

Berghmans L C, Hendriks H J, Bø K et al 1998 Conservative treatment of stress urinary incontinence in women: a systematic review of randomized clinical trials. British Journal of Urology 82(2):181–191

Blanker M H, Bohnen A M, Groenveld F P 2000 Normal voiding patterns and determinants of increased diurnal and nocturnal voiding frequency in elderly men. The Journal of Urology 164:1201–1205

Blok B F M, Sturms L M, Holstege G 1997 A PET study on cortical and subcortical control of pelvic floor musculature in women. The Journal of Comparative Neurology 389:535–544

Bø K, Sherburn M 2005 Evaluation of female pelvic-floor muscle function and strength. Physical Therapy 85(3):269–282

Bogner H R 2004 Urinary incontinence and psychological distress in community-dwelling older African Americans and whites. Journal of the American Geriatrics Society 52(11):1870–1874

Bonita R (ed) 1998 Women, Ageing and Health. Achieving health across the life span. World Health Organization, Geneva. Online. Available: http://www.who.int/hpr/ageing/womenandageing.pdf

Brown W J, Miller Y D 2001 Too wet to exercise? Leaking urine as a barrier to physical activity in women. Journal of Science and Medicine in Sport 4(4):373–378

Burgio K L, Locher J L, Goode P S et al 1998 Behavioral vs drug treatment for urge urinary incontinence in older women: a randomized controlled trial. JAMA 280(23):1995–2000

Burns P A, Pranikoff K, Nochajski T et al 1990 Treatment of stress incontinence with pelvic floor exercises and biofeedback. Journal of the American Geriatrics Society 38(3):341–344

Camilleri M, Lee J S, Viramontes B et al 2000 Progress in geriatrics. Insights into the pathophysiology and mechanisms of constipation, irritable bowel syndrome, and diverticulosis in older people. Journal of the American Geriatrics Society 48(9):1142–1150

Chiarelli P, Brown W, McElduff P 1999 Leaking urine: prevalence and associated factors in Australian women. Neurourology and Urodynamics 18:567–577

Constantinou C E, Hvistendahl G, Ryhammer A et al 2002 Determining the displacement of the pelvic floor and pelvic organs during voluntary contractions using magnetic resonance imaging in younger and older women. BJU International 90(4):408–414

Corcos J, Schick E (eds) 2001 The urinary sphincter. Marcel Dekker, New York, p 194–196

Cundiff G W, Nygaard I, Bland D R et al 2000 Proceedings of the American Urogynecologic Society Multidisciplinary Symposium on Defecatory Disorders. American Journal of Obstetrics and Gynecology 182(1 Pt 1):S1–S10

Davila G W, Karapanagiotou I, Woodhouse S et al 2001 Are women with urogenital atrophy symptomatic? Obstetrics and Gynaecology 97(4):S48

Davila G W, Singh A, Karapanagiotou I et al 2003 Are women with urogenital atrophy symptomatic? American Journal of Obstetrics and Gynecology 188(2):382–388

De Ridder D, Vermeulen C, De Smet E et al 1998 Clinical assessment of pelvic floor dysfunction in multiple sclerosis: urodynamic and neurological correlates. Neurourology and Urodynamics 17(5):537–542

Dimpfl T, Jaeger C, Mueller-Felber W et al 1998 Myogenic changes of the levator ani muscle in premenopausal women: the impact of delivery and age. Neurourology and Urodynamics 17:197–205

Diokno A C, Brock B M, Brown M B et al 1986 Prevalence of urinary incontinence and other urological symptoms in the noninstitutionalized elderly. The Journal of Urology 136:1022–1025

Diokno A C, Sampselle C M, Herzog A R et al 2004 Prevention of urinary incontinence by behavioral modification program: a randomized, controlled trial among older women in the community. The Journal of Urology 171(3):1165–1171

Duong T H, Korn A P 2001 A comparison of urinary incontinence among African American, Asian, Hispanic, and white women. American Journal of Obstetrics and Gynecology 184(6):1083–1086

Eekhof J A H, De Bock G H, Schoopveld K et al 2000 Effects of screening for disorders among the elderly: an intervention study in general practice. Family Practice 17:329–333

Esler M, Lambert G, Kaye D et al 2002 Influence of aging on the sympathetic nervous system and adrenal medulla at rest and during stress. Biogerontology 3:45–49

Eustice S, Roe B, Paterson J 2000 Prompted voiding for the management of urinary incontinence in adults. Cochrane Database of Systematic Reviews 2: CD002113

Falconer C, Ekman-Ordeberg G, Ulmsten U 1996 Changes in para-urethral connective tissue at menopause are counteracted by oestrogen. Maturitas 24:197–204

Fantl J A, Wyman J F, McClish D K et al 1991 Efficacy of bladder training in older women with urinary incontinence. JAMA 265(5):609–613

Fiatarone M A, O'Neill E F, Ryan N D et al 1994 Exercise training and nutritional supplementation for physical frailty in very elderly people. New England Journal of Medicine 330(25):1769–1775

Fonda D 1992 The billion dollar question: can incontinence be reduced in nursing homes? Medical Journal of Australia 156:6–7

Fonda D, Benvenuti F, Cottenden A et al 2002 Urinary incontinence and bladder dysfunction in older persons. In: Abrams P, Cardozo L, Khoury S et al (eds) Incontinence. 2nd edn. Plymbridge Distributors, Plymouth, UK, p 636

Fonda D, Resnick N M, Colling J et al 1998 Outcome measures for research of lower urinary tract dysfunction in frail older people. Neururology and Urodynamics 17:273–281

Fonda D, Woodward M, D'Astoli M, Chin W F 1995 Sustained improvement of subjective quality of life in older community-dwelling people after treatment of urinary incontinence. Age Ageing 24(4):283–286

Frankel V H, Nordin M 1980 Basic biomechanics of the skeletal system. Lea & Febiger, Philadelphia, p 101

Gariballa S E 2003 Potentially treatable causes of poor outcome in acute stroke patients with urinary incontinence. Acta Neurologica Scandinavica 107(5):336–340

Gnanadesigan N, Saliba D, Roth C P et al 2004 The quality of care provided to vulnerable older community-based patients with urinary incontinence. Journal of the American Medical Directors Association 5(3):141–146

Grimby A, Milsom I, Molander U et al 1993 The influence of urinary incontinence on the quality of life of elderly women. Age and Ageing 22:82–89

Grodstein F, Fretts R, Lifford K et al 2003 Association of age, race, and obstetric history with urinary symptoms among women in the Nurses' Health Study. American Journal of Obstetrics and Gynecology 189(2):428–434

Gunnarsson M, Mattiasson A 1999 Female stress, urge and mixed urinary incontinence are associated with a chronic and progressive pelvic floor/vaginal neuromuscular disorder: an investigation of 317 healthy and incontinent women using vaginal surface electromyography. Neurourology and Urodynamics 18:613–621

Hannestad Y S, Rortveit G, Sandvik H et al 2000 A community-based epidemiological survey of female urinary incontinence: the Norwegian EPINCONT study. Journal of Clinical Epidemiology 53:1150–1157

Hannestad Y S, Rortveit G, Hunskaar S 2002 Help-seeking and associated factors in female urinary incontinence. The Norwegian EPINCONT study. Epidemiology of incontinence in the county of Nord-Trondelag. Scandinavian Journal of Primary Health Care 20(2):102–107

Harari D, Coshall C, Rudd A G et al 2003 New-onset fecal incontinence after stroke: prevalence, natural history, risk factors, and impact. Stroke 34(1):144–150

Hay-Smith E J C, Bø K, Berghmans L C M et al 2001 Pelvic floor muscle retraining for urinary incontinence in women. Cochrane Database of Systematic Reviews 1:CD001407

Hay-Smith E J, Herbison P, Morkved S 2002 Physical therapies for prevention of urinary and faecal incontinence in adults. The Cochrane Database of Systematic Reviews (2):CD003191

Herzog A R, Diokno A C, Brown M B et al 1990 Two-year incidence, remission, and change patterns of urinary incontinence in noninstitutionalized older adults. Journal of Gerontology 45(2): M67–M74

Holroyd-Leduc J M, Straus S E 2004 Management of urinary incontinence in women: scientific review. Journal of the American Geriatrics Society 291(8):986–995

Jackson R A, Vittinghoff E, Kanaya A M et al 2004 Urinary incontinence in elderly women: findings from the Health, Aging, and Body Composition Study. Obstetrics and Gynecology 104(2):301–307

Jenkins K R, Fultz N H 2005 Functional impairment as a risk factor for urinary incontinence among older Americans. Neurourology and Urodynamics 24:51–55

Kok A L, Voorhoost F J, Burger C W et al 1992 Urinary and faecal incontinence in community residing elderly women. Age and Aging 21:211–215

Klauser A, Frauscher F, Strasser H et al 2004 Age-related rhabdosphincter function in female urinary stress incontinence: assessment of intraurethral sonography. Journal of Ultrasound in Medicine 23(5):631–663

Kushner L, Chen Y, Desautel M et al 1999 Collagenase activity is elevated in conditioned media from fibroblasts of women with pelvic floor weakening. International Urogynecology Journal and Pelvic Floor Dysfunction 10(S1):34

Lose G, Alling-Moller L, Jennum P 2001 Nocturia in women. American Journal of Obstetrics and Gynecology 185(2): 514–521

Madersbacher S, Pycha A, Klingler C H et al 1999 Interrelationships of bladder compliance with age, detrusor instability, and obstruction in elderly men with lower urinary tract symptoms. Neurourology and Urodynamics 18(1):3–15

Maggi S, Minicuci N, Langlois J et al 2001 Prevalence rate of urinary incontinence in community-dwelling elderly individuals: the Veneto study. Journals of Gerontology. Series A, Biological Sciences and Medical Sciences 56(1):M14–M18

McDowell B J, Engberg S, Sereika S et al 1999 Effectiveness of behavioural therapy to treat incontinence in homebound older adults. Journal of the American Geriatrics Society 47(3):309–318

McGrother C W, Donaldson M M K, Shaw C et al 2003 Storage symptoms of the bladder: prevalence, incidence and the need for services in the UK. BJU International 93(6):763–769

Miller M 2000 Nocturnal polyuria in older people: pathophysiology and clinical implications. Journal of the American Geriatrics Society 48(10):1321–1329

Miller Y D, Brown W J, Smith N et al 2003 Managing urinary incontinence across the lifespan. International Journal of Behavioral Medicine 10(2):143–161

Nilsson K, Risberg B, Heimer G 1995 The vaginal epithelium in the postmenopause – cytology, histology and pH as methods of assessment. Maturitas 21(1):51–56

Notelovitz M 1995 Estrogen therapy in the management of problems associated with urogenital ageing: a simple diagnostic test and the effect of the route of hormone administration. Maturitas 22(suppl):S31–S33

Ostaszkiewicz J, Johnston L, Roe B. 2004a Habit retraining for the management of urinary incontinence in adults. The Cochrane Database of Systematic Reviews 2:CD002801

Ostaszkiewicz J, Johnston L, Roe B 2004b Timed voiding for the management of urinary incontinence in adults. The Cochrane Database of Systematic Reviews 1:CD002802

Ouslander J G 2000 Intractable incontinence in the elderly. BJU International 85(suppl 3):72–78, discussion 81–72

Palmer M H 2002 Urinary incontinence in nursing homes [editorial]. Journal of Wound, Ostomy and Continence Nursing 29:4–5

Perucchini D, DeLancey J O L, Ashton-Miller J A et al 2002a Age effects on urethral striated muscle. I. Changes in number and diameter of striated muscle fibres in the ventral urethra. American Journal of Obstetrics and Gynaecology 186:351–355

Perucchini D, DeLancey J O L, Ashton-Miller J A et al 2002b Age effects on urethral striated muscle. II. Anatomic location of muscle loss. American Journal of Obstetrics and Gynaecology 186:356–360

Peters T J, Horrocks S, Stoddart H et al 2003 Factors associated with variations in older people's use of community-based continence services. Health & Social Care in the Community 12(1):53–62

Podsiadlo D, Richardson S 1991 The timed 'up & go': a test of basic functional mobility for frail elderly persons. Journal of the American Geriatrics Society 39(2):142–148

Powers S K, Howley E T 2001 Exercise physiology and application to fitness and performance. 4th edn. McGraw-Hill, New York, p 145

Rociu E, Stoker J, Eijkemans M J et al 2000 Normal anal sphincter anatomy and age- and sex-related variations at high-spatial-resolution endoanal MR imaging. Radiology 217(2):395–401

Samsioe G 1998 Urogenital aging – a hidden problem. American Journal of Obstetrics and Gynecology 178(5):S245–S249

Sarkar P K, Ritch A E 2000 Management of urinary incontinence. Journal of Clinical Pharmacy and Therapeutics 25(4):251–263

Schafer W 1999 Urodynamics of micturition. Current Opinion in Urology 2:252–256

Schaffer J, Fantl J A 1996 Urogenital effects of the menopause. In: Barlow D H (ed) The menopause: key issues. Clinical Obstetrics and Gynaecology 10(3):401–417

Schnelle J F, Alessi C, Simmons S F et al 2002 Translating clinical research into practice: a randomized controlled trial of exercise and incontinence care with nursing home residents. Journal of the American Geriatrics Society 50:1476–1483

Seynnes O, Singh M A F, Hue O et al 2004 Physiological and functional responses to low-moderate versus high-intensity progressive resistance training in frail elders. Journals of Gerontology. Series A, Biological Sciences and Medical Sciences 59(5):503–509

Sherburn M, Guthrie J R, Dudley E C et al 2001 Is incontinence associated with menopause? Obstetrics and Gynecology 98:628–633

Simeonova Z, Milsom I, Kullendorff A M et al 1999 The prevalence of urinary incontinence and its influence on the quality of life in women from an urban Swedish population. Acta Obstetricia et Gynecologica Scandinavica 78(6):546–551

Spruijt J, Vierhout M, Verstraeten R et al 2003 Vaginal electrical stimulation of the pelvic floor: a randomized feasibility study in urinary incontinent elderly women. Acta Obstetricia et Gynecologica Scandinavica 82:1043–1048

Stein C, Moritz I 1999 A life course perspective of maintaining independence in older age. World Health Organization, Geneva. Online. Available: www.who.int/hpr/ageing/lifecourse.pdf

Subak L L, Quesenberry C P, Posner S F et al 2002 The effect of behavioral therapy on urinary incontinence: a randomized controlled trial. Obstetrics and Gynecology 100(1):72–78

Swithinbank L, Abrams P 2001 Lower urinary tract symptoms in community dwelling women: defining diurnal and nocturnal frequency and 'the incontinence case'. BJU International 88(suppl 2):18–22

Szonyi G, Collas D M, Ding Y Y et al 1995 Oxybutynin with bladder retraining for detrusor instability in elderly people: a randomized controlled trial. Age and Ageing 24(4):287–291

Tannenbaum C, Mayo N 2003 Women's health priorities and perceptions of care: a survey to identify opportunities for improving preventative health care delivery for older women. Age and Ageing 32(6):626–635

Teunissen T A, van den Bosch W J, van den Hoogen H J et al 2004 Prevalence of urinary, fecal and double incontinence in the elderly living at home. International Urogynecology Journal and Pelvic Floor Dysfunction 15(1):10–13, discussion 13

Thom D 1998 Variations in estimates of urinary incontinence prevalence in the community: effects of differences in definition, population characteristics and study type. Journal of the American Geriatrics Society 46(4):473–480

Timiras P S, Leary J 2003 The kidney, the lower urinary tract, body fluids and the prostate. In: Timiras P S (ed) Physiological basis of aging and geriatrics, 3rd edn. CRC Press, Boca Raton, FL, p 347–351

Truijen G, Wyndaele J J, Weyler J 2001 Conservative treatment of stress urinary incontinence in women: who will benefit? International Urogynecology Journal and Pelvic Floor Dysfunction 12(6):386–390

Vaillant G E, Mukamal K 2001 Successful aging. The American Journal of Psychiatry 158(6):839–847

Verelst M, Maltau J M, Orbo A 2002 Computerised morphometric study of the paraurethral tissue in young and elderly women. Neurourology and Urodynamics 21(6):529–533

Wallace S A, Roe B, Williams K et al 2000 Bladder training for urinary incontinence in adults. The Cochrane Database of Systematic Reviews 1:CD001308

Weinberger M W, Goodman B M, Carnes M 1999 Long-term efficacy of nonsurgical urinary incontinence treatment in elderly women. Journals of Gerontology. Series A, Biological Sciences and Medical Sciences 54(3):M117–M121

Wells T J, Brink C A, Diokno A C et al 1991 Pelvic muscle exercise for stress urinary incontinence in elderly women. Journal of the American Geriatrics Society 39(8):785–791

Wyman J F, Fantl J A, McClish D K et al 1998 Comparative efficacy of behavioral interventions in the management of female urinary incontinence. American Journal of Obstetrics and Gynecology 179:999–1007

Yoshida M, Homma Y, Inadome A et al 2001 Age-related changes in cholinergic and purinergic neurotransmission in human isolated bladder smooth muscles. Experimental Gerontology 36(1):99–109

Yoshida M, Miyamae K, Iwashita H et al 2004 Management of detrusor dysfunction in the elderly: changes in acetylcholine and adenosine triphosphate release during aging. Urology 63(3 Suppl 1):17–23

Chapter 13

Pelvic floor physical therapy in elite athletes

Kari Bø

INTRODUCTION

Because of its location inside the pelvis, the pelvic floor muscles (PFM) are the only muscle group in the body capable of giving structural support for the pelvic organs and the pelvic openings (urethra, vagina and anus) (see Fig. 9.21, p. 241). Ultrasound and MRI studies have shown that the PFM is 'stiffer' and has a more cranial position in nulliparous compared to parous women (Miller et al 2001, Peschers et al 1996, Peschers 1997), and in continent versus incontinent women (Haderer et al 2002).

Lack of co-contraction or delayed or weak co-contraction of the PFM may lead to urinary and fecal incontinence, prolapse of the anterior vaginal wall (cystocoele), posterior vaginal wall (rectocoele), vaginal apex (enterocoele), and uterus, or constipation, pain and sexual dysfunction (Bump & Norton 1998). Although there are anecdotal reports of pelvic organ prolapse in young, nulliparous marathon runners and weight lifters, no studies have been found on this topic. So far, the focus within the sports literature has been on urinary incontinence (UI) during physical activity (Bø 2004a). Well-established aetiological factors for urinary incontinence include older age, obesity, gynaecological surgery, and pregnancy and vaginal childbirth (instrumental deliveries increase the risk). Other factors are less clear, such as strenuous work or exercise, constipation with straining on stool, chronic coughing, or other conditions that increase abdominal pressure chronically (Bump & Norton 1998, Hunskaar et al 2002, Wilson et al 2002).

The aim of this chapter is to give a systematic review of the literature on urinary incontinence in connection with participation in sport and fitness activities with a special emphasis on prevalence and treatment of female elite athletes.

METHODS

This is a systematic review of the literature covering incidence, prevalence, treatment and prevention of female urinary incontinence in sport and fitness activities, with focus on stress urinary incontinence (SUI) (see Ch. 9). For epidemiological studies computerized search on 'Sport' and 'Pub Med' were done. Mesh words of 'urinary incontinence' or 'pelvic organ prolapse' combined with 'exercise', 'fitness', 'physical activity' and 'sport' were used. In addition, the chapter on epidemiology from the 2nd International Consultation on Incontinence (ICI, Paris) was consulted (Hunskaar et al 2002). All studies found on prevalence and incidence was included in this chapter.

For treatment the same computerized search was conducted, together with a manual search of abstracts from International Continence Society Annual Meetings from 1984 to 2001, and the Cochrane library (Hay-Smith et al 2001). Only results from randomized controlled trials (RCTs) are reported.

PREVALENCE OF URINARY INCONTINENCE AND PARTICIPATION IN SPORT AND FITNESS ACTIVITIES

Urinary incontinence is more common in women than in men and may affect women of all ages. Prevalence rates in the general population of women aged between 15 and 64 years vary between 10 and 55% (Fantl et al 1996, Hunskaar et al 2002). The most common type of urinary incontinence in women is SUI, followed by urge and mixed incontinence. Urinary incontinence is often regarded as a problem affecting older, postmenopausal, multiparous women. However, several epidemiological studies have demonstrated that symptoms of SUI are frequent in populations of nulliparous young females (Bø et al 1989a, Brown & Miller 2001, Nygaard et al 1994, Nygaard et al 1990).

Urinary incontinence is not a life-threatening nor dangerous condition. However, it is socially embarrassing, and may cause withdrawal from social situations and reduced quality of life (Fantl et al 1996, Hunskaar & Vinsnes 1991, Norton et al 1988). In the elderly it is a significant cause of disability and dependency. SUI implies that urine loss occurs during increases in abdominal pressure. If present, it is therefore likely that urine loss will occur during physical activity. Thus, sedentary women who are less exposed to physical exertion may not manifest SUI, though the underlying condition may be present. SUI has shown to lead to withdrawal from participation in sport and fitness activities (Bø et al 1989b, Nygaard et al 1990) and may be considered a barrier for lifelong participation in health and fitness activities in women (Brown & Miller 2001). Hence, although urinary incontinence itself does not cause significant morbidity or mortality, it may lead to inactivity. A sedentary lifestyle is an independent risk factor for several diseases and conditions (e.g. high blood pressure, coronary hearth disease, type II diabetes mellitus, obesity, colon and breast cancer, osteoporosis, depression and anxiety [Bouchard et al 1993, Physical Activity and Health a Report of the Surgeon General 1996]).

Prevalence of urinary incontinence in female elite athletes

An overview of published studies on prevalence of urinary incontinence in elite athletes is shown in Table 13.1. There is a high prevalence of symptoms of both SUI and urge incontinence in young nulliparous as well as parous elite athletes. Only one study has compared the prevalence of incontinence in elite athletes with that of age-matched controls. Bø & Borgen (2001) found equal prevalences of overall SUI and urge incontinence in both groups. However, the prevalence of leakage during physical activities was significantly higher in the elite athletes.

None of these studies characterized incontinence with urodynamic testing (simultaneous measurement of urethral and bladder pressures during increase in abdominal pressure), and it is therefore not possible to confirm whether the leakage represents SUI or urge or mixed incontinence. However, in a study by Sandvik et al (1993), questions used in a survey were validated against the diagnosis made by a gynaecologist after urodynamic evaluation. The diagnosis of SUI increased from 51 to 77%, mixed incontinence decreased from 39 to 11%, and urge incontinence increased from 10 to 12% after urodynamic assessment. In another study of nulliparous physical education students, six of seven who underwent ambulatory urodynamic assessment showed evidence of urodynamic SUI (Bø et al 1994).

As seen from Table 13.1, the question on incontinence was posed in a general way with no time restrictions (e.g. leakage during past week or month). Eliasson et al (2002) is the only research group adding clinical measurements to the study. They measured urinary leakage in all elite trampolinists who reported the leakage to be a problem during trampoline training. The leakage was verified in all participants with a mean leakage of 28 g (range 9–56) in a 15-minute test on the trampoline. PFM function was measured in a subgroup of ten women. They were all classified as having strong voluntary contractions by vaginal palpation.

Unlike the current ICS definition of urinary incontinence, the former ICS definition required that the

Table 13.1 Prevalence of urinary incontinence in elite female athletes

Author	Bø & Sundgot Borgen 2001
Design	Cross-sectional, case control. Postal questionnaire
Population/sample	All female elite athletes on national team or recruiting squad in Norway (n = 660) and age-matched controls (n = 765). Age 15–39 years. Parity: 5% in elite athletes, 33% in controls
Response rate	Athletes: 87% Controls: 75%
Question	Do you currently leak urine during coughing, sneezing and laughter, physical activity (running and jumping, abrupt movements and lifting) or with urge to void (problems in reaching the toilet without leaking)?
Results	**SUI** Athletes: 41% Controls: 39% Range between sports: 37.5–52.2% **Urge** Athletes: 16% Controls: 19% Range between sports: 10–27.5% **Social/hygienic problem** Athletes: 15% Controls: 16.4% **Moderate/severe problem** Athletes/controls: 5%
Author	Eliasson et al 2002
Design	Cross-sectional. Postal survey Clinical assessment: Pad test during trampoline training (n = 18), measurement of pelvic floor muscle strength (n = 10)
Population/sample	All 35 female Swedish trampolinists at national level 1993–1996. Mean age 15 (range 12–22). Nulliparous
Response rate	100% on survey 51.4% on pad test 28.6% on strength measurement
Question	Do you leak urine during trampoline training/competition/daily life?
Results	80% reported leak during trampoline training/competition and sport. None leaked during coughing, sneezing or laughing 51.4 % reported the leakage to be embarrassing. Mean leakage on pad testing: 28 g (range 9–56)
Author	Nygaard et al 1994
Design	Cross-sectional. Postal survey
Population/sample	All women participating in competitive varsity athletics at a large state university in USA (n = 156). Mean age 19.9 years ± 3.3 (SD). Nulliparous
Response rate	92%
Question	Have you ever experienced unanticipated urinary leakage during participation in your sport, coughing, sneezing, heavy lifting, walking to the bathroom, sleeping, and upon hearing the sound of running water?

Table 13.1 Prevalence of urinary incontinence in elite female athletes—cont'd

Results	28% reported at least one episode of urinary incontinence while practising or competing in their sport: Gymnastics: 67% Tennis: 50% Basketball: 44% Field hockey: 32% Track: 26% Volleyball: 9% Swimming: 6% Softball: 6% Golf: 0% 42% experienced urine loss during daily activities. 38% felt embarrassed
Author	Nygaard 1997
Design	Retrospective and cross-sectional. Postal survey
Population/sample	Former American female Olympians (between 1960 and 1976) participating in gymnastics and track and field compared to swimmers (n = 207). Mean age 44.3 years (range 30–63). Mean number of years since beginning training: 30
Response rate	51.2%
Question	Do you now/did you while being Olympian participant experience urinary leakage related to feeling of urgency, or related to activity, coughing or sneezing
Results	**While Olympians** Swimming: 4.5% Gymnastics/track and field: 35.0% (p < 0.005) **Now** Swimming: 50% Gymnastics/track and field: 41% (NS)
Author	Thyssen et al 2002
Design	Cross-sectional. Postal survey
Population/sample	8 Danish sport clubs (including ballet) competing at national level (n = 397). Mean age 22.8 years (range 14–51). 8.6% were parous
Response rate	73.7%
Question	Do you experience urine loss while participating in your sport or in daily life?
Results	51.9% experienced urine loss during sport or in daily life. 43% while participating in their sport: Gymnastics: 56% Ballet: 43% Aerobics: 40% Badminton: 31% Volleyball: 30% Athletics: 25% Handball: 21% Basketball: 17%

leakage had to be considered a hygienic or social problem. The reported prevalence is reduced when this definition is used (Hunskaar et al 2002). Nevertheless a high proportion of elite athletes report that the leakage is embarrassing, affects their sport performance, or is a social or hygienic problem. There is no report of how many of the athletes seek help for their problems.

There is limited knowledge about associated factors. In a study of college athletes, Nygaard et al (1994) found no significant association between incontinence and amenorrhoea, weight, hormonal therapy or duration of athletic activity. In a study of former Olympians they found that among factors such as age, body mass index (BMI), parity, Olympic sport group, and incontinence during Olympic sport 20 years ago, only current BMI was significantly associated with regular SUI or urge incontinence symptoms (Nygaard 1997). Bø & Borgen (2001) reported that significantly more elite athletes with eating disorders had symptoms of both SUI and urge incontinence, and Eliasson et al (2002) showed that incontinent trampolinists were significantly older (16 versus 13 years), had been training longer and more frequently and were less able to interrupt the urine flow stream by voluntarily contracting the PFM than the non-leaking group.

PELVIC FLOOR AND STRENUOUS PHYSICAL ACTIVITY

There are two hypotheses about the pelvic floor in elite athletes, going in opposite directions.

Hypothesis one: female athletes have strong PFM

The rationale would be that any physical activity that increases abdominal pressure will lead to a simultaneous or pre-contraction of the PFM, and the muscles will be trained. Based on this assumption general physical activity would prevent and treat SUI. However, women leak during physical activity, and they report worse leakage during high-impact activities. No sports involve a voluntary contraction of the PFM. Many women do not demonstrate an effective simultaneous or pre-contraction of the PFM during increased abdominal pressure (Bø et al 2003). In nulliparous women this may be due to genetically weak connective tissue, location of the PFM at a lower, caudal level inside the pelvis, lower total number of muscle fibres (especially fast-twitch fibres), or untrained muscles in those leaking.

To date there is little knowledge about PFM function in elite athletes. Bø et al (1994) measured PFM function in sport and physical education students with and without urinary incontinence and did not find any difference in PFM strength. The increase in PFM pressure during a voluntary contraction was 16.2 cmH$_2$O (SD 8.7) in the group with SUI and 14.3 cmH$_2$O (SD 8.2) in the continent group. However, this study was limited by its small sample size, and no strong conclusion can be drawn. Statistically significant differences in PFM function and strength between continent and incontinent women have been shown in the adult population (Gunnarsson 2002, Hahn et al 1996, Mørkved et al 2002). Bø (unpublished data) assessed PFM strength in four elite female power lifters and compared them to 20 physical therapy students. Mean muscle strength during voluntary contraction in power lifters was 22.6 cmH$_2$O (SD 9.1) and in the physical therapy students 19.3 cmH$_2$O (SD 6.8) (NS). Only one of the elite athletes in the above-mentioned ongoing study had exercised the PFM systematically. She reported to have trained her PFM regularly to increase low back stability and abdominal pressure during lifting. Her mean PFM strength was 36.2 cmH$_2$O. She was totally continent even when competing in World championships, but so were those who had not trained the PFM.

Hypothesis two: female athletes may overload, stretch and weaken the pelvic floor

Heavy lifting and strenuous work have been listed as risk factors for the development of pelvic organ prolapse and SUI (Bump & Norton 1998, Hunskaar et al 2002, Wilson et al 2002). Nichols & Milley (1978) suggested that the cardinal and uterosacral ligaments, PFM, and the connective tissue of the perineum might be damaged chronically because of repeatedly increase in abdominal pressure due to hard manual work and chronic cough. To date, there are still few data to support the hypothesis. In a study of Danish nursing assistants it was found that they were 1.6 times more likely to undergo surgery for genital prolapse and incontinence than women in the general population (Jørgensen et al 1994). However, the study did not control for parity. Hence, it is difficult to conclude whether heavy lifting is an aetiological factor. Fig. 13.1 shows urinary leakage in a weight lifter.

In the United States Air Force female crew 26% of women capable of sustaining up to 9 G reported urinary incontinence (Fischer & Berg 1999). However, more women had incontinence off duty than while flying and it was concluded that flying high-performance military aircraft did not affect the rate of incontinence. Davis & Goodman (1996) found that nine of 420 nulliparous female soldiers entering the airborne infantry training programme developed severe incontinence. Hence, most women were not negatively affected by this high

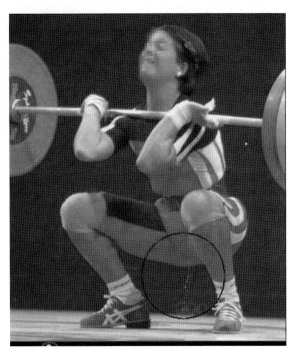

Fig. 13.1 Weightlifting increases abdominal pressure and leakage may occur.

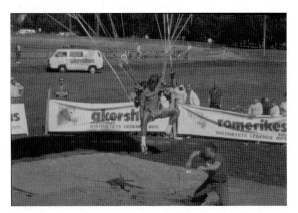

Fig. 13.2 The reaction force during landing in parachute jumping must be counteracted by the pelvic floor muscles.

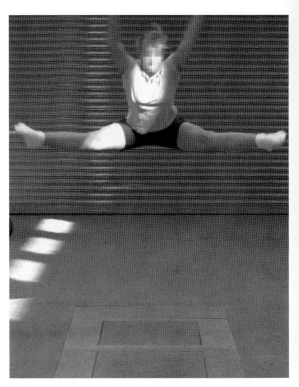

Fig. 13.3 Stress urinary incontinence is common in gymnasts during high impact (jumping and running) activities.

impact activity. Fig. 13.2 shows a parachute jumper in the landing phase.

Hay (1993) reported the maximum vertical ground reaction forces during different sport activities to be 3–4 times body weight for running, 5–12 times for jumping, 9 times for landing from front somersault, 14 times for landing after double back somersault, 16 times during landing in long jumps, and 9 times body weight in the lead foot in javelin throwing. Thus, one would anticipate that the pelvic floor of athletes needs to be much stronger than in the normal population to counteract these forces. Fig. 13.3 shows a gymnast performing a jump.

To date it has been concluded that there is no evidence that strenuous exercise causes SUI or pelvic organ prolapse (Wilson et al 2002). Although the prevalence is high, most athletes do not leak during strenuous activities and high increases in abdominal pressure. However, from a theoretical understanding of functional anatomy and biomechanics, it is likely that heavy lifting and strenuous activity may promote these conditions in women already at risk (e.g. those with benign hypermobility joint syndrome). Physical activity may unmask and exaggerate the condition.

PREVENTION

There are no studies applying PFM training (PFMT) for primary prevention for SUI. Theoretically, one could argue that strengthening the PFM by specific training would have the potential to prevent SUI and pelvic organ prolapse. Strength training may increase PFM volume, and 'lift' the levator plate to a more cranial level inside the pelvis. If the pelvic floor possesses a certain 'stiffness' (Ashton-Miller et al 2001, Harderer et al 2002), it is likely that the muscles could counteract the increases in abdominal pressures occurring during physical exertion.

Preventive devices

Devices that involve external urinary collection, intra-vaginal support of the bladder neck or blockage of urinary leakage by occlusion are available, and have shown to be effective in preventing leakage during physical activity (Wilson et al 2002). A vaginal tampon can be such a simple device. In a study by Glavind (1997) six women with SUI demonstrated total dryness when using a vaginal device during 30 minutes of aerobics. For smaller leakage, specially designed protecting pads can be used during training and competition.

TREATMENT OF SUI IN ELITE ATHLETES

SUI can be treated with bladder training, PFMT with or without resistance devices, vaginal cones or biofeedback, electrical stimulation, drug therapy or surgery (Fantl et al 1996, Wilson et al 2002). One would assume that the elite athletes would respond in the same way to treatment as other women do. However, to this author's knowledge, to date, there are no studies on the effect of any treatment of SUI in female elite athletes. In addition, there are methodological problems assessing bladder and urethral function during physical activity before and after treatment (James 1978, Kulseng-Hanssen & Klevmark 1988).

Surgery

Elite athletes are young and mostly nulliparous, and it is therefore recommended that PFMT should be the first choice of treatment, and always tried before surgery (Wilson et al 2002). The leakage in athletes seems to be related to strenuous high-impact activity, and elite athletes do not seem to have more urinary incontinence than others later in life when the activity is reduced (Nygaard 1997). Therefore, surgery seems inappropriate in elite athletes who have incontinence only during exercise and sport.

Bladder training

Most elite athletes empty their bladder before practice and competition. Therefore, it is unlikely that any of them would exercise with a high bladder volume. However, as in the rest of the population elite athletes may have a non-optimal toilet behaviour and the use of frequency–volume chart may be an important first step to improve this.

Oestrogen

The role of oestrogen in incidence, prevalence, and treatment of SUI is controversial. Two meta-analyses of the effect have concluded that there is no change in urine loss after oestrogen replacement therapy (Andersson et al 2002). Oestrogen given alone therefore does not seem to be an effective treatment for SUI. There is a higher prevalence of eating disorders in athletes compared to non-athletes, and these athletes may be low in oestrogen (Bø & Borgen 2001). However, most amenorrhoeic elite athletes would be on oestrogen replacement therapy because of the risk of osteoporosis. Oestrogen has adverse effects such as a higher risk of coronary heart disease and cancer.

PFMT

Based on systematic reviews and meta-analysis of RCTs it has been stated that conservative treatment should be first-line treatment for SUI (Fantl et al 1996, Wilson et al 2002). The Cochrane review 'Pelvic floor muscle training for urinary incontinence' (Hay-Smith et al 2001) concludes that PFMT is an effective treatment for adult women with SUI or mixed incontinence, and consistently better than no treatment or placebo treatments. Subjective cure and improvement rates after PFM for SUI or mixed incontinence reported in RCTs vary between 56 and 70 % (Hay-Smith et al 2001). Cure rates, defined as ≤2 g of leakage on pad tests, vary between 44 and 70% in SUI (Bø et al 1999, Dumoulin et al 2004, Mørkved et al 2002). Adverse effects have only been reported in one study (Lagro-Janssen et al 1992). One woman out of 54 reported pain with PFM contractions; three had an uncomfortable feeling during exercise and two felt that they did not want to be continually occupied with the problem.

No RCTs have been conducted with elite athletes. However, Bø et al (1999, 1990) and Mørkved et al (2002) used tests involving high-impact exercise (running and jumping) before and after treatment, and showed that it is possible to cure or reduce urinary leakage during physical activity. Bø et al (1989b) demonstrated that after specific strength training of the PFM, 17 of 23 women reported improvement during jumping and running, and 15 during lifting. Significant improvement was also obtained while dancing, hiking, during general group exercise, and in an overall score on ability to participate in different activities. Measured with a pad test with standardized bladder volume during activities comprising running, jumping jacks and sit ups, there was a significant reduction in urine loss from mean 27 g (95% CI 8.8, 45.1, range 0–168) to 7.1 g (95% CI: 0.8, 13.4, range 0–58.3), p < 0.01 (Bø et al 1990). Mørkved et al (2002) demonstrated a 67% cure rate in a test involving physical activity after individual biofeedback-assisted strength training of the PFM.

Sherman et al (1997) randomized 39 female soldiers, mean age 28.5 years (SD 7.2), with exercise-induced urinary incontinence to PFMT with or without biofeedback. All improved subjectively and showed normal readings on urodynamic assessment after treatment. Only eight subjects desired further treatment after 8 weeks of training.

Elite athletes are accustomed to regular training and are highly motivated for exercise. Adding three sets of 8–12 close to maximum contractions, 3–4 times a week (Pollock et al 1998) of the PFM to their regular strength-training programme does not seem to be a big task. However, there is no reason to believe that they are more able than the general population to perform a correct PFM contraction. Therefore, thorough instruction and assessment of ability to contract is mandatory. Because most elite athletes are nulliparous, there are no ruptures of ligaments, fascias, muscle fibres, or peripheral nerve damage. Therefore, it is expected that the effect would be equal or even better in this specific group of women. On the other hand, the impact and increase in abdominal pressure that has to be counteracted by the PFM in athletes performing high-impact activities is much higher than what is required in the sedentary population. The pelvic floor therefore probably needs to be much stronger in elite athletes.

There are two different theoretical rationales for the effect of PFMT (Bø 2004b). Miller et al (1998) found that a voluntary contraction of the PFM before and during cough reduced leakage by 98 and 73% during a medium and deep cough, respectively. Kegel (1948) first described the PFMT method in 1948 as 'tightening' of the pelvic floor. The rationale behind a strength-training regimen is to increase muscle tone and cross-sectional area of the muscles and increase stiffness of connective tissue, thereby lifting the pelvic floor into a higher pelvic position.

It is unlikely that continent elite athletes or participants in fitness activities think about the PFM or pre-contract them voluntarily. A contraction of the PFM most likely occurs automatically and simultaneously or even before the impact or abdominal pressure increase (Constantinou & Govan 1981). It seems impossible to voluntarily pre-contract the PFM before and during every increase in abdominal pressure while participat-

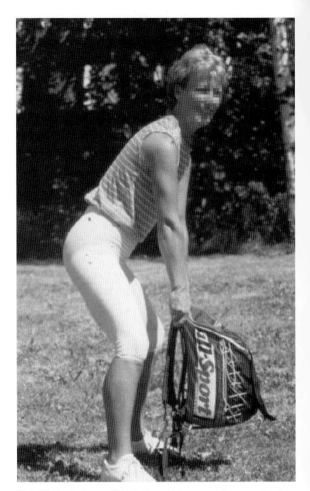

Fig. 13.4 It is possible to learn to pre- and co-contract the pelvic floor muscles before and during single task activities such as lifting.

ing in sport and leisure activities (Fig. 13.4). The aim of the training programme therefore would be to build up the PFM to a firm structural base where such contractions occur automatically.

Most likely very few, if any, athletes have learned about the PFM, and one could assume that none have tried to train them systematically. The potential for improvement in function and strength is therefore huge. PFMT has proved to be effective when conducted intensively and with a close follow-up in the general population (Hay-Smith et al 2002). It is a functional and physiological non-invasive treatment with no known serious adverse effects and it is cost-effective compared to other treatment modalities. However, there is a need for high-quality RCTs to evaluate the effect of PFM strength training in female elite athletes.

CONCLUSION

SUI may be a barrier to women's participation in sport and fitness activities and may therefore be a threat to women's health, self-esteem and well-being. Its prevalence among young, nulliparous elite athletes is high, with the highest prevalence found in those involved in high-impact activities such as gymnastics, track and field, and some ball games. There are no RCTs or reports on the effect of any treatment in female elite athletes. PFMT has been shown to be effective in RCTs, has no serious adverse effects, and has been recommended as first-line treatment in the general population. There is a need for more basic research on PFM function during physical activity and the effect PFMT in female elite athletes.

CLINICAL RECOMMENDATIONS

- Suggest use of preventive devices or tampons to prevent leakage during physical activity.
- Follow general recommendations for PFMT for SUI (see Ch. 9).

REFERENCES

Andersson K, Appell R, Awad S et al 2002 Pharmacological treatment of urinary incontinence. In: Abrams P, Cardozo L, Khoury S et al (eds). Incontinence. Plymbridge Distributors, Plymouth, p 479–511

Ashton-Miller J, Howard D, DeLancey J 2001 The functional anatomy of the female pelvic floor and stress continence control system. Scandinavian Journal of Urology and Nephrology Supplementum (207):1–7

Bø K 2004a Urinary incontinence, pelvic floor dysfunction, exercise and sport. Sports Medicine 34(7):451–464

Bø K 2004b Pelvic floor muscle training is effective in treatment of stress urinary incontinence, but how does it work? International Urogynecology Journal and Pelvic Floor Dysfunction 15:76–84

Bø K, Borgen J 2001 Prevalence of stress and urge urinary incontinence in elite athletes and controls. Medicine and Science in Sports and Exercise 33:1797–1802

Bø K, Hagen R, Kvarstein B et al 1989b Female stress urinary incontinence and participation in different sport and social activities. Scandinavian Journal of Sports Sciences 11(3):117–121

Bø K, Hagen R H, Kvarstein B et al 1990 Pelvic floor muscle exercise for the treatment of female stress urinary incontinence: III. Effects of two different degrees of pelvic floor muscle exercise. Neurourology and Urodynamics 9:489–502

Bø K, Mæhlum S, Oseid S et al 1989a Prevalence of stress urinary incontinence among physically active and sedentary female students. Scandinavian Journal of Sports Sciences 11(3):113–116

Bø K, Sherburn M, Allen T 2003 Transabdominal ultrasound measurement of pelvic floor muscle activity when activated directly or via transverses abdominal muscle contraction. Neurourology and Urodynamics 22:582–588

Bø K, Stien R, Kulseng-Hanssen S et al 1994 Clinical and urodynamic assessment of nulliparous young women with and without stress incontinence symptoms: a case control study. Obstetrics and Gynecology 84:1028–1032

Bø K, Talseth T, Holme I 1999 Single blind, randomised controlled trial of pelvic floor exercises, electrical stimulation, vaginal cones, and no treatment in management of genuine stress incontinence in women. BMJ 318:487–493

Bouchard C, Shephard R J, Stephens T 1993 Physical activity, fitness, and health. Consensus Statement. Human Kinetics, Champaign, IL

Brown W, Miller Y 2001 Too wet to exercise? Leaking urine as a barrier to physical activity in women. Journal of Science and Medicine in Sport 4(4):373–378

Bump R, Norton P 1998 Epidemiology and natural history of pelvic floor dysfunction. Obstetrics and Gynecology Clinics of North America 25(4):723–746

Constantinou C E, Govan D E 1981 Contribution and timing of transmitted and generated pressure components in the female urethra. Female incontinence. Allan R Liss, New York, p 113–120

Davis G D, Goodman M 1996 Stress urinary incontinence in nulliparous female soldiers in airborne infantry training. Journal of Pelvic Surgery 2(2):68–71

Dumoulin C, Lemieux M, Bourbonnais D et al 2004 Physiotherapy for persistent postnatal stress urinary incontinence: a randomized controlled trial 104:504–510

Eliasson K, Larsson T, Mattson E 2002 Prevalence of stress incontinence in nulliparous elite trampolinists. Scandinavian Journal of Medicine and Science in Sports 12:106–110

Fantl J A, Newman D K, Colling J et al 1996 Urinary incontinence in adults: acute and chronic management. 2, update [96–0682]. U.S. Department of Health and Human Services, Public Health Service, Agency for Health Care Policy and Research. Clinical Practice Guideline, Rockville, MD, p 1–154

Fischer J, Berg P 1999 Urinary incontinence in United States air force female aircrew. Obstetrics and Gynecology 94:532–536

Glavind K 1997 Use of a vaginal sponge during aerobic exercises in patients with stress urinary incontinence. International Urogynecology Journal and Pelvic Floor Dysfunction 8:351–353

Gunnarsson M 2002 Pelvic floor dysfunction. A vaginal surface EMG study in healthy and incontinent women [thesis]. Faculty of Medicine, Department of Urology, Lund University

Haderer J, Pannu H, Genadry R et al 2002 Controversies in female urethral anatomy and their significance for understanding urinary continence: observations and literature review. International Urogynecology Journal and Pelvic Floor Dysfunction 13:236–252

Hahn I, Milsom I, Ohlson B L et al 1996 Comparative assessment of pelvic floor function using vaginal cones, vaginal digital palpation and vaginal pressure measurement. Gynecological and Obstetrical Investigation 41:269–274

Hay J 1993 Citius, altius, longius (faster, higher, longer): The biomechanics of jumping for distance. Journal of Biomechanics 26(suppl 1):7–21

Hay-Smith E, Bø K, Berghmans L et al 2001 Pelvic floor muscle training for urinary incontinence in women [Cochrane review]. The Cochrane Library, Oxford

Hunskaar S, Burgio K, Diokno A et al 2002 Epidemiology and natural history of urinary incontinence (UI). In: Abrams P, Cardozo L, Khoury S et al (eds) Incontinence. Plymbridge Distributors, Plymouth, p 165–201

Hunskaar S, Vinsnes A 1991 The quality of life in women with urinary incontinence as measured by the sickness impact profile. Journal of the American Geriatrics Society 39:378–382

James E D 1978 The behaviour of the bladder during physical activity. British Journal of Urology 50:387–394

Jørgensen S, Hein H, Gyntelberg F 1994 Heavy lifting at work and risk of genital prolapse and herniated lumbar disc in assistant nurses. Occupational Medicine (Oxford) 44(1):47–49

Kegel A H 1948 Progressive resistance exercise in the functional restoration of the perineal muscles. American Journal of Obstetrics and Gynecology 56:238–249

Kulseng-Hanssen S, Klevmark B 1988 Ambulatory urethro-cystorectometry: a new technique. Neurourology and Urodynamics 7:119–130

Lagro-Janssen A, Debruyne F, Smiths A et al 1992 The effects of treatment of urinary incontinence in general practice. Family Practice 9(3):284–289

Miller J M, Ashton-Miller J A, DeLancey J 1998 A pelvic muscle precontraction can reduce cough-related urine loss in selected women with mild SUI. Journal of the American Geriatrics Society 46:870–874

Miller J, Perucchini D, Carchidi L et al 2001 Pelvic floor muscle contraction during a cough and decreased vesical neck mobility. Obstetrics and Gynecology 97:255–260

Mørkved S, Bø K, Fjørtoft T 2002 Is there any additional effect of adding biofeedback to pelvic floor muscle training? A single-blind randomized controlled trial. Obstetrics and Gynecology 100(4):730–739

Nichols D H, Milley P S 1978 Functional pelvic anatomy: the soft tissue supports and spaces of the female pelvic organs. The human vagina. Elsevier/North-Holland Biomedical Press, Amsterdam, p 21–37

Norton P, MacDonald L D, Sedgwick P M et al 1988 Distress and delay associated with urinary incontinence, frequency, and urgency in women. BMJ 297:1187–1189

Nygaard I E 1997 Does prolonged high-impact activity contribute to later urinary incontinence? A retrospective cohort study of female olympians. Obstetrics and Gynecology 90:718–722

Nygaard I, DeLancey J O L, Arnsdorf L et al 1990 Exercise and incontinence. Obstetrics and Gynecology 75:848–851

Nygaard I, Thompson F L, Svengalis S L et al 1994 Urinary incontinence in elite nulliparous athletes. Obstetrics and Gynecology 84:183–187

Peschers U, Schaer G, Anthuber C et al 1996 Changes in vesical neck mobility following vaginal delivery. Obstetrics and Gynecology 88:1001–1006

Physical activity and health; a report of the Surgeon General 1996 U.S Department of Health and Human Services, Center for Disease Control and Prevention, National Center for Chronic Disease Prevention and Health Promotion, Atlanta, GA

Pollock M L, Gaesser G A, Butcher J D et al 1998 The recommeneded quantity and quality of exercise for developing and maintaining cardiorespiratory and muscular fitness and flexibility in healthy adults. Medicine and Science in Sports and Exercise 30(6):975–991

Sandvik H, Hunskaar S, Seim A et al 1993 Validation of a severity index in female urinary incontinence and its implementation in an epidemiological survey. Journal of Epidemiology and Community Health 47:497–499

Sherman R A, Wong M F, Davis G D 1997 Behavioral treatment of exercise induced urinary incontinence among female soldiers. Military Medicine 162(10):690–694

Thyssen H H, Clevin L, Olesen S et al 2002 Urinary incontinence in elite female athletes and dancers. International Urogynecology Journal and Pelvic Floor Dysfunction 13:15–17

Wilson P D, Bø K, Nygaard I et al 2002 Conservative treatment in women. In: Abrams P, Cardozo L, Khoury S et al (eds) Incontinence. Plymbridge Distributors, Plymouth, UK, p 571–624

Chapter **14**

Evidence for pelvic floor physical therapy in men

Marijke Van Kampen

INTRODUCTION

It is since the end of the 90s that randomized controlled studies (RCTs) considering physical therapy for men with incontinence have been published (Bales et al 2000, Dorey 2001, Floratos et al 2002, Franke et al 2000, Mathewson-Chapman 1997, Moore et al 1999, Parekh et al 2003, Paterson et al 1997, Porru et al 2001, Sueppel et al 2001, Van Kampen et al 2000, Wille et al 2003).

Prostate surgery is one of the major causes of urinary incontinence in the male population. Besides urinary incontinence, men may suffer from other lower urinary tract symptoms (LUTS), including:

- filling or irritative symptoms: frequency, urgency, urgency incontinence and nocturia;
- voiding or obstructive symptoms: hesitancy, weak stream, straining, incomplete emptying, intermittency, terminal and postvoiding dribble (Abrams et al 2003, Dorey 2001).

Terminal dribbling is the prolonged final part of micturition when the flow has slowed to a dribble, while postvoiding dribble is the involuntary loss of urine immediately after finishing passing urine, usually after leaving the toilet in men. Postvoiding dribble is a minor pathological condition caused by pooled urine in the bulbous urethra (Dorey 2002).

Although physical therapy should have the potential to alleviate LUTS, there are few studies concerning male urinary problems and physical therapy. Only the efficacy of physical therapy for incontinence after prostatectomy and for terminal and postvoid dribble has been investigated in RCTs (Chang et al 1998, Hunter et al 2004, Paterson 1997).

Postprostatectomy incontinence

Urinary incontinence is a common consequence in many men undergoing prostate surgery (Diokno 1998, Dorey 2000, Peyromaure et al 2002). The prostate gland is part of the male sex gland and is composed of two zones: a central or transition zone and a peripheral zone. The transition zone is the site of the development of benign prostatic hyperplasia (Fig. 14.1). Prostate hyperplasia can be treated by transurethral resection (TUR) or transvesical resection of the prostatic adenoma (Fig. 14.2). The peripheral zone is most often the site of origin of prostatic adenocarcinoma. Localized prostate cancer can be treated by radical prostatectomy and this treatment is commonly thought to be the most effective (Baert et al 1996).

Removal of the prostate can lead to leakage of urine. The occurrence of incontinence, especially in the early recovery period after surgery is hard to accept for all patients. Patients express fear of odour, shame, self-consciousness and embarrassment and there is evidence that incontinent patients appear to benefit from support (Moore et al 1999).

Pelvic floor muscle training (PFMT), biofeedback and electrical stimulation with a transcutaneous or a rectal electrode have been suggested to improve incontinence after prostate surgery (Hunter et al 2004). The rationale for this treatment is that pelvic floor contraction may improve the strength of the external urethral sphincter during periods of increased abdominal pressure. PFMT results in hypertrophy of the striated muscles increasing the external mechanical pressure on the urethra. Moreover, contraction of the pelvic floor leads to inhibition of detrusor contraction, therefore incontinence can be improved (Berghmans et al 1998).

INCIDENCE OF INCONTINENCE

The incidence of incontinence after TUR and open adenectomy is low and incontinence resolves in a few days or months. In a small proportion of patients it is a troubling long-term problem (Van Kampen et al 1997). The incidence after radical prostatectomy varies widely. Immediately after catheter removal an incidence of 91% has been described (Van Kampen et al 2000). One year after radical prostatectomy several reports from prestigious academic centres claim that 95% of patients are continent (Myers 1995, Poon et al 2000, Walsh et al 1994). However, several studies cast a rather more pessimistic light on the problem, reporting that 30–40% of patients were wearing an incontinence pad 1 year or more after surgery (Bishoff et al 1998, Boccon-Gibod 1997, Braslis et al 1995). Variation in reported frequency of incontinence depends on the definition of incontinence, the difference in outcome measures, various follow-up periods and the person (patient, physician, urologist or therapist) who makes the assessment (Donnellan et al 1997, Fowler et al 1995, Moore et al 1999).

PATHOPHYSIOLOGY

Incontinence after adenectomy for prostate hyperplasia is mostly due to bladder dysfunction as bladder overactivity or poor compliance more than sphincter injury.

After radical prostatectomy, intrinsic sphincter deficiency is the primary cause (60 to 97%) of incontinence (Baert et al 1996). An overlooked cause is detrusor overactivity. Outlet obstruction that results in overflow incontinence is rare (Baert et al 1996, Foote et al 1991, Grise & Thurman 2001, Gudziak et al 1996, Haab et al 1996).

A small group of patients reported terminal and post-micturition dribble in the early postoperative period (Chang et al 1998, Porru et al 2001). This is due to urethral dysfunction as a result of decreased or absent postvoid urethral milking resulting in residual unexpelled urine in the bulbous urethra (Wille et al 2000).

Many risk factors have been described that increase the possibility of urinary incontinence after radical prostatectomy: previous TUR, shortened functional urethral length, no preservation of the bladder neck, no preservation of the neurovascular bundles, higher age, less surgical expertise and more advanced clinical and pathological stage of the tumour (Aboseif et al 1994, Eastham et al 1996, Van Kampen et al 1998).

TREATMENT: EVIDENCE FOR EFFECT (PREVENTION AND TREATMENT)

We analysed literature on urinary incontinence in men to generate clinical recommendations. Overall effective-

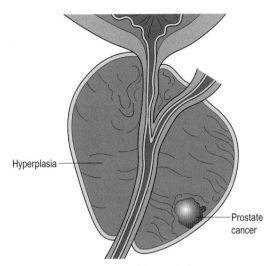

Fig. 14.1   The prostate gland, hyperplasia, prostate cancer.

ness of conservative management of postprostatectomy urinary incontinence has been widely investigated (Burgio 1989, Ceresoli et al 1995, Dorey 2000, Meaglia et al 1990, Moul 1998). Symptoms of incontinence after prostatectomy tend to improve over time without intervention. The specific effectiveness of a physiotherapeutic approach for incontinence after prostatectomy can only be evaluated in RCTs. Different types of intervention are described. PFMT involves any method of training the PFM including PFM exercises (PFME), biofeedback and electrical stimulation. Biofeedback involves the use of a device to provide visual or auditory feedback. Electrical stimulation involves any type of stimulation by using a rectal probe or transcutaneous electrodes (Fig. 14.3). This method is used to facilitate awareness of contraction of the PFM or to inhibit detrusor contraction.

Although relaxation of the PFM is as important as contraction, up to now no study gives attention to that part of the therapy.

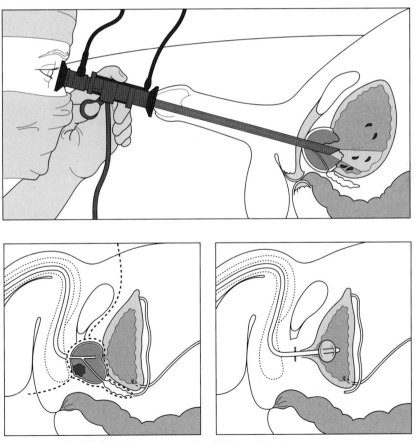

Fig. 14.2   Transurethral resection (TUR) of the prostate and radical prostatectomy.

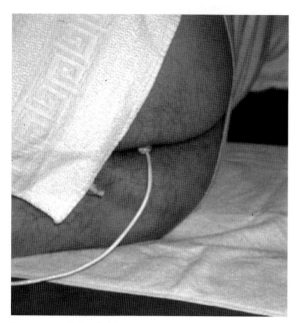

Fig. 14.3   Biofeedback and electrical stimulation of the pelvic floor with an anal probe.

A Cochrane review concerning conservative management for post-prostatectomy urinary incontinence was written by Moore et al (2003) and Hunter et al (2004).

There was a wide variation in outcome measures of incontinence. Assessment of incontinence was mostly based on the number of pads where 0 and 1 pad was defined as continent. Different pad tests (20-, 40-, 60-minute and 24- and 48-hour pad tests) were used to assess incontinence objectively (Hunter et al 2004, Moore et al 2003). Other assessments were voiding diaries for incontinent episodes, strength of the pelvic floor by digital test, visual analogue scale (VAS) and quality of life (QoL) questionnaires for incontinence (Emberton et al 1996, Herr 1994, Laycock 1994). The American Urological Association Symptom Score (AUA) and the International Prostate Symptom Score (IPSS) assess LUTS (Barry et al 1992).

Evidence-based medicine

We identified 11 eligible trials considering physical therapy for men with incontinence after prostatectomy, two on physical therapy and incontinence after TUR of the prostate and nine on physical therapy and incontinence after radical prostatectomy (Table 14.1). No abstracts were included. In one study (Chang et al 1998), patients of the control and the experimental group were not randomized. All other trials were randomized (Bales et al 2000, Floratos et al 2002, Franke et al 2000, Mathewson-Chapman 1997, Moore et al 1999, Parekh et al 2003, Porru et al 2001, Sueppel et al 2001, Van Kampen et al 2000, Wille et al 2003).

The methodological quality of all identified studies concerning incontinence after prostatectomy based on PEDro ranges between 3 and 7 out of 10 (Table 14.2).

The following hypotheses were tested in alleviating urinary incontinence after adenectomy or radical prostatectomy.

Is PFMT is better than no treatment or placebo (three trials)?

In two trials (Chang et al 1998, Van Kampen et al 2000) a significant difference in incontinence was found between the experimental and control group. In the first study, treatment was given after TUR of the prostate, the second study showed significant difference after radical prostatectomy. In both studies, pelvic floor exercises were started immediately after catheter withdrawal. The treatment of Chang et al (1998) took 4 weeks. In the study of Van Kampen et al (2000) patients were treated once a week for as long as any degree of incontinence persisted with a time frame of 1 year.

In one trial, Franke et al (2000) could not find a significant difference between the experimental and control group. They started 6 weeks postoperatively with pelvic floor exercises and biofeedback and five sessions were given. There is a remarkably high rate of drop-outs in this study.

Is preoperative and postoperative PFMT better than postoperative PFMT only (two trials)?

Sueppel et al (2001) showed improved outcomes in the group of patients who receive instructions for PFME and biofeedback training with rectal pressure probe before surgery against another group who started training 6 weeks after radical prostatectomy. Limitations of the study are the small sample size (n = 16) and the use of descriptive statistics only. Parekh et al (2003) found a significant difference in incontinence at 3 months after radical prostatectomy in favour of the early start of PFMT but not at 1 year.

Is preoperative PFMT and biofeedback better than preoperative information about PFMT only (1 trial)?

Bales et al (2000) could not find a significant difference in incontinence postoperatively by adding one session

Table 14.1 (Randomized) controlled studies of physiotherapy for incontinence after prostatectomy

Study	Bales et al 2000
Design	2-arm RCT: experimental group (E), preoperative PFMT + EMG BFB; control group (C), preoperative information about PFMT
n	100 men (E = 50, C = 50), mean age 59.3 in E and 60.9 year in C
Diagnosis	Questionnaire UI Number of pads
Training protocol	E: one 45-min treatment preoperatively BFB with surface electrodes + home exercises pre- and postoperatively C: information (written and brief verbal information) pre- and postoperatively + same home exercises as E Home: 10–15 contractions of 5–10 s, 4×/day
Drop-outs	3%
Results	No significant difference in incidence of incontinence (number of pads) between E and C group at 1–6 months after surgery (p 0.271–0.648)
Study	Chang et al 1998
Design	2-arm CT not randomized: experimental (E), PFME; control (C), no treatment
n	50 men after TUR prostate (E = 25, C = 25) mean age 65 years in E (range 51–74) and 66 years in C (range 45–79)
Diagnosis	Digital evaluation for strength of pelvic floor (0–4) Questionnaires Voiding dairy Uroflow
Training protocol	E: PFMT 4 weeks; home 30 exercises 4×/day C: no treatment
Drop-outs	Not mentioned
Results	Significant difference in strength of pelvic floor between E and C group only at week 4 (p < 0.05) Significant difference in duration of between void interval between E and C group at weeks 1 until 4 (p < 0.01) Significant difference in incontinence between E and C group at weeks 3 and 4 (p < 0.05) Significant difference in terminal dribbling between E and C group at week 4 (p < 0.05) Significant difference in QoL between E and C group at week 4 (p < 0.01) No significant difference in uroflow between E and C group at week 4
Study	Floratos et al 2002
Design	2-arm RCT: experimental group (E), FMT + EMG BFB; control group (C), verbal instructions about PFMT
n	42 men (E = 28, C = 14), mean age 63.1 in E (SD = 4) and 65.8 year in C (SD = 4.3)
Diagnosis	ICS 1-h pad-test Questionnaire

Table 14.1 (Randomized) controlled studies of physiotherapy for incontinence after prostatectomy—cont'd

Training protocol	E: 15 sessions EMG biofeedback with surface electrodes, 3×/week, 30-min; home: 50–100 contractions/day C: verbal instructions on PFMT, 1 session anal control: home 80–100 contractions/day 3–5 s with submaximal strength of 70%
Drop-outs	0
Results	No significant difference in incontinence (ICS 1-h pad test and number of pads) between E and C group at baseline 1, 2, 3 and 6 months after surgery (p > 0.05)
Study	Franke et al 2000
Design	2-arm RCT: experimental (E), PFMT + BFB; control (C), no treatment
n	30 men (E = 15, C = 15), mean age E = 62.3, C = 60.7
Diagnosis	Voiding diary 48-h pad test
Training protocol	E: 5 sessions of 45-min BFB behavioural therapy C: no therapy
Drop-outs	6 at 6 weeks, 7 at 12 weeks, 15 at 24 weeks
Results	No significant difference between E and C group in pad test and incontinence episodes at 6 weeks, 3 and 6 months
Study	Mathewson-Chapman 1997
Design	2-arm RCT: experimental group (E) 30-min preoperative information about PFMT and perineal muscle evaluation (not defined), postoperatively home exercises with biofeedback; control group (C), 30-min preoperative information about PFMT and perineal muscle evaluation (not defined)
n	53 men (E = 27, C = 26), mean age 60 years
Diagnosis	Voiding diary Perineal muscle strength Number of pads
Training protocol	E: information preoperatively PFME, home exercises with BFB C: information preoperatively PFME; home 15 contractions of few seconds daily increasing by 10 contractions every 4 days
Drop-outs	4%
Results	No significant difference between E and C group in number of pads
Study	Moore et al 1999
Design	3-arm RCT: experimental group 1 (E1) PFMT; experimental group 2 (E2): PFMT + ES; control group (C) verbal and written information about PFMT
n	63 men (E1 = 21, E2 = 21, C = 21), mean age 67 years (range 49–77)
Diagnosis	24-h pad test Questionnaires (Incontinence Impact Questionnaire IIQ7 and EORTC QLQ C30)

Table 14.1 (Randomized) controlled studies of physiotherapy for incontinence after prostatectomy—cont'd

Training protocol	E1: information (written and brief verbal information) pre- and postoperatively, 30-min PFMT in outpatient clinic twice a week for 12 weeks + home exercises E2: information (written and brief verbal information) pre- and postoperatively, 30-min PFME in outpatient clinic twice a week for 12 weeks + ES – surface anal electrode, 50 Hz, biphasic pulse shape with 1-s bursts, a 1-s pulse width and 1-s pulse trains + home exercises C: information (written and brief verbal information) pre- and postoperatively + same home exercises Home exercises: 12–20 contractions of 5–10 s, 8–10 contractions of 20–30 s and repetitive contractions in 10 s 3×/day
Drop-outs	8%
Results	No significant difference in incontinence between E1, E2 and C group for all assessments
Study	Parekh et al 2003
Design	2-arm RCT: experimental group (E) pre- and postoperative PFMT + BFB; control group (C) no formal PFE instructions
n	38 men (E = 19, C = 19), mean age 61.6 years in E and 55.5 years in C
Diagnosis	Number of pads/day at 6, 12, 16, 20, 28 and 52 weeks
Training protocol	E: two treatments pre- and postoperatively 1×/3 weeks for 3 months PFM (+ BFB depending on the patient) exercises described C: no formal education on PFMT Home: 6 months or longer functional re-training (2×/day)
Drop-outs	5% (week 28 and 52)
Results	Significant difference in achievement of continence between E and C group at week 12 (p < 0.05) Significant difference in median time to regain continence between E and C group (p < 0.05)
Study	Porru et al 2001
Design	2-arm RCT: experimental group (E) PFMT + BFB; control group (C) information (written and verbal) postoperatively + same home exercises
n	58 men after TUR (E = 30, C = 28), mean age 67.5 years in E (range 55–73) and 66 years in C (range 53–71)
Diagnosis	Questionnaires of LUTS and QoL Voiding diary Postmicturition dribble Digital test for strength of PFM
Training protocol	E: 4 treatments postoperatively 1×/week PFMT + home exercises C: information (written and verbal) postoperatively + same home exercises Home: 15 contractions on strength and endurance, 3×/day
Drop-outs	3/58 (5%)

Table 14.1 (Randomized) controlled studies of physiotherapy for incontinence after prostatectomy—cont'd

Results	AUA symptom score: both significantly improved pre-compared with 4 weeks postoperatively, no significant difference between E and C group QoL: significant difference in E group only between preoperatively and week 4 postoperatively (p < 0.001) Strength of PFM: significant difference in E group only between preoperatively and week 4 postoperatively (p < 0.01) Incontinent episodes: significant difference between E and C group (p < 0.01) Postmicturition dribble: significant difference between E and C group (p < 0.01)
Study	Sueppel et al 2001
Design	2-arm RCT: experimental group (E) preoperative instructions about PFMT and one session PFMT + BFB with rectal probe + PFMT + BFB 6 weeks postoperatively and 3, 6, 9 12 months after surgery + home exercises; control group (C): PFMT + BFB 6 weeks postoperatively and 3, 6, 9 12 months after surgery + home exercises
n	16 men (E = 8, C = 8), mean age 61.8 years in E (range 45–69) and 61.1 years in C (range 55–69)
Diagnosis	45-min pad test Bladder diary Number of incontinence episodes Number of pads/day QoL AUA and leakage index before surgery and at 6 weeks, 3, 6, 9 12 months after surgery
Training protocol	E: information on PFMT (written and brief verbal information) and PFMT + BFB with rectal pressure probe pre- and postoperatively 6 weeks, 3, 6, 9, 12 months after surgery + home exercises C: PFMT + BFB with rectal pressure probe 6 weeks, 3, 6, 9, 12 months after surgery + same home exercises 3×/day
Drop-outs	Not mentioned
Results	Only descriptive statistics but better improvement in incontinence in E group
Study	Van Kampen et al 2000
Design	2-arm RCT: experimental group (E) PFMT + BFB; control group (C) placebo treatment
n	102 men (E = 50, C = 52), mean age 64.36 years in E (SD 0.81) and 66.58 years in C (SD 0.80)
Diagnosis	24-h and ICS 1-h pad test VAS Voiding volume charts IPSS Number of pads/day (0 pads = continent)
Training protocol	E: treatment 30-min PFME and BFB in outpatient clinic once a week until continence + home exercises C: 30-min placebo ES, once a week until continence Home: total of 90 contractions/day, 40 contractions of 1 s and 50 contractions of 10 s/day in supine, sitting or standing position
Drop-outs	4%
Results	Significant difference between E and C group in duration and degree of incontinence at 1, 6 and 12 months after radical prostatectomy

Table 14.1   (Randomized) controlled studies of physiotherapy for incontinence after prostatectomy—cont'd

Study	Wille et al 2003
Design	3-arm RCT: experimental group 1 (E1) information + PFMT and ES; experimental group 2 (E2) information + PFMT + ES + BFB; control group (C): information about PFME
n	139 men (E1 = 46, E2 = 46, C = 47), mean age 64.6 years in E1 and E2 and 65.9 years in C
Diagnosis	20-min pad test Diary with number of pads/day($\geq$1 pad/day = continent) Urine symptom inventory at baseline, 3, 12 months
Training protocol	Started after catheter withdrawal, duration 3 months E1: PFMT + ES, ES = surface electrodes, 27 Hz, biphasic 1-s bursts, 5-s pulse width and 2-s pulse trains, 15 min 2×/day home device E2: PFMT, ES (5-s stimulation time, 5-s contracting and 15-s relaxing), BFB: 15 min 2×/day same home device, C: information (written and brief verbal information) and 3 days of therapy 20–30 min + home exercises (2×/day for 3 months)
Drop-outs	?
Results	No significant difference between E1, E2 and C group in incontinence at 3 and 12 months Questionnaire: p = 0.8 at 3 months, 0.5 at 12 months Pad test: p = 0.5 at 3 months, 0.2 at 12 months

AUA, American Urological Association; BFB, biofeedback; EMG, electromyography; ES, electrical stimulation; IPSS, International Prostate Symptom Score; LUTS, lower urinary tract symptoms; PFME, pelvic floor muscle exercise; PFMT, pelvic floor muscle training; QoL, quality of life; TUR, transurethral resection; UI, urinary incontinence; VAS, Visual analogue scale.

of EMG biofeedback 2–4 weeks before surgery. In the control group only information on PFMT was given. Both groups had to do home exercises as well pre- as postoperatively. The author suggested that instead of one biofeedback training, more intensive biofeedback training might have led to a better outcome.

Is postoperative PFMT better than information only about PFMT before and after surgery (2 trials)?

In one study (Porru et al 2001), one group received PFMT after TUR of the prostate for 4 weeks. The control group was only given information about PFMT before and after surgery. A significant difference in incontinence episodes was found between the experimental and control group at 1, 2 and 3 weeks after surgery, but not at 4 weeks. They concluded that early pelvic floor exercises should be recommended to all cooperative patients after TUR of the prostate.

Moore et al (1999) could not find any difference in duration of incontinence between a group of incontinent men given information of therapy before surgery and another group treated with PFMT 2 months after catheter withdrawal.

Is adding biofeedback to PFMT better than PFMT alone or information alone (three trials)?

Three trials (Floratos et al 2002, Mathewson-Chapman 1997, Wille et al 2003) could not prove an additional effect by adding biofeedback to exercises alone or verbal instructions only.

Is adding rectal stimulation to PFMT better than PFMT alone or information alone (two trials)?

Two trials (Moore et al 1999, Wille et al 2003) could not prove any additional effect by adding electrical stimulation to exercises alone or instructions only.

Table 14.2 PEDro quality score of (R)CTs in systematic review of physiotherapy for incontinence after prostatectomy

E – Eligibility criteria specified
1 – Subjects randomly allocated to groups
2 – Allocation concealed
3 – Groups similar at baseline
4 – Subjects blinded
5 – Therapist administering treatment blinded
6 – Assessors blinded
7 – Measures of key outcomes obtained from over 85% of subjects
8 – Data analysed by intention to treat
9 – Comparison between groups conducted
10 – Point measures and measures of variability provided

Study	E	1	2	3	4	5	6	7	8	9	10	Total score
Bales et al 2000	+	+	–	–	–	–	+	+	+	+	–	5
Chang et al 1998	+	–	–	–	–	–	–	+	–	+	+	3
Floratos et al 2002	+	+	–	–	–	–	–	+	+	+	+	5
Franke et al 2000	+	+	–	+	–	–	–	–	–	+	+	4
Mathewson-Chapman 1997	–	+	–	–	–	–	–	+	–	+	+	4
Moore et al 1999	+	+	+	–	–	–	–	+	–	+	+	5
Parek et al 2003	+	+	–	–	–	–	–	+	+	+	+	5
Porru et al 2001	+	+	–	+	–	–	+	+	–	+	+	6
Sueppel et al 2001	+	–	–	+	–	–	–	+	–	–	–	2
Van Kampen et al 2000	+	+	+	+	–	–	–	+	+	+	+	7
Wille et al 2003	+	+	–	+	–	–	–	+	–	+	+	5

+, criterion is clearly satisfied; –, criterion is not satisfied; ?, not clear if the criterion was satisfied. Total score is determined by counting the number of criteria that are satisfied, except that scale item one, eligibility criteria specified is not used to generate the total score. Total scores are out of 10.

Adverse effects

In one study (Moore et al 1999), one patient complained of rectal pain by contracting the PFM and discontinued the therapy. No other author described adverse effects of PFMT after prostatectomy.

Health economics

Information on the total cost of the intervention of physical therapy after prostatectomy was never given. One study (Wille et al 2003) gives details of the costs of a home biofeedback and electrical stimulation device. In another study (Van Kampen et al 2000), the number of physical therapy sessions (an average of eight in the experimental and 16 in the control group) were calculated and the authors concluded that the cost of treatment was low.

Discussion

Urinary incontinence is a common problem after prostatectomy and the role of physical therapy as a first-line treatment option provides has a small supportive role. A lack of good studies means that few data show the effect of pelvic floor training after TUR of the prostate. Only two studies describe a clear benefit on the recovery of incontinence with PFMT (Chang et al 1998, Porru et al 2001).

Three trials show that PFMT with biofeedback is significantly more effective after radical prostatectomy than no treatment or sham treatment in the postoperative period immediately after catheter withdrawal (Parekh et al 2003, Sueppel et al 2001, Van Kampen et al 2000).

The results of preoperative PFMT on incontinence were inconsistent. Two trials found a positive effect on incontinence whereas one trial concluded the opposite.

Analysis of a possible additional effect of biofeedback or electrical stimulation to PFMT alone or information alone does not demonstrate an advantage in men undergoing radical prostatectomy: five trials could not find a positive effect (Bales et al 2000, Floratos et al 2002, Mathewson-Chapman 1997, Moore et al 1999, Wille et al 2003).

Several limitations should be considered in the different studies. A variety of outcome measurements are used to assess urinary incontinence. The most widely used assessment is the number of pads (Bales et al 2000, Floratos et al 2002). In most studies 0 or 1 pad/24 hours is defined as continent. Clinical experience showed that some men wear 1 pad but have a loss of more than 10 g. The severity of incontinence was objectively assessed by the ICS 1-hour pad test (Floratos et al 2002, Van Kampen et al 2000) or during 24 hours (Moore et al 1999, Van Kampen et al 2000). In most studies no effort was made to assess PFM strength before surgery. At present, we do not know if men with a weaker pelvic floor might have more benefit from biofeedback or electrical stimulation. Some studies described a limited number of treatments. We do not know whether positive effects

might be found if patients were treated more frequently.

Many hypotheses have not been investigated so conclusions on male incontinence after prostatectomy are limited. The effect of lifestyle changes such as weight loss, smoking cessation, adequate fluid intake and regular bowel movements on incontinence after prostatectomy remains undetermined because no trial involves these interventions. Other questions are the effect of the quality of the physiotherapist, a training programme specifically for endurance of muscles and functional exercises, motivation and compliance of the patient. No studies were found that investigated these questions.

CLINICAL RECOMMENDATIONS BASED ON CURRENT EVIDENCE

The value of PFMT for the treatment of incontinence after prostatectomy remains unclear. There may be some benefit offering PFMT and biofeedback immediately after catheter withdrawal after prostatectomy. The therapy is noninvasive and avoids the side-effects that can occur with medical or surgical treatments. There is no consensus on the efficacy of PFMT preoperatively. Information on PFMT in comparison with effective treatment should be sufficient to reduce or shorten incontinence after prostatectomy. The efficacy of additional biofeedback or electrical stimulation PFMT has not been proved. These methods increase economic cost and positive effects have not been found.

Terminal and postvoid dribble

A prolonged final part of micturition when the flow has slowed to a dribble is a troublesome and common problem in older men. In a recent Australian survey, 12% of older men reported frequent terminal dribble (Sladden et al 2000) mostly associated with obstruction of the urethra. Postvoiding dribble is the involuntary loss of urine usually after leaving the toilet in men, or after rising from the toilet in women. Authors suggested that the condition is caused by pooling of urine in the bulbar urethra for unknown reasons (Denning 1996, Millard 1989) or because of failure of the bulbocavernosus muscle to empty the urethra (Dorey 2002). A small group of patients report post-micturition dribble in the early postoperative period after prostatectomy because

of urethral dysfunction (Wille et al 2000). A decreased or absent postvoid urethral milking results in residual unexpelled urine in the bulbar urethra (Wille et al 2000).

Bulbar urethral massage, with the finger behind the scrotum and moving in a forwards and upwards direction to evacuate the remaining urine from the urethra is not perceived as the optimal long-term treatment strategy by many men. Pelvic floor muscle training (PFMT) can eliminate the urine left in the bulbar urethra after voiding and provide men with a more acceptable option for management (Paterson et al 1997).

A systematic review of treatment of post-micturition dribble in men was carried out by Dorey (2002). Effectiveness of a physiotherapeutic approach for terminal and post-micturition dribble has only been investigated in four controlled studies (Chang et al 1998, Dorey 2001, Paterson et al 1997, Porru et al 2001). One study (Paterson et al 1997) recruited participants with pure post-micturition dribble without a history of surgery of bladder, prostate or urethra or a history of urgency or stress incontinence. Two other studies investigated the efficacy of PFME after TUR of the prostate on terminal (Chang et al 1998) and post-micturition dribble (Porru et al 2001).

Paterson et al (1997) compared PFMT, bulbar urethral massage and counselling on drinking and toileting. Assessment was done by less than 4-hour pad test stored in two sealed plastic bags over 72 hours and improvement in pad weight gain was measured. The best results were obtained by PFMT eliminating an average of 4.9 g

urine while the effect of urethral massage was 2.9 g. The group with counselling showed no improvement. The outcome measure was strongly influenced by the degree of urine loss at the start of the study ($p < 0.001$); if initial loss is too small then it would not be possible to detect a treatment effect.

Chang et al (1998) and Porru et al (2001) investigated the efficacy of PFMT after TUR of the prostate for 4 weeks. The control group was given information about PFMT before and after surgery only. Both studies have already been discussed in the section on post-prostatectomy. A significant difference for post-micturition dribble was found in favour of the experimental group 4 weeks after surgery. The others concluded that early PFMT should be considered in alleviating the problem of post-micturition dribble after TUR of the prostate (Tables 14.3 and 14.4).

Table 14.3 Randomized controlled studies of physiotherapy for incontinence for terminal and postmicturition dribble

Study	Chang et al 1998
Design	2-arm CT not: randomized experimental (E) PFME; control (C) no treatment
n	50 men after TUR prostate (E = 25, C = 25) mean age 65 years in E (range 51–74) and 66 years in C (range 45–79)
Diagnosis	Digital evaluation for strength of pelvic floor (0–4) Questionnaires Voiding dairy Uroflow
Training protocol	E: PFMT 4 weeks, home, 30 exercises 4×/day C: no treatment
Drop-out	Not mentioned
Results	Significant difference in strength of pelvic floor between E and C group only at week 4 ($p < 0.05$) Significant difference in duration of between void interval between E and C group at week 1 until 4 ($p < 0.01$) Significant difference in incontinence between E and C group at week 3 and 4 ($p < 0.05$) Significant difference in terminal dribbling between E and C group at week 4 ($p < 0.05$) Significant difference in QoL between E and C group at week 4 ($p < 0.01$) No significant difference in uroflow between E and C group at week 4
Study	Paterson et al 1997
Design	3-arm RCT: experimental group 1 (E1) PFMT; experimental group 2 (E2) urethral milking by bulbar massage; control group (C) counselling about drinking and toileting, relaxation therapy
n	49 men (E1 = 14, E2 = 15, C = 15), mean age 70.8 in E1 (SD 2.7), 69.3 years in E2 (SD 3.1) and 69.5 years in C (SD 2.4)
Diagnosis	Pad test Pelvic muscle strength by Oxford Grading System 0–4 Bladder chart

Table 14.3 Randomized controlled studies of physiotherapy for incontinence for terminal and postmicturition dribble—cont'd

Training protocol	E1: PFMT for 12 weeks with control at 5, 7, 13 weeks, home exercises 5 contractions of 1 s, 5 contractions of endurance gradually extending the number of repetitions, spread exercise sessions throughout the day in lying, sitting and standing position E2: urethral milking by bulbar massage C: counselling about drinking and toileting, relaxation therapy
Drop-out	12%
Results	Significant difference in incontinence between E1 and C group for small pad test (p < 0.01) Significant difference in incontinence between E2 and C group for small pad test (p < 0.01)
Study	Porru et al 2001
Design	2-arm RCT: experimental group (E)PFMT + BFB; control group (C) preoperative information about PFMT
n	58 men after TUR (E = 30, C = 28), mean age 67.5 years in E (range 55–73) and 66 years in C (range 53–71)
Diagnosis	Voiding diary
Training protocol	E: 4 treatments postoperatively 1×/week PFMT + home exercises C: information (written and verbal) postoperatively + same home exercises Home: 15 contractions on strength and endurance, 3×/day
Drop-out	3/58 (5%)
Results	Post-micturition dribble significant difference between E and C group (p < 0.01)

BFB, biofeedback; TUR, transurethral resection; PFMT, pelvic floor muscle training; QoL, quality of life.

Table 14.4 PEDro quality score of (R)CTs of physiotherapy for postmicturition dribble

E – Eligibility criteria specified
1 – Subjects randomly allocated to groups
2 – Allocation concealed
3 – Groups similar at baseline
4 – Subjects blinded
5 – Therapist administering treatment blinded
6 – Assessors blinded
7 – Measures of key outcomes obtained from over 85% of subjects
8 – Data analysed by intention to treat
9 – Comparison between groups conducted
10 – Point measures and measures of variability provided

Study	E	1	2	3	4	5	6	7	8	9	10	Total score
Chang 1998	+	–	–	–	–	–	–	+	–	+	+	3/10
Paterson 1997	+	+	–	–	–	–	+	+	–	+	+	5/10
Porru 2001	+	+	–	+	–	–	+	+	–	+	+	6/10

+, criterion is clearly satisfied; –, criterion is not satisfied; ?, not clear if the criterion was satisfied. Total score is determined by counting the number of criteria that are satisfied, except that scale item one, eligibility criteria specified is not used to generate the total score. Total scores are out of 10.

CLINICAL RECOMMENDATIONS AND CONCLUSION

- Evaluation of the efficacy of physical therapy for men with postvoid dribble was hampered by the paucity and the methodological quality of published reports in the field.

- At present, we can consider that PFMT is effective for post-micturition dribble based on three studies reporting positive results in comparison with information only. Bulbar massage gave an additive effect with PFMT for post-micturition dribble in one study.

CONCLUSIONS

Many male patients with incontinence and LUTS are referred for physical therapy based on the results of pelvic floor physical therapy in women. Despite the high number of referrals, evidence for using physical therapy in men is focused only on incontinence after prostatectomy and postvoid dribble.

Physical therapy is a non-invasive treatment modality and adverse effects or complications of physical therapy are very rare in contrast with pharmacological treatment and surgery.

Conclusions about incontinence and physical therapy after TUR of the prostate are limited because of the lack of studies. However, two studies describe a positive effect on incontinence when patients are treated with PFMT for 4 weeks postoperatively.

After radical prostatectomy there was support from three trials that PFMT with biofeedback is significantly more effective than information on PFMT, no treatment or sham treatment in the postoperative period immediately after catheter withdrawal. Six studies concluded there was limited benefit or no benefit of guided PFMT, additional biofeedback or additional electrical stimulation. In only one of the six studies, the patients of the control group were not informed of PFMT.

Preoperative PFMT had a positive effect in two studies, but another study could not confirm this finding.

A treatment programme of additional ES and/or additional BFB-enhanced PFMT did not affect continence after radical prostatectomy. At present three studies confirm no additional benefit from these approaches to reduce urinary incontinence.

For post-micturition dribble, physical therapy is effective, as shown in three studies. All reported positive results with PFMT in comparison with bulbar massage or no treatment.

Our knowledge on the effect of physical therapy for urinary incontinence and lower urinary tract dysfunction remains limited. Considering the absence of side-effects, the low cost and no risk level, pelvic floor re-education continues to be debated as an option in alleviating the problem of incontinence after prostatectomy. Future research is required to determine when men are most likely to benefit from which type/treatment modality of physical therapy.

REFERENCES

Aboseif S R, Konety B, Schmidt R A et al 1994 Preoperative urodynamic evaluation: does it predict the degree of urinary continence after radical retropubic prostatectomy? Urologia Internationalis 53:68–73

Abrams P, Cardozo L, Fall M et al 2003 The standardisation of terminology in lower urinary function: report from the Standardisation Sub-committee of the International Continence Society. Urology 61(1):37–49

Baert L, Elgamal A A, Van Poppel H 1996 Complications of radical prostatectomy. In: Petrovich Z, Baert L, Brady L W (eds) Carcinoma of the prostate. Springer–Verlag, Berlin, p 139–156

Bales G T, Gerber G S, Minor T X et al 2000 Effect of preoperative biofeedback/pelvic floor training on continence in men undergoing radical prostatectomy. Urology 56:627–630

Barry M J, Fowler F J, O'Leary M P et al 1992 The American Urological Association symptom index for benign prostatic hyperplasia. The Measurement Committee of the American Urological Association. The Journal of Urology 148:1549–1557

Berghmans L C, Hendriks H J, Bø K et al 1998 Conservative treatment of stress urinary incontinence in women: a systematic review of randomised clinical trials. British Journal of Urology 82(2):181–191

Bishop J T, Motley G, Optenberg S A et al 1998 Incidence of fecal and urinary incontinence following radical perineal and retropubic prostatectomy in a national population. Journal of Urology 160(2):454–458

Boccon-Gibod L 1997 Urinary incontinence after radical prostatectomy. European Urology 6:112–116

Braslis K G, Santa-Cruz C, Brickman A L et al 1995 Quality of life 12 months after radical prostatectomy. British Journal of Urology 75:48–53

Burgio K L, Stutzman R E, Engel B T 1989 Behavioral training for post-prostatectomy urinary incontinence. Journal of Urology 141:303–306

Ceresoli A, Zanetti G, Trinchieri A et al 1995 Stress urinary incontinence after perineal radical prostatectomy. Archivio Italiano di Urologia, Andrologia 67(3): 207–210

Chang P L, Tsai T H, Huang S T et al 1998 The early effect of pelvic floor muscle exercise after transurethral prostatectomy. The Journal of Urology 160: 402–405

Denning J 1996 Male urinary incontinence. In: Norton C (ed) Nursing for continence, 2nd edn. Beaconsfield Publishers, Beaconsfield, p 163

Diokno A C 1998 Post prostatectomy urinary incontinence. Ostomy/Wound Management 44(6):54–60

Donnellan S M, Duncan H J, MacGregor R J et al 1997 Prospective assessment of incontinence after radical retropubic prostatectomy: objective and subjective analysis. Urology 49:225–230

Dorey G 2000 Male patients with lower urinary tract symptoms. 2: Treatment. British Journal of Nursing 9(9):553–558

Dorey G 2001 Conservative treatment of male urinary incontinence and erectile dysfunction. Whurr Publishers, London, p 5–32

Dorey G 2002 Prevalence, aetiology and treatment of post-micturition dribble in men: literature review. Physiotherapy 88:225–234

Eastham J A, Kattan M W, Rogers E et al 1996 Risk factors for urinary incontinence after radical prostatectomy. The Journal of Urology 156:1707–1713

Emberton M, Neal D E, Black N et al 1996 The effect of prostatectomy on symptom severity and quality of life. British Journal of Urology 77:233–247

Floratos D L, Sonke G S, Rapidou C A et al 2002 Biofeedback versus verbal feedback as learning tools for pelvic muscle exercises in the early management of urinary incontinence after radical prostatectomy. BJU International 89:714–719

Foote J, Yun S, Leach G E 1991 Postprostatectomy incontinence. Pathophysiology, evaluation and management. Urologic Clinics of North America 18(2):229–241

Fowler F J, Barry M J, Lu-Yao G et al 1995 Effects of radical prostatectomy for prostate cancer on patient quality of life: results from a Medicare survey. Urology 45:1007–1014

Franke J J, Gilbert W B, Grier J et al 2000 Early post prostatectomy pelvic floor biofeedback. The Journal of Urology 163:191–193

Grise P, Thurman S 2001 Urinary incontinence following treatment of localized prostate cancer. Cancer Control 8(6):532–539

Gudziak M R, McGuire E J, Gormley E A 1996 Urodynamic assessment of urethral sphincter function in post-prostatectomy incontinence. The Journal of Urology 156:1131–1135

Haab F, Yamaguchi R, Leach G E 1996 Postprostatectomy incontinence. Urologic Clinics of North America 23:447–457

Hadley H R, Zimmern P E, Raz S 1986 The treatment of male urinary incontinence. In: Walsh P C, Gittes R F, Perlmutter A D et al (eds) Campbell's Urology, 5th edn. W B Saunders, Philadelphia, p 2668–2669

Herr H W 1994 Quality of life of incontinent men after radical prostatectomy. The Journal of Urology 151:652–654

Hunter K F, Moore K N, Cody D J et al 2004 Conservative management for post prostatectomy urinary incontinence [Cochrane review]. The Cochrane Database of Systematic Reviews 2:CD001843

Laycock J 1994 Clinical evaluation of the pelvic floor. In: Schüssler B, Laycock J, Norton P et al (eds) Pelvic floor re-education. Springer–Verlag, London, p 42–48

Mathewson-Chapman M 1997 Pelvic floor exercise/biofeedback for urinary incontinence after prostatectomy. Journal of Cancer Education 12:218–223

Meaglia J P, Joseph A C, Chang M et al 1990 Post-prostatectomy urinary incontinence: response to behavioral training. The Journal of Urology 144:674–676

Millard R J 1989 After dribble. In: Bladder control. A simple self-help guide. William and Wilkins, NSW, Australia, p 89–90

Moore K N, Cody D J, Glazener C M A 2003 Conservative management for post prostatectomy urinary incontinence [Cochrane Review]. The Cochrane Library, Issue 1. Update Software, Oxford

Moore K N, Griffiths D, Hughton A 1999 Urinary incontinence after radical prostatectomy: a randomised controlled trial comparing pelvic muscle exercises with or without electrical stimulation. BJU International 83:57–65

Moul J W 1998 Pelvic muscle rehabilitation in males following prostatectomy. Urologic Nursing 18:296–300

Myers R P 1995 Radical retropubic prostatectomy: balance between preserving urinary continence and achievement of negative margins. European Urology 27:32–33

Parekh A R, Feng M I, Kirages D et al 2003 The role of pelvic floor exercises on post-prostatectomy incontinence. The Journal of Urology 170:130–133

Paterson J, Pinnock C B, Marshall V R 1997 Pelvic floor exercises as a treatment for post-micturition dribble. British Journal of Urology 79:892–897

Peyromaure M, Ravery V, Boccon-Gibod L 2002 The management of stress urinary incontinence after radical prostatectomy. BJU International 90:155–161

Poon M, Ruckle H, Bamshad B R, Tsai C, Webster R, Lui P 2000 Radical retropubic prostatectomy: bladder neck preservation versus reconstruction. Journal of Urology 163(1):194–198

Porru D, Campus G, Caria A et al 2001 Impact of early pelvic floor rehabilitation after transurethral resection of the prostate. Neurourology and Urodynamics 20:53–59

Sladden M J, Hughes A M, Hirst G H et al 2000 A community study of lower urinary tract symptoms in older men in Sydney Australia. Australian and New Zealand Journal of Surgery 70:322–328

Sueppel C, Kreder K, See W 2001 Improved continence outcomes with preoperative pelvic floor muscle exercises. Urologic Nursing 21:201–210

Van Kampen M, De Weerdt W, Van Poppel H et al 1997 Urinary incontinence following transurethral, transvesical and radical prostatectomy. Retrospective study of 489 patients. Acta Urologica Belgica 65:1–7

Van Kampen M, De Weerdt W, Van Poppel H et al 1998 Prediction of urinary incontinence following radical prostatectomy. Urologia Internationalis 60:80–84

Van Kampen M, De Weerdt W, Van Poppel H et al 2000 Effect of pelvic-floor re-education on duration and degree of incontinence after radical prostatectomy: a randomised controlled trial. Lancet 355:98–102

Walsh P C, Partin A W, Epstein J I 1994 Cancer control and quality of life following anatomical radical retropubic prostatectomy: results at 10 years. The Journal of Urology 152:1831–1836

Wille S, Mills R D, Studer U E 2000 Absence of urethral post-void milking: an additional cause of incontinence after radical prostatectomy? European Urology 37(6):665–669

Wille S, Sobotta A, Heidenrich A et al 2003 Pelvic floor exercises, electrical stimulation and biofeedback after radical prostatectomy: results of a prospective randomized trial. The Journal of Urology 170:490–493

Chapter **15**

Evidence for pelvic floor physical therapy in children

Wendy F Bower

Dysfunction of bladder control

Lower urinary tract dysfunction can be classified as either congenital or acquired. Acquired dysfunction is often secondary to an underlying abnormality or the result of learned behaviours, such as during the toilet training process or in response to dysuria or an unacceptable voiding environment (Ellsworth et al 1995, Greenfield & Wan 2000).

CLASSIFICATION: URINARY INCONTINENCE DURING THE DAY

Urinary incontinence is most often associated with underlying detrusor overactivity and accompanied by the symptoms of an overactive bladder (OAB), such as frequency of micturition, urgency to find a toilet, posturing to prevent leakage during urgency, small volume voids, nocturnal enuresis or nocturia (Chiozza 2002). On bladder ultrasound the detrusor wall may be thickened; a cross-section of over 3–4 mm at 50% of the expected bladder capacity is suspicious of detrusor overactivity (Nijman et al 2005). On uroflowmetry a high flow rate early in the void and an overall shortened flow is often seen, and referred to as the 'tower' pattern. If urodynamic investigation is carried out a small bladder capacity can be confirmed and detrusor overactivity noted during filling (Van Gool & de Jonge 1989), towards end of fill only, or just preceding the voiding contraction.

Recently, incontinence in a subgroup of children has been attributed to volitional voiding postponement and found to be associated with a significant number of behavioural symptoms (Lettgen et al 2002). Postvoid leakage in the presence of a normal foreskin or adequate labial separation is likely to indicate dysfunctional voiding mechanics. In some children laughter triggers partial to complete bladder emptying and although various hypotheses have been proposed to explain the symptom, no definitive aetiology is yet accepted (Nijman et al 2005).

Alteration in the frequency of micturition is another common symptom of bladder dysfunction. Although increased frequency is often associated with an underlying OAB, it is also a hallmark of sensitivity of the urothelium. Current bacteriuria, post-infection inflammation, chronic inflammatory changes, oestrogen and prostaglandin swings, elevated caffeine and acidic urine can all precipitate increased voiding frequency (Martini & Guignard 2001). A less common presentation relates to the sudden onset of extraordinary urinary frequency, with voiding intervals as short as 15 minutes. This self-limiting condition is not associated with incontinence, nocturnal enuresis or nocturia, but may be linked to alterations in renal solute handling (Parekh et al 2000).

VOIDING DYSFUNCTION

Dysfunctional voiding refers to an inability to fully relax the bladder neck, urinary sphincter or pelvic floor during voiding. Alternatively it may be associated with dyssynergia of the external urinary sphincter, engendering an inappropriate response to a detrusor contraction. Once urethral resistance is encountered, the detrusor may:

1. continue to contract and effect emptying;
2. reduce contractile activity and prolong bladder emptying; or
3. be completely inhibited by urethral or pelvic floor muscle (PFM) activity, with bladder emptying achieved by abdominal straining.

A child with either of the last two presentations is said to have detrusor underactivity (Neveus et al 2005).

Altered patterns of voiding are independent of underlying neurological impairment, and may be learned during the toilet training years, adopted following episodes of dysuria or constipation, or occur secondary to sexual abuse. The child's environment, in particular toilet conditions and privacy issues, can trigger or exacerbate voiding anomalies (Cooper et al 2003, Meulwaeter et al 2002). Because no true structural obstruction can be identified the intermittent incomplete pelvic floor relaxation that occurs during abnormal voiding is termed a functional disorder (Nijman et al 2005).

Significant morbidity results in up to 40% of patients with dysfunctional voiding (Yang & Mayo 1997). This ranges from filling phase anomalies (OAB, urethral instability) to urinary tract infections, vesicoureteric reflux, kidney damage, detrusor overdistension, urinary retention and bladder decompensation.

Urinary symptoms associated with dysfunctional voiding range from urgency to complex incontinence patterns during the day and night (Chiozza 2002). Urgency and incontinence of urine may result from detrusor overactivity and thus be seen in conjunction with increased urinary frequency. Alternatively, infrequent or poor bladder emptying may precipitate symptoms. Micturition is often achieved with significant abdominal activity and simultaneous perineal EMG and uroflowmetry may show an interrupted or staccato flow pattern that coincides with rises in abdominal activity (Nijman et al 2005).

Signs of dysfunctional voiding may include small bladder capacity, increased detrusor thickness, low detrusor contractility, impaired relaxation of the external urinary sphincter during voiding, weak or interrupted urinary stream, large postvoid residual volumes of urine, and fecal soiling (Cvitkovic-Kuzmic et al 2002, Hellerstein & Linebarger 2003, Hoebeke et al 2001, Mazzola et al 2003). There may also be secondary vesicoureteric reflux, constipation or obstipation.

The optimal diagnosis of voiding dysfunction is gained from urodynamic investigation, with simultaneous perineal electromyographic (PF EMG) monitoring. The detrusor pressure preceding and during micturition can be clearly monitored and the lag time between detrusor pressure rise and initiation of urine flow quantified. The findings of note are:

- the PF EMG trace is silent until the void is initiated and then becomes active;
- the PF EMG is intermittently active during the void; or
- the abdomen is used to generate voiding pressure.

In conjunction with a significant volume of urine remaining in the bladder postvoid, such a trace would indicate voiding dysfunction. A videourodynamic study will further elucidate whether there is specific dysfunction at the bladder neck (Grafstein et al 2005).

PHYSICAL THERAPY INTERVENTION FOR CHILDREN WITH URINARY INCONTINENCE OR DYSFUNCTIONAL VOIDING

Children with bladder dysfunction require a multidisciplinary approach for both investigation and intervention. Box 15.1 outlines the components of a physical therapy programme for children with bladder dysfunction during the day. Treatment efficacy can be evaluated by reduction in number of wet episodes, improvement in bladder emptying and resolution of associated symptoms.

A systematic review of randomized controlled trials (RCTs) of non-pharmacological intervention in children with urinary incontinence of any non-neurological/structural aetiology identified two studies (Sureshkumar et al 2003), one reporting the efficacy of daytime alarms (Halliday et al 1987) and the other

---

included an arm that used biofeedback therapy for children with proven urgency syndrome (Van Gool et al 1999).

From the details in Table 15.1 it appears that:

- there was no difference between the proportions of children with persistent wetting in either alarm group;
- there was no decrease in the frequency of wetting episodes in children receiving clinic-based biofeedback; and
- anal electrical stimulation (ES) may be effective in the treatment of daytime incontinence and OAB in girls.

A review of non-pharmacological intervention for dysfunctional voiding revealed two randomized uncontrolled trials of biofeedback training (Klijn et al 2003, van Gool et al 1999). Other therapies described in cohort studies included PFM awareness training, ES and electromagnetic stimulation and clean intermittent catheterization. From the trial summaries in Table 15.2 it appears that:

- home-based uroflow training for 8 weeks significantly increased daytime continence at 6-month follow-up;
- clinic-based biofeedback did not improved daytime wetting when compared to standard therapy alone (Van Gool et al 1999).

Quality aspects of the RCT or non-randomized controlled trials are reported in Table 15.3. Clearly further controlled studies of the various interventions for both incontinence and voiding dysfunction in children are needed. The techniques reported favourably in cohort studies may be effective, but to date have been incompletely evaluated.

NOCTURNAL ENURESIS

Nocturnal enuresis is defined as emptying of the bladder during sleep (Neveus et al 2005). Enuresis in children without any other lower urinary tract symptoms (LUTS) or history of bladder dysfunction is further defined as monosymptomatic. Where the symptoms of increased or decreased voiding frequency, incontinence, urgency, hesitancy, straining, weak or intermittent urine flow, incomplete emptying, postvoid dribble or dysuria coexist with nocturnal enuresis, the condition is defined as non-monosymptomatic (Neveus et al 2005). A child with primary nocturnal enuresis (PNE) has never been dry for at least 6 months, whereas secondary enuresis implies initial reliable night dryness that has been lost.

Box 15.1: Components of a physiotherapy programme for children with bladder dysfunction during the day

- Educate normal bladder behaviour and specific changes underlying the child's symptoms
- Implement voiding routine so that child passes urine at regular intervals
- Teach pelvic floor muscle (PFM) awareness (±mirror, surface perineal EMG/anal probe EMG, transabdominal or perineal ultrasound) and coordination to achieve PFM recruitment and relaxation with minimal accessory muscle activity
- Train optimal voiding mechanics and posture (±biofeedback during voiding)
- Bowel management and optimal defecation dynamics if indicated
- Normalize PFM capabilities if necessary
- Adjunctive neuromodulation for overactive bladder symptoms
- Consider clean intermittent catheterization if large postvoid residual volumes of urine persist (Pohl et al 2002).

Table 15.1 RCTs for intervention in children with incontinence

Study	Halliday et al 1987
Design	RCT: contingent vs non-contingent alarm system
n	50
Diagnosis	'Troublesome' day wetting
Protocol	Alarm when wet versus alarm every 2 h for 3 months
Drop-outs/adherence	89% follow-up
Results	16/22 persistent wetting vs 13/22 on 2-hourly alarm RR 0.67 (0.29–1.56)
Study	Trsinar & Kralj 1996
Design	Anal ES vs sham anal plug electrode
n	73 ES, 21 sham
Diagnosis	Day incontinence ± nocturia/enuresis in girls
Protocol	ES/sham 20-min daily for 1–2 months
Drop-outs/adherence	100% completed study; 49% drop-out at 14-month review
Results	ES: 31.5% cured, 44% improved by 50%+, 25% no benefit Sham: 0 cured, 14.20% improved, 86% no benefit
Study	Van Gool & de Jonge 1989
Design	Biofeedback vs placebo
n	60
Diagnosis	U/D proven urge syndrome
Protocol	Ongoing with 9-month evaluation
Drop-outs/adherence	Unspecified
Results	15/33 biofeedback vs 11/27 placebo RR 0.92 (0.59–1.43)

ES, electrical stimulation; U/D, urodynamically.

As can be seen from Table 15.4, prevalence of nocturnal enuresis differs by gender in children under 12 years of age, but shows no gender bias in older adolescents and adults. From the age of 16 years onward, prevalence remains constant at around 2.3%, but most sufferers wet more than three nights per week (Yeung et al 2004a). Recent findings indicate that underlying urinary tract pathology (OAB, functional bladder outlet obstruction, congenital obstructive lesions) is associated with up to 93% of cases of enuresis in adulthood (Yeung et al 2004b).

Detrusor overactivity is implicated in nocturnal enuresis because enuretic children who do not respond to first-line therapy have been shown to have reduced nocturnal bladder capacity (Yeung et al 2004c). It is well known that overactivity during the day is associated with small voided volumes and a reduced functional bladder capacity (Kruse et al 1999). Asian researchers have identified the presence of nocturnal detrusor overactivity in up to one-third of all enuretic children (Watanabe 1995, Watanabe et al 1997) and 44% of patients whose nocturnal enuresis failed to respond to standard

Table 15.2   Trial details for intervention in children with dysfunctional voiding

Study	Klijn et al 2003
Design	1. Standard therapy vs 2. additional personalized home video vs 3. standard therapy, home video and home uroflowmeter
n	143
Diagnosis	U/D proven voiding dysfunction of non-neurogenic origin
Protocol	8 weeks, 4-month outpatient follow-up
Drop-outs/adherence	Not stated
Results	Daytime continence: 1. 46% 2. 54% 3. 61% PVR < 10% 1. 60% 2. 77% 3. 73% NS
Study	Van Gool & de Jonge 1989
Design	1. Biofeedback and standard therapy vs 2. standard therapy
n	104
Diagnosis	U/D proven dysfunctional voiding
Protocol	Ongoing with 6- and 9-month evaluation
Drop-outs/adherence	Not stated
Results	Improved at 6 months: 1. 20/34 2. 18/25 RR 1.47 (0.67–1.79) 9 months: 1. 25/45 2. 25/42 RR 1.10 (0.67–1.79)

NS, not significant; PVR, post-void residual volume of urine; U/D, urodynamically

treatment (Yeung et al 1999, 2002). Recent findings correlate low functional bladder capacity with high sleep arousal threshold and less frequent arousal episodes (Yeung et al 2005). Thus the bladder–brain dialogue is clearly impaired.

Renal urine production and its circadian rhythm contributes to nocturnal enuresis. Diuresis during sleep should be approximately 50% of daytime levels (Rittig et al 1995) and be regulated by free water excretion (arginine vasopressin, AVP) or solute excretion (angiotensin II and aldosterone) (Rittig et al 1999). Scandinavian studies have demonstrated that two-thirds of patients with monosymptomatic nocturnal enuresis produce large amounts of nocturnal urine, exceeding bladder capacity (Norgaard et al 1985, Rittig et al 1989). It is not known whether these patients have impaired renal sensitivity to vasopressin or require supranormal levels to achieve a circadian rhythm of urine production. Recently children with nocturnal enuresis and nocturnal polyuria were shown to have sodium retention

Table 15.3 PEDro table of levels of evidence for non-pharmacological treatment of paediatric bladder dysfunction

E – Eligibility criteria specified
1 – Subjects randomly allocated to groups
2 – Allocation concealed
3 – Groups similar at baseline
4 – Subjects blinded
5 – Therapist administering treatment blinded
6 – Assessors blinded
7 – Measures of key outcomes obtained from over 85% of subjects
8 – Data analysed by intention to treat
9 – Comparison between groups conducted
10 – Point measures and measures of variability provided

Study	E	1	2	3	4	5	6	7	8	9	10	Total score
Halliday et al 1987	+	+	+	?	+	+	?	+	+	+	–	7
Van Gool & de Jonge 1989 (Branch 1)	+	+	+	+	+	+	?	+	?	+	Ongoing	7
Trsinar & Kralj 1996	+	–	+	+	–	–	?	–	?	+	–	3
Klijn et al 2003	+	+	?	?	?	–	?	?	?	+	–	2
Van Gool & de Jonge 1989 (Branch 2)	+	+	+	+	+	+	?	+	?	+	Ongoing	7

+, criterion is clearly satisfied; –, criterion is not satisfied; ?, not clear if the criterion was satisfied. Total score is determined by counting the number of criteria that are satisfied, except that scale item one, eligibility criteria specified is not used to generate the total score. Total scores are out of 10.

Table 15.4 Prevalence of enuresis by gender at different ages

	5 years (%)	7 years (%)	9 years (%)	Mid–late teens (%)
Boys	13–19	15–22	9–13	1–2
Girls	9–16	7–15	5–10	1–2

that generated hypovolaemia and inhibited vasopressin production (Kamperis et al 2004, Vande Walle et al 2004). An additional finding is that children with nocturnal enuresis and nocturnal polyuria are also likely to have reduced functional bladder capacity for age (Yeung et al 2004d) when the formula (age + 2) × 30 is applied (Koff 1983).

In summary, the interplay of pathological changes in children with nocturnal enuresis remains elusive. There is clearly a mismatch between nocturnal urine production volume, bladder functional capacity and a distur-

bance of arousal mechanisms. Not all disturbances are present in each child and the relative vulnerability to each remains largely undetermined. The only independent variables conclusively associated with nocturnal enuresis are non-pathophysiological and include gender (males more at risk) (Cher et al 2002), a positive family history (Fergusson et al 1986), and co-existing behavioural problems.

Children with nocturnal enuresis can be classified into one of three groups, facilitating a treatment approach that targets each child's underlying pathology.

1. Polyuria will be proven when there is a monosymptomatic presentation. It is likely that no bladder wall changes will be demonstrated on ultrasound and that normal bladder emptying will be observed. Polyuric children with nocturnal enuresis may have either age-expected or reduced bladder capacity.

2. Underlying bladder dysfunction will be suggested by a small bladder capacity revealed on ultrasound,

and confirmed functionally by the frequency–volume chart (FVC). The bladder will empty appropriately and with a normal flow, but commonly displays hypertrophy. Specific urodynamic findings in this group may include moderate or severe OAB, sphincter and pelvic floor discoordination during voiding and a small cystometric capacity. There is generally no evidence of polyuria.

3. In the third diagnostic group, children show normal day FVC, acceptable voiding dynamics and appropriate ultrasound parameters. However there is nocturnal onset of covert detrusor overactivity and an associated reduction in nocturnal bladder capacity. This category of patients has recently been shown to comprise enuretics with persistent non-response to therapy (Yeung et al 2002).

PHYSICAL THERAPY INTERVENTION FOR CHILDREN WITH NOCTURNAL ENURESIS

Because nocturnal enuresis is either monosymptomatic or associated with underlying bladder dysfunction, optimal care of the child involves multidisciplinary evaluation and multimodal management. Physical therapy strategies offer adjunctive intervention and are best used as part of a combined and tailored therapeutic approach. Box 15.2 outlines the treatment strategies available to the therapist treating children with nocturnal enuresis who have proven filling or emptying bladder dysfunction.

Three Cochrane reviews have evaluated behavioural, physical and alarm interventions. To date no trials have been identified that evaluate the effect of musculoskeletal/pelvic floor motor control therapy on resolution of

> **Box 15.2: Components of a physiotherapy programme for children with nocturnal enuresis**
>
> - Retrain age-appropriate bladder storage ability
> - Institute regular voiding schedule and appropriate hydration
> - Teach the sensation of a full bladder
> - Teach strategies to prevent urge leak (±neuromodulation)
> - Train unopposed bladder emptying and normalize voiding mechanics
> - Develop pelvic floor muscle (PFM) proprioception, awareness and timing (±biofeedback)
> - Train specific PFM muscle relaxation during voiding
> - Treat underlying bowel dysfunction
> - Teach and supervise use of enuretic alarm (12–16-week trial)

nocturnal enuresis in children with coexisting voiding dysfunction.

The bedwetting alarm is the most effective intervention for monosymptomatic nocturnal enuresis (Glazener et al 2003, 2004). Children are 13 times more likely to become dry with an alarm than without treatment, with a 43% lasting cure rate (Houts et al 1994, Nijman et al 2005). Optimal results appear to be associated with high levels of motivation of the child and family and a high initial frequency of wet nights (Nijman et al 2005), whereas failure was associated with a low functional bladder capacity and an inability to be woken by the alarm (Butler & Robinson 2002).

Constipation in children

Children with bladder dysfunction often present with bowel symptoms and until recently this was considered coincidental. It is now accepted that in the absence of anatomical/neurological anomaly, dysfunction of emptying in both systems is inter-related. Chronic constipation requires two or more of the following characteristics over the preceding 8 weeks (Benninga et al 2005):

- frequency of defecation less than 3/week;
- more than one episode of fecal incontinence/week;

- large stools in the rectum or palpable on abdominal examination;
- passing of stools so large that they obstruct the toilet;
- retentive posturing and withholding behavior;
- painful defecation.

The frequently used terms in childhood bowel dysfunction are presented in Box 15.3. Within the population of children with constipation 64% fulfill the criteria

> **Box 15.3:** Definitions of childhood bowel dysfunction (Benninga et al 2005, Rasquin-Weber et al 1999)
>
> - Fecal impaction: fecal mass in rectum/abdomen that cannot be passed on demand
> - Organic constipation: congenital/anatomical structural defects that obstruct the colon, metabolic and endocrine disorders, connective tissue disease, neurological causes, slow colonic transit, infections and degenerative conditions
> - Functional constipation: no underlying organic cause; subclassified into functional constipation, functional fecal retention and constipation-predominant irritable bowel syndrome
> - Fecal incontinence: passage of stools in an inappropriate place for at least 8 weeks; sub-classified into organic or functional
> - Functional fecal incontinence is further classified depending on the presence or absence of associated constipation
> - Pelvic floor dyssynergia: lack of pelvic floor relaxation during attempts to defecate – paediatric physiotherapists have much to offer the child with this dysfunction

for functional constipation, 18% functional fecal retention and 21% functional non-retentive fecal soiling (Voskuijl et al 2004). Organic causes account for around 2% of all presentations of childhood constipation.

PATHOPHYSIOLOGY OF CONSTIPATION

In the newborn, meconium is passed within the first 24 hours, with lower birth weight children having delayed passage of stool (Weaver & Lucas 1993). Bowel actions occur up to six times daily for the first few weeks of life, but decline in frequency and increase in size and weight until by 4 years a child will defecate once daily (Weaver 1988). Defecation frequency is highly variable, with a 4-year-old being as likely as an adult to pass stool three times daily to three times a week (Hatch 1988).

Stool arriving in the rectum distends rectal and pelvic floor stretch receptors leading to relaxation of the internal anal sphincter and movement of stool into the anal canal. Contraction of the external anal sphincter follows perception of the call to stool. At a convenient time and place the external anal sphincter and pelvic floor are voluntarily relaxed, intra-abdominal pressure is generated and defecation follows. Many children achieve

bowel control around 18 months, but the age at which complete control is evidenced varies widely.

Up to 70% of constipated children have blunted or absent rectal sensitivity (Benninga et al 2004b, Loening-Baucke 1984), related to increased rectal compliance, a lack of daily routine, unacceptable toilets or inadequate privacy. Poor perception of rectal filling can trigger increased rectal capacity, impaired stool quality, an increased rectoanal inhibitory reflex threshold and incomplete emptying at eventual defecation. Although stool consistency in constipation is generally assumed to be hard and dry, it may be soft and unformed, and therefore difficult to perceive and fully evacuate.

Children can voluntarily suppress the urge to defecate, a behaviour that may be due to an impairment of learning, distress, trauma, a disruption of routine, inattention, or cognition difficulties. Toilet refusal is often associated with the memory or expectation of pain at defecation. Causes include having passed a large or hard stool, the presence of an anal fissure, an anal streptococcal infection, anxiety or irrational fears associated with the toilet (Chase et al 2004). Recent longitudinal studies of toilet training have identified that constipation precedes both stool withholding and hiding before defecation (Blum et al 2004, Taubman et al 2003). The signs of stool withholding in a toddler include squatting, crossing of the legs, stiffening of the body, forcefully contracting the gluteal muscles, hiding and holding onto furniture. During this time of stool urge, the rectum accommodates stool content until the urge to defecate passes. Over time the stool accumulates, becoming harder and drier (Chase et al 2004).

Constipation can be broadly considered to be due to an abnormal contraction pattern of colonic motor function or to an inability to relax the pelvic floor and anal sphincter during defecation. One recent study reported these underlying causes to coexist in 13% of adolescent subjects (Chitkara et al 2004), while other researchers reported no overlap (Gutierrez et al 2002).

In a Dutch sample normal colonic transit time was found in 56% of children with chronic constipation, with the remainder showing both significantly longer segmental and total transit time when compared to children with either non-retentive soiling or abdominal pain (Benninga et al 2004a). The presence of a postprandial gastrocolonic response implies normal colonic motility. It has been suggested that increased colonic transit time may be secondary to chronic fecal retention in the rectum (Benninga et al 2004a).

Abnormal contraction of the external anal sphincter was observed during attempted defecation in 64% of children with chronic constipation (Gutierrez et al 2002). There may also be a lack of increased intra-abdominal pressure or a partial or non-relaxation of the internal anal sphincter in children with pelvic floor dyssynergia.

PHYSICAL THERAPY INTERVENTION FOR FUNCTIONAL CONSTIPATION

It is recommended that physiotherapists who treat children with constipation are part of a specialized medical team. A comprehensive evaluation process will identify the presence or absence of pelvic floor dyssynergia and impaired colonic transit. Multidisciplinary behavioural and medical therapy is more likely to succeed when the child complies with treatment. Box 15.4 outlines the steps in a multidisciplinary intervention for functional constipation.

Biofeedback has been proposed as the treatment of choice for retraining defecation dyssynergia and is of interest to physiotherapists. Treatment sessions involve anal mamometry with a rectal balloon used to produce

> **Box 15.4:** Intervention cascade for functional incontinence in children
>
> - Comprehensive bowel history including 2-week stool chart
> - Abdominal palpation to identify fecal mass
> - Perineal inspection to confirm anal position, identify any descent, soiling, dermatitis, fissures, haemorrhoids or excoriation
> - Neurological screen, including inspection of lumbar region
> - Rectal emptying of impacted stool
> - Maintenance of regular soft stools (often requires stool softeners/laxatives for a prolonged period of time)
> - Toilet habit training, desensitization of toilet phobias, environmental management
> - Training optimal defecation mechanics

Table 15.5   RCTs for biofeedback intervention in children with constipation

Study	Loening-Baucke 1990
Design	1. Coordination biofeedback plus medical care vs 2. Medical care
n	43
Diagnosis	Contraction of EAS and pelvic floor during defecation Fecal incontinence
Protocol	6 sessions of weekly EMG anal sphincter and rectal biofeedback
Drop-outs/adherence	2 patients lost to follow-up
Results	Symptoms resolved at 7 and 12 months 1. 55%, 50% 2. 5%, 16% **Normal defecation dynamics** 1. 77% 2. 13%
Study	Nolan et al 1998
Design	1. Standard medical management with biofeedback 2. Standard medical management
n	29
Diagnosis	Soiling resistant to treatment with proven pelvic floor dysfunction
Protocol	3–4 sessions of weekly anal EMG biofeedback
Drop-outs/adherence	3 lost to repeat manometry at 6 months

Table 15.5 RCTs for biofeedback intervention in children with constipation—cont'd

Results	**Symptom improvement** 1. 4/14 2. 6/15 NS **Normal defecation dynamics** 1. 7/13 2. 2/13
Study	Sunic-Omejc et al 2002
Design	1. Standard medical management with biofeedback 2. Standard medical management
n	49
Diagnosis	Non-organic chronic constipation in children <5 years Abnormal defecation in 57%
Protocol	Biofeedback in clinic and home pelvic floor exercises for 12 weeks
Drop-outs/adherence	Not stated
Results	**Improved constipation** 1. 84% 2. 62.5%
Study	Van der Plas et al 1996
Design	1. Standard medical management with biofeedback 2. Standard medical management
n	192
Diagnosis	<3 stools/week Soiling >2×/month Laxative use 60% abnormal defecation dynamics
Protocol	5 clinic visits for both groups
Drop-outs/adherence	5 and 8 patients lost to follow-up at 6 months and 1 year respectively
Results	**Symptom resolution** 1. 32% 2. 33% **Normal defecation dynamics** 1. 86% 2. 52% (p < 0.001)
Study	Wald et al 1987
Design	1. Pressure biofeedback 2. Mineral oil therapy
n	50
Diagnosis	Fecal soiling 18 had abnormal defecation dynamics

Table 15.5   RCTs for biofeedback intervention in children with constipation—cont'd

Drop-outs/adherence	Not stated
Results	No difference in soiling 1 vs 2 post treatment or at follow-up **Normal defecation dynamics** 1. 6/9 2. 3/9

EAS, external anal sphincter; EMG, electromyography; NS, not significant.

Table 15.6   PEDro quality evaluation of trials of biofeedback treatment for functional childhood constipation

E – Eligibility criteria specified
1 – Subjects randomly allocated to groups
2 – Allocation concealed
3 – Groups similar at baseline
4 – Subjects blinded
5 – Therapist administering treatment blinded
6 – Assessors blinded
7 – Measures of key outcomes obtained from over 85% of subjects
8 – Data analysed by intention to treat
9 – Comparison between groups conducted
10 – Point measures and measures of variability provided

Study	E	1	2	3	4	5	6	7	8	9	10	Total score
Loening-Baucke 1990	+	+	?	+	−	?	?	+	?	+	+	5
Nolan et al 1998	+	+	?	+	?	−	+	+	+	+	+	7
Sunic-Omejc et al 2002	+	+	?	+	−	?	?	+	+	+	−	5
Van der Plas et al 1996	+	+	?	+	−	−	?	+	−	+	+	5
Wald et al 1987	+	+	?	?	−	?	+	+	?	+	−	4

+, criterion is clearly satisfied; −, criterion is not satisfied; ?, not clear if the criterion was satisfied. Total score is determined by counting the number of criteria that are satisfied, except that scale item one, eligibility criteria specified is not used to generate the total score. Total scores are out of 10.

rectal distension and train appropriate volume sensation. Perianal EMG electrodes record external anal sphincter activity and feedback can assist the patient to improve proprioception and control of the external anal sphincter. As a stand-alone treatment biofeedback has not been shown to be efficacious for constipation that is not associated with dysfunctional defecation (Poenaru et al 1997). A recent review of the efficacy of biofeedback for anorectal disorders (Palsson et al 2004) identified five randomized trials of biofeedback in children with constipation and pelvic floor dyssynergia (Table 15.5). Biofeedback in the overall group of children with constipation has a varied outcome, however in the subset of children with identified pelvic floor dyssy-

nergia, improvement is accelerated and may be associated with resolution of abnormal defecation dynamics. Clearly an accurate diagnostic process that allows the therapist to select adjunctive biofeedback for only those children with proven pelvic floor dyssynergia, is vital. Quality aspects of the studies are shown in Table 15.6.

No studies have been identified that compare physical therapy training of optimal defecation dynamics and pelvic floor relaxation without biofeedback with other forms of intervention for children with constipation. Trials investigating postural correction, optimal positioning and coordinated abdominopelvic relaxation known to increase both the anorectal angle and rectal funneling are eagerly awaited.

REFERENCES

Benninga M A, Candy D, Catto-Smith A G et al 2005 The Paris Consensus on Childhood Constipation Terminology (PACCT) Group. Journal of Pediatric Gastroenterology and Nutrition 40(3):273–275

Benninga M A, Voskuijl W P, Akkerhuis G W et al 2004a Colonic transit times and behaviour profiles in children with defecation disorders. Archives of Disease in Childhood 89(1):13–16

Benninga M A, Voskuijl W P, Taminiau J A 2004b Childhood constipation: Is there new light in the tunnel? Journal of Pediatric Gastroenterology and Nutrition 39(5):448–464

Blum N J, Taubman B, Nemeth N 2004 During toilet training, constipation occurs before stool toileting refusal. Pediatrics 113(6):e520–522

Butler R J, Robinson J C 2002 Alarm treatment for childhood nocturnal enuresis: an investigation of within-treatment variables. Scandinavian Journal of Urology and Nephrology 36(4):268–272

Chase J W, Homsy Y, Siggaard C et al 2004 Functional constipation in children: Proceedings of the 1st International Children's Continence Society Bowel Dysfunction Workshop. The Journal of Urology 171(6 Pt 2):2641–2643

Cher T W, Lin G J, Hsu K H 2002 Prevalence of nocturnal enuresis and associated familial factors in primary school children in Taiwan. The Journal of Urology 168(3):1142–1146

Chiozza M L 2002 Dysfunctional voiding. La Pediatria Medica e Chirurgica 24(2):137–140

Chitkara D K, Bredenoord A J, Cremonini F et al 2004 The role of pelvic floor dysfunction and slow colonic transit in adolescents with refractory constipation. The American Journal of Gastroenterology 99(8):1579–1584

Cooper C S, Abousally C T, Austin J C et al 2003 Do public schools teach voiding dysfunction? Results of an elementary school teacher survey. The Journal of Urology 170(3):956–958

Cvitkovic-Kuzmic A, Brkljacic B, Ivankovic D et al 2002 Ultrasound assessment of detrusor muscle thickness in children with non-neuropathic bladder/sphincter dysfunction. European Urology 41(2):214–218

Ellsworth P I, Merguerian P A, Copening M E 1995 Sexual abuse: another causative factor in dysfunctional voiding. The Journal of Urology 153(3 Pt 1):773–776

Fergusson D M, Horwood L J, Shannon F T 1986 Factors related to the age of attainment of nocturnal bladder control: an 8-year longitudinal study. Pediatrics 78(5):884–890

Glazener C M, Evans J H, Peto R E 2003 Alarm interventions for nocturnal enuresis. Cochrane Database Systematic Reviews 2: CD002911

Glazener C M, Evans J H, Peto R E 2004 Complex behavioural and educational interventions for nocturnal enuresis in children. Cochrane Database Systematic Reviews 1:CD004668

Grafstein N H, Combs A J, Glassberg K I 2005 Primary bladder neck dysfunction: an overlooked entity in children. Current Urology Reports 6(2):133–139

Greenfield S P, Wan J 2000 The relationship between dysfunctional voiding and congenital vesicoureteral reflux. Current Opinion in Urology 10(6):607–610

Gutierrez C, Marco A, Nogales A et al 2002 Total and segmental colonic transit time and anorectal manometry in children with chronic idiopathic constipation. Journal of Pediatric Gastroenterology and Nutrition 35(1):31–38

Halliday S, Meadow S, Berg I 1987 Successful management of daytime enuresis using alarm procedures: a randomly controlled trial. Archives of Disease in Childhood 62(2):132–137

Hatch T F 1988 Encopresis and constipation in children. Pediatric Clinics of North America 35(2):257–280

Hellerstein S, Linebarger J S 2003 Voiding dysfunction in pediatric patients. Clinical Pediatrics 42(1):43–49

Hoebeke P, Van Laecke E, Van Camp C et al 2001 One thousand video-urodynamic studies in children with non-neurogenic bladder sphincter dysfunction. BJU International 87(6):575–580

Houts A C, Berman J S, Abramson H 1994 Effectiveness of psychological and pharmacological treatments for nocturnal enuresis. Journal of Consulting and Clinical Psychology 62(4):737–745

Kamperis K, Rittig S, Jorgensen K A et al 2004 Osmotic diuresis in children with monosymptomatic nocturnal enuresis and DDAVP resistant nocturnal polyuria. Proceedings of ICCS-ESPU, Gent, Belgium, p 30–31

Klijn A J, Winkler-Seinstra P L, Vijverberg M A et al 2003 Results of behavioural therapy combined with home biofeedback for non-neuropathic bladder sphincter dysfunction, a prospective randomized study in 143 patients [abstract 272]. Proceedings of AAP Section on Urology

Koff S A 1983 Estimating bladder capacity in children. Urology 21(3):248

Kruse S, Hellstrom A L, Hjalmas K 1999 Daytime bladder dysfunction in therapy-resistant nocturnal enuresis. A pilot study in urotherapy. Scandinavian Journal of Urology and Nephrology 33(1):49–52

Lettgen B, von Gontard A, Olbing H et al 2002 Urge incontinence and voiding postponement in children: somatic and psychosocial factors. Acta Paediatrica 91(9):978–984, discussion 895–896

Loening-Baucke V A 1990 Modulation of abnormal defecation dynamics by biofeedback treatment in chronically constipated children with encopresis. The Journal of Pediatrics 116(2):214–222

Loening-Baucke V A 1984 Sensitivity of the sigmoid colon and rectum in children treated for chronic constipation. Journal of Pediatric Gastroenterology and Nutrition 3(3):454–459

Martini S, Guignard J P 2001 Polyuria, pollakiuria, and nocturia in children: diagnostic and therapeutic approach. Revue Médicale de la Suisse Romande 121(3):197–204

Mazzola B L, von Vigier R O, Marchand S et al 2003 Behavioral and functional abnormalities linked with recurrent urinary tract infections in girls. Journal of Nephrology 16(1):133–138

Meulwaeter J, Vandewalle C, Segaert A et al 2002 Hygienic facilities in schools. Proceedings of the International Children's Continence Society p 39

Neveus T, von Gontard A, Hoebeke P et al 2005 The standardization of terminology of lower urinary tract function in children and adolescents. Report of the International Children's Continence Society

Nijman R J M, Bower W, Elsworth P et al 2005 Diagnosis and management of urinary incontinence and encopresis in childhood. In: Abrams P, Cardozo L, Khoury S et al (eds) Incontinence, 3rd edn. Health Publication, Plymouth, p 965–1057

Nolan T, Catto-Smith T, Coffey C et al 1998 Randomised controlled trial of biofeedback training in persistent encopresis with anismus. Archives of Disease in Childhood 79(2):131–135

Norgaard J P, Matthiesen T B, Pedersen E B 1985 Diurnal antidiuretic hormone levels in enuretics. The Journal of Urology 134:1029–1031

Palsson O S, Heymen S, Whitehead W E 2004 Biofeedback treatment for functional anorectal disorders: a comprehensive efficacy review. Applied Psychophysiology and Biofeedback 29(3):153–174

Parekh D J, Pope J C IV, Adams M C et al 2000 The role of hypercalciuria in a subgroup of dysfunctional voiding syndromes of childhood. The Journal of Urology 164(3 Pt 2):1008–1010

Poenaru D, Roblin N, Bird M et al 1997 The pediatric bowel management clinic: initial results of a multidisciplinary approach to functional constipation in children. Journal of Pediatric Surgery 32(6):843–848

Pohl H G, Bauer S B, Borer J G et al 2002 The outcome of voiding dysfunction managed with clean intermittent catheterization in neurologically and anatomically normal children. BJU International 89(9):923–927

Rasquin-Weber A, Hyman P E, Cucchiara S et al 1999 Childhood functional gastrointestinal disorders. Gut 45(suppl 2): II60–II68

Rittig S, Matthiesen T B, Hunsballe J M 1995 Age related changes in the circadian control of urine output. Scandinavian Journal of Urology and Nephrology. Supplementum 173:71–74

Rittig S, Matthiesen T B, Pedersen E B 1999 Sodium regulating hormones in enuresis. Scandinavian Journal of Urology and Nephrology. Supplementum 202:45–46

Rittig S, Knudsen U B, Norgaard J P et al 1989 Abnormal diurnal rhythm of plasma vasopressin and urinary output in patients with nocturnal enuresis. The American Journal of Physiology 256:664–667

Sunic-Omejc M, Mihanovic M, Bilic A et al 2002 Efficiency of biofeedback therapy for chronic constipation in children. Collegium Antropologicum 26(suppl):93–101

Sureshkumar P, Bower W, Craig J C et al 2003 Treatment of daytime urinary incontinence in children: a systematic review of randomized controlled trials. The Journal of Urology 170(1):196–200

Taubman B, Blum N J, Nemeth N 2003 Children who hide while defecating before they have completed toilet training: a prospective study. Archives of Pediatrics & Adolescent Medicine 157(12):1190–1192

Trsinar B, Kraij B 1996 Maximal electrical stimulation in children with unstable bladder and nocturnal enuresis and/or daytime incontinence: a controlled study. Neurourology and Urodynamics 15(2):133–142

Van der Plas R N, Benninga M A, Buller H A et al 1996 Biofeedback training in treatment of childhood constipation: a randomised controlled study. Lancet 348(9030):776–780

Van Gool J D, de Jonge G A 1989 Urge syndrome and urge incontinence. Archives of Disease in Childhood 64:1629–1634

Van Gool J D, de Jong T P V M, Winkler-Seinstra P et al 1999 A comparison of standard therapy, bladder rehabilitation with biofeedback, and pharmacotherapy in children with non-neuropathic bladder sphincter dysfunction. Proceedings of the 2nd International Children's Continence Society, Denver

Vande Walle J, Raes A, Dehoorne J et al 2004 Abnormal nycthemeral rhythm of diuresis (nocturnal polyuria) is related to increased sodium and water-retention during daytime. Proceedings of ICCS-ESPU, Gent, Belgium, p 29

Voskuijl W P, Heijmans J, Heijmans H S et al 2004 Use of Rome II criteria in childhood defecation disorders: applicability in clinical and research practice. The Journal of Pediatrics 145(2):213–217

Wald A, Chandra R, Gabel S et al 1987 Evaluation of biofeedback in childhood encopresis. Journal of Pediatric Gastroenterology and Nutrition 6(4):554–558

Watanabe H 1995 Sleep patterns in children with nocturnal enuresis. Scandinavian Journal of Urology and Nephrology. Supplementum 173:55–58

Watanabe H, Imada N, Kawauchi A et al 1997 Physiological background of enuresis Type 1: a preliminary report. Scandinavian Journal of Urology and Nephrology. Supplementum 183:7–10

Weaver L T 1988 Bowel habit from birth to old age. Journal of Pediatric Gastroenterology and Nutrition 7(5):637–640

Weaver L T, Lucas A 1993 Development of bowel habit in preterm infants. Archives of Disease in Childhood 68(3):317–320

Yang C C, Mayo M E 1997 Morbidity of dysfunctional voiding syndrome. Urology 49(3):445–448

Yeung C K, Chiu H N, Sit F K Y 1999 Sleep disturbance and bladder dysfunction in enuretic children with treatment failure: fact or fiction? Scandinavian Journal of Urology and Nephrology. Supplementum 202:20–23

Yeung C K, Diao M, Sihoe J D Y et al 2004c Treatment of refractory nocturnal enuresis in children with reduced bladder capacity: a prospective randomized study comparing desmopressin plus enuretic alarm versus desmopressin plus oxybutynin hydrochloride. International Paediatric Nephrology Association, Adelaide:

Yeung C K, Diao M, Sreedhar B et al 2005 Sleep pattern and cortical arousal in enuretic children: a comparison with non-enuretic normal children. Proceedings of ESPU-AAP Joint Meeting, Upsalla, Sweden

Yeung C K, Diao M, Sreedhar B et al 2004d Treatment implications of nocturnal polyuria in enuretic children. Proceedings of ICCS-ESPU, Gent, Belgium, p 45–46

Yeung C K, Sihoe J D Y, Sit F K Y et al 2004a Characteristics of primary nocturnal enuresis in adults: an epidemiological study. BJU International 93(3):341–345

Yeung C K, Sihoe J D Y, Sit F K Y et al 2004b Urodynamic findings in adults with primary nocturnal enuresis. The Journal of Urology 171(6 Pt 2):2595–2598

Yeung C K, Sit F K Y, To L K et al 2002 Reduction in nocturnal functional bladder capacity is a common factor in the pathogenesis of refractory nocturnal enuresis. BJU International 90:302–307

Chapter 16

The development of clinical practice guidelines in physical therapy

Bary Berghmans, Erik Hendriks, Nol Bernards and Rob de Bie

INTRODUCTION

Quality assurance and cost-effectiveness are, worldwide, issues of great concern in modern-day health care. The development of clinical practice guidelines (CPGs) is considered to be a strategy to guarantee and improve the quality and efficiency of care. Also the development and implementation of CPGs constitute an important part of the quality of physical therapy care (policy) for both national and international physical therapy associations (Van der Wees et al 2003). The interest in CPGs is due to pressure on physiotherapists from society (policy-makers, healthcare managers, financiers and patients) to ensure quality of care and to justify their position in the health care system (Hendriks et al 2000a) as well as from physiotherapists themselves to embed evidence-based practice into their profession (Van der Wees et al 2003).

A useful working definition of CPGs is derived from the Institute of Medicine of the United States Agency for Health Care Policy and Research (AHCPR) (Field & Lohr 1992). CPGs are defined as 'systematically, on the basis of (best) evidence and consensus developed recommendations, drafted by experts, field-tested, and directed at performing diagnostic and therapeutic interventions in persons with definitive, suspected or health-threatening conditions, or directed at areas which have to do with good management and administration of the profession(al)' (Field & Lohr 1992, Grol et al 2005, Hendriks et al 1995).

CPGs can be considered as important state-of-the-art documents that can guide professionals in their daily practice and make explicit what professionals can do in a certain situation or with a specific condition, and why they do it. CPGs should not be applied rigidly, but are intended to be more flexible; however, in most cases, they can and should be followed. Yet, it is important to realise that CPGs only reflect the current state of knowledge at the time of publication, and expertise on effective and appropriate care with respect to certain health problem(s). They are subject to a continuous process of integration of new views, based on inevitable changes in the state of scientific information and technology. New evidence is mostly gathered in systematic reviews. However, this kind of research is not a panacea for the problems associated with reviews of the literature. Due to its non-experimental nature it is prone to the flaws that apply to all non-experimental research (de Bie 1996).

The reader should therefore always keep these facts in mind while studying both systematic reviews and CPGs and must be critical in appraising the information. Statements about efficacy and efficiency of interventions in particular that are only based on clinical practice or experience or reflecting opinions of so-called experts in the field might be biased.

GUIDING PRINCIPLES IN THE DEVELOPMENT OF CPGS

Important guiding principles in the development of CPGs are (Hendriks et al 2000b):

- the subject matter is clearly delineated on the basis of a clear medical diagnosis of health problems and related conditions that can be addressed by physical therapy;

- structuring should be according to the phases of the physical therapy process (Fig. 16.1) as laid down in CPGs by the professional organization (Herbert et al 2005).

- use of a uniform professional language is used – whenever indicated, use is made of available (international) classifications and accepted terminology, in particular the International Classification of Functioning, Disability and Health (WHO 2001) but also the International Classification of Diseases (WHO 1993), and Medical Terms for Health Professionals (Heerkens et al 1998) (see Fig. 16.1);

- uniform and valid diagnostic and responsive outcome measurements are used;

- based on the best available clinical evidence, and on consensus between experts if no evidence is available;

- clinical considerations have priority over cost-effectiveness;

- consistency with CPGs produced by other professions or groups of professions;

- based on integration and coherence of care – physical therapy may be one of the possible interventions in the total care of a patient and it should be evident at which point and why physical therapy is appropriate.

- patient-orientation and in agreement with the policies of patient organizations – individual patients also need to have a voice in determining care (Newman et al 2002) – are the expectations and treatment goals of patients the same as those of physiotherapists?

- the necessary expertise and knowledge required of physiotherapists should be made clear.

THE DEVELOPMENT OF CPGS

The bases for every physiotherapeutic CPG are the different stages of its process (Berghmans et al 1998b,c), the available clinical evidence, and, if evidence is lacking, expert consensus. In the development of CPGs priority should be given to a cost-effective approach and multidisciplinary consensus on diagnosis, intervention and secondary prevention. Recommendations need to be based on the results of new or recorded systematic reviews or meta-analysis.

Five groups may contribute to the development of the CPGs (Fig. 16.2):

- national and/or international physical therapy societies or associations and relevant collaborating or allied (scientific) parties/institutions;
- the steering group that plans and coordinates the activities;
- the task group that develops the CPGs;
- a group of clinical experts in the subject matter of the CPGs that comments on the guidelines or parts of it during the development; and
- a randomly selected group of physiotherapists who pilot test the guidelines in clinical practice.

Phases in CPG development

The four important phases in the development of clinical practice guidelines are:

- the preparatory phase;
- the design phase, encompassing the draft guidelines and the authorization phase;
- the implementation phase;
- the evaluation and updating phase.

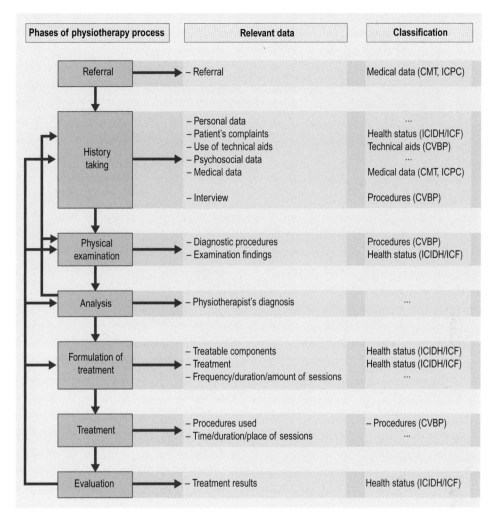

Fig. 16.1 The physical therapy process, relevant data and necessary classifications. CMT, Classification of Medical Terms; CVBP, Classification of Interventions and Procedures (for the allied health professions); ICF, International Classification of Functioning, Disability, and Health; ICIDH International Classification of Impairment, Disability and Handicap; ICPC, International Classification of Primary Care.

Method of CPG development

The preparatory phase

The preparatory phase involves the selection of a topic based on certain criteria (Field & Lohr 1992, Grimshaw et al 1995a, Grol et al 2005, Hendriks et al 2000b) (Box 16.1).

The design phase

This design phase should guide the task group in the development of the guidelines and is, for educational reasons, based on the different stages of the physical

therapy process (Box 16.2 and see Fig. 16.1). In the process of physical therapy practice a number of inter-related stages can be distinguished (Berghmans et al 1998b,c, Hendriks et al 2000a): a physiotherapist sees a patient, with a medical referral and a request for professional help. The physiotherapist takes the patient's history, examines the patient, draws conclusions, and finally, informs the patient about the findings and conclusions. Together with the patient the physiotherapist formulates a treatment plan and, if indicated, the treatment goals.

Following the formulation of a plan of activities and basic algorithms, systematic literature searches, reviews

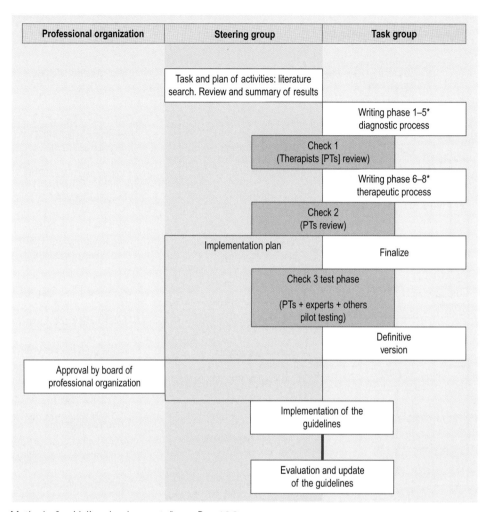

Fig. 16.2 Method of guideline development. *, see Box 16.2.

and/or meta-analysis are conducted into the efficacy of possible interventions, diagnostic procedures and measurements, prognoses, prevention, patient preferences, and current practice (Grol et al 2005, Sackett et al 1991, 2000).

The strategy described in Box 16.3 is used. The purpose of these rigorous literature reviews is to document the evidence to justify the recommendations (Sackett et al 2000, van Tulder et al 2003). See for an example on stress urinary incontinence Berghmans et al (1998a) or Hay-Smith et al (2001).

When scientific evidence from systematic reviews or primary trials is not available, the task group and the clinical experts formulate CPGs on the basis of consensus.

The task group first develops the diagnostic part of the CPG, which may include an algorithm of the process

of care and clinical decision-making, to formulate the management goals and an intervention plan. Randomly selected pelvic physiotherapists with practical expertise in the specific health problem review the content and applicability for clinical practice of the CPG's diagnostic part.

Following the plan of activities the task group continues with the therapeutic part of the guidelines, which if indicated and possible should include the recommended intensity, frequency and duration of the intervention(s). The same group of therapists who were consulted in the previous phase also reviews this part.

When both diagnostic and therapeutic parts of the guidelines are completed, another selection of pelvic physiotherapists use the CPG in their clinical practice. Critical analysis and evaluation will finalize this pilot testing phase. Additional comments are obtained from

Box 16.1: Possible criteria to select a subject for the development of a guideline

- Subject concerns a problem or controversy in health care for which health care providers are seeking a solution
- It is anticipated that consensus about the procedure/intervention is possible
- Health care providers are awaiting guidelines because they need a state-of-the-art document about a subject/topic
- The subject is relevant because it has an impact on the costs of health care in terms of prevention of health problems or saving of costs
- There is enough scientific evidence
- There is a genuine expectation that the guidelines fit within existing norms, values and routines
- The subject matter can be reasonably delineated
- It is possible to collect data about the care

Box 16.2: The different phases of the process of physiotherapy practice

1. Examination of the referral data
2. History taking
3. Physical examination and evaluation of the patient's (functional) status
4. Formulating the physiotherapist's diagnosis and deciding whether or not physiotherapy treatment is indicated
5. Formulating the treatment plan
6. Providing the treatment
7. Evaluating the (changes in) a patient's (functional) status and one's own course of action
8. Concluding the treatment period and reporting to the referring discipline

Box 16.3: Guides for selecting articles that are most likely to provide valid results

THERAPY
- Was the assignment of patients to treatments randomized?
- Were all patients who entered the trial properly accounted for and attributed at its conclusion?

DIAGNOSIS
- Was there an independent, blind comparison with a reference standard?
- Did the patient sample include an appropriate spectrum of the sort of patients to whom the diagnostic test will be applied in clinical practice?

HARM
- Were there clearly identified comparison groups that were similar with respect to important determinations of outcome (other than the one of interest)?
- Were outcomes and exposures measured in the same way in groups being compared?

PROGNOSIS
- Was there a representative patient sample at a well-defined point in the course of disease?
- Was the follow-up sufficiently long and complete?

1. The practice guidelines themselves.
2. A summary or algorithm on an A4 laminated quick reference card.
3. Qualitative and quantitative assessment of relevant studies used to assess levels of evidence of efficacy and efficiency and scientific justification with references.
4. A specific strategy and instruments for implementation of the guidelines (e.g. a knowledge check to test for discrepancies between the actual and the recommended practice as stated in the guidelines).

During and after the course of treatment, the therapeutic process and results are evaluated. Data obtained during the care process are recorded according to the CPGs for documentation that have been developed to ensure systematic and uniform record keeping (Bekkering et al 2005, Herbert et al 2005)

clinical experts in relevant professions. Based on the comments and experiences of the physiotherapists and the clinical experts, the draft is rewritten. The modified draft is then discussed by an 'authorization committee' (see Fig. 16.2). Following approval of this committee the guidelines are published in a scientific journal and introduced and implemented in the field.

The final product, as a result of the method of development, consists of four parts.

Table 16.1 Four groups of factors that determine the uptake and use of clinical guidelines (Grol & Jones 2000, with permission)

Features of	To improve the uptake and use of clinical guidelines:
The guidelines	The guidelines should be feasible, scientifically justifiable, specific and yet differentiated, flexible, clear, readable, didactic and attractive
The target group	The physiotherapists should have sufficient knowledge and skills, have a positive attitude towards guidelines, and be aware of their knowledge, skills and attitudes
The social context or setting	The routines of the physiotherapists and the expectations of the patients and colleagues should conform to the recommendations in the guidelines
The organizational context	The guidelines should not have negative financial consequences, give problems in organizing the care or require big structural changes related to staff or equipment

The implementation phase

This implementation phase comprises the dissemination and specific strategy to implement the developed CPGs according to the general method of implementation (Bekkering et al 2005).

In physical therapy CPGs are implemented by postal dissemination and by drawing attention to them in an article published in a physical therapy journal.

As it was well known that passive implementation strategies are usually not effective (Grimshaw et al 2001), a new and active implementation strategy was developed. The strategy aimed to reduce perceived barriers for implementation that may be related to specific features of the guidelines, features of the target group, features of the social context or setting, or features of the organizational context (Table 16.1) (Grol & Jones 2000).

The strategy was further constructed using a model for improving professionals' knowledge and influencing the management of primary care clinicians (Grol 2001). This model consists of four steps that have to be taken by the clinicians in order to change practice (Table 16.2):

1. orientation;
2. insight;
3. acceptance; and
4. change.

For each step specific activities or interventions can be chosen to implement guidelines, preferably using evidence-based interventions.

As to date there are no studies describing implementation interventions for guidelines on physical therapy, literature about implementation interventions in other health care professions has been used. The effectiveness

Table 16.2 Steps in the model for changing behaviour of a health care professional (Grol 2001, with permission)

Step	Goals with respect to professional
Orientation	To be informed To arouse interest
Insight	To understand content of guidelines To get insight in own way of working
Acceptance	To get a positive attitude towards guidelines To be inclined to change
Change	To implement in practice To maintain the change

of an implementation strategy probably depends on the health profession at issue, the topic of the guidelines and the setting that they refer to (Grol 2001).

Systematic reviews on the effectiveness of implementation interventions show that:

- information transfer is an essential part of the implementation process, but multiple interventions are usually needed to achieve changes in practice (Wensing et al 1998);
- reminders, multifaceted interventions and interactive educational meetings are consistently effective (Bero et al 1998);
- that strategies that are closely linked to the level of clinical decision-making process are more likely to have good results (Davis et al 1995, Grimshaw et al 1995a, b).

Clinical guidelines on physical therapy are considered to be important tools with which to close the gap between theory and practice and facilitate evidence-based practice in physical therapy. Systematic reviews have included studies from various countries conducted in various health care settings. Therefore, recommendations of the guidelines are universal and may be useful for physiotherapists worldwide. The applicability of the evidence-based recommendations is, however, not universal and may depend on the health care system. In the Dutch health care system, patients do not have direct access to physical therapy, but need a referral from a primary care physician (or a medical specialist). However, the content of the guidelines would not be changed if physiotherapists were the first-contact practitioners.

Investigating perceived barriers, and linking these to implementation interventions that have been shown to be effective is a useful way to obtain insight into the most appropriate implementation strategies.

The most important discrepancy between current practice and recommendations in CPGs is related to the knowledge or skills of physiotherapists and stress the importance of continuing education and postgraduate education for physiotherapists. The guidelines should help physiotherapists realise which type of education they need to keep their knowledge and skills up to date. In our survey physiotherapists frequently reported a lack of knowledge with respect to the use of behavioural principles in exercise therapy.

Collaboration with referring practitioners and the expectations of patients are important barriers to the implementation of the guidelines. Good collaboration is vital to ensure consistency across professions and to provide optimal quality of care. Changing the expectations of patients may take some time because some patients may have received traditional treatment for several years. It is the responsibility of the physiotherapist, as a professional, to provide good-quality treatment, but to do so it may be necessary to change the expectations of the patient. Because physiotherapists have difficulties changing patients' expectations, learning how to deal with expectations that are not consistent with the guidelines is an important part of the implementation strategy.

Passive approaches of implementation are unlikely to produce positive results and there are no interventions that are effective under all circumstances; reminders are a promising intervention; and multifaceted interventions targeting at different barriers to change are more likely to be effective than single interventions (Grimshaw et al 2001).

In the opinion of the authors, essential elements in the development of an implementation strategy for guidelines are:

1. a survey to identify barriers of the implementation of guidelines;
2. a model for changing professionals' behavior;
3. a systematic review of the literature to identify effective interventions for implementation.

Understanding the outcome of implementation in terms of changing physiotherapeutic management, health outcomes and costs are important because this is more likely to appeal to a change in physical therapy practice. Therefore, at present, in the Netherlands a randomized trial is being conducted to evaluate the cost-effectiveness of this implementation strategy.

The evaluation and updating phase

The effectiveness of the guidelines needs to be evaluated at the level of professionals and patients (see Fig. 16.2). The CPGs should be updated every 3–5 years after the guidelines are put into practice, or whenever new scientific insights make an update necessary.

DISCUSSION

Changing practice

An important strategy to improve the quality of physical therapy and to minimize undesirable variability in clinical practice is the development and implementation of evidence-based CPGs. In general, it can be concluded that the provision of explicit CPGs, supported by reinforcement strategies, will improve physiotherapist performance and, in certain situations as a main goal, patients' health outcomes.

It is clear that just developing and disseminating of CPGs is not sufficient! No matter how well established guidelines are, they will not contribute to an improved quality unless they are embedded in effective implementation programmes (Davis & Taylor-Vaisey 1997, Field & Lohr 1992, Grimshaw et al 2001, Grol & Grimshaw 2003, Grol et al 2005, Hendriks et al 2000a,b, Wensing et al 1998). Implementation implies the introduction of a change or innovation such that it becomes a normal component of clinical practice for individual physiotherapists and is no longer considered new. In other words, a vital element of successful CPG implementation is changing the individual physiotherapist's behavioural process that has to take place in the constantly changing environment of evidence-based practice and lifelong learning.

CPG implementation is often laborious and has proven to be the weakest link in the whole process (Field & Lohr 1992, Grol et al 2005, Hendriks et al 2000b). Therefore, next to publication, dissemination and implementation of CPGs, a set of (postgraduate) courses and tools should be developed and published to facilitate and promote practical use of the guidelines in clinical practice (Bekkering et al 2005).

A number of systematic reviews by Grimshaw et al (1995a,b) described 91 studies and showed that the effect of introducing guidelines, especially in terms of their impact on clinical practice, is greater than had been previously assumed. Also on the basis of the studies of Grimshaw & Russel (1993), Grimshaw et al (1995a,b) and Davis et al (1997) it can be concluded that thoroughly developed guidelines can alter clinical practice patterns and lead to positive changes in patient outcomes. However, the studies also showed that acceptance and use of guidelines are closely connected with the way in which they are developed and introduced. These findings were confirmed by recent reviews (Grimshaw et al 2001, Grol & Grimshaw 2003).

To optimize the development of CPGs, it is recommended that future users are involved as much as possible in the developmental process (Grimshaw et al 2001, Grol et al 2005) and that physiotherapists are able to exert a great deal of influence on guideline implementation. The use of a top-down approach will engender resistance and have an adverse effect. However, adopting a bottom-up approach is often inefficient in terms of making the best use of the time invested and of avoiding ambiguity. To increase the acceptance and use of CPGs it might therefore be helpful to adapt centrally produced guidelines with the help of a local team to deal specifically with the local situation or to add a number of complimentary agreements or criteria if necessary.

Although guidelines can be put into practice immediately, they may also be adapted to individual situations. Converting guidelines into a locally used protocol is possible and, at times, desirable. The conversion of centrally produced guidelines into a local protocol ensures that there is a local investment in, or 'buying into' the guidelines. This will speed up acceptance and therefore implementation of the guidelines.

THE FUTURE

Evaluation of the effect of the implementation process of CPGs is needed to draw conclusions about how CPGs can be effectively and efficiently implemented in future. Only by evaluating carefully the effect of developing and implementing the centrally produced guidelines is it possible to identify specific barriers and impediments that need to be overcome in the successful implementation of guidelines or to identify innovations.

REFERENCES

Bekkering G E, van Tulder M W, Hendriks E J et al 2005 Implementation of clinical guidelines on physical therapy for patients with low back pain: randomized trial comparing patient outcomes after a standard and active implementation strategy. Physical Therapy 85(6):544–555

Berghmans L C, Bernards A T, Bluyssens A M et al 1998b Clinical practice guidelines for physical therapy in patients with stress urinary incontinence. KNGF-guidelines for physical therapy. Nederlands Tijdschrift voor Fysiotherapie 108(4)(suppl):1–33

Berghmans L C, Bernards A T, Hendriks H J et al 1998c Physiotherapeutic management for genuine stress incontinence. Physical Therapy Reviews 3:133–147

Berghmans L C, Hendriks H J, Bo K et al 1998a Conservative treatment of stress urinary incontinence in women. A systematic review of randomized controlled trials. British Journal of Urology 82:181–191

Bero L A, Grilli R, Grimshaw J M et al 1998 Closing the gap between research and practice: an overview of systematic reviews of interventions to promote the implementation of research findings. The Cochrane Effective Practice and Organization of Care Review Group. BMJ 317:465–468

Davis D A, Taylor-Vaisey A 1997 Translating guidelines into practice. A systematic review of theoretic concepts, practical experience and research evidence in the adoption of clinical practice guidelines. Canadian Medical Association Journal 157:408–416

Davis D A, Thomson M A, Oxman A D et al 1995 Changing physician performance. A systematic review of the effect of continuing medical education strategies. JAMA 274: 700–705

De Bie R A 1996 Methodology of systematic reviews: an introduction. Physical Therapy Reviews 1:47

Field M J, Lohr K N (eds) 1992 Guidelines for clinical practice: from development to use. Institute of Medicine, National Academy Press, Washington DC

Grimshaw J, Eccles M, Russell I 1995a Developing clinically valid practice guidelines. Journal of Evaluation in Clinical Practice 1(1):37–48

Grimshaw J, Freemantle N, Wallace S et al 1995b Developing and implementing clinical practice guidelines. International Journal of Health Care Quality Assurance Incorporating Leadership in Health Services 4:55–64

Grimshaw J M, Russell I T 1993 Effect of clinical guidelines on medical practice: a systematic review of rigorous evaluations. Lancet 342:1317–1322

Grimshaw J M, Shirran L, Thomas R et al 2001 Changing provider behavior. An overview of systematic reviews of interventions. Medical Care 39(8 suppl 2):II2–II45

Grol R 2001 Successes and failures in the implementation of evidence-based guidelines for clinical practice. Medical Care 39:46–54

Grol R, Grimshaw J 2003 From best evidence to best practice: effective implementation of change in patient's care. Lancet 362:1225–1230

Grol R, Jones R 2000 Twenty years of implementation research. Family Practice 17(suppl 1):S32–S35

Grol R, Wensing M, Eccles M 2005 Improving patient care. The implementation of change in clinical practice. Elsevier Butterworth Heinemann, London

Hay-Smith E, Bø K, Berghmans L et al 2001 Pelvic floor muscle training for urinary incontinence in women [Cochrane review]. The Cochrane Library, Oxford

Hendriks H J, Bekkering G E, van Ettekoven H et al 2000b Development and implementation of national practice guidelines: a prospect for continuous quality improvement in physiotherapy. Physiotherapy 86(10):535–547

Hendriks H J, Oostendorp R A, Bernards A T et al 2000a The diagnostic process and indication for physiotherapy: a prerequisite for treatment and outcome evaluation. Physical Therapy Reviews 5:29–47

Hendriks H J, Reitsma E, van Ettekoven H 1995 Improving the quality of physical therapy by national (central) guidelines: introduction of a method of guideline development and implementation. Proceedings of the World Confederation for Physical Therapy Congress, Washington DC

Heerkens Y F, Hevvel van den J, Klaveren van A A, Ravensberg van C D 1998 Ontwerp Classification Medische Termen (CMT) voor Paramedische Beroepen. Amerstoort: Nederlands Paramedisch Instituut (NPI)

Herbert R D, Bø K 2005 Analysis of quality of interventions in systematic reviews. British Medical Journal 331(7515):507–509

Newman D K, Denis L, Gartley C B et al 2002 Promotion, education and organization for continence care. In: Abrams P, Cardozo L, Khoury S et al (eds) Incontinence. Health Publication, Plymouth, p 937–966

Sackett D L, Haynes R B, Guyatt G H et al 1991 Clinical epidemiology. A basic science for clinical epidemiology, 2nd edn. Little, Brown and Company, Boston

Sackett D L, Straus S E, Richardson W S et al 2000 Evidence based medicine. How to practice and teach EBM, 2nd edn. Churchill Livingstone, Edinburgh

Van der Wees P J, Hendriks E J, Veldhuizen R J 2003 Quality assurance in the Netherlands: from development to implementation and evaluation. Dutch Journal of Physical Therapy 3(WCPT special):3–6

Van Tulder M, Furlan A, Bombadier C et al 2003 Updated method guidelines for systematic reviews in the Cochrane collaboration group. Spine 28:1290–1299

Wensing M, Van der Weijden T, Grol R 1998 Implementing guidelines and innovations in general practice: which interventions are effective? British Journal of General Practice 48:991–997

World Health Organization 1993 International statistical classification of disease and related health problems (ICD-10). World Health Organization, Geneva

World Health Organization 2001 International classification of functioning disability and health. World Health Organization, Geneva

Appendix: Useful URLs

PATIENT ADVOCACY GROUPS

American Foundation for Urologic Disease
www.afud.org
Foundation providing, education, research information and support groups to patients and their families

Canadian Continence Foundation
www.continence-fdn.ca
Information and resources for those with incontinence and their families

Interstitial Cystitis Association
www.ichelp.org
Organization offering information and support to patients, educating the medical community and promoting research

Interstitial Cystitis Network
www.ic-network.com
Information resource developed by patients for patients, physicians and researchers

National Association for Continence
www.nafc.org
Educational site about causes, diagnosis and treatments of incontinence

New Zealand Continence Association
www.continence.org.nz
Charitable organization that assesses and manages bladder control problems

Simon Foundation
www.simonfoundation.org
Foundation providing discussion groups, education and resources for those with incontinence and their families

Prostate.org
www.prostate.org
Support group for men with prostatitis and their families

The Prostatitis Foundation
www.prostatitis.org
Support group for men with prostatitis and their families

UROlog
www.urolog.nl
General urology information for physicians and the general public

UrologyHealth.org
AUA site providing a step-by-step guide to treating incontinence

WebMD
my.webmd.com/living_better/her
Patient Website providing information about personal questions regarding women's health

CLINICAL GROUPS

American Academy of Family Physicians
www.aafp.org
Association providing medical information, educational opportunities and resources to physician members

American College of Sports Medicine
www.acsm.org
As the largest sports medicine and exercise science organization in the world the ACSM puts into practice strategic efforts to advancing the health of all

American Foundation for Urologic Disease
www.afud.org
Foundation providing research, education and patient support services

American Urogynecologic Association
www.augs.org
Society dedicated to research and education in urogynecology

American Urological Association
www.auanet.org
Organization providing education and research information in urology

British Association of Urological Surgeons
www.baus.org.uk
Association dedicated to advancing urology research and education in the UK

Canadian Urological Association
www.cua.org
Association dedicated to the study of urology, the improvement of its practice, the elevation of its standards, the promotion of research and the encouragement to secure higher qualifications in Urology

European Association of Urology
www.uroweb.org
The Association represents more than 16,000 urology professionals across Europe and worldwide. Its mission is to raise the level of urological care in Europe

The International Continence Society
www.continet.org
Society to study storage and voiding function of the lower urinary tract as well as the diagnosis and management of dysfunction

International Urogynaecological Association
www.iuga.org
An international organization committed to promoting and exchanging knowledge regarding the care of women with urinary and pelvic floor dysfunction

National Bladder Foundation
www.bladder.org
NIH site with research and information for physicians and patients

National Institute of Digestive & Diabetes & Kidney Diseases
www.niddk.nih.gov
Clinical research site with information on serious diseases affecting public health

Society of Urologic Nurses and Associates
www.suna.org
Organization committed to urologic education for excellence in patient care

World Confederation of Physical Therapy
www.wcpt.org
Confederation of national physical therapy associations, one organisation per country, representing physical therapists

Wound, Ostomy and Continence Nurses Society
www.wocn.org
Association providing educational, clinical and research opportunities for members

GENERAL SITES

Agency for Healthcare Research and Quality
www.ahcpr.gov
U.S. Dept. of Health and Human Services site translating research findings into clinical practice guidelines

Dr. Koop
www.drkoop.com
Patient and consumer health information center

HealthCentral
www.healthcentral.com
Health news and information; Dr. Dean column

Mayo Clinic
www.mayo.edu
Health information and publications for patients and physicians

Obgyn.net
www.obgyn.net
Medical information for women, medical professionals and industry

Physiotherapy Evidence Database
www.pedro.fhs.usyd.edu.au
An initiative of the Centre for Evidence-Based Physiotherapy (CEBP). It has been developed to give rapid access to bibliographic details and abstracts of randomised controlled trials, systematic reviews and evidence-based clinical practice guidelines in physiotherapy

Urology Channel
www.urologychannel.com
Provides information on urinary disorders, research and education, as well as a chat room, Q&A and doctor locator

MEDICAL JOURNALS

Contemporary Urology
www.conturo.com
Urology publication

Digital Urology Journal
www.duj.com
Urology publication

Journal of the American Medical Association
www.ama-assn.org
General medical publication

Medline and other resources
www.medportal.com
Medical journal resource site

New England Journal of Medicine
www.nejm.org
General medical publication

SEARCH ENGINES

Doctor's Guide to the Internet
docguide.com

Medexplorer: Health and medical information center
www.medexplorer.com

Index